PHARMACOVIGILANCE

PHARMACOVIGILANCE

Edited by

RONALD D. MANN

ELIZABETH B. ANDREWS

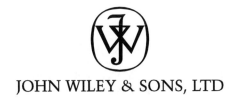

JOHN WILEY & SONS, LTD

Copyright © 2002   John Wiley & Sons Ltd, The Atrium, Southern Gate, Chichester,
                        West Sussex PO19 8SQ, England

                        Telephone   (+44) 1243 779777

Email (for orders and customer service enquiries): cs-books@wiley.co.uk
Visit our Home Page on www.wileyeurope.com or www.wiley.com

This publication is designed to provide accurate and authoritative information in regard to the subject
matter covered. It is sold on the understanding that the Publisher is not engaged in rendering
professional services. If professional advice or other expert assistance is required, the services of a
competent professional should be sought.

Other Wiley Editorial Offices

John Wiley & Sons Inc., 111 River Street, Hoboken, NJ 07030, USA

Jossey-Bass, 989 Market Street, San Francisco, CA 94103-1741, USA

Wiley-VCH Verlag GmbH, Boschstr. 12, D-69469 Weinheim, Germany

John Wiley & Sons Australia Ltd, 33 Park Road, Milton, Queensland 4064, Australia

John Wiley & Sons (Asia) Pte Ltd, 2 Clementi Loop #02-01, Jin Xing Distripark, Singapore 129809

John Wiley & Sons Canada Ltd, 22 Worcester Road, Etobicoke, Ontario, Canada M9W 1L1

British Library Cataloguing in Publication Data

A catalogue record for this book is available from the British Library

ISBN 0-470-49441-0

Typeset in 10/12pt Times by Mathematical Composition Setters Ltd, Salisbury, Wiltshire
Printed and bound in Great Britain by Antony Rowe Ltd, Chippenham, Wiltshire
This book is printed on acid-free paper responsibly manufactured from sustainable forestry
in which at least two trees are planted for each one used for paper production.

Contents

Contributors

SYED R. AHMAD, MB, BS, MPH   Medical Epidemiologist, Division of Drug Risk Evaluation, Office of Drug Safety, Center for Drug Evaluation and Research, US Food and Drug Administration, 5600 Fishers Lane, HFD-400, Rm 15B-32, Rockville, MD 20857, USA, AHMADS@cder.fda.gov

GURUPRASAD P. AITHAL, MD, MRCP, PhD   Consultant Hepatobiliary Physician, Queen's Medical Centre, University Hospital, D Floor, South Block, Nottingham NG7 2UH, UK, guru.aithal@mail.qmcuh-tr.trent.nhs.uk

SUSAN E. ANDRADE, ScD   Senior Research Associate, Meyers Primary Care Institute, Fallon Healthcare System, and University of Massachusetts, Worcester, MA 01605, USA, susaneandrade@aol.com

ELIZABETH B. ANDREWS, MPH, PhD   Vice President, RTI Health Solutions, Research Triangle Institute, 3040 Cornwallis Road, PO Box 12194, Research Triangle Park, NC 27709-2194, USA, Adjunct Associate Professor, School of Public Health and School of Pharmacy, University of North Carolina at Chapel Hill, NC, USA, eandrews@rti.org

PETER ARLETT, BSc, MBBS, MRCP   Senior Medical Assessor and CPMP Delegate, Post-Licensing Division, Medicines Control Agency, Market Towers, 1 Nine Elms Lane, London SW8 5NQ, UK, peter.arlett@mca.gsi.gov.uk

PRIYA BAHRI, PhD   Scientific Administrator, Sector Pharmacovigilance and Post-Authorisation Safety and Efficacy of Human Medicines, European Agency for the Evaluation of Medicinal Products (EMEA), 7 Westferry Circus, London E14, 4HB, UK, priya.bahri@emea.eu.int

ANDREW BATE, MA   Programme Leader, Signal Research Methodology, Uppsala Monitoring Centre, Stora Torget 3, 753 20 Uppsala, Sweden, andrew.bate@who-umc.org

BERNARD BÉGAUD, MD   Professor of Pharmacology, Départment de Pharmacologie Clinique—Unité de Pharmaco-épidémiologie, ARME-Pharmacovigilance, Université Victor Segalen, 33076 Bordeaux, France, Bernard.Begaud@pharmaco.u-bordeaux2.fr

DONNA A. BOSWELL, JD, PhD   Partner, Hogan & Hartson, L.L.P., Columbia Square, 555 Thirteenth Street, NW, Washington, DC 20004-1109, USA, daboswell@hhlaw.com

ROBERT P. BRADY, Esq.	Partner, Hogan & Hartson, L.L.P., Columbia Square, 555 Thirteenth Street, NW, Washington, DC 20004-1109, USA, rpbrady@hhlaw.com
CHRISTINA D. CHAMBERS, MPH, PhD	Assistant Professor of Pediatrics, Department of Pediatrics, UCSD Medical Center MC8446, 200 W Arbor Drive, San Diego, CA 92103, USA, chchambers@ucsd.edu
K. ARNOLD CHAN, MD, ScD	Assistant Professor, Department of Epidemiology, Harvard School of Public Health, Boston, MA 02215, USA, kachan@hsph.harvard.edu
JOHN A. CLARK, MD, MSPH	Vice President, Safety Services, Galt Associates, Inc., 21240 Ridgetop Circle, Ste 140, Sterling, VA 20166, USA, johnc@galt-assoc.com
DAVID M. COULTER, MB, ChB (NZ), DTM&H (Sydney)	Head, Centre for Adverse Drug Reactions Monitoring, Director, Intensive Medicines Monitoring Programme, Department of Preventive and Social Medicine, University of Otago, PO Box 913, Dunedin, New Zealand, david.coulter@stonebow.otago.ac.nz
PAULINE CUREL, MPS	Team Leader, Drug Information Pharmacists, Clineanswers, Clear Centre, Smales Farm Office Park, PO Box 33-1548, Takapuna, Auckland 1332, New Zealand, pauline.curel@clineanswers.com
ALBAN DAHNANI, PharmD	Assistant to the Head of the Pharmacovigilance Unit, Agence Française de Sécurité Sanitaire des Produits de Santé (AFSSAPS), 143/147 Bd Anatole, France 93 285 St Denis, France, alban.dahnani@afssaps.sante.fr
ROBERT L. DAVIS, MD, MPH	Associate Professor, Department of Pediatrics and Epidemiology, University of Washington, and Group Health Cooperative Center for Health Studies, Seattle, WA 98101, USA, rdavis@u.washington.edu
SARAH DAVIS, BSc (Hons), PhD	Scientific Assessor, Pharmacovigilance Group, Post-Licensing Division, Medicines Control Agency, Market Towers, 1 Nine Elms Lane, London SW8 5NQ, UK, sarah.davis@mca.gsi.gov.uk
CHRISTOPHER P. DAY, FRCP, MD, PhD	Professor of Liver Medicine and Honorary Consultant Hepatologist, Centre for Liver Research, The Medical School, Framlington Place, Newcastle upon Tyne NE2 4HH, UK, c.p.day@ncl.ac.uk
FRANK DESTEFANO, MD, PhD	Project Director, Vaccine Safety Datalink, National Immunization Program, Centers for Disease Control and Prevention, Atlanta, GA 30333, USA, fxd1@cdc.gov
PAULE DROUAULT-GARDRAT, LL.M, CEIPI, Avocat	Pharmacist, Lovells, 37 Avenue Pierre-1er-De Serbie, 75008 Paris, France, pdg@lovells.com
J. GUY EDWARDS, MB, BCh, FRCPsych, DPM	Visiting Professor, Khon Kaen University, Khon Kaen and Prince of Songkla University, Hat Yai, Thailand
I. RALPH EDWARDS, MB, ChB, FRCP, FRACP	Director, Uppsala Monitoring Centre, Stora Torget 3, 753 20 Uppsala Sweden, ralph.edwards@who-umc.org
JOSIE M. M. EVANS, MA (Oxon) MPH, PhD	Lecturer in Epidemiology, Department of Epidemiology and Public Health, Ninewells Hospital and Medical School, Dundee DD1 9SY, UK, j.m.m.stansfield@dundee.ac.uk
STEPHEN EVANS, BA, MSc, CStat, FRCP (Ed)	Professor of Pharmacoepidemiology, Medical Statistics Unit, The London School of Hygiene and Tropical Medicine, Keppel Street, London WC1E 7HT, UK, stephen.evans@lshtm.ac.uk

RICHARD E. FERNER, MD, MSc, FRCP	Director, West Midlands Centre for Adverse Drug Reaction Reporting, City Hospital, Birmingham B18 7QH, UK, r.e.ferner@bham.ac.uk
JONATHAN A. FINKELSTEIN, MD, MPH	Associate Professor, Department of Ambulatory Care and Prevention and of Pediatrics, Harvard Medical School and Harvard Pilgrim Health Care, Boston, MA 02215, USA, Jonathan_Finkelstein@hphc.org
F. T. FRAUNFELDER, MD	Professor of Ophthalmology, Casey Eye Institute, Oregon Health Sciences University, 3375 SW Terwilliger Blvd, Portland, OR 97035, USA, fraunfel@ohsu.edu
F. W. FRAUNFELDER, MD	Assistant Professor, Cornea and External and Disease Director of the National Registry of Drug-Induced Ocular Side Effects, Casey Eye Institute, Oregon Health Sciences University, 3375 SW Terwilliger Blvd, Portland, OR 97035, USA, fraunfer@ohsu.edu
SIR CHARLES GEORGE, BSc, MD, FRCP	Medical Director, British Heart Foundation, 14 Fitzhardinge Street, London W1H 6DH, UK, cawdrong@bhf.org.uk
ALAN S. GO, MD, MPH	Physician Scientist, Division of Research, Kaiser Foundation Research Institute, Oakland, CA 94611, USA
MICHAEL J. GOODMAN, PhD	Senior Research Investigator, HealthPartners Research Foundation, Minneapolis, MN 55440, USA, Michael.J.Goodman@HealthPartners.com
DAVID J. GRAHAM, MD, MPH	Associate Director for Science and Medicine, Office of Drug Safety, Centre for Drug Evaluation and Research, US Food and Drug Administration, 5600 Fishers Lane, HFD-400, Rm 15B-32, Rockville MD 20857, USA, GRAHAMD@cder.fda.gov
A. C. VAN GROOTHEEST, MD	Director, Netherlands Pharmacovigilance Centre Lareb, Goudsbloem vallei 7, 5273 MH's-Hertogenbosch, The Netherlands, ac.vangrootheest@lareb.nl
THOMAS GROSS, MD, MPH	Director, Division of Postmarket Surveillance, Office of Surveillance and Biometrics, Center for Devices and Radiological Health, US Food and Drug Administration, 1350 Piccard Drive, Room 300P, Rockville, MD 20850, USA, TPG@CDRH.FDA.GOV
JERRY H. GURWITZ, MD	The Dr John Meyers Professor of Primary Care Medicine, University of Massachusetts Medical School and Executive Director, Meyers Primary Care Institute, Fallon Healthcare System, and University of Massachusetts Medical School, Worcester, MA 01605, USA
CHRISTOPH HILTL, Dr.jur.	Partner, Lovells Boesebeck Droste, Marstallstrasse 8, 80539 Munchen, Germany, christoph.hiltl@lovells.com
NORMA KELLETT, BSc, MBChB, MRCGP, FFPM	Director Clinical Services, Inveresk Research, Tranent EH33 2NE, UK, norma.kellett@inveresk.com
LARRY G. KESSLER, ScD	Office Director, Office of Surveillance and Biometrics, Centre for Devices and Radiological Health, US Food and Drug Administration, 1350 Piccard Drive, Rockville MD 20850, USA igk@cdrh.fda.gov
JUDITH L. KINMAN, MA	Project Manager, Center for Clinical Epidemiology and Biostatistics, University of Pennsylvania School of Medicine, 824 Blockley Hall, 423 Guardian Drive, Philadelphia, PA 19104-6021, USA, jkinman@

cceb.med.upenn.edu, Regional Managing Editor, *Pharmacoepidemiology and Drug Safety*

STEPHEN L. KLINCEWICZ, DO, MPH, JD — Global Safety Officer, Drug Safety and Surveillance, Johnson and Johnson Pharmaceutical Research and Development LLC, 1125 Trenton-Harbourtown Road, Titusville, NJ 08560-0200, USA, sklincew@prdus.jnj.com

CARMEN KREFT-JAIS, MD — Head, Pharmacovigilance Unit, Agence Française de Sécurité Sanitaire des Produits de Santé (AFSSAPS), 143/147 Bd Anatole France, 93 285 St Denis, France, carmen.kreft-jais@afssaps.sante.fr

PAOLA LA LICATA, JD — Lawyer, Lovells, Via Dei Due Marcelli 66, 00187 Roma, Italy, Paola.LaLicata@lovells.com

DAVID H. LAWSON, CBE, MD, FRCP — Head of Department of Clinical Pharmacology, Royal Infirmary, Glasgow, UK, ann.rodden@northglasgow.scot.nhs.uk

MARK D. LEARN, Esq. — Associate, Hogan & Hartson, L.L.P., Columbia Square, 555 Thirteenth Street, NW, Washington, DC 20004-1109, USA, MDLearn@HHLAW.com

MARIE LINDQUIST, MSc Pharm — Head of Data Management & Research, General Manager, Uppsala Monitoring Centre, Stora Torget 3, 753 20 Uppsala, Sweden, marie.lindquist@who-umc.org

THOMAS M. MACDONALD, BSc, MD, FRCP, FESC — Professor of Clinical Pharmacology and Pharmacoepidemiology, Director, MEdicines MOnitoring Unit (MEMO), Department of Clinical Pharmacology and Therapeutics, University of Dundee, Ninewells Hospital and Medical School, Dundee DD1 9SY, UK, tom@memo.dundee.ac.uk

NICHOLAS MACFARLANE, BA — Partner, Lovells, 65 Holborn Viaduct, London EC1A 2DY, UK, nicholas.macfarlane@lovells.com

STUART J. MAIR, MBChB, DRCOG, DCPSA — Medical Advisor, Inveresk Research, Tranent EH33 2NE, UK, stuart.mair@inveresk.com

PENELOPE K. MANASCO, MD — Chief Medical Officer, First Genetic Trust, 3 Parkway North Center Suite 150N, Deerfield, IL 60015, USA, pmanasco@firstgenetic.net

RONALD D. MANN, MD, FRCP, FRCGP, FFPM — Professor Emeritus, University of Southampton, UK, and 42 Hazleton Way, Waterlooville, Hampshire PO8 9BT, UK, DrMann@manorcottage.fsbusiness.co.uk

UNA MARTIN, BSc, PhD, FRCPI — Senior Lecturer in Clinical Pharmacology, Division of Medical Sciences, The University of Birmingham, Queen Elizabeth Hospital, Edgbaston, Birmingham B15 2TH, UK, u.martin@bham.ac.uk

BRIAN C. MARTINSON, PhD — Research Investigator, HealthPartners Research Foundation, Minneapolis, MN 55440, USA, Brian.C.Martinson@HealthPartners.com

RONALD MEYBOOM, MD, PhD — Medical Adviser, Uppsala Monitoring Centre, Stora Torget 3, 753 20 Uppsala, Sweden, R.Meyboom@who-umc.org

CAROLINE MOORE, BA (Oxon) — Barrister, Lovells, 65 Holborn Viaduct, London EC1A 2DY, UK, caroline.moore@lovells.com

NICHOLAS MOORE, MD, PhD — Professor of Clinical Pharmacology, Département de Pharmacologie, Université Victor Segalen—CHU de Bordeaux, 33076 Bordeaux cedex, France, nicholas.moore@pharmaco.u-bordeaux2.fr

MICHAEL MOSTELLER, MS, PhD	Statistical Geneticist, Population Genetics, Genetics Research, Glaxo SmithKline, 5 Moore Drive, Research Triangle Park, NC 27709, USA, mm41601@gsk.com
WALTER S. NIMMO, BSc, MD, FRCP, FRCA, FANZCA, FFPM, FRSE	Chief Executive, Inveresk Research, Tranent EH33 2NE, UK, walter. nimmo@inveresk.com
STEN OLSSON, MSci, Pharm	Head, External Affairs, Uppsala Monitoring Center, Stora Torget 3, 753 20 Uppsala, Sweden, sten.olsson@who-umc.org
ROLAND ORRE, MSc	Department of Mathematical Statistics, Stockholm University S-10691 Stockholm, Sweden, orre@mathematic.su.se
B. KEVIN PARK, BSc (Hons), PhD, Hon MRCP	Professor of Pharmacology, Department of Pharmacology and Therapeutics, The University of Liverpool, Ashton Street, Liverpool L69 3GE, UK, bkpark@liverpool.ac.uk
TONI PIAZZA-HEPP, PharmD	Deputy Director, Division of Surveillance, Research and Communication Support, Office of Drug Safety, Center for Drug Evaluation and Research, US Food and Drug Administration, 5600 Fishers Lane, HFD-400, Rm 15B-32, Rockville, MD 20857, USA, PIAZZAHEPPT@ cder.fda.gov
GRAHAM A. PIPKIN, BSc (Hons)	Communications Manager, GI, Neurology and GI GCS, GlaxoSmith-Kline, Stockley Park West, Uxbridge, Middlesex UB11 1BU, UK, gp5771@gsk.com
MUNIR PIRMOHAMED, PhD, FRCP, FRCP (Ed)	Professor of Clinical Pharmacology/Consultant Physician, Department of Pharmacology and Therapeutics, The University of Liverpool, Ashton Street, Liverpool L69 3GE, UK, munirp@liv.ac.uk
RICHARD PLATT, MD, MSc	Professor of Ambulatory Care and Prevention, Harvard Medical School, Director of Research, Harvard Pilgrim Health Care, 133 Brookline Avenue, 6th Floor, Boston MA 02215, USA, richard.platt@channing. harvard.edu
E. P. VAN PUIJENBROEK, MD, PhD	Head, Science Department, Netherlands Pharmacovigilance Centre Lareb, Goudsbloemvallei 7, 5273 MH's-Hertogenbosch, The Netherlands, e.vanpuijenbroek@lareb.nl
MARSHA A. RAEBEL, PharmD	Pharmacotherapy Research Manager, Kaiser Permanente Colorado, and Adjoint Associate Professor of Pharmacy, University of Colorado School of Pharmacy, Denver, CO 80231, USA, Marsha.A.Raebel@kp.org
JUNE M. RAINE, MA, MSc, FRCP (Ed)	Director, Post-Licensing Division, Medicines Control Agency, Market Towers, 1 Nine Elms Lane, London SW8 5NQ, UK, june.raine@ mca.gov.uk
GAILE RENEGAR, JD, RPh	Director, Genetics Education and External Relations, Genetics Research, GlaxoSmithKline, 5 Moore Drive, Research Triangle Park, NC 27709, USA, glr42379@gsk.com
PAOLO RICCI, JD	Partner, Lovells, Via Dei Due Marcelli 66, 00187 Roma, Italy, paolo.ricci@lovells.com
PATRICIA RIESER, BSN, RN, CFNP	Consultant, Genetics Education and External Relations, Genetics Research, GlaxoSmithKline, 5 Moore Drive, Research Triangle Park, NC 27709, USA, pr63544@gsk.com

DOUGLAS ROBLIN, PhD	Research Scientist, Kaiser Permanente Georgia, Atlanta, GA 30305, USA, douglas.roblin@kp.org
SUSAN RODEN, BSc, MSc, MRPS	Director, Global Pharmacovigilance and Risk Management, GCSP, GlaxoSmithKline Research and Development Ltd, Greenford Road, Greenford, Middlesex UB6 0HE, UK, SMR4761@gsk.com
DENNIS ROSS-DEGNAN, ScD	Associate Professor, Department of Ambulatory Care and Prevention, Harvard Medical School, and Harvard Pilgrim Health Care, Boston, MA 02215, USA, dennis_ross-degnan@hphc.org
JOHN-CLAUDE ROUJEAU, MD	Assistant, Service de Dermatologie, Hôpital Henri Mondor, Université Paris XII, 94010 Créteil, France, jean-claude.roujeau@hmn.ap-hop-paris.fr
RASHMI R. SHAH, BSc, MBBS, MD, FRCP, FFPM	Senior Medical Officer, Medicines Control Agency, Market Towers, 1 Nine Elms Lane, Vauxhall, London SW8 5NQ, UK, clin.safety@lineone.net
SAAD A.W SHAKIR, FRCP (Glas & Ed), FFPM, MRCGP	Director, Drug Safety Research Unit, Bursledon Hall, Blundell Lane, Southampton SO31 1AA, UK, saad.shakir@dsru.org
DAVID H. SMITH, RPh, PhD	Investigator, Kaiser Permanente Center for Health Research, Portland, OR 97227, USA, david.h.smith@kpchr.org
STEPHEN B. SOUMERAI, ScD	Professor of Ambulatory Care and Prevention, Department of Ambulatory Care and Prevention, Harvard Medical School and Director of Drug Policy Research Group, Harvard Pilgrim Health Care, Boston, MA 02215, USA, stephen_soumerai@hphc.org
PAUL E. STANG, PhD	Executive Vice-President, Galt Associates, Inc., 1744 DeKalb Pike, Suite 175, Blue Bell, PA 19422-3352, USA, Adjunct Associate Professor of Epidemiology, University of North Carolina School of Public Health, Chapel Hill, NC, USA, pstang@galt-assoc.com
ROSIE STATHER, MA (Cantab)	Editor, *Drug Safety*; Consulting Editor, *Reactions Weekly*, Adis International Ltd, 41 Centorian Drive, Private Bag 65901, Mairangi Bay, Auckland 10, New Zealand, rosie.stather@adis.co.nz
DOUGLAS STEINKE, BSc (Pharm), MSc, PhD	Research Pharmacist, Primary Care Information Group, Information and Statistics Division, Room BO12, Trinity Park House, South Trinity Road, Edinburgh EH5 3SQ, UK, douglas.steinke@isd.csa.scot.nhs.uk
PETER D. STONIER, PhD, MRCPsych, FRCP, FFPM	Medical Director, HPRU Medical Research Centre, University of Surrey, Egerton Road, Guildford GU2 5XP, UK, peterstonier@btinternet.com
BRIAN STROM, MD, MPH	Director, Center for Clinical Epidemiology and Biostatistics, University of Pennsylvania School of Medicine, 824 Blockley Hall, 423 Guardian Drive, Philadelphia PA 19104-6021, USA, bstrom@cceb.med.upenn.edu
MIRIAM C.J.M. STURKENBOOM PHD, MSc, PharmD	Assistant Professor, Pharmaco-epidemiology Unit, Department of Epidemiology and Biostatistics and Medical Informatics. Erasmus University Medical Centre., PO Box 1738, 3000 DR Rotterdam, The Netherlands; International Pharmacoepidemiology and Pharmacoeconomics Research Centre (IPPRC), Via Mantova 11, 20033 Desio (MI), Italy, sturkenboom@epib.fgg.eur.nl

PATRICIA TENNIS, PhD

Senior Director of Safety Epidemiology, Worldwide Epidemiology, GlaxoSmithKline, 5 Moore Drive, Research Triangle Park, NC 27709, USA, pst49347@gsk.com

MARGARET THOROGOOD, PhD

Reader in Public Health and Preventative Medicine, Research Degrees Director, Health Promotion Research Unit, Department of Public Health and Policy, London School of Hygiene and Tropical Medicine, Keppel Street, London WC1E 7HT, UK, margaret.thorogood@lshtm.ac.uk

GABRIELLE TURNER, LL.M

Solicitor, Lovells, 65 Holborn Viaduct, London EC1A 2DY, UK, Gabrielle.turner@lovells.com

MARIANNE ULCICKAS-YOOD, DSc, MPH

Senior Epidemiologist, Henry Ford Health Systems, Detroit, MI 48202, USA, marianne.yood@yale.edu

LAURENCE VALEYRIE, MD

Chef de Clinique, Service de Dermatologie, Hôpital Bichat, 46 Ave Henri Huchard, 75877 Paris Cedex 18, France, laurence.valeyrie@bch.ap-hop-paris.fr

PATRICK C. WALLER, MD, FRCP (Ed), FFPM, MPH

Post-Licensing Division, Medicines Control Agency, Market Towers, 1 Nine Elms Lane, London SW8 5NQ, UK, patrick.waller@mca.gsi.gov.uk

R. M. WHITTINGTON

Former HM Coroner for Birmingham and Solihull Districts, Coroner's Court, Newton Street, Birmingham B4 6NE, UK

RICHARD N. WILD, MB, ChB, DCH, FFPM, FRCP (Ed)

Medical Director, Arakis Ltd, Chesterford Research Park, Little Chesterford, Saffron Walden, Essex CB10 1XL, UK, richardwild@arakis.com

JOHN R. WOOD, MB, BSc, PhD

Managing Director, Wood and Mills Limited, The Mill House, Framewood Road, Fulmer, Bucks SL2 4QS, UK, DrJRWood@cs.com

LOUISE WOOD, BSc (Hons), PhD

Director, GPRD Division, Medicines Control Agency, Room 15-103 Market Towers, 1 Nine Elms Lane, Vauxhall, London SW8 5NQ, UK, louise.wood@gprd.com

Preface

The editors of this volume have looked upon pharmacovigilance as being the study of the safety of marketed drugs under the practical conditions of clinical usage in large communities. However, some aspects of this definition need qualification: safety cannot be considered apart from efficacy in most situations. For example, an ineffective drug used in a serious and life-threatening disease would be unsafe. Those individuals conducting pharmacovigilance are concerned not only with marketed drugs but also with their pre-marketing data—but our working definition serves a practical purpose.

Spontaneous reporting of suspected adverse drug effects is central to pharmacovigilance—which is the systematic search for signals of drug toxicity. When such a signal is detected it has to be verified, explored, and understood—realising that the drug may be acceptably safe if used by individuals who are not at especially high risk by virtue of genetic constitution, metabolism, or other characteristics that could alter individual risk.

Pharmacovigilance is conducted by a very large number of people concerned with protecting populations from serious unintended adverse consequences of medication exposure. It is important to recognise that most medications carry some risk due to their pharmacologic properties or to other factors. The evaluation of risk must be conducted in the context of the patient benefit derived from treatment, the severity of the condition being treated, and other objective and subjective factors (such as the patient's values). Each of the stakeholders—the patient, physician, pharmaceutical company, academic investigator, government—may have a different perspective on the same set of evidence. For example, a patient may be willing to accept a high risk of side-effects for benefits of the treatment for a condition that might be considered trivial by others. A regulatory agency may consider the burden of the same side-effects to be too high, given their view of the risk–benefit equation. A governmental or third-party payer might see the issue from an even different perspective, since a payer may not wish to bear the cost of the treatment or the cost of treating an adverse event. It is perhaps not surprising that each group may take a different view of the same evidence. In addition, each group may also be swayed by intense external pressures to take action to protect specific interests, for example to protect the public against potential harm or to protect against legal liability. These pressures may lead to early decisions based on incomplete scientific data.

There have been mistakes and errors in the field of pharmacovigilance: some drugs have been withdrawn when the benefit to large numbers of patients has not been properly balanced against the harm done to very few highly susceptible subjects. Identifying the patients most susceptible to risk and finding ways to channel medications to the appropriate patients would have been more rational. It is always highly desirable to subject the signal to the formal processes of pharmacoepidemiology (such as case–control, cohort, large simple randomised trial, etc.) before taking gross action on a weak or questionable signal. We have to weigh benefit against risk and the benefit may be to a large population affected by a serious disease and the risk may be to a small population of susceptibles.

This book intends to help bring more rigorous considerations of scientific evidence to the various sectors that face critical decisions about how to act in the face of incomplete information. Our hope is that future decisions will be improved, and that public policy decisions can be made more transparent in the process.

The tension between regulator (government oversight agencies) and regulated (pharmaceutical industry) that was apparent in earlier years must be viewed in a more complex environment in which additional sectors also have considered opinions of the evidence, and possess strong interests as well. All sectors must grapple with the evidence and the pros and cons of decisions and the consequences of these decisions. The subject is not easy and its participants are frequently highly exposed. If this book is of any help to those exposed to political pressure, media pressure, their own indecision and anxieties, etc., then it will have been worth the effort taken to produce it.

The book falls into four parts: the basis of pharmacovigilance, signal generation, pharmacovigilance and the system–organ classes, and, finally, lessons and directions. We have eliminated some duplication but not all of it: people come at the same thing from different directions and some-times those different viewpoints need to be preserved. Some subjects, for a variety of reasons, have been inadequately covered (signal generation in important countries and developing areas of the world; dictionaries and MedDRA; pharmacovigilance as conducted by some of the big companies, other than those already reviewed; non-US medical devices legislation; renal, cardiovascular and respiratory adverse drug reactions, etc.). Some of these subjects have been left for expansion in our second edition; some have been omitted this time round because, for example, we do not intend to cover all the system–organ classes in each edition but will choose different themes as time goes by.

A large number of people are concerned with pharmacovigilance but they are a very small number compared with the populations that they set out to protect. We hope that this volume will be of help to them and we thank our many authors for their contributions.

The editors wish to express their considerable appreciation to John and Celia Hall who took over the management of the production of this book in difficult circumstances and whose contribution is much appreciated. Professor Mann also wishes to acknowledge the considerable support of his personal assistant, Mrs Susan Jerome.

Ronald D. Mann
Elizabeth B. Andrews

Foreword

My introduction to the world of drug toxicity took place in 1965 when a patient attending our Hypertension Clinic at Hammersmith Hospital in London donated blood for transfusion and problems in cross matching the blood sample were encountered. This was found to be due to a positive direct Coombs' test (DCT). The hypertensive patient in question was being treated with α-methyldopa, which at that time was one of the most widely used antihypertensive drugs in the world and had been so for several years. When a possible connection between α-methyldopa and a positive DCT was postulated, initial hilarity and scepticism were rapidly replaced by curiosity and interest when blood samples from a further 202 patients treated with the same drug revealed 40 (20%) patients with the same haematological abnormality, while none of a control group of 76 hypertensive patients on other forms of therapy demonstrated a positive DCT. This led to a series of investigations to document the clinical epidemiology of the adverse effect and to investigate the underlying immunological abnormality. We learned several lessons from this episode. The first was that careful observation and high clinical suspicion are of crucial importance in order to identify a drug toxicity problem. The second lesson was that even though a drug has been on the market for several years and is widely used, unusual adverse reactions may still be identified, stressing the importance of continuing watchfulness. The term "post-marketing drug surveillance" had not been introduced in 1965.

The history of drug safety, pre- and post-thalidomide, has been documented many times. In many respects, this history parallels the development of what we now call rational, or evidence-based, therapeutics. One of the editors of this book, Ronald Mann, elsewhere describes how the United Kingdom in 1914 was on the point of adopting a drug regulatory system very akin to that which we have today. This occurred because around the turn of the last century there was widespread public concern and professional scepticism about the therapeutic value and the safety of patent medicines which were widely promoted and used. In 1909 the British Medical Association published a booklet entitled *Secret Remedies* detailing the excesses and shortcomings of these medicines; this proved to be a best seller which was reprinted several times in quick succession. Such was the level of public anxiety caused by this publication that a Parliamentary Select Committee was established to examine the whole topic of patent medicines. The Committee, which took evidence over three years, pulled no punches in interviewing the purveyors of these products, and its final report recommended in considerable detail how the public should be protected from the frequently unjustifiable and often fraudulent claims of the manufacturers of proprietary medicines. These recommendations included the creation of a Commission whose role was to oversee drug quality, safety and efficacy, drug advertising should be controlled and the Ministry of Health should regulate the field. The publication of the report of the Select Committee on 4 August 1914 was totally overshadowed by *force majeure*, namely the outbreak of the First World War, and the report sat gathering dust on the Ministry's shelves with no action being taken. As Ronald Mann succinctly states, "It is not altogether fanciful to look on the children of the thalidomide disaster as late and unwilling victims of World War One."

Post thalidomide there was a worldwide realisation that the introduction of new therapies and the continuing use of existing therapies had to be regulated based on sound scientific principles. As part of this, systems for doctors to report adverse reactions to drugs were set up; in the United Kingdom a yellow card was used to file the reports. But by the 1980s there was an increasing realisation that all was not well with the methods available to assess adverse drug reactions, and while spontaneous reporting using yellow cards or their like continued to make a valuable contribution to drug safety, other methods had to be devised to help attribute adverse effects to specific drugs. It was suggested that the methodology being pioneered by epidemiologists might make a contribution to study the response of the population to both the adverse and beneficial effects of drugs, thus obtaining a better assessment of risk and benefit. In particular, prospective and retrospective cohort studies, case–control studies, and linked data bases might help unravel the problems of drug safety surveillance. Thus, pharmacoepidemiology arose as a new discipline. The limitations of applying the techniques of the epidemiologist to drug surveillance are, of course, widely appreciated. The clinical data used can rarely be as robust as those from the laboratory and the introduction of bias is a constant risk. Furthermore, the pharmacology of the drugs used and the pathophysiology of the diseases involved have to be understood.

In general, scientists involved in drug safety have espoused the adoption of the principles of pharmacoepidemiology into pharmacovigilance with enthusiasm. However, from time to time, post-marketing safety surveillance studies fall below the required standards, usually due to poor trial design or the total lack of a comparator group. If sound principles are not followed, then such studies are worthless in scientific terms and make no meaningful contribution to pharmacovigilance.

The concept of balancing risk and benefit is now firmly embedded in modern drug treatment. Doctors, patients and the public are familiar with the concept of iatrogenic disease. Large-scale randomised control trials (a particular example of a prospective cohort study) are particularly valuable in defining the balance of risk and benefit and few modern medicines are introduced without being subjected to this form of analysis. One weakness of this approach is that risks and benefits usually have different end points. For example, a trial of an angiotensin converting enzyme inhibitor to investigate the beneficial reduction of stroke, heart failure or myocardial infarction in patients with hypertension has to be balanced against increasing the incidence of cough and rash. Formal decision analysis is one way of dealing with issues like this, but medicine is often uncomfortable with this approach. Another problem is that in any clinical trial there may be a cohort of patients who may show great benefit, but the overall risk–benefit balance of the trial may be negative. Unless one can clearly define the population who will show a beneficial response, perhaps using pharmacogenetic methodology, a drug may be discarded by a developer or rejected by a regulatory authority.

No branch of science stands still. It either makes significant advances or sinks back and becomes irrelevant, and pharmacovigilance is no exception. Looking to the future, perhaps we should be less focused on finding evidence of harm and more interested in extending our knowledge of safety. A specification of what is known about a medicine at the time of licensing should form the basis of what is required to extend understanding of its safety as it is introduced into the community. Risk–benefit decisions in clinical practice and drug regulation are often complex, but other disciplines have also struggled with these problems and medicine should be more prepared to adopt techniques such as formal decision analysis to improve its decision making. Outcome measures should be classified on a hierarchical basis; hard end points such as mortality and morbidity are not always available and imaginative work on surrogate end points of drug safety should be encouraged and validated. As in all branches of medicine, the systematic audit of the processes involved and the outcomes measured should be mandatory and should form the basis of the milestones to be set for the development of the medicine once it becomes widely used. Finally, on perhaps a more mundane level, increasing emphasis should be placed on the provision of comprehensive, and at the same time comprehensible, information on the medicine for the prescriber and the patient. One currently sees an unfortunate tendency for such documentation to become more legalistic and less user friendly. Unless the house physician prescribing for a patient at 3 a.m. has easy access to the essential information he requires, or a patient can understand why he is taking a medicine and what the outcomes are likely to be, all the work that has gone into the development of the drug is valueless. A new approach to providing relevant information on medicines is urgently needed, but sadly this sometimes seems to become more distant as the practice of medicine becomes more complex.

I know of no book with a remit as extensive as this. As the editors say in their preface, repetitions are bound to occur and omissions (some of which they have already defined) are inevitable. The book is a *tour de force* and is a great tribute to the driving energy, enthusiasm and professionalism of Ronald Mann and Elizabeth Andrews, and I am extremely proud to be associated with it.

Alasdair Breckenridge
Chairman of the Committee
on Safety of Medicines

Part I

BASIS OF PHARMACOVIGILANCE

1

Introduction

RONALD D. MANN
Waterlooville, Hampshire, UK

ELIZABETH B. ANDREWS
RTI Health Solutions, Research Triangle Institute, Research Triangle Park, NC, USA, and School of Public Health
and School of Pharmacy, University of North Carolina at Chapel Hill, NC, USA

"Not all hazards can be known before a drug is marketed."

Pharmacovigilance—the study of the safety of marketed drugs under the practical conditions of clinical usage in large communities—involves a paradox. The nature of the paradox is best explained by glancing back to the very early 1960s and then looking at contemporary experience.

The greatest of all drug disasters was the thalidomide tragedy of 1961–1962. Thalidomide had been introduced, and welcomed, as a safe and effective hypnotic and anti-emetic. It rapidly became popular for the treatment of nausea and vomiting in early pregnancy. Tragically, the drug proved to be a potent human teratogen that caused major birth defects in an estimated 10 000 children in the countries in which it was widely used in pregnant women. Figure 1.1 shows such a child fitted with the kind of prostheses available at that time. The story of this disaster has been reviewed elsewhere (Mann, 1984).

The thalidomide disaster led to the establishment of the drug regulatory mechanisms of today. These mechanisms require that new drugs shall be licensed by the well-established regulatory authorities before being introduced into clinical usage. This, it might be thought, would have made medicines safe—or, at least, acceptably safe. But Table 1.1 shows a list of over 30 licensed medicines withdrawn, after marketing, and for drug safety reasons, over the last 25 years in the United Kingdom.

What is the explanation for the paradox that the highly regulated pharmaceutical industry should need, or be compelled, to withdraw licensed medicines for drug safety reasons? Why do these withdrawals continue despite the accumulated experience of more than 40 years since the thalidomide tragedy?

Partly, the problem is one of numbers. To take but one example: the median number of patients contributing data to the clinical safety section of new drug licensing applications in the United Kingdom is only just over 1500 (Rawlins and Jefferys, 1991). Increasing regulatory demands for additional information prior to approval have presumably increased the average numbers of patients in applications, especially for new chemical entities. Nevertheless, the numbers remain far

---

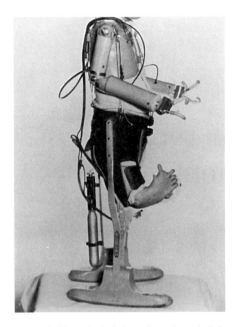

Figure 1.1. Child with thalidomide-induced deformities of upper and lower limbs fitted with pneumatic prostheses.

too small to detect uncommon or rare adverse drug reactions, even if these are serious.

The size of the licensing applications for important new drugs cannot be materially increased without delaying the marketing of new drugs to an extent damaging to diseased patients. Thus, drug safety depends very largely on the surveillance of medicines once they have been marketed.

A second reason for difficulty is that the kinds of patients who receive licensed medicines are very different from the kinds of volunteers and patients in whom pre-marketing clinical trials are undertaken. The patients in formal clinical trials almost always have only one disease being treated with one drug. The drug, once licensed, is likely to be used in an older group of patients, many of whom will have more than one disease and be treated by means of polypharmacy. The formal clinical trials may be a better test of efficacy than they are of safety under the practical conditions of everyday clinical usage.

A third problem is that doctors may be slow or ineffective in detecting and reporting adverse drug effects. Many of the drugs shown in Table 1.1

were in wide-spread, long-term use before adverse reactions were detected and, even now, hospital admissions due to adverse drug reactions have shown an incidence of between 2.4% and 3.6% of all admissions in Australia with similar or greater figures in France and the United States (Pouyanne *et al.*, 2000). Even physicians astute in detecting adverse drug effects are unlikely to identify effects of delayed onset.

An underlying reason is that drugs are often withdrawn from the market for what may be very rare adverse effects—too infrequent by far to have shown up in the pre-licensing studies—and we just do not have effective means in place for monitoring total post-marketing safety experience. The methodological problem is fundamental and its recognition widespread amongst those who have devoted long periods to the issue of drug safety monitoring.

Some of these difficulties were recognized from quite early on. The Committee on Safety of Drugs in the United Kingdom (established after the thalidomide disaster, originally under the chairmanship of Sir Derrick Dunlop, to consider drug safety whilst the Medicines Act of 1968 was being written) said—quite remarkably—in its last report (for 1969 and 1970) that "no drug which is pharmacologically effective is without hazard. Furthermore, not all hazards can be known before a drug is marketed." This then has been known for over 30 years. Even so, many prescribers still seem to think that licensed drugs are "safe"—and they are surprised when a very small proportion of licensed drugs have to be withdrawn due to unexpected drug toxicity. And patients themselves may have expectations that licensed drugs are "completely safe" rather than having a safety profile that is acceptably safe in the context of the expected benefit and nature of the underlying health condition.

The methodological problems have been long recognized. The Committee on Safety of Medicines, the successor in the United Kingdom to the Dunlop Committee, investigating this and related problems, established a Working Party on Adverse Reactions. This group, under the chairmanship of Professor David Grahame-Smith, published its second report in July 1985. The report supported

Table 1.1. Drugs withdrawn in the United Kingdom by the marketing authorization holder or suspended or revoked by the Licensing Authority.

Brand name (drug substance)	Year action taken	Major safety concerns
Secholex (polidexide)	1975	Safety concerns due to impurities
Eraldin (practolol)	1975	Oculomucocutaneous syndrome
Opren (benoxaprofen)	1982	Hepatotoxicity, serious skin reactions
Devryl (clomacran phosphate)	1982	Hepatotoxicity
Flosint (indoprofen)	1982	Gastrointestinal toxicity
Zomax (zomepirac)	1983	Anaphylaxis
Osmosin (indomethacin-modified release)	1983	Small instestine perforations
Zelmid (zimeldine)	1983	Neurotoxicity
Flenac (fenclofenac)	1984	Lyell's syndrome
Methrazone (feprazone)	1984	Serious skin reactions Multi-system toxicity
Althesin (alphaxolone plus alphadolone)	1984	Anaphylaxis
Pexid (perhexilene)	1985	Hepatotoxicity, neruotoxicity
Suprol (suprofen)	1986	Nephrotoxicity
Merital (nomifensine)	1986	Haemolytic anaemia
Unicard (dilevalol)	1990	Hepatotoxicity
Glauline eye drops 0.6% (metipranolol)	1990	Uveitis
Halcion (triazolam)	1991	Psychiatric reactions
Micturin (terodiline)	1991	Arrhythmias
Teflox (temafloxacin)	1992	Multi-system toxicity
Centoxin (nebacumab)	1993	Mortality
Roxiam (remoxipride)	1994	Aplastic anaemia
Volital (pemolin)	1997	Hepatotoxicity
Romazin (troglitazone)	1997	Hepatotoxicity
Serdolect (sertindole)	1998	Arrhythmias
Tasmar (tolcapone)	1998	Hepatotoxicity
Ponderax (fenfluramine)	1998	Cardiac valvular disease
Adifax (dexfenfluramine	1998	Cardiac valvular disease
Posicor (mibefradil)	1998	Drug interactions
Trovan (trovafloxacin)	1999	Hepatotoxicity
Grepafloxacin (Raxar)	1999	QT prolongation
Prepulsid (cisapide)	2000	QT prolongation

continuation of methods of spontaneous reporting by professionals but recommended that post-marketing surveillance (PMS) studies should be undertaken on "newly-marketed drugs intended for widespread long-term use"; the report also mentioned record-linkage methods and prescription-based methods of drug safety surveillance as representing areas of possible progress (see Mann, 1987).

Similar reviews and conclusions have emerged from the United States over the last 30 years. A series of events in the United States recently created a resurgence of interest in drug safety evaluation and management. The Prescription Drug User Fee Act (PDUFA) of 1992 provided additional resources at the Food and Drug Administration (FDA) for drug reviews through user fees, and established target timelines for FDA reviews. The shorter approval times lead to some medications being approved sooner in the United States than in Europe, in contrast to the pre-PDUFA experience. A few highly visible drug withdrawals led to a perception that perhaps drugs were being approved too quickly. In 1998, Lazarou *et al.* published the results of a meta-analysis that estimated that 106 000 fatal adverse reactions occurred in the United States in 1994 (Lazarou *et al.*, 1998). This and other papers (Wood *et al.*, 1998) stimulated considerable public, Congressional, and regulatory attention on reducing the societal burden of drug reactions and medication errors (FDA, 1999; Institute of

Medicine, 1999; US General Accounting Office, 2000). As a result, greater attention and resources are currently being devoted to signal generation and evaluation by the FDA, industry, and academic centers. Moreover, efforts are underway to develop better tools to manage recognized risks, through a variety of interventions, such as communications with healthcare providers and patients, restricted product distribution systems, and other mechanisms. Additional effort is being focused on measuring the success of these risk management interventions. This new initiative represents a fundamental shift in the safety paradigm in the United States, and offers new challenges to pharmacovigilance professionals.

We have long recognized then that the safety of patients depends not only drug licensing by regulatory bodies but also on post-marketing drug safety surveillance, pharmacovigilance. It is also important to note that the same post-marketing information needed to confirm new safety signals is also needed to refute signals and protect patients' ability to benefit from needed medicines that may be under suspicion due to spurious signals.

DIAGNOSING ADVERSE DRUG REACTIONS (ADRS)

There are two types of adverse drug reactions (ADRs). Type A are common, predictable, usually dose-dependent and appear as excessive manifestations of the normal pharmacology/toxicology of the drug; they are seldom fatal. Type B are uncommon, unpredictable, often independent of dose and usually represent abnormal manifestations of the drug's pharmacology/toxicology; they involve relatively high rates of serious morbidity and mortality.

ADRs frequently mimic ordinary diseases and, if they are uncommon, may easily be overlooked. They tend to affect the skin, haematopoietic system and lining of the gut (situations in which there is rapid cell multiplication) or the liver or kidneys (where drugs are detoxified and excreted). These special sites are frequently involved in iatrogenic (doctor-induced), type B illnesses, such

as toxic epidermal necrolysis, aplastic anaemia, pseudomembranous colitis, drug-induced hepatitis or nephritis.

A high index of suspicion is needed if ADRs are to be successfully diagnosed. The clinician always has to think: "Could this be drug-induced—is this an ADR?" The question is important, for withdrawal of the cause of an ADR is usually essential.

Iatrogenic ADRs are usually uncommon or rare—and this adds to the difficulty of diagnosis. Some are avoidable, such as skin rashes in patients with glandular fever given ampicillin. Some are accidental, such as the non-iatrogenic disaster of an asthmatic given a beta-adrenergic blocking agent by another member of the family. It is a truism that the detection of common or uncommon ADRs requires vigilance. Many of the known serious ADRs have been recognized by astute clinicians with a high level of awareness—and such awareness is likely to be just as important, as new methods of pharmacovigilance are developed, as it has been in the past.

Linked with this problem of diagnosing ADRs is the problem of understanding them. Why does one patient in 10 000 get some bizarre Type B reaction—and the rest of this cohort not get it? Clearly our increasing knowledge of clinical pharmacology, drug metabolism and genetics will contribute to our understanding of these things—and these subjects are explored in many of the chapters in this book.

CURRENT METHODS OF PHARMACOVIGILANCE

Pharmacoepidemiology is the study of the use of, and effects of, drugs in large numbers of people. As the term implies, this form of enquiry uses the methods of epidemiology; it is concerned with all aspects of the benefit–risk ratio of drugs in populations. Pharmacovigilance is a branch of pharmacoepidemiology but is restricted to the study, on an epidemiological scale, of drug events or ADRs.

"Events", in this context, are happenings recorded in the patient's notes during a period of drug monitoring; they may be due to the disease for which the drug is being given, some other intercurrent disease or infection, an adverse reaction to the drug being monitored or the activity of a drug being given concomitantly. They can also be due to drug–drug interactions.

Public health surveillance methods are used to identify new signals of possible ADRs. Studies in pharmacoepidemiology are intended to be either "hypothesis-generating" or "hypothesis-testing", or to share these objectives. Hypothesis-generating studies, with a recently marketed drug, aim to detect unexpected ADRs; hypothesis-testing studies aim to prove whether any suspicions that may have been raised are justified.

HYPOTHESIS-GENERATING METHODS

Spontaneous ADR Reporting

Doctors (in some countries other health care professionals or patients as well) are provided with forms upon which they can notify a central authority of any suspected ADRs that they detect. In the United Kingdom the "yellow card" has been used for this purpose since 1964. Similar forms are provided in the FP10 prescriptions pads, the British National Formulary, and other sources. In the United States, the MedWatch form is used, and is made broadly available to health professionals to encourage reporting.

The great strength of spontaneous reporting is that it operates for all drugs throughout the whole of their lifetime; it is the only affordable method of detecting really rare ADRs. The main weaknesses are that there is gross under-reporting and the data provide a "numerator" (the number of reports of each suspected reaction) only. Nevertheless, the scheme is invaluable and it is essential that health professionals should be provided with the means of reporting their suspicions.

Spontaneous reporting has led to identification and verification of many unexpected and serious ADRs. These findings have resulted in a number of marketed drugs being withdrawn, or additional information being provided to guide safer use of the product.

A variety of formal epidemiologic studies can be undertaken to generate or test hypotheses.

Prescription Event Monitoring (PEM)

PEM, as conducted in the United Kingdom and New Zealand, represents a "hybrid" method, combining aspects of public health surveillance and spontaneous reporting with aspects of formal epidemiologic studies. This important technique in the United Kingdom takes advantage of a number of features of the British National Health Service (NHS). Within the NHS, prescriptions written by general practitioners are sent, once they have been dispensed, to a central Prescription Pricing Authority (the PPA). The PPA provides confidential copies of certain prescriptions for newly-introduced drugs that are being monitored to the Drug Safety Research Unit (DSRU) at Southampton. Six or 12 months after the first prescription for an individual drug in an individual patient, the DSRU sends a "green form" questionnaire to the general practitioner who wrote the original prescription. Changing requirements regarding confidentiality and the effect that these have had on PEM is discussed in the appropriate chapter of this volume.

Thus, the prescriptions provide the "exposure data" showing which patients have been exposed to the drug being monitored and the green forms provide the "outcome data" showing any events noted during the period of monitoring. Pregnancies, deaths, or events of special interest can be followed up by contact between the DSRU and the prescribing doctor who holds, within the NHS, the lifetime medical record of all of his or her registered patients.

The great strengths of this method are that it provides a numerator (the number of reports) and a denominator (the number of patients exposed), both being collected over a precisely known period of observation. Furthermore, nothing happens to interfere with the doctor's decision regarding which drug to prescribe for each individual patient—and this avoids selection biases, which can make data interpretation difficult. The main weakness of PEM is that only 50%–70% of the green forms are returned, and the experience of the patients whose forms are not returned may differ from those returned. Thus, it is of great importance that doctors should continue to support the scheme by returning those green forms that they receive.

So far, some 80 drugs have been studied by PEM and the average number of patients included in each study (the cohort size) has been over 10 000. This is a substantial achievement and a tribute to the general practitioners who have participated. PEM in the United Kingdom and a similar program in New Zealand are unique in providing a monitored-release program that can detect or help refute new signals in the early life of a medicine. The pressures to protect confidentiality of patient-specific medical information has precluded this type of program in countries that do not consider such programs worthy of strong legal and public health enablement. More will be discussed in this book about the ethical framework for pharmacovigilance.

HYPOTHESIS-TESTING METHODS

Case–Control Studies

Studies of this type compare cases with a disease with controls susceptible to the disease but free of it. Using this method, the research compares the exposure rate in the cases with the exposure rate in the controls, adjusting statistically for factors that may confound the association. As with any formal epidemiology study, great care has to be taken in the design. Special attention is needed in case definition so that the cases truly represent the specific outcome of interest (e.g. Stevens–Johnson Syndrome, and not all cases of rash). It is also important to select an appropriate control group that represents the population that gave rise to the cases. Careful design can minimize the amount of bias in a study; adequate control in the analysis is also important. Case–control studies have provided a substantial body of evidence for major drug safety questions. Two notable examples are studies that demonstrated the association between aspirin and Reyes Syndrome (Hurwitz et al., 1987), and the evaluation of DES and vaginal cancer in the offspring of mothers who took DES in pregnancy (Herbst et al., 1974, 1975). Moreover, a case–control study established the protective effects of prenatal vitamin supplementation on the develop-

ment of neural tube defects (Werler et al., 1993) The final results of these studies present a measure of the risk of the outcome associated with the exposure under study—expressed as the Odds Ratio. Only in very special circumstances can the absolute risk be determined. Clearly, a fairly small increase in the risk of a common, serious condition (such as breast cancer) may be of far greater public health importance than a relatively large increase in a small risk (such as primary hepatic carcinoma).

Case–control studies are more efficient than cohort studies, because intensive data need only be collected on the cases and controls of interest. Case–control studies can often be nested within existing cohort or large clinical trial studies. A nested case–control study affords the ability to quantify absolute risk while taking advantage of the inherent efficiency of the case–control design.

Cohort Studies

These studies involve a large body of patients followed up for long enough to detect the outcome of interest. Cohort studies generally include an exposed and an unexposed group, but there are also single-exposure, disease, or general population follow-up studies and registries. Studies must be designed to minimize potential biases. An advantage of the cohort study is its ability to quantify both an absolute risk and a relative risk. Cohort studies can be conducted prospectively, but such studies are usually expensive and time-consuming. Retrospective cohort studies can be conducted within large existing databases, providing the advantage of the cohort study design and the efficiencies inherent in studies using existing records.

Case–control studies are particularly useful to confirm a safety signal relating to a rare event (less than 1/1000). Cohort studies are useful when the outcome has not already been identified or when multiple outcomes are of interest. Both case–control and cohort studies can be conducted within large existing databases, assuming the required information is available.

An example of a large existing database can be found in the Medicines Evaluation and Monitoring Organization (MEMO). MEMO achieves "record-linkage" by joining together general practitioner prescription data (the exposure data) with hospital discharge summaries (the outcome data). This activity takes place in Tayside, Scotland where (uniquely in the United Kingdom) all patients have a personal Community Health Number (CHNo) which is widely used by National Health Service facilities of all types. Advantages include completeness, freedom from study-introduced bias in data collection, and timely availability of data for analysis. MEMO is an example of the types of databases that have been established over the last 30 years that utilize data collected systemmatically for other purposes. These databases have been used to detect and quantitatively evaluate hypotheses regarding safety signals.

Data resources now exist in many countries, especially in North America and Western Europe. Some examples of these data resources and application of these databases to answer important safety questions will be described in further chapters.

Randomized Controlled Trials (RCTs)

In this method of study a group of patients is divided into two in strictly random order; one group is then exposed and the other not exposed, so that the outcomes can be compared. The method is of great importance because of its resistance to biases. It is, however, of only limited (but important) use as a pharmacoepidemiological tool because most serious ADRs are relatively uncommon; RCTs used in such contexts can, therefore, become unmanageably large and expensive. Large simple trials have become common in evaluating safety and efficacy in special circumstances, such as vaccine development.

CONCLUSION

The identification of signals of drug reactions is a complex and daunting task, especially since some reactions mimic common illnesses and may therefore be difficult to identify. Constant awareness is needed if signals are to be detected. The diagnosis and reporting of suspected ADRs are needed to protect both individual patients and the community. Present methods are indispensable but inadequate.

The pharmacovigilance professional is best able to place potential safety signals into appropriate context with a full appreciation of methods for surveillance, epidemiology and critical appraisal. This book intends to present the regulatory and ethical framework for drug safety evaluation, some of the key clinical outcomes of frequent interest, and a variety of approaches that have been used over time. This book is intended as a prompt for further development in this important field. Physicians and patients will be better served with richer information on appropriate medication use. More comprehensive and accurate definition of medication safety can help regulators and industry take appropriate action to improve safety—from removal of unsafe products to protection of useful products from unwarranted removal.

REFERENCES

Food and Drug Administration (1999) *Managing the Risks from Medical Product Use: Creating a Risk Management Framework*. Washington: US Food and Drug Administration, http://www.fda.gov/oc/tfrm/riskmanagement.pdf.

Herbst AL, Poskanzer DC, Robboy SJ, Friedlander L, Scully RE (1975) Prenatal exposure to stilbestrol: A prospective comparison of exposed female offspring with unexposed controls. *New Engl J Med* **292**: 334–9.

Herbst AL, Robboy SJ, Scully RE, Poskanzer DC (1974) Clear-cell adenomcarcinoma of the vagina and cervix in girls: An analysis of 170 registry cases. *Am J Obstet Gynecol* **119**: 713–24.

Hurwitz ES, Barrett MJ, Bregman D, Gunn WJ, Pinsky P, Schonberger LB, Drage JS, Kaslow RA, Burlington DB, Quinnan GV, *et al.* (1987) Public Health Service study of Reye's syndrome and medications. Report of the main study [published erratum appears in *J Am Med Assoc* **257**(24): 3366, June 26]. *J Am Med Assoc* **257**(14): 1905–11.

Institute of Medicine, Kohn LT, Corrigan JM, Donaldson MS, eds. (1999) *To Err is Human: Building a Safer Health System*. Washington, DC: National Academy Press.

Lazarou JB, Pomeranz H, Corey PN (1998) Incidence of adverse drug reactions in hospitalized patients: A meta-analysis of prospective studies. *J Am Med Assoc* **279**: 1200–5.

Mann RD (1984) *Modern Drug Use-An Enquiry on Historical Principles*. Lancaster, UK: MTP Press (Kluwer Academic), pp. 597–619.

Mann RD (1987) The yellow card data: The nature and scale of the adverse drug reactions problem. In: Mann RD, ed., *Adverse Drug Reactions*. Carnforth, UK: Parthenon Publishing, pp. 59–63.

Pouyanne P, Haramburu F, Imbs JL, Begaud B for the French Pharmacovigilance Centres (2000) Admissions to hospital caused by adverse drug reactions: Cross sectional incidence study. *Br Med J* **320**: 1036.

Rawlins MD, Jefferys DB (1991) Study of United Kingdom product licence applications containing new active substances, 1987–9. *Br Med J* **302**: 223–5.

United States General Accounting Office (2000) *Adverse Drug Events: The Magnitude of Health Risk is Uncertain Because of the Limited Incidence Data.* Report GAO/HEHS-00–21. Washington, DC: US General Accounting Office.

Werler MM, Shapiro S, Mitchell AA (1993) Periconceptional folic acid exposure and risk of occurrent neural tube defects. *J Am Med Assoc* **269**(10): 1257–61.

Wood AJ, Stein CM, Woosley RL (1998) Making medicines safer—the need for an independent drug safety board. *New Eng J Med* **339**: 1851–4.

2

Legal Basis—EU

NICHOLAS MACFARLANE, GABRIELLE TURNER AND CAROLINE MOORE
Lovells, 65 Holborn Viaduct, London, UK

WITH CONTRIBUTIONS BY

CHRISTOPH HILTL
Lovells, Munich, Germany

PAULE DROUAULT-GARDRAT
Lovells, Paris, France

PAOLO RICCI AND PAOLA LA LICATA
Lovells, Rome, Italy

INTRODUCTION

Within the European Union (EU), the pharmaceutical industry is a highly regulated sector. The level of regulation reflects the potential hazards associated with the use of medicinal products. Subject to a limited number of exceptions, all medicinal products placed on the market within the EU must have a marketing authorisation. The grant of a marketing authorisation signifies that a medicinal product complies with the quality, safety and efficacy criteria set out in European medicinal product regulatory law.

Marketing authorisations for products to be placed on the EU market are granted:

- on a national basis by the competent authority of a Member State (where the product will be marketed in one Member State only); or

- through the mutual recognition procedure, where a marketing authorisation granted by the competent authority of an original Reference Member State is accepted by the competent authorities of other Member States;
- since 1 January 1995, on a EU basis by the European Commission (the Commission) under the centralised procedure, in accordance with the provisions of Regulation (EEC) No. 2309/93.

Pharmacovigilance requirements apply to all authorised medicinal products on the market in the EU and EFTA states (Iceland, Liechtenstein and Norway). Both human use and veterinary medicinal products are subject to these requirements; this chapter outlines the requirements for human use medicinal products only.

The need for pharmacovigilance arises from the fact that, despite extensive clinical trials at the

Pharmacovigilance. Edited by R.D. Mann and E.B. Andrews
© 2002 John Wiley & Sons, Ltd

pre-licensing stage in support of a marketing authorisation application for a medicinal product, some safety hazards are only identified after wider use in the general population. The aim of establishing pharmacovigilance systems is to safeguard public health by monitoring medicinal products once authorised and by removing any from the market which are found to present an unacceptable level of risk under normal conditions of use.

The key legal requirements for pharmacovigilance for human use medicinal products are set out in European legislation. For medicinal products authorised under national or mutual recognition procedures, the relevant legislation is Directive 2001/83/EC of 6 November 2001 on the Community Code relating to medicinal products for human use. Directive 2001/83/EC is a codifying text, in which numerous previous Directives have been assembled into a single document. References throughout this chapter are to the codified text, as published in the *Official Journal of the European Communities* on 28 November 2001 and currently in force. For medicinal products authorised under the centralised procedure, the relevant legislation is Regulation (EEC) No. 2309/93 laying down Community procedures for the authorisation and supervision of medicinal products for human and veterinary use and establishing a European Agency for the Evaluation of Medicinal Products (the Agency).

GUIDANCE

Both Article 106 of Directive 2001/83/EC and Article 24 of Regulation (EEC) No. 2309/93 require the Commission, in consultation with the Agency, the Member States and interested parties, to produce guidance on the collection, verification and presentation of adverse reaction reports, so as to facilitate the exchange of pharmacovigilance information within the EU. All Commission guidance must take account of international harmonisation work on pharmacovigilance terminology and classification.

In accordance with this requirement, the Commission provides guidance on the interpretation and implementation of pharmacovigilance requirements in Volume 9 of *The Rules Governing Medicinal Products in the European Union* (Volume 9 (see Appendix 4)). For ease of reference, it should be noted that although Volume 9 was recently updated and replaces all pharmacovigilance guidance published by the Commission prior to 30 September 2001, it has yet to be revised to take account of the codification in Directive 2001/83/EC (and Directive 2001/82/EC which relates to veterinary medicinal products).

The Agency is advised by a scientific committee, the Committee for Proprietary Medicinal Products. A sub-division of this committee is the Pharmacovigilance Working Party, which has a mandate to provide a forum for discussion, consensus development and co-ordination of pharmacovigilance issues at EU level with which Member States are required to co-operate. The Pharmacovigilance Working Party produces documents which supplement the guidance in Volume 9; these are identified in Part IV of Volume 9.

DEFINITIONS

The definitions of key pharmacovigilance concepts apply to all European pharmacovigilance and are set out in Title I of Directive 2001/83/EC. The Commission provides guidance on their interpretation in Volume 9.

An "adverse reaction" is a response to a medicinal product which is noxious and unintended and which occurs at doses normally used in man for the prophylaxis, diagnosis or therapy of disease or for the restoration, correction or modification of physiological function. Volume 9 advises that an adverse reaction, contrary to an adverse event, is characterised by the fact that a causal relationship between the drug and the occurrence is suspected.

A "serious adverse reaction" means an adverse reaction which results in death, is life-threatening, requires inpatient hospitalisation or prolongation of existing hospitalisation, results in persistent or significant disability or incapacity or is a congenital anomaly/birth defect. Volume 9 advises that this includes congenital anomalies or birth defects, serious adverse clinical consequences associated with use outside the terms of the Summary of Product Characteristics, overdoses or abuse. Important adverse reactions that are not immediately life-threatening or do not result in death or hospitalisation, but may jeopardise the patient, should be considered as "serious".

An "unexpected adverse reaction" means an adverse reaction, the nature, severity or outcome of which is not consistent with the Summary of Product Characteristics. Volume 9 advises that this includes reactions related to the class of products within which the particular product falls, which are mentioned in the Summary of Product Characteristics but which are not specifically described as occurring with the product.

For nationally authorised products, the relevant Summary of Product Characteristics is that approved by the competent authority in the Member State to whom the reaction is being reported. For centrally authorised products, the relevant Summary of Product Characteristics is that authorised by the European Commission.

"Abuse of medicinal products" means the persistent or sporadic, intentional excessive use of medicinal products which is accompanied by harmful physical or psychological effects.

EUROPEAN PHARMACOVIGILANCE FOR MEDICINAL PRODUCTS AUTHORISED BY NATIONAL OR MUTUAL RECOGNITION LICENSING PROCEDURES—DIRECTIVE 2001/83/EC

Title IX of Directive 2001/83/EC deals with pharmacovigilance obligations imposed on the Agency, the Commission, marketing authorisation holders and the Member States for medicinal products authorised through national and mutual recognition procedures. Article 102 explains that:

In order to ensure the adoption of appropriate regulatory decisions concerning the medicinal products authorized within the Community, having regard to information obtained about adverse reactions to medicinal products under normal conditions of use, the Member States shall establish a pharmacovigilance system. This system shall be used to collect information useful in the surveillance of medicinal products, with particular reference to adverse reactions in human beings, and to evaluate such information scientifically.

Such information shall be collated with data on consumption of medicinal products.

This system shall also take into account any available information on misuse and abuse of medicinal products which may have an impact on the evaluation of their benefits and risks.

THE AGENCY

Article 105 requires the Agency, in collaboration with the Member States and the Commission, to set up a data-processing network to facilitate the exchange of pharmacovigilance information in order to enable all the competent authorities to share pharmacovigilance information at the same time. The development of the EudraNet facility is discussed further below.

THE COMMISSION

As discussed previously, the Commission has obligations under Article 106 in relation to the publication of pharmacovigilance guidance.

MARKETING AUTHORISATION HOLDERS

Article 104 of Directive 2001/83/EC sets out the obligations of marketing authorisation holders.

Marketing authorisation holders must maintain detailed records of all suspected adverse reactions occurring either in the Community or in a third country. All suspected serious adverse reactions brought to the attention of marketing authorisation holders by health care professionals must be recorded and reported to the competent authority of the Member State where the incident occurred within 15 days.

In addition, marketing authorisation holders are required to record and report suspected serious adverse reactions of which they can reasonably be expected to have knowledge which meet the reporting criteria set out in Volume 9. This addresses the fact that, in addition to adverse reactions reported by health care professionals, others will be identified in worldwide scientific literature or during post-authorisation studies.

Marketing authorisation holders must ensure that all suspected serious and unexpected adverse reactions that are brought to their attention by health care professionals and have occurred in a third country must be reported to the Agency and the competent authorities of the Member States where the product is authorised, within 15 days. The format for these reports is set out in Volume 9.

Where a medicinal product has been authorised through the mutual recognition procedure, the marketing authorisation holder must ensure that all suspected serious adverse reactions occurring in the Community are reported to the competent authority that first authorised the product (known as the Reference Member State) in a format and at a frequency to be agreed with that competent authority.

All suspected adverse reactions must be submitted to the competent authorities in the form of a periodic safety update report (accompanied by a risk/benefit scientific evaluation):

- immediately upon request; or
- at least every six months during the two years after a medicinal product has been granted a marketing authorisation; or
- once a year between the second and fifth years following the grant of the marketing authorisation.

At the end of the five-year period following authorisation, periodic safety update reports must be submitted every five years with each marketing authorisation renewal application.

QUALIFIED PERSON

Article 103 of Directive 2001/83/EC requires marketing authorisation holders to have an appropriately qualified person, responsible for pharmacovigilance, permanently and continuously at their disposal. Volume 9 confirms that the qualified person must be located in the European Economic Area (EEA). The qualified person is responsible for:

- establishing and maintaining a system which ensures that information about all suspected adverse reactions, reported to people within the company and medical representatives, is collected and collated at a single point within the EU;
- preparing reports (in accordance with Article 104, see below) for the competent authorities, in accordance with national guidelines and Volume 9;
- ensuring a full and prompt response to any request from a competent authority for additional information (including information about volume of sales or prescriptions) necessary for a risk/benefit evaluation of a medicinal product.

MEMBER STATES

Article 101 of Directive 2001/83/EC requires Member States to take all appropriate measures to encourage health care professionals to report suspected adverse reactions to the competent authorities. Member States can impose specific reporting requirements on health care professionals, particularly where reporting is a condition of the marketing authorisation.

Once notified of suspected serious adverse reactions, Article 105 requires Member States to ensure that they are brought to the attention of the Agency, the other Member States and the marketing authorisation holder within 15 days, using the Agency's data-processing network. Where, following an evaluation of adverse reaction reports, a Member State decides that a marketing authorisation should be varied, suspended or withdrawn, Article 107 imposes an obligation to notify the Agency and the marketing authorisation holder immediately. In urgent cases, a Member State may suspend the marketing of a medicinal product, on condition that the Agency is informed the following working day at the latest.

EUROPEAN PHARMACOVIGILANCE FOR CENTRALLY AUTHORISED MEDICINAL PRODUCTS— REGULATION (EEC) NO. 2309/93

Article 51c of Regulation (EEC) No. 2309/93 makes the Agency responsible for the co-ordination of the supervision of medicinal products which have been authorised within the Community and for providing advice on the measures necessary to ensure the safe and effective use of these products. Chapter 3 of Regulation (EEC) No. 2309/93 deals specifically with pharmacovigilance.

THE AGENCY

Article 20 requires the Agency to co-operate with the national pharmacovigilance systems, in order to receive all relevant information about suspected adverse reactions to authorised medicinal products in the EU. If necessary, the Agency's Committee for Proprietary Medicinal Products will provide opinions on the measures necessary to ensure the safe and effective use of particular medicinal products.

The EudraNet system, an electronic data-processing network, has been developed to enable the rapid transmission of data between the competent EU authorities in the event of an alert relating to faulty manufacture, serious adverse reactions and other pharmacovigilance data. Although at this stage, not all competent authorities are using EudraNet for pharmacovigilance reporting, it is envisaged that this will eventually replace paper reporting. The Agency is required to evaluate the pharmacovigilance information it receives and to make this information available through a database (Article 51c). To meet this requirement, the EudraVigilance system is currently being developed within EudraNet, following International Conference on Harmonisation (ICH) guidelines and recommendations.

The Agency is also responsible for collaboration with the World Health Organisation (WHO) on international pharmacovigilance, and to take any steps necessary to submit appropriate and adequate information promptly to the WHO regarding the measures taken in the EU which may have a bearing on public health protection in third countries (Article 25). The Pharmacovigilance Working Party of the Committee on Proprietary Medicinal Products produces guidance documents on a wide range of pharmacovigilance issues, including the principles of providing the WHO with pharmacovigilance information (see Chapter 2.6 of Volume 9 and CPMP/PhVWP/053/98 at Appendix 5).

THE COMMISSION

The Commission's obligations under Article 24 in relation to the publication of guidance are discussed above.

MARKETING AUTHORISATION HOLDERS

Article 20 requires marketing authorisation holders to ensure that all relevant information about suspected adverse reactions to centrally authorised products is brought to the attention of the Agency.

Article 22 requires holders of centralised marketing authorisations to ensure that all suspected serious adverse reactions occurring within the EU to one of their products, that are brought to their attention by a health care professional, are recorded and reported within 15 days to the Member States where the incidents have taken place. Marketing authorisation holders must also ensure that all suspected serious unexpected adverse reactions occurring in the territory of a third country are reported immediately to the Agency in addition to all the Member States, within 15 days. Commission Regulation (EC) No. 540/95 sets out the arrangements for reporting suspected unexpected adverse reactions to centrally authorised medicinal products for human (or veterinary) use which are not serious, whether occurring in the EU or a third country; see Appendix 3.

As with holders of marketing authorisations granted under national or mutual recognition procedures, marketing authorisation holders for centrally authorised products are required to maintain detailed records of all suspected adverse reactions occurring within or outside the EU reported to them by health care professionals.

Subject to the specific terms of a marketing authorisation, periodic safety update reports (accompanied by a scientific evaluation) must be submitted to both the Agency and Member States:

- immediately upon request; or
- at least every six months during the two years after a medicinal product has been granted a marketing authorisation; or
- once a year between the second and fifth years following the grant of a marketing authorisation.

At the end of the five-year period following authorisation, periodic safety update reports must be submitted every five years together with each marketing authorisation renewal application.

QUALIFIED PERSON

Article 21 of Regulation (EEC) No. 2309/93 is similar to Article 103 of Directive 2001/83/EC and requires holders of centralised marketing authorisations to have an appropriately qualified person, responsible for pharmacovigilance, permanently and continuously at their disposal. This qualified person is responsible for:

- establishing and maintaining a system which ensures that information about all suspected adverse reactions, reported to people within the company and medical representatives, is collected, evaluated and collated so that it may be accessed at a single point within the EU;
- preparing reports (in accordance with Article 22, see below) for the competent authorities and the Agency;
- ensuring a full and prompt response to any request from the competent authorities for additional information (including information about volume of sales or prescriptions) necessary for a risk/benefit evaluation of a medicinal product.

MEMBER STATES

Article 20 requires the competent authorities of Member States to ensure that all relevant informa-

tion about suspected adverse reactions to centrally authorised products are brought to the attention of the Agency. Where the suspected adverse reactions are classified as serious, Article 23 requires the competent authorities to record and report them to the Agency and the marketing authorisation holder within 15 days. The Agency is then responsible for informing the competent authorities of the other Member States.

EUROPEAN PHARMACOVIGILANCE LEGISLATION—MEMBER STATE IMPLEMENTATION

European Council Directives are not directly binding on Member States, but must be implemented nationally through domestic legislation. Council Regulations have a direct effect on Member States and no further procedural action is required for them to bind Member States.

UNITED KINGDOM

The UK competent authority responsible for medicinal product pharmacovigilance is the Medicines Control Agency (MCA), an executive agency of the Department of Health. European pharmacovigilance requirements are implemented into UK law by the Medicines for Human Use (Marketing Authorisations Etc.) Regulations 1994 (the 1994 Regulations), as amended (see Appendix 6). Schedule 3 of the 1994 Regulations creates certain criminal offences for non-compliance with European pharmacovigilance requirements.

The MCA's post-licensing division, together with the Committee on Safety of Medicines, runs the "Yellow Card" scheme for the reporting of all suspected adverse drug reactions (the name of the scheme derives from the colour of the standardised reporting forms, see Appendix 8). Voluntary reports are accepted by the Committee on Safety of Medicines/MCA from doctors, dentists, coroners and, since November 1999, community pharmacists. Reports are not accepted from members of the public. In addition, reports are received from marketing authorisation holders in accordance with their legal obligations. All reports are entered into the MCA's Adverse Drug Reactions On-Line Information Tracking (ADROIT) database. Marketing authorisation holders may subscribe to the MCA's ADROIT Electronically Generated Information Service (AEGIS), enabling electronic exchange of pharmacovigilance data.

The Committee on Safety of Medicines/MCA encourages reporting of all suspected reactions to newer products. These products are identified with an inverted black triangle symbol ▼ in the relevant professional publications. In addition, the Committee on Safety of Medicines/MCA has a particular interest in adverse reactions in children, the elderly, delayed drug effects, congenital abnormalities and herbal remedies.

In accordance with the requirements of the Data Protection Directive 95/46/EEC (as implemented by Member States) and with common law confidentiality requirements, personal details, such as name and date of birth of patients, are no longer requested for completion of the Yellow Card. Instead, reporters include the patient's age, sex and a reference number, to enable identification of the particular report in any further correspondence. In light of developments in the law of data protection and confidentiality, the UK General Medical Council publishes guidance on confidentiality to assist members of the medical profession when submitting Yellow Card reports (see Appendix 7).

To provide feedback and adverse reaction warnings, the MCA sends doctors and pharmacists *Current Problems in Pharmacovigilance*, a quarterly bulletin providing alerts to problems identified with particular medicines. For urgent medicinal product hazard warnings, "Dear Healthcare Professional" letters are sent to all doctors and pharmacists by post or electronic cascade.

ITALY

The European pharmacovigilance requirements have been implemented in Italy by Legislative Decree no. 178 of 29 May 1991 and Legislative Decree no. 44 of 18 February 1997.

The Italian authority responsible for pharmacovigilance is the Department for the Evaluation of Medicinal Products and Pharmacovigilance of the Ministry of Health (the Department of Pharmacovigilance). The Department of Pharmacovigilance liaises with regional health authorities, with the national pharmacovigilance authorities of other Member States, with the Agency and with international institutions, such as the WHO.

In accordance with European requirements, all pharmaceutical companies must appoint, a "qualified person" responsible for pharmacovigilance, on a continuous and permanent basis. Pharmaceutical companies must notify local health authorities of any serious adverse reaction relating to their products of which they have been informed within three to six days (depending on the seriousness of the reaction). Local health authorities must pass this information to the Department of Pharmacovigilance.

Medical doctors and pharmacists are required to provide the same notification, within the same deadline, whether or not they have prescribed or dispensed the product, and even for products which are undergoing clinical trials. Local private or public authorities must inform the Department of Pharmacovigilance within three to five days and give notice to the product's marketing authorisation holder and to the regional authorities. As from 30 April 2002, adverse event reports may be submitted online. A copy of the reporting form is included at Appendix 10.

Non-compliance with the regulatory requirements constitutes a criminal offence. Marketing authorisation holders and "qualified persons" breaching the regulatory requirements are liable on conviction to a fine between 15 494 and 92 962 Euros. Medical doctors and pharmacists are liable on conviction to a fine between 516 and 5165 Euros.

FRANCE

The European pharmacovigilance requirements are implemented into French law by decree No. 95–278, dated 13 March 1995, as codified in the French Public Health Code. The competent authorities responsible for pharmacovigilance are the French Agency for the Sanitary Safety of Health Products (AFSSAPS), the National Pharmacovigilance Commission (Commission

Nationale de Pharmacovigilance) and the Technical Committee (Comité Technique).

The French Public Health Code requires medical doctors, dental surgeons and midwives to report any serious or unexpected adverse reaction in relation to a medicinal product, whether or not they have actually prescribed the product. Pharmacists are also obliged to report serious or unexpected adverse reactions relating to products that they have dispensed. Reports are filed in a prescribed form (see Appendix 9) at the nearest regional centre, which forwards the data to the AFSSAPS. Voluntary reporting for adverse reactions which are not serious or unexpected may also be filed at the nearest regional centre. The Technical Committee is responsible for co-ordinating and evaluating the data provided by regional centres. Regional centres are obliged to forward information relating to serious adverse reactions to the AFSSAPS directly.

In accordance with the European regulatory requirements, the French Public Health Code requires the "pharmacien responsable" (qualified person) of all pharmaceutical companies to report every serious adverse reaction in relation to its products to the Director of the AFSSAPS. All pharmaceutical companies must maintain a pharmacovigilance department and the directors' names must be registered with the AFSSAPS.

The requirements in Volume 9 were implemented into the French Public Health Code by Article 23 of Law No. 2002-303, dated 4 March 2002. In particular, Article 23 inserts a new Article L.1413-14, requiring health care professionals and health establishments to report any suspected adverse reactions that they become aware of to the competent authority.

GERMANY

The EU pharmacovigilance requirements have been implemented in the German Drug Act (*Arzneimittelgesetz*, AMG). All individuals or businesses involved in the marketing of medicinal products, including manufacturers, wholesalers, physicians and pharmacists, are bound by an ongoing pharmacovigilance duty to ensure that no unsafe drugs enter the market (s. 5 AMG).

According to the legal definition, a drug is to be considered "unsafe" if the current state of scientific knowledge suggests and gives rise to reasonable concerns that the adverse side-effects of the properly applied drug outweigh its benefits. This ban on the marketing of (purportedly) unsafe drugs applies irrespective of whether a marketing authorisation for the product concerned has been granted but not yet revoked. Possible legal sanctions for violations of this duty can be severe, with fines and terms of imprisonment of up to three years, or one year in the case of simple negligence (s. 95 AMG).

The holder of a German national marketing authorisation must report any serious adverse reactions within 15 days of learning of the effects to the Federal Authority for Medicinal Products and Medical Devices, *Bundesinstitut für Arzneimittel und Medizinprodukte* (BfArM). This is the competent authority responsible for pharmacovigilance in Germany.

The applicant must also make all related documentation available together with a scientific evaluation of the adverse reactions (s. 29 (1) AMG). All adverse reactions, other than serious ones, must be recorded and reported at regular intervals. The reporting form is at Appendix 11.

Both BfArM and the district governments of the German states are vested with far-reaching powers to protect public health against hazards resulting from medicinal products by imposing certain restrictions on a medicinal product and/or withdrawing the product from the market. BfArM may restrict, suspend or revoke the marketing authorisation of the drug in question, whereas the state authorities have competence for all other issues. As always in German public law, each acting authority must establish that the measure taken is appropriate and reasonable under the particular circumstances of the case.

In cases where practical experience or scientific research leads to a new risk–benefit assessment of medicinal products on the market, BfArM may order a so-called "Phased Plan Procedure" (PPP, *Stufenplanverfahren;* ss. 62 and 63 AMG). The goal of the PPP is to arrive at an amicable solution for addressing and responding to health risks which come to light after the medicinal product concerned has been approved for circulation on the market.

If the available data and information support reasonable concerns that a certain drug is creating a health hazard, the competent authority must initiate the PPP by calling meetings where all parties concerned (including the manufacturers) are represented and can put forward their arguments. If no consensus can be reached, or if the majority recommendations are not voluntarily complied with, the authority may revert to its general supervisory powers and impose the above-mentioned measures, including informing the public of health hazards caused by certain medicinal products.

Each pharmaceutical company is legally obliged to appoint a PPP Officer (*Stufenplanbeauftragter*) whose duty is to comply with the reporting requirements of the AMG and to co-ordinate and implement pharmacovigilance activities within the company.

PHARMACEUTICAL LEGISLATION 2001 REVIEW

A major review of European pharmaceutical legislation was carried out on behalf of the Commission by independent consultants and published in October 2000. Following this, the Commission announced proposals for legislative reform in July 2001. The Commission identified seven main goals, including guaranteeing tighter surveillance of the market, in particular by strengthening pharmacovigilance procedures.

The proposed changes to existing regulatory requirements include an obligation to prepare and review periodic safety update reports more frequently than at present. After the initial two-year period, post-authorisation reports will be submitted on an annual basis for the following two (rather than three) years and at three (rather than five) yearly intervals from then on. Marketing authorisation holders will be required to use the medical terminology accepted at international level for the transmission of adverse reaction reports (as set out in Volume 9).

There will be new obligations for the Agency; it will be required to ensure the dissemination of

information on adverse reactions to centrally authorised products by means of a database permanently accessible to all Member States and to distribute pharmacovigilance information to the general public. The role of the Committee for Proprietary Medicinal Products will be replaced with a newly established Committee for Human Medicinal Products, with responsibilities that specifically include pharmacovigilance. Following receipt of pharmacovigilance information concerning centrally authorised products, the Committee for Human Medicinal Products will be able to formulate opinions on the measures necessary, which may include amendments to the marketing authorisation.

The proposed amendments have been drafted as a recasting of Regulation (EEC) No. 2309/93 and as amendments to the codifying Directives 2001/83/EC (and 2001/82/EC for veterinary medicinal products). The draft legislation was sent to the European Parliament and Council on 26 November 2001. However, the amendments are unlikely to be adopted before 2003, with implementation in early 2004.

PHARMACOVIGILANCE AND PRODUCT LIABILITY

Consumers who claim to have been injured by medicinal products have various remedies in law against those who manufactured or supplied the products in question. Until 1988 patients in the United Kingdom who wished to bring civil claims for compensation in the absence of a contractual relationship with the supplier, were generally restricted to any claim they might have in negligence.

In 1985, Directive 85/374/EEC (the Directive) introduced the principle of strict liability for defective products, including pharmaceuticals, in the EU. The Directive has now been implemented by national legislation in all the Member States. In the United Kingdom it was incorporated in the Consumer Protection Act 1987 (the 1987 Act), Part 1 of which adds, in theory, a strict liability remedy to those which may be available at common law in contract and tort. Liability is strict in the sense that it is not necessary to prove that a manufacturer or other defendant failed to take reasonable care to avoid injury to those likely to use the product. A claimant still has to prove that the product was defective and that that defect caused his injury or other loss.

The 1987 Act defines those against whom proceedings under Part 1 can be brought. These are a producer (manufacturer), own brander, importer of a product from outside the EU or the supplier (retailer or distributor) if he fails upon request to identify the producer, own brander or importer. Such a person may be liable for injuries caused by a defective medicinal product put into circulation in the United Kingdom after 1 March 1988.

Clearly, a medicinal product is not defective simply because it is capable of producing adverse reactions. Unavoidable side-effects and those in respect of which warnings are given do not render a medicine defective under the 1987 Act. The claimant must prove that the product was defective in that its safety was "not such as persons generally are entitled to expect" (section 3(1); Directive 85/374/EEC, Article 6.1). In determining what persons generally are entitled to expect, all the circumstances should be taken into account including the marketing, packaging, labelling, instructions for use and warnings, foreseeable use or misuse and the time when a product was supplied (see section 3(2)).

Section 3(2) concludes "and nothing in this section shall require a defect to be inferred from the fact alone that the safety of a product which is supplied after that time is greater than the safety of the product in question" (Article 6.2). Thus the mere fact that an improved, lower risk formulation of a medicine has been put on the market since the date the product complained of was supplied, is not enough to render that product defective. However, pharmacovigilance will often bring to light new information about a medicine, rendering certain risks to patients avoidable. Since "persons generally" are entitled to expect that a less risky formulation or presentation of a product will replace an earlier version with riskier characteristics, a product that could not be proved to have been defective under the 1987 Act in 1990 might

have been rendered defective by 1995 through the accumulation of information resulting from post-marketing surveillance. It is not enough for a manufacturer to show that a marketing authorisation has been properly obtained in respect of any given product. The 1987 Act does not apply to medicinal products supplied in the course of clinical trials.

The Directive provides for a number of statutory defences. The most important for the pharmaceutical industry is the "development risks" defence, set out in Article 7(e), which provides that a producer is not liable if he proves "that the state of scientific and technical knowledge at the time when he put the product into circulation was not such as to enable the existence of the defect to be discovered". Article 15(1)(b) of the Directive makes its inclusion in implementing legislation optional for each Member State. In the United Kingdom it is enacted in Section 4(1)(e) of the 1987 Act, the wording of which is to be construed to bring it in line with that of Article 7(e). (See *European Commission v. United Kingdom* [1997] AER (EC) 481; paragraph 21.)

The circumstances in which a medicinal product may be rendered defective by reason of information acquired through pharmacovigilance have yet to be explored fully in any reported cases under Part 1 of the UK 1987 Act of which there are currently fewer than 10. Across the EU, there is a general paucity of reported cases under the national legislation implementing the Directive. The provisions of the Directive were, however, reviewed in depth by the English High Court in the Hepatitis C case (*A and others v. The National Blood Authority and others* [2001] All ER (D) 298 (MAR)), in which 114 claimants sought damages under the 1987 Act after being infected with Hepatitis C virus through blood transfusions. Mr Justice Burton held that the unavoidability of the harmful characteristic of the product was irrelevant to whether it was defective. He also held that the medical profession's knowledge of the risk of infection, which was not shared by the public at large, did not assist the Defendants. If the "learned intermediary" doctrine is to be rejected in strict liability cases, it will be necessary for pharmaceutical companies to warn the actual product users of risks, including those detected through pharmacovigilance, and not to rely on warnings given by the doctor or pharmacists, even where the product is only available from a health care professional.

Failure to meet post-marketing obligations may of course render a pharmaceutical manufacturer liable to a claim in negligence brought by a patient whose injuries can be attributed to that failure.

APPENDICES OF REFERENCE MATERIALS

EUROPEAN COMMISSION

1. Directive 2001/83/EC of 6 November 2001 on the Community Code relating to medicinal products for human use, available at `http://pharmacos.eudra.org`
2. Regulation (EEC) No. 2309/93 laying down Community procedures for the authorisation and supervision of medicinal products for human and veterinary use and establishing a European Agency for the Evaluation of Medicinal Products, available at `http://europa.eu.int/`
3. Commission Regulation (EC) No 540/95 laying down the arrangements for reporting suspected unexpected adverse reactions which are not serious, whether arising in the Community or in a third country, to medicinal products for human or veterinary use authorised in accordance with the provisions of Council Regulation (EEC) No. 2309/93, available at `http://europa.eu.int/`
4. *The Rules Governing Medicinal Products in the European Union*, Volume 9: *Pharmacovigilance*,

available at `http://pharmacos.eudra.org/F2/eudralex`

EUROPEAN AGENCY FOR THE EVALUATION OF MEDICINAL PRODUCTS

5. Principles of providing the WHO with pharmacovigilance information (CPMP/PhVWP/053/98), available at `http://www.emea.eu.int/htms/human/phvwpfin.htm` or at `http://www.emea.eu.int/htms/human/phv/phvpaper.htm`

UNITED KINGDOM

6. The Medicines for Human Use (Marketing Authorisations Etc.) Regulations 1994, as amended, available at `http://www.butterworths.co.uk/legislation/index.htm`
7. UK General Medical Council guidance on confidentiality (June 2000), available at `http://www.gmc.uk.org/`
8. UK Yellow Card reporting form.

FRANCE

9. Pharmacovigilance reporting form, also available at `http://afssaps.sante.fr/`.

ITALY

10. Pharmacovigilance reporting form.

GERMANY

11. Pharmacovigilance reporting form.

APPENDIX 8

In Confidence

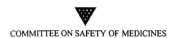

COMMITTEE ON SAFETY OF MEDICINES

M C A
MEDICINES CONTROL AGENCY

SUSPECTED ADVERSE DRUG REACTIONS

If you are suspicious that an adverse reaction may be related to a drug or combination of drugs please complete this Yellow Card. For reporting advice please see over. Do not be put off reporting because some details are not known.

PATIENT DETAILS   Patient Initials: _____   Sex: M / F   Weight if known (kg): _____

Age (at time of reaction): _____   Identification number (Your Practice / Hospital Ref.)*: _____

SUSPECTED DRUG(S)
Give brand name of drug and
batch number if known

	Route	Dosage	Date started	Date stopped	Prescribed for
_____	_____	_____	_____	_____	_____
_____	_____	_____	_____	_____	_____

SUSPECTED REACTION(S)
Please describe the reaction(s) and any treatment given:

Outcome
Recovered ☐
Recovering ☐
Continuing ☐

Date reaction(s) started: _____   Date reaction(s) stopped: _____   Other ☐

Do you consider the reaction to be serious?   Yes / No

If *yes*, please indicate why the reaction is considered to be serious (please tick all that apply):

Patient died due to reaction ☐   Involved or prolonged inpatient hospitalisation ☐

Life threatening ☐   Involved persistent or significant disability or incapacity ☐

Congenital abnormality ☐   Medically significant; please give details: _____

OTHER DRUGS (including self-medication & herbal remedies)
Did the patient take any other drugs in the last 3 months prior to the reaction?   Yes / No

If *yes*, please give the following information if known:

Drug (Brand, if known)	Route	Dosage	Date started	Date stopped	Prescribed for
_____	_____	_____	_____	_____	_____
_____	_____	_____	_____	_____	_____
_____	_____	_____	_____	_____	_____
_____	_____	_____	_____	_____	_____

Additional relevant information   e.g. medical history, test results, known allergies, rechallenge (if performed), suspected drug interactions. For congenital abnormalities please state all other drugs taken during pregnancy and the last menstrual period.

REPORTER DETAILS	**CLINICIAN (if not the reporter)**
Name and Professional Address: _____	Name and Professional Address: _____
	_____ Post code: _____
Post code: _____ Tel No: _____	Tel No: _____ Speciality: _____
Speciality: _____	If you would like information about other adverse reactions
Signature: _____ Date: _____	associated with the suspected drug, please tick this box ☐

* This is to enable you to identify the patient in any future correspondence concerning this report

Please attach additional pages if necessary

APPENDIX 9

RÉPUBLIQUE FRANÇAISE

DÉCLARATION D'EFFET INDÉSIRABLE SUSCEPTIBLE D'ÊTRE DÛ À UN MÉDICAMENT OU PRODUIT MENTIONNÉ À L'ART. R. 5144-1

N° 10011*01

Art. L. 5121-20 13°, R. 5144-7 à 35 du Code de la Santé publique

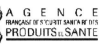
A G E N C E
FRANÇAISE DE SÉCURITÉ SANITAIRE DES
PRODUITS et SANTE

PHARMACOVIGILANCE

| DÉCLARATION À ADRESSER AU |
| Centre de Pharmacovigilance : |

Les informations recueillies seront, dans le respect du secret médical, informatisées et communiquées au centre régional de pharmacovigilance et à l'AFSSAPS. Le droit d'accès du patient s'exerce auprès du centre régional de pharmacovigilance auquel a été notifié l'effet indésirable, par l'intermédiaire du praticien déclarant ou de tout médecin désigné par lui. Le droit d'accès du praticien déclarant s'exerce auprès du centre régional de pharmacovigilance auquel a été notifié l'effet indésirable, conformément aux dispositions de la loi du 6 janvier 1978.

Patient traité

Nom (3 premières lettres)

Prénom (première lettre)

Sexe ☐ F ☐ M

Département de résidence

Date de naissance

ou

Age

Poids

Taille

S'il s'agit d'un nouveau-né, les produits ont été pris :

☐ par le nouveau-né

☐ lors de l'allaitement

☐ par la mère durant sa grossesse
Trimestre de grossesse

☐ *indiquer : 1, 2 ou 3*

Cachet du Praticien déclarant

ou du Médecin désigné par le patient

Produits

	Nom	Voie	Posologie	Début	Fin	Indication
1						
2						
3						
4						
5						
6						

Un ou des produits ont-ils été arrêtés ?

Sans information ☐ Non ☐ Oui ☐ N° ☐ N° ☐ N° ☐ N° ☐ N° ☐ N° ☐

Disparition de la réaction après arrêt d'un ou des produits ?

Sans information ☐ Non ☐ Oui ☐ N° ☐ N° ☐ N° ☐ N° ☐ N° ☐ N° ☐

Un ou des produits ont-ils été réintroduits ?

Sans information ☐ Non ☐ Oui ☐ N° ☐ N° ☐ N° ☐ N° ☐ N° ☐ N° ☐

Réapparition de la réaction après réintroduction ?

Sans information ☐ Non ☐ Oui ☐ N° ☐ N° ☐ N° ☐ N° ☐ N° ☐ N° ☐

En cas d'administration de : **médicament dérivé du sang** ➔ *indiquer son N°* ☐

Nom du prescripteur

Service hospitalier dans lequel le produit a été administré

Numéro de lot du produit

Pharmacie qui a délivré le produit

En cas d'administration de : **produits sanguins labiles** ➔ *préciser leur Dénomination, ainsi que leur Numéro de lot*

Effet

Département de survenue

Date de survenue

Durée de l'effet

Nature et description de l'effet :
utiliser le cadre page 2

Gravité

☐ Hospitalisation ou prolongation d'hospitalisation

☐ Incapacité ou invalidité permanente

☐ Mise en jeu du pronostic vital

☐ Décès

Evolution

☐ Guérison sans séquelle

☐ Décès dû à l'effet

☐ Décès sans rapport avec l'effet

☐ Sujet non encore rétabli

☐ Guérison avec séquelles

☐ Décès auquel l'effet a pu contribuer

☐ Inconnue

Page 1/2

APPENDIX 10

ALLEGATO 5

N.B.:E' OBBLIGATORIA SOLTANTO LA COMPILAZIONE DEI SEGUENTI CAMPI: 2; 4; 7; 8; 12; 22; 24; 25.

SCHEDA DI SEGNALAZIONE DI SOSPETTA REAZIONE AVVERSA
(Da compilarsi a cura del medico o farmacista)

1. INIZIALI DEL PAZIENTE	2.ETA'	3. SESSO	4.DATA INSORGENZA REAZIONE	5. ORIGINE ETNICA	6. CODICE MINISTERO SANITA':

7. DESCRIZIONE DELLE REAZIONI ED EVENTUALE DIAGNOSI*	8. GRAVITA' DELLA REAZIONE

8. GRAVITA' DELLA REAZIONE

MORTE ☐
HA PROVOCATO O HA PROLUNGATO L'OSPEDALIZZAZIONE ☐
HA PROVOCATO INVALIDITA' GRAVE O PERMANENTE ☐
HA MESSO IN PERICOLO LA VITA DEL PAZIENTE ☐

* NOTA: SE IL SEGNALATORE E' UN FARMACISTA, RIPORTI SOLTANTO LA DESCRIZIONE DELLA REAZIONE AVVERSA, SE E' UN MEDICO ANCHE L'EVENTUALE DIAGNOSI.

10. ESITO:

RISOLTA ☐

9. ESAMI STRUMENTALI E/O DI LABORATORIO RILEVANTI

RISOLTA CON POSTUMI ☐

PERSISTENTE ☐

11. SPECIFICARE SE LA REAZIONE E' PREVISTA NEL FOGLIO ILLUSTRATIVO

MORTE:
DOVUTA ALLA REAZIONE AVVERSA ☐

SI ☐   NO ☐

IL FARMACO POTREBBE AVER CONTRIBUITO ☐

COMMENTI SULLA RELAZIONE TRA FARMACO E REAZIONE:

NON DOVUTA AL FARMACO ☐

CAUSA SCONOSCIUTA ☐

INFORMAZIONI SUL FARMACO

12. FARMACO(I) SOSPETTO(I) (NOME SPECIALITA' MEDICINALE)* A) B) C)	13. LA REAZIONE E' MIGLIORATA DOPO LA SOSPENSIONE DEL FARMACO? SI ☐ NO ☐

*NEL CASO DI PRODOTTI BIOLOGICI INDICARE IL NUMERO DEL LOTTO.

14. DOSAGGIO(I) GIORNALIERO(I) A) B) C)	15. VIA DI SOMMINISTRAZIONE A) B) C)	16. DURATA DELLA TERAPIA DAL AL A) B) C)	17. RIPRESA DEL FARMACO SI ☐ NO ☐ RICOMPARSA DEI SINTOMI SI ☐ NO ☐

18. INDICAZIONI PER CUI IL FARMACO E' STATO USATO

19. FARMACO(I) CONCOMITANTE(I) E DATA(E) DI SOMMINISTRAZIONE

20. CONDIZIONI CONCOMITANTI E PREDISPONENTI	21. LA SCHEDA E' STATA INVIATA ALLA: AZIENDA PROD. ☐ USL ☐ DIR. SANITARIA ☐ MINISTERO DELLA SANITÀ ☐

INFORMAZIONI SUL SEGNALATORE

22. FONTE: OSPEDALIERO ☐ MEDICO DI BASE ☐ FARMACISTA ☐ SPECIALISTA ☐ ALTRO ☐	23. NOME ED INDIRIZZO DEL MEDICO O FARMACISTA -NUMERO ISCRIZIONE ORDINE PROFESSIONALE - PROVINCIA

24. DATA DI COMPILAZIONE	25. FIRMA
26. CODICE USL	27. FIRMA RESPONSABILE

(Confidenziale)

APPENDIX 11

BERICHT ÜBER UNERWÜNSCHTE ARZNEIMITTELWIRKUNGEN (auch Verdachtsfälle)

Bundesinstitut für Arzneimittel und Medizinprodukte, Friedrich-Ebert-Allee 38, D-53113 Bonn, Tel.: (0228) 207 - 30, FAX: (0228) 207 - 5207

BfArM

Firmen Code Nr.	Pat. Init. N-name ⊔ V-name ⊔	Geburtsdatum	Geschlecht m ☐ w ☐	Größe	Gewicht	Schwangerschafts- woche:

Beobachtete unerwünschte Wirkungen   aufgetreten am   Dauer

Arzneimittel / Darreichungsform	Tagesdosis	Applikation	gegeben von / bis	wegen (Indikation)
1. Chrg.-Nr:				
2. Chrg.-Nr:				
3. Chrg.-Nr:				
4. Chrg.-Nr:				

Vermuteter Zusammenhang mit Arznei- mittel Nr. 1 2 3 4	dieses früher gegeben ja ☐ nein ☐	vertragen ja ☐ nein ☐	ggf. Reexposition neg. ☐ pos. ☐

Grunderkrankung: Begleiterkrankungen:

Anamn. Besonderheiten: Nikotin ☐   Alkohol ☐   Kontrazeptiva ☐   Schrittmacher ☐
Implantate ☐   Strahlentherapie ☐   physikal. Therapie ☐   Diät ☐   Allergien* ☐
Stoffwechseldefekte* ☐   Arzneimittelabusus* ☐   Sonstige:

* weitere Erläuterungen

Veränderung von Laborparametern in Zusammenhang mit der unerwünschten Arzneimittelwirkung: (ggf. Befund beifügen)

Verlauf und Therapie der unerwünschten Arzneimittelwirkung: lebensbedrohend <br> ja ☐ nein ☐

Ausgang der unerwünschten Arzneimittelwirkung:
wiederhergestellt ☐   bleibender Schaden ☐   noch nicht wiederhergestellt ☐   unbekannt ☐
Exitus ☐   Sektion ja ☐   nein ☐   (ggf. Befund beifügen)
Todesursache:

a) behand. Arzt b) Hersteller c) Arzneim.- Komm.	**Beurteilung des Kausalzusammenhanges:** gesichert ☐ wahrscheinlich ☐ möglich ☐ unwahrscheinlich ☐ unbeurteilt ☐ nicht zu beurteilen ☐ **Weitere Bemerkungen:** (ggf. Anlage verwenden)

Wer wurde informiert: BfArM ☐   Hersteller ☐   Arzneim.-Komm.-Ärzte ☐   Sonstige:

Name des Arztes: Hersteller: Datum:
Fachrichtung:
PLZ:

Klinik: ja ☐ nein ☐   (ggf. Stempel)   Unterschrift:

BfArM 643 / I (10.99)

3

Legal Basis—US

ROBERT P. BRADY AND MARK D. LEARN

Hogan & Hartson L.L.P., Washington, DC, USA

INTRODUCTION

From a pharmaceutical regulatory perspective in the United States, the decade of the 1990s was primarily about user fees, accelerated approvals and fast-track drugs. There was an unusual confluence of Congress, patient groups, the Food and Drug Administration (FDA) and industry all focused on a more timely and efficient drug approval process. The first decade of the twenty-first century will focus on drug safety, in part a reaction to what occurred in the 1990s. Risk management plans, restricted access, product monitoring and accelerated withdrawals will be the focus of that same confluence of interests. While innovative solutions will be discussed and embraced, pharmacovigilance has been, and will remain, at the heart of drug safety. This chapter will describe the legal basis and requirements for pharmacovigilance in the United States with regard to drugs and biological products. The chapter will then review how the FDA enforces these requirements and the penalties for non-compliance. For purposes of this chapter, pharmacovigilance means the collection, analysis and submission to the FDA of adverse experiences and other safety information related to drugs and biological products.

BACKGROUND

The legal requirements for the development, approval and marketing of drugs in the United States are contained in the Federal, Food, Drug and Cosmetic Act (FDCA). Pub. L. No. 75–717, 52 Stat. 1040 (1938), as amended (codified as amended at 21 U.S.C. §§ 301 *et seq.*). Biological products (for example, vaccines, blood, and cellular derived products and most products derived from biotechnology) are approved (licensed) pursuant to the Public Health Service Act (PHSA). Ch. 288, 37 Stat. 309 (1912), as amended (codified as amended at 42 U.S.C. § 262). Biological products are also subject to the legal requirements for drugs during the developmental stage as well as the post-approval marketing stage. For purposes of this chapter, when there is a discussion of drugs, the reader must assume that the same requirements apply to biological products unless specifically identified as different.

A pharmaceutical company must look to three sources of information to determine the legal standards for pharmacovigilance in the United States: laws, regulations and guidances. If a manufacturer, sponsor or individual violates the standard in the law, then they are subject to the

Pharmacovigilance. Edited by R.D. Mann and E.B. Andrews

© 2002 John Wiley & Sons, Ltd

penalties described in such laws. Laws, however, are often relatively general (i.e. manufacturers shall keep records and make reports). Often the FDA must publish regulations that further define the more generalized standards in the law. The FDA develops regulations by publishing a proposed regulation in the *Federal Register*; taking public comment; and then publishing a final rule that takes into account comments received. Once a final regulation takes effect, it is published in the US government's Code of Federal Regulations (CFR). If the FDA regulations are properly developed, then they set legally binding standards. If a company violates a regulation, it is the same as if the company has violated the law itself and the company is subject to the penalties described in the law. Guidances are a third source of information about what the standards are. These are informal communications from the FDA which provide the agency's current thinking about how to comply with various legal requirements. Guidances, how-ever, do not have the force and effect of law. Therefore, if a company violates the conduct described in a guidance or otherwise does not comply, the company is not automatically violating the law and subject to penalties. The FDA adds the following disclaimer to all guidances it publishes:

> This guidance has been prepared by the Center for Drug Evaluation and Research at the Food and Drug Administration (FDA). This guidance represents the Agency's current thinking on [the topic of the respective guidance]. It does not create or confer any rights for or on any person and does not operate to bind FDA or the public. An alternative approach may be used if such approach satisfies the requirements of the applic-able statutes, regulations, or both.

Conduct that is contrary to an FDA Guidance represents a risk however that the FDA will consider it a violation of law and attempt to bring an enforcement action.

LAW

The specific law that governs pharmacovigilance requirements in the United States for drugs is section 505 of the FDCA. 21 U.S.C. § 355. Section 505(i) of that law gives the FDA the authority to regulate investigational drugs. As part of that authority the FDA must, by regulation, require "the establishment and maintenance of such records, and the making of such reports to the Secretary, by the manufacturer or the sponsor of the investigation of such drug ... as the Secretary finds will enable him to evaluate the safety and effectiveness of such drug in the event of the filing of an application ..." 21 U.S.C. § 355(i)(1)(C). As discussed above, biological products are regulated as drugs during the investigational stage and therefore this is the legal basis for safety reporting for biological products as well. 21 C.F.R. § 312.2(a); § 601.21. The specifics of what must be reported are set forth in the regulations and guidances discussed below.

For approved drugs, the basis in law for pharmacoviligance is section 505(k) of the FDCA. 21 U.S.C. § 355(k). That provision states, in part, for approved drugs that: "... the appli-cant shall establish and maintain such records, and make such reports to the Secretary, of data relating to clinical experience and other data or information, received or otherwise obtained ... as the Secretary may by general regulation, or by order with respect to such application, pre-scribe ..." in order to determine, among other things, whether the drug should be withdrawn from the market due to safety concerns. As with investigational drugs, the law merely gives the FDA the authority to require such records and make such reports, but it is the regulation and guidances, as discussed below, which set forth the specific standards.

For biological products approved under the PHSA, the FDA has been given the legal authority to set standards for such products that "... insure the continued safety, purity and potency of such products ..." 42 U.S.C. § 262(d). The standards, according to the law, must be set forth in regulations. The FDA gathers further legal support for these legal requirements from the drug misbranding provi-sions of the FDCA (21 U.S.C. §§ 352(a) and (f)(1)). As with drugs, there is a general legal authority to require pharmacovigilance activities for biological products but the specific standards, as discussed below, are set forth in regulations and guidances.

REGULATIONS

The FDA regulations contain provisions establishing a system for reviewing reports of adverse events and submitting them to the FDA. Only certain reports must be sent to the FDA, depending on the nature of the event and the source of the information. Before 1997, there were several differences in the regulatory requirements for the reporting of adverse events between investigational and marketed products. Those changes have largely disappeared as a result of a final rule designed to create consistency in pre- and post-marketing adverse event reporting and to bring the FDA requirements more in-line with international standards.

FDA REPORTING STANDARDS FOR INVESTIGATIONAL DRUGS AND BIOLOGICAL PRODUCTS

Review of Adverse Events

A sponsor must "promptly review all information relevant to the safety of [a] drug obtained or otherwise received by the sponsor from any source, foreign or domestic, including information derived from any clinical or epidemiological investigations". 21 C.F.R. § 312.32(b). The safety information that sponsors receive from clinical investigations often is in the form of reports relating to experiences of the clinical study subjects.

In contrast to the criteria for sponsor reporting of adverse events to the FDA, the regulations specify different criteria for what investigators must report to the Investigational New Drug (IND) sponsors. An investigator has no obligation to report adverse events to the FDA. Under FDA regulations, investigators must only evaluate adverse experiences based on two criteria: whether the event is serious and whether it was caused by the drug. FDA regulations require

investigators to "promptly report to the sponsor any adverse effect that may reasonably be regarded as caused by, or probably caused by, the drug. If the adverse effect is alarming, the investigator shall report the adverse effect immediately." *Id.* at § 312.64(b).

Depending on several criteria discussed below, FDA regulations provide two mechanisms for reporting adverse event and other safety information about investigational drugs to the Agency. Sponsors report adverse experiences to the FDA either as (1) an expedited report, or (2) as part of an IND annual report. 21 C.F.R. §§ 312.32–33. Adverse experiences that are not reported to the FDA under one of these two mechanisms are usually included in listings submitted to FDA as part of a final study report.

Expedited Reports—Telephone and Written IND Safety Reports

The goal of expedited safety reporting is to ensure timely communication to the FDA of the most important new information about the safety of investigational drugs. 52 Fed. Reg. 8798, 8815 (1987). There are two types of expedited reports: telephone IND safety reports and written IND safety reports. 21 C.F.R. § 312.32(c). Sponsors must make a telephone IND safety report to the FDA as soon as possible, but in no event later than seven calendar days after the sponsor's initial receipt of the reportable information. *Id.* at § 312.32(c)(2). IND sponsors must submit written IND safety reports within 15 calendar days after the sponsor's initial receipt of the reportable information. *Id.* at § 312.32(c)(1).

Expedited reports are required for adverse events experienced by subjects taking investigational drugs if the event is (1) serious, (2) associated with the use of the drug, *and* (3) unexpected. The regulatory standards for these three criteria are discussed below. Expedited safety reports also are required when the sponsor receives reports of pre-clinical findings that suggest significant risk for human subjects including reports of mutagenicity, teratogenicity or carcinogenicity. 21 C.F.R. § 312.32(c)(1)(i)(B).

Serious Adverse Events

The type of expedited safety report that is required depends on the seriousness of the event. A telephone IND safety report is required when an adverse event is fatal or life-threatening. A written IND safety report is required if the event is serious. *Id.* at § 312.32(c). FDA regulations define a serious adverse event for subjects receiving investigational drugs as one that

> results in any of the following outcomes: death, a life-threatening adverse drug experience, inpatient hospitalization or prolongation of existing hospitalization, a persistent or significant disability/incapacity, or a congenital anomaly/birth defect. Important medical events that may not result in death, be life-threatening, or require hospitalization may be considered a serious adverse drug experience when, based upon appropriate medical judgment, they may jeopardize the patient ... and may require medical or surgical intervention to prevent one of the outcomes listed in this definition. 21 C.F.R. § 312.32(a).

Because adverse events that are fatal or life-threatening are included in the definition of a "serious" event, they must be submitted to the FDA as a written report in addition to a telephone report.

Unexpected Adverse Events

Telephone and/or written IND safety reports are required only for adverse events that are unexpected. FDA regulations define an unexpected adverse drug experience with an investigational drug as one for which

> the specificity or severity ... is not consistent with the current investigators' drug brochure or, if an investigator brochure is not required or available, the specificity or severity of which is not consistent with the risk information described in the general investigational plan or elsewhere in the current application, as amended. *Id.*

Associated with the Use of the Drug

Neither telephone nor written IND safety reports are required for an adverse event unless it is associated with the use of the drug. For purposes of IND safety reporting, an event is associated with the use of a drug if "there is a reasonable possibility that the experience may have been caused by the drug". *Id.* at § 312.32(a).

Follow-up Reports

In addition to reviewing promptly adverse safety information that it receives, an IND sponsor also must "promptly investigate" all safety information. *Id.* at § 312.32(d). If the investigation reveals additional "relevant" follow-up information, the information must be submitted to the FDA as soon as it is available. *Id.*

> Determining the relevance of information is invariably a matter of judgment. In this case, relevant information is information that explains or clarifies the circumstances of the reported adverse experience. For example, each follow-up might include reports of autopsy findings or reports of their results of additional blood tests. 52 Fed. Reg. 8798, 8818 (1987).

If a sponsor initially determines that safety information does not meet the criteria for an expedited report to the FDA, but a subsequent investigation reveals that the information should be reported to the FDA, the sponsor must report it as soon as possible "and in no event later than 15 calendar days after the determination is made." 21 C.F.R. § 312.33(d).

Annual Reports

Sponsors also report adverse experiences with investigational drugs and preclinical findings suggesting a significant risk for human subjects to the FDA as part of the IND annual reports. FDA regulations require the IND sponsors to submit a summary of the status and progress of investigations each year within 60 days of the anniversary date on which the IND went into effect. *Id.* at § 312.33. A purpose of the requirement for submitting annual reports is to provide both sponsors and the FDA with insight into the status and progress of the studies conducted under an IND. 52 Fed. Reg. at 8819. In furtherance of this purpose,

> FDA believes it is important periodically to aggregate all [adverse] experiences, whether or not the individual events are thought to be drug related, for review and analysis. Such groupings may show an increased incidence of an adverse experience or other problem that would not be readily ascertainable in a review of single, discrete adverse events. *Id.*

The regulations require that annual reports include a brief summary of the status of each clinical study that is in progress or completed. The information must at least include the total number of subjects who initially planned the study, entered into the study, completed the study as planned, and dropped out of the study for any reason.

The regulations also require that annual reports include a narrative or tabular summary of the most frequent and most serious adverse experiences by body system and a list of pre-clinical studies completed or in progress during the previous year. *Id.* at § 312.33(b). FDA regulations and the preamble to those regulations provide no guidance about what the Agency expects sponsors to include among the most frequent and most serious events. Sponsors also must list all patients who died during participation in the investigation and all who discontinued the study in association with any adverse experience, regardless of any conclusions regarding whether or not the event was related to the drug. *Id.* at §§ 312.33(b)(3)-(4). Annual reports also include a summary of all IND safety reports submitted during the preceding year. *Id.* at § 312.33(b)(2).

FDA REPORTING STANDARDS FOR MARKETED DRUGS AND BIOLOGICAL PRODUCTS

Collection, Review, and Recordkeeping of Adverse Product Experience Information

There are three separate regulatory provisions governing the review and reporting of safety information related to marketed drugs and biologics. Separate provisions govern the review and reporting of (1) drugs marketed pursuant to a New Drug Application (NDA) and an Abbreviated New Drug Application (ANDA), (2) biological products, and (3) drugs that are lawfully marketed without an approved NDA. 21 C.F.R. §§ 314.80, 314.98, 600.80, 310.305, respectively. Physicians or other healthcare professionals have no legal obligation to report safety information to either the manufacturer, sponsor or FDA.

As with investigational drugs, any applicant or licensed manufacturer having an approved application or a biologics license must promptly review all adverse product experience information regarding its product. 21 C.F.R. §§ 314.80(b), 314.98, 600.80(b). This requirement covers information obtained or received from any foreign or domestic source, including information derived from commercial marketing experience, post-marketing clinical investigations, post-marketing epidemiological/surveillance studies, reports in the scientific literature, and unpublished scientific papers. *Id.* Prescription drug products marketed for human use without an approved drug application must meet the same requirements as well. 21 C.F.R. § 310.305.

Applicants or licensed manufacturers also must establish and follow written procedures for the surveillance, receipt, evaluation and reporting of post-marketing adverse product experiences. 21 C.F.R. §§ 310.305(a), 314.80(b), 314.98, 600.80(b). The regulations require applicants or licensed manufacturers to retain records of all adverse product experiences, including raw data and any related correspondence, for 10 years. 21 C.F.R. §§ 310.305(f), 314.80(i), 314.98, 600.80(i).

While licensed biological products are generally covered by these standards (21 C.F.R. 600.80), there are some product-specific differences. Licensed blood and blood components (as defined in 21 C.F.R. § 606.3(c)) are exempt from these requirements. Rather, these products must keep adverse reactions records and make those available to the FDA upon request. 21 C.F.R. § 606.170(a). With regard to a "complication of blood collection or transfusion" that is fatal, this information must be communicated to the FDA as soon as possible, followed by a written report within seven days. 21 C.F.R. § 606.170(b). With regard to vaccines, such products must comply with the requirements of 21 C.F.R. § 600.80 as set forth below. In addition, certain childhood vaccines are also regulated by the National Childhood Vaccine Injury Act of 1986 (NCVIA) (Section 2125 of the PHSA). 42 U.S. § 300aa-25. This law requires manufacturers of certain vaccines and healthcare providers who administer such vaccines to report to a separate reporting system known as the Vaccine Adverse Event Reporting System (VAERS). This VAERS program is co-administered by FDA and the Centers for Disease Control (CDC) which is a separate unit of the Federal Department of Health and Human Services. If a vaccine falls under the jurisdiction of NCVIA, then any adverse event is to be reported only to the VAERS program. These manufacturers must meet the other requirements of 21 C.F.R. § 600.80.

REPORTING ADVERSE PRODUCT EXPERIENCES FROM MARKETED PRODUCTS

The regulations require two specific types of post-marketing reports for post-marketing adverse product experiences: 15-day Alert reports and periodic reports.

All adverse product experience reports for both drugs and biological products (unless treated differently as discussed above) should include a completed FDA Form 3500A for each individual patient or publication, unless the adverse product experience is foreign, in which case either a Form 3500A or a CIOMS I is acceptable. 21 C.F.R. §§ 314.80(f), 600.80(f). If the product is a vaccine, a VAERS form should be used. Applicants or licensed manufacturers may use computer-generated forms or use an alternative format, such as a computer-generated tape or tabular listing, if the alternative format contains the same content as Form 3500A and the appropriate FDA department agrees to the alternate format in advance. *Id.*

The FDA has proposed a regulation requiring the reporting of adverse product experiences in electronic form, but has not taken final action on the matter. 63 Fed. Reg. 59,746 (1998).

15-DAY ALERT REPORTS

Applicants and licensed manufacturers must submit a "15-day Alert report" for each domestic or foreign adverse product experience that is both "serious" and "unexpected" to the FDA within 15 calendar days of the receipt of information about the experience. 21 C.F.R. §§ 310.305(d), 314.80(c)(1)(i), 600.80(c)(1)(i).

The definition of "serious" for post-marketing adverse product experiences is identical to that for IND adverse product experiences discussed above. 21 C.F.R. §§ 310.305(b), 314.80(a), 314.98, 600.80(a).

The definition of "unexpected" for post-marketing adverse product experiences is similar to that for the IND adverse product experiences. An adverse product experience is "unexpected" if the experience is not listed in the current labeling for that product. 21 C.F.R. §§ 310.305(b), 314.80(a), 314.98, 600.80(a). An adverse product experience is "unexpected" even if it could have been anticipated from the pharmacological properties of the product so long as it is not listed in the labeling. *Id.* This definition includes events that are symptomatically and pathophysiologically related to events listed in the labeling, but differ due to greater severity or specificity. *Id.* As an example of an event that is "unexpected" due to greater severity, the regulations cite hepatic necrosis when the labeling refers only to elevated hepatic enzymes or hepatitis. *See id.* As an example of an event that is "unexpected" due to greater specificity, the regulations cite cerebral thromboembolism and cerebral vasculitis when the labeling refers only to cerebral vascular accidents. *Id.*

Unlike the expedited reporting of adverse events to the INDs, spontaneous post-marketing events do not require an assessment of causality. It is the FDA's view that when a report is spontaneously made regarding a drug, there is implied causality, because the reporter would otherwise not have taken the time to transmit the information to the applicant or a regulatory authority.

15-day Alert Report Follow-Ups

Applicants or licensed manufacturers also are required to perform promptly a "follow-up" investigation into the adverse product experience and separately to report any new information to the FDA as a "15-day Alert report follow-up" within 15 calendar days of the receipt of that information. 21 C.F.R. §§ 310.305(c)(2), 314.80(c)(1)(ii), 314.98, 600.80(c)(1)(ii). If the applicant or licensed manufacturer performs an investigation but is unable to uncover any additional information, then the applicant or licensed manufacturer should maintain records of the steps taken but need not submit a follow-up report. *Id.*

15-day Alert Reports Based on Scientific Literature

Fifteen-day Alert reports must be filed when "serious" or "unexpected" adverse product experiences are reported in case reports or in the results of formal clinical trials published in scientific or medical journals. 21 C.F.R. §§ 314.80(d), 314.98, 600.80(d). When a 15-day Alert report is based on information obtained from scientific or medical journals, a copy of the article must be included with the report. *Id.*

Exceptions to the 15-day Alert Report Requirements

No 15-day Alert report is required for information regarding an adverse product experience that was obtained from a post-marketing study, including those conducted under an IND application, unless the applicant or licensed manufacturer concludes that there is a "reasonable possibility" that the product caused the experience. 21 C.F.R. §§ 310.305(c)(1)(ii), 314.80(e), 314.98, 600.80(e). When reports of adverse product experiences obtained during a post-marketing study are reported in any context, they should be marked to indicate that they were so obtained. *Id.*

PERIODIC REPORTS

Any adverse product experience that is not "serious" and "unexpected" must be reported to the FDA in a periodic report. 21 C.F.R. §§ 314.80(c)(2)(i), 314.98, 600.80(c)(2)(i). Periodic reports must contain a "narrative summary and

analysis" of the information in the report, including an analysis of all 15-day Alert reports filed during that period. 21 C.F.R. §§ 314.80(c)(2)(ii), 314.98, 600.80(c)(2)(ii). Periodic reports must also contain a completed FDA Form 3500A for each adverse product experience not reported in a 15-day Alert report during the period as well as an index consisting of a line listing of the patient identification number and adverse reactions terms. *Id.* Finally, periodic reports must contain a history of actions taken in response to adverse product experiences during the period, such as labeling changes or initiation of studies. *Id.*

Follow-up Investigations for Periodic Reports

Follow-up investigations for adverse product experiences that are not "serious" and "unexpected" are not required. If the applicant or licensed manufacturer chooses to perform an investigation, then it may submit any information that it discovers in the next periodic report, rather than filing a separate "follow-up" report. 21 C.F.R. §§ 314.80(c)(2)(i), 314.98, 600.80(c)(2)(i).

Quarterly v. Annual Periodic Reports

During the first 3 years after the date of approval or licensing of a product, periodic reports must be submitted quarterly. 21 C.F.R. §§ 314.80(c)(2)(i), 314.98, 600.80(c)(2)(i). For the purposes of quarterly reports, the first quarter begins on the date of approval of the application. *Id.* Each quarterly report must be filed within 30 days of the close of the quarter. *Id.* After 3 years, applicants or licensed manufacturers need only submit annual reports, which must be filed within 60 days of the anniversary of approval or licensing. *Id.* The FDA may require quarterly reports for a period longer than three years. *Id.*

Exceptions to Periodic Reporting Requirements

Periodic reports need not contain adverse product experience information obtained from reports in scientific literature, foreign marketing experience, or post-marketing studies, including studies conducted under IND applications. 21 C.F.R. §§ 314.80(c)(2)(iii), 314.98, 600.80(c)(2)(iii). Thus, the only adverse product experiences that must be included in periodic reports are those that have not been included in a 15-day Alert report that were reported as spontaneous reports from domestic sources.

ANNUAL REPORTS

In addition to the periodic safety reports that applicants submit to the FDA, annual reports also are required for drugs that include other safety information. Annual reports include a variety of information including distribution data and manufacturing changes, but they also include safety information in the form of copies of unpublished reports of new clinical and preclinical findings. 21 C.F.R. §§ 314.81(b)(2).

MULTIPLE REPORTS, APPLICATIONS, OR PRODUCTS

Applicants and licensed manufacturers are not required to report adverse product experience information that has already been reported to the FDA. Thus, no report should contain adverse product experiences that occurred in clinical trials if those experiences were previously submitted as part of an approved application. 21 C.F.R. §§ 314.80(g), 314.98, 600.80(g). Similarly, an applicant or licensed manufacturer is not required to file a report if the FDA was the source of the adverse product experience information and no additional information was uncovered during the "follow-up" investigation. 21 C.F.R. §§ 310.305(c)(5), 314.80(b), 314.98, 600.80(b).

The reporting requirements apply to all entities identified on the product's label as manufacturers, packers, or distributors. 21 C.F.R. §§ 310.305(c)(1)(i), 314.80(c)(1)(iii), 314.98, 600.80(c)(1)(iii). In order to avoid duplication in reporting, however, these entities may submit any adverse product experience information to the applicant or licensed manufacturer for inclusion in the applicant or licensed manufacturer's 15-day Alert report. 21 C.F.R. §§ 310.305(c)(3), 314.80(c)(1)(iii), 314.98,

600.80(c)(1)(iii). This submission must occur within five calendar days of the entities' receipt of the information. *Id.* If the entity elects this method, it must keep a record that includes a copy of each adverse product experience report, the date that it received the report, the date that the report was submitted to the applicant or licensed manufacturer, and the name and address of the applicant or licensed manufacturer. *Id.*

PATIENT PRIVACY

The names and addresses of patients should not be included in any reports submitted to the FDA. 21 C.F.R. §§ 310.305(e), 314.80(h), 314.81(c)(2), 314.98, 600.80(h). Instead, the applicant or licensed manufacturer should create a unique code number of less than eight characters for each report. *Id.* The applicant or licensed manufacturer must include the name of the person who reported the adverse product experience. *Id.* The applicant or licensed manufacturer also must maintain sufficient patient identification information to permit the FDA to identify the name and address of individual patients. *Id.*

GUIDANCES

Over the last decade, FDA has published a series of guidances that further articulate its views about how IND sponsors and NDA or Biologics License Application (BLA) applicants can comply with the regulations and statutes governing adverse event review and reporting. Unlike the statutes and regulations, however, guidances do not have the force and effect of law. Thus, if a company does not comply with the conduct described in a guidance, the company is not automatically violating the law and therefore subject to penalties. Conduct that is contrary to an FDA Guidance represents a risk however that the FDA will consider it a violation of law and attempt to bring an enforcement action. It is important, therefore, that companies understand these guidances and make carefully informed judgments that actions that differ from a guidance meet the requirements of the applicable law and regulations. Regardless, the guidances do provide IND sponsors and NDA applicants a clear idea of what FDA considers lawful conduct and, therefore, familiarity with them is critical.

INVESTIGATIONAL PRODUCTS

There are several guidances/guidelines applicable to the review and reporting of adverse events prior to product approval. The most important, but not all, of these guidances are

- ICH, *Guidance on Data Elements for Transmission of Individual Case Safety Reports* (1998)
- ICH, *Guideline for Industry—E2A Clinical Safety Data Management: Definitions and Standards for Expedited Reporting* (1995)

The first guidance addresses issues such as the specific and minimal data necessary or advisable for reporting of adverse events to the FDA. The second guidance addresses issues including how to manage blinded studies, adverse reactions occurring on placebo, reporting time frames, and post-study events.

MARKETED PRODUCTS

There also are numerous guidances regarding the review and reporting of adverse events for marketed products. The most important, but not all, of these guidances are

- CBER, *Guidance for Industry—How to Complete the Vaccine Adverse Event Reporting System Form (VAERS-1)*
- CDER/CBER, *Guidance for Industry—Postmarketing Adverse Experience Reporting for Human Drug and Licensed Biological Products: Clarification of What to Report* (1997)
- ICH, *Guidance for Industry—E2C Clinical Safety Data Management: Periodic Safety Update Reports for Marketed Drugs* (1996)
- CBER, *Guideline for Adverse Experience Reporting for Licensed Biological Products* (1993).
- CDER, *Guidance for Industry—Guideline for Postmarketing Reporting of Adverse Drug Experiences* (1992)

The guidances address issues such as how and when to submit safety reports and how FDA expects applicants to manage such issues as foreign reports, reports of deaths, overdoses, or lack of effect, and how to submit reports associated with multiple drugs.

INTERNATIONAL CONFERENCE ON HARMONIZATION

The FDA recently published a draft consolidated guidance for post-marketing safety reporting. CDER/CBER, *Draft Guidance for Industry—Postmarketing Safety Reporting for Human Drug and Biological Products Including Vaccines* (March 2001). This guidance covers many of the topics addressed in the previous post-marketing guidances discussed above. This guidance was prepared, however, under the auspices of the International Conference on Harmonization. In general, FDA's policy on international standards states that

> [w]here a relevant international standard exists or completion is imminent, it will generally be used in preference to a domestic standard, except when the international standard would be, in FDA's judgment, insufficiently protective, ineffective, or otherwise inappropriate. 60 Fed. Reg. 53077, 53084 (1995).

Physician/Consumer Reporting: The FDA Medical Products Reporting Program (MedWatch)

In addition to receiving mandatory adverse event information from drug manufacturers and distributors, the FDA also receives voluntary adverse event reports from the medical community and consumers through its MedWatch program. The program provides a system for healthcare professionals and consumers to report adverse events to the FDA about drugs, biologics, medical devices, and nutritional products such as medical foods, dietary supplements and infant formulas. The FDA has a web site on the internet that permits healthcare professionals voluntarily to transmit adverse event information electronically and the FDA also has designed a specific MedWatch adverse event reporting form that can be submitted through the mail or fax. Internet reports can be submitted through the FDA's Web page at `http://www.accessdata.fda.gov/scripts/medwatch/`. The MedWatch forms are available on the internet, through the the FDA, and also appear, for example, in the Physicians' Desk Reference. Additionally, the FDA has a toll-free telephone number for reporting adverse experiences.

ENFORCEMENT

Generally the FDA evaluates compliance with these safety reporting standards through inspections of manufacturers, sponsors, and clinical investigators and relevant records maintained by each entity. FDCA § 704; 21 U.S.C. § 374; PHSA § 351(c); 42 U.S.C. § 262(c). Under the law, it is a prohibited act to fail to "... establish or maintain any record, or make any report, required under section ... 505(i) or (k) ... or the refusal to permit access to or verification or copying of any such required record." FDCA § 301(e); 21 U.S.C. § 331(e). Committing this prohibited act or causing someone else to do so, makes the manufacturer, sponsor (including any culpable individuals) and clinical investigators liable either under the civil or criminal penalties of the FDCA and the PHSA. FDCA § 303(a); 21 U.S.C. § 333(a); PHSA § 351; 42 U.S.C. § 262.

If the FDA determines that anyone is either not submitting required safety information, submitting false information or otherwise not in compliance with the applicable laws and regulations, then there are generally several enforcement steps that the FDA will take, although they are not required to take them sequentially. The first would be to send the entity or person a Warning Letter which briefly describes what the FDA investigation has found and concludes that the conduct violates one or more provisions of the law. The FDA asks for prompt action to correct the conduct described by the FDA. The agency routinely states that if prompt action is not taken, then further regulatory action by the FDA may result. In most such letters, the FDA identifies product seizure, FDCA § 304; 21 U.S.C. § 334, or injunction, FDCA § 302; 21 U.S.C. § 332, as two possible actions that could be taken without further warning. In the decade of the 1990s, there were a dozen or more Warning

Letters issued on this topic by the FDA. In virtually every instance, the entity or person took the necessary corrective action to ensure future compliance with the safety reporting standards. These Warning Letters are available on the FDA Website at `http://www.fda.gov/foi/warning.htm`. In addition, if a manufacturer does not comply with its safety reporting obligations, then the FDA may revoke an approved NDA for a drug (21 C.F.R. § 314.150(b)(1)) or the approved license for a biological product (21 C.F.R. § 601.5(b)(iv)).

Another serious step that could occur, even if the recipient of the letter corrects the actions that the FDA objects to, is the initiation of a criminal prosecution. Violations of the FDCA subject any culpable entity or individual to both misdemeanor and felony criminal convictions that can involve substantial fines and prison sentences. If there are records kept or submitted which are knowingly false and they are material to the FDA's compliance assessment, then there are also potential violations of several provisions of the general federal criminal code, including the False Statements Act. 18 U.S.C. § 1001. Such criminal violations are felony violations with substantial monetary penalties and jail sentences. In the late 1980s, the FDA brought several criminal prosecutions against pharmaceutical companies for violations of pharmacovigilance reporting laws and regulations.

CONCLUSION

Compliance with the FDA requirements for pharmacovigilance reporting is essential. It is also complex. As this brief summary makes clear, there are laws, regulations and guidances that must be understood and met. These standards, especially the regulations and guidances, change with relative frequency. Thus, it is important that any company and/or individual must ensure that they have available the most current versions of all applicable standards. Therefore, while this Chapter provides a reasonable framework of the legal requirements, it, alone, cannot be the basis upon which up-to-date compliance with the FDA requirements is established.

4

Ethical Oversight, Consent, and Confidentiality

Hogan & Hartson, L.L.P., Washington, DC, USA

ELIZABETH B. ANDREWS

RTI Health Solutions, Research Triangle Institute, Research Triangle Park, NC, USA, and School of Public Health
and School of Pharmacy, University of North Carolina at Chapel Hill, NC, USA

INTRODUCTION

We put the money that we do not spend in the bank—not under the mattress or in a hole in the back yard. We are not bankers, and neither of the authors has any special expertise in economics or bank regulation. Sometime early in childhood, however, we learned to believe that the bank would safeguard every penny, would pay a modest rate of interest, and would give our money back to us on request. Eventually (probably by watching Jimmy Stewart save the Bailey Savings and Loan each Christmas), we figured out that our money is not in the vault and that people who receive loans are being given "our" money. At some level, we recognized that by collecting and circulating the money of significant numbers of people, banks provided the critical infrastructure for a sound and fluid economy. At some level we recognized that our money is the lifeblood of the US economy. The US economy is a system in which a public good is created and sustained while protecting the very personal financial interests of the individuals whose investments are a critical component of the economy.

This chapter is not about the economy, but it is about something that is just as vital to our quality of life: the epidemiologic and outcomes research that sustains quality and fuels innovation in our health care system. Information is the lifeblood of twenty-first century health care, whether the information and analyses that researchers provide clinicians and public health officials, or information about individuals' health and health care made available to researchers for analysis. However, we lack a model or metaphor that enables ordinary citizens to appreciate the critical role played by their health information—maintained and used in confidence—for sustaining quality and innovation in our health care system.

The new US privacy regulations, promulgated by the Department of Health and Human Services,[1] were authorized as part of the "administrative

---

[1] Department of Health and Human Services, Standards for Privacy of Individually Identifiable Health Information, 65 Federal Register 82 463 (Dec. 28, 2000) *hereinafter* "privacy regulations", adding parts 160 and 164 to Title 45 of the Code of Federal Regulations ("CFR").

simplification" section of the Health Insurance Portability and Accountability Act (HIPAA).[2] They establish the infrastructure for protecting individuals' personal privacy interests while "banking" their medical information to make it available for determining their course of treatment and for administration health benefits. With respect to research, however, and particularly with respect to epidemiology and outcomes research, the approach to individual privacy taken by this regulation (and by most state laws affecting research) is comparable to telling each individual to protect his or her financial interests by stuffing money in a mattress or digging a hole, and lending very, very carefully.[3]

The HIPAA approach to data-only research is irrevocably, and we argue, mistakenly, rooted in the authorization of each individual for each research use of his or her health information.[4] The same is true of the European Union's Data Privacy Directive[5] although the Directive arguably allows for more flexibility in implementation than the HIPAA regulations. The consent/authorization model is grounded in a system of ethics that values autonomy over community.[6] Given the level of debate that has characterized virtually all of the public policy discussion of how to achieve the objective of both privacy and sound epidemiologic and outcomes research, an analysis grounded in autonomy seems little more than a natural

outgrowth of American individualism. As discussed more fully below, with respect to archival or records research, a consent-based model is entirely unsuited to protecting individuals' privacy interests. This chapter reviews the roots of the current regulatory approach and offers preliminary thoughts regarding the parameters of a model more suited to protecting the privacy interests of individuals while encouraging the secure use of medical archives in epidemiologic and outcomes research.

RESEARCH ETHICS

ROOTS IN INTERVENTION AND MANIPULATION

Almost every paper or book on research ethics includes a cautionary reference to atrocities committed in the name of science or abuses resulting from a researcher's crass objectification of research subjects. Lurking in the background of the calls for more laws protecting human subjects are memories of the abuses at Auschwitz, and in the Tuskegee and Willowbrook studies. Contemporary research ethics is grounded in the desire to protect the individual from unknown, and at some level unknowable risks. Both the Declaration of Helsinki[7] and the "Common Rule"[8] (that forms the basis for laws protecting human subjects in the United States) reflect a philosophical framework that prioritizes individual autonomy, well-being,

---

[2] Pub. L. No. 104–191 (Aug. 21, 1996), amending the Social Security Act ("SSA") by adding Part C of Subchapter XI, codified at 42 U.S.C. §§ 1320d et seq. ("HIPAA").

[3] By comparison, the laws for protecting our personal financial interests from banking risks appear to build on a recognition that it is possible to create something good for our society by collecting and investing money, while protecting individuals' interests by insuring deposits and establishing strong incentives for banks to comply with strict regulations.

[4] As discussed more fully below, the regulation establishes specific criteria that a committee, after debating the relative value of the specific research proposal and the privacy risk to the individual, may apply to decide whether or not to waive individual consent as to the specific research project. 45 C.F.R. § 164.514(b)(1).

[5] European Union Directive 95/46/EC on the protection of individuals with regard to the processing of personal data and on the free movement of such data. July 25, 1995. http://www.ecommerce.gov/eudir.htm

[6] See Barefoot (1998) (describing the argument that respect for individual autonomy demands a consent/authorization model, even when there is a societal need for access to personal health information).

[7] Declaration of Helsinki, World Medical Association, Inc, adopted by the 18th World Medical Association General Assembly in June 1964, and revised most recently in October 2000. The Declaration is a statement of ethical principles to provide guidance to physicians and other participants in medical research involving human subjects, including research on identifiable data.

[8] The federal regulatory framework for the protection of human research subjects is known as the Common Rule. It has been codified, in some cases with slight modifications, by 17 different federal agencies at 7 C.F.R. Part 1c; 10 C.F.R. Part 745; 14 C.F.R. Part 1230; 15 C.F.R. Part 27; 16 C.F.R. Part 1028; 21 C.F.R. Part 56; 22 C.F.R. Part 225; 28 C.F.R. Part 46; 32 C.F.R. Part 219; 34 C.F.R. Part 97; 38 C.F.R. Part 16; 40 C.F.R. Part 26.; 45 C.F.R. Part 46; 45 C.F.R. Part 690; and 49 C.F.R. Part 11. See 56 Fed. Reg. 28 002 (June 18, 1991), implementing Pub. L. No. 95–622, 92 Stat. 3412, Title III, Section 301 (Nov. 9, 1978).

and just distribution of burdens and benefits in the conduct of research.

Under the Common Rule, there are two different types of protection for research participants:

1. review of specific research protocols by an Institutional Review Board (IRB) to identify the risks to participants presented by the specific research protocol, and
2. informed consent of each research participant.

The two protections become co-mingled because our regulations assign the IRB two different tasks. In addition to identifying and weighing the risks presented by the protocol, the IRB reviews the forms and documents used to obtain informed consent, *and* under certain limited circumstances, is authorized to waive the consent requirement with respect to a given research protocol.

Review Boards and Risk

As clinical interventions become more complex and involve newer scientific approaches, it is increasingly clear that competent and independent IRB analysis and review is indispensable for identifying and evaluating the desirability of subjecting individuals to the known and unknown risks of a researcher's proposed protocol.

With respect to research using medical archives, however, the risks are essentially the same in every study: all of the risks stem from the privacy interests of a data subject and the potential damage from potential *non*-research misuses of personal information in our society. The risk to the data subject from the research, therefore, is a direct function of the arrangements for data security and the potential for breaches of the security arrangements and dishonest behavior by a researcher in using or disclosing information for non-research purposes. Assuming that the researcher is obliged to use information only for research and to maintain adequate security to protect it from further disclosure or unauthorized use, none of the privacy risks stems from any specific research protocol itself. Rather, to the extent that different data analyses *appear* to involve more or less risk, the differences can be traced to social values and attitudes toward the *subject matter* of the investigation.

For example, most people would say that research relating to HIV or genetics involves greater privacy risk than research on the common cold. This perceived difference in the risk of the research is an illusion. Assume that a single database, maintained under tight security arrangements, is made available to two different researchers under confidentiality agreements that bind the two investigators to the same obligations regarding use and protection of the data. One is studying HIV infection and the other is studying staphylococcus infection. The privacy risks in both cases are the same; they stem from the adequacy of data security arrangements and the obligations imposed on the investigators. The appearance of differential risk stems from the current cultural perceptions of HIV, and the fact that people or institutions—other than the researcher—might misuse the information to embarrass or harm the data subject, *if* they were to gain access to the information. Similarly, test results from the various breast cancer genes only appear to be more sensitive than information about a family history of breast cancer. In fact, both could be misused in precisely the same way *if* they were to fall into the wrong hands. The fact that there are persons in our society who, if unchecked, might discriminate against individuals in violation of the law, or misuse information to disadvantage or harm a data subject, does not vary based on the subject matter of the research. Rather, the perceived differences among data projects reflect differences in the potential for social, psychological, or financial *damage* to the data subject in our society, *assuming* that there is a negligent or intentional failure of data security arrangements.[9]

---

[9] Consideration of the danger from external factors rather than the research itself also has crept into agency interpretations of the concept of risk under the Common Rule. In 1998, in discussing revisions to the categories of research eligible for "expedited review", the Department (through both the Food and Drug Administration (FDA) and the National Institute of Health (NIH)) stated that expedited review was impermissible where "identification of subjects or their responses would place them at risk of criminal or civil liability or be damaging to the subjects' financial standing, employability, insurability, reputation, or be stigmatizing, unless reasonable and appropriate protections will be implemented so that risks related to invasions of privacy and breach of confidentiality are not greater than minimal". 63 Fed. Reg. 60 355, 60 366.

Unlike interventional research involving physical manipulation or intervention in the subject's care, nothing in the research design in a data-analysis project can control, eliminate, or mitigate these societal damages. In a data study, one cannot modify the dosing, the subject selection criteria, or the laboratory tests used to monitor the effect of the research manipulation on the individual. The events to be examined in the research have already occurred. The epidemiologic or outcomes researcher is an active observer of natural processes that have been recorded in the history of an individual's health care and health benefits interactions. An epidemiologic study, by definition, seldom can be shown to have a potential benefit to the individuals who are the data subjects. Rather, because the observed events and interventions have already occurred in the natural course of events, any benefit of the *research* is to the public health in general, or to succeeding generations that may benefit from innovations that may be developed. Accordingly, when, as is required by the Common Rule, the Review Board attempts to determine whether the "[r]isks to subjects are reasonable in relation to anticipated benefits, if any, to subjects, and the importance of the knowledge that may reasonably be expected to result from the research",[10] the Review Board is not being asked to weigh the risks the protocol poses to an individual in relation to the importance of the knowledge to be gained. Rather, the Review Board is being asked to consider the potential socio-psychological damage to an individual in our society based on the fact that he or she evidences the characteristic under investigation, *assuming* that there is a breach of data security that results in a disclosure of data outside the research context where the data are used for an impermissible purpose.[11]

As a result, the "weighing" question posed to the Review Board misses the mark entirely. It largely becomes a philosophical question about the importance of the knowledge that might be gained in comparison with how badly our society discriminates or misuses the particular characteristics that are under study. By comparison, for interventional research the Review Board evaluates the risk of the research protocol and proposes modifications to minimize the risk posed by the research. The Board evaluates the *research* risk in relation to benefits to the participant and the importance of the potential knowledge. The risk equation does *not* include consideration of the possibility that a negligent or intentional action that is *not* a part of the research protocol could result in the death or serious bodily harm of a participant.

The critical problem is that as formulated, the Common Rule's risk equation—when applied in review of a data-only project—is almost certain to devolve into a referendum on the value of the researcher's hypothesis. In fact, the vast majority of IRBs appear to avoid such tangled debates by establishing procedures under which most data-only studies fall into the category posing "minimal risk" to data subjects. The categories of studies eligible for expedited review under the Common Rule are specified in a guidance document promulgated by the Office for Human Research Protections.[12] Under this guidance, where there is a risk of discrimination based on disclosure of the subject's responses or data, the research is *not* eligible for expedited review, *unless* "reasonable and appropriate protections will be implemented".[13]

The Department's introduction of "reasonable and appropriate protections" in evaluating the risks inherent in data-only studies hints at the underlying issue that, in our view, *should* be of concern in any Board Review of a data study: does the study design appropriately limit use and disclosure of personal identifying information? And, does the researcher have adequate arrangements for data security?[14] However, as currently

---

[10] 45 C.F.R. § 46.111(a)(2).
[11] Under the Common Rule, data security is a separate issue from the issue of the relative risk and value of interventional research. *Compare* 45 C.F.R. § 46.111 (a)(1) & (2) *with* § 46.111(a)(7).

[12] Categories of Research That May Be Reviewed by the Institutional Review Board (IRB) through an Expedited Review Procedure, 63 Fed. Reg. 60 355–67 (Nov. 9, 1998).
[13] 63 Fed. Reg. 60 355, 60 366.
[14] See, for example, Lowrance, (1997).

formulated, this decision is made in considering whether or not to *have* a full Board review of a study. In other words, the review itself is still premised on a risk-value inquiry that does not address the real questions about the risk posed by the research, i.e. the risk that identifying data might be used or disclosed for non-research purposes.

Informed Consent and Control

The concept of consent is critical in interventional research because the physical risks and rigors of the research will directly affect the individual and his or her health and well-being. The informed consent process helps to minimize the potential for coercion and for ensuring that the individual maintains control over what is done to him or her in the research protocol. In effect, it is a recognition of the value our society places on an individual's physical integrity and autonomy. A properly informed individual may decide to accept fairly significant risks. However, only in rare circumstances where the risk is judged to be minimal would our values and our current laws permit a researcher or Board to decide to subject others to physical risks without their knowledge; never would we expect an IRB to permit experimentation on human beings against their will.

In the context of archival research, where the researcher will access only information in existing records, the role of informed consent is conceptually different from consent to physical participation. As discussed above, assuming adequate data security arrangements and protection of direct identifiers, the research itself does not pose a risk to the data subject. Epidemiologic and outcomes research is concerned not with a specific individual, but with populations.

At best, therefore, any "informed consent" discussion with individual data subjects is little more than an explanation of the researcher's hypotheses and research interests, and his or her promises and arrangements regarding the safeguarding of data. Because epidemiologic researchers are concerned with populations and not individuals, both of these discussions could be addressed in a more general manner, such as a

researcher's data practices, and more effective communication to the public regarding research topics and how data archives are used in investigating them. A discussion between a researcher and an individual data subject may elicit sympathy or the "beneficence" of the data subject and a motivation to permit the records to be used. However, to the extent that the data subject dislikes the topic or the philosophical underpinnings of the research question, consent is little more than an invitation for the data subject to exert control over the researcher's inquiry by denying access to data.[15] If this very natural exercise of power can be expected to occur fairly systematically (e.g. those who favor the researcher's point of view consent to use of their records and those who do not, decline to consent), then the records sample available for analysis of any kind is systematically biased and may not meet the criteria to be considered a valid sample for conducting the research.

Suppose that the discussion of the research topic is more neutral to minimize adverse selection, and the informed consent documents seek merely to inform the individual of the risks. As discussed above, the risks to the individual from data-only studies are from the potential misuses of information by *non*-researchers who obtain it through

---

[15] Some have maintained that an individual's privacy interests justify his or her refusal to allow information to be used in research. To once again make the analogy to the banking world, this is analogous to the argument that I don't want you to lend my money to industries or activities that I find morally repugnant. In the financing case, the objection is rooted in the concept of unjust enrichment. Arguably, the situation is somewhat different where the researcher's endeavor is designed to contribute to the quality and innovation in health care and health care delivery. In this context, the reason that data pertaining to an individual are in the archives is because the individual already has availed him or herself from the resources of the health care system, and is, therefore, an unwitting, direct beneficiary of the quality improvement and innovation that has gone before. In this case, the equities, benefits, and distribution of burdens of the research process arguably warrant secure use of data without each individual's authorization. To say "I do not what to know about that subject, and I do not want anyone else to learn about that subject", runs counter to the freedom of inquiry on which our research and scholarly activities are based. Particularly where the researcher does not know or have access to information identifying individual subjects, it is difficult to make the case for the opposition other than as a differential value for free scientific inquiry.

illegal or negligent activities. A full statement of
the risks might very well detail the various possible
illegal acts that could cause damage to the
individual's reputation, employment, insurability,
etc. The individual has little or no way of
estimating or evaluating the probability of these
occurrences. Arguably, this is what the review
Board should have done. The prudent individual,
when confronted with a catalog of abuses that
might occur if the information found its way
outside of the research lab, would be hard pressed
to find a reason why she or he *should* authorize the
information to go to the lab in the first place.

As a practical matter, in institutions where
data-only studies are subject to the Common
Rule, it is widely understood that the rule
"works" only because these studies typically are
considered eligible for expedited review, and the
reviewer decides to waive the requirement for
obtaining the consent of data subjects. Any
additional requirement that threatens to disrupt
this accommodation, either by requiring the
Board to debate and review the relative merits
of the research question and society's potential
for discrimination and privacy invasion, can do
little more than increase the probability that the
existing regulatory scheme may threaten the
viability of valid epidemiologic and outcomes
research. This is precisely the new requirement
put in place by the medical privacy regulation for
waiver of individual authorization.

CONFIDENTIALITY ISSUES IN EPIDEMIOLOGY STUDIES

For some of the epidemiologic challenges we are
likely to face, such as anticipating the spread of
new viral strains and drug-resistant bacteria,
consent-based models are scientifically inappropriate for the research questions being asked. Validity
depends on the characteristics of the sampling
criteria used in compiling the database: if data
subjects are self-selected, each epidemiologic analysis will likely require a separate analysis of the
impact of the self-selection factors on the research
findings. In some cases, this will mean that it is not
possible to obtain a valid answer to an important
research question.

Research using information collected for other
purposes, such as health care delivery or health
benefits administration, is critically important as
we enter into the century of discoveries based on
genomic science. Pinpointing differences in health
or health care quality based on geography,
demography, health history, or co-morbidities will
become ever more important for clinical research,
for public health planning, and for ensuring access
to appropriate care. We do not have the luxury of
time and resources to collect consents and obtain
data from volunteers, and evaluate the validity of
the sample for testing every unique data hypothesis.

Public health surveillance is typically conducted
under specific laws authorizing or requiring the
collection of certain types of data in the public
interest. (See, for example, Chapter 3 this volume.)
The new medical privacy regulations, for example,
have explicit exemptions from the prohibitions
on disclosure where the data are being collected
under various public health surveillance laws.[16] In
enacting the mandatory reporting laws the legis-
lature has been persuaded that the individual's
interest in privacy can be achieved in other ways
that are not anathema to the public interest in
pharmacovigilance and other public health surveillance. They have required public health authorities and regulated entities to simultaneously
protect the privacy interests of individuals while
making the requisite reports and appropriately
using and safeguarding the collected data.

But most epidemiologic studies do not have the
legislative protections of public health surveillance. Follow-up studies of drug safety, confidentiality issues generally are covered by different
laws and regulations than spontaneous reporting
aspects of pharmacovigilance. The challenge in
North America and the European Union is to
create a system in which patient needs for
confidentiality protections can be achieved while
also facilitating important public health research.
If society moves too far in the direction of
providing absolute protection to seal off access
to health information from secondary uses, such as

---

[16] 45 C.F.R. § 164.512(b).

formal studies of drug safety, then we are at risk of eroding the information foundation that supports public health planning and health care quality, including societal judgements on the benefits and risks of medications.

Follow-up studies of drug or devise safety fall into the broad general category of "research", which is defined in the Common Rule as "a systematic investigation ... designed to develop or contribute to generalizable knowledge".[17] Instead of an exemption from the prohibitions on use or disclosure of patient data, the regulation subjects disclosure or use of information for research purposes to an entirely new patient authorization process.[18] In other words, the same attention to the public interest in *both* privacy and research results that is seen in event reporting laws is not evident in US laws regulating data access for epidemiologic and outcomes research.

Admittedly, the "worst case" damage to a given individual from the disclosure and misuse of personal information may be highly significant. This potential damage or risk from the non-research misuse of personal information is precisely the same risk that adheres in pharmacovigilance and public health reporting. Indeed, with respect to the types of conditions that often are the subject of mandatory public health reporting—sexually transmitted diseases (STDs), child abuse, substance abuse—the potential damage from stigmatization or prejudice arguably is at its greatest.

EXISTING LAW

Three separate categories of laws govern confidentiality issues in epidemiologic and outcomes research: the Federal Common Rule, state laws, and the new federal medical privacy regulations promulgated under "HIPAA".

COMMON RULE

As discussed above, the Federal Common Rule was designed to be a mechanism for protecting the

interests of human subjects in federally funded or regulated research. Congress did not enact a law regulating research under its power to regulate matters affecting interstate commerce or even under its authority to safeguard the rights and liberties of individuals under the Constitution. Rather, the law is an expression of a federal policy not to spend federal money on research that is not consistent with certain social values. As a result, the applicability of the Common Rule, and the regulatory authority of the agency administering it, is somewhat odd. It applies to:

- research conducted by the 17 agencies that have adopted the rule;
- recipients of federal research grants as a condition of awarding the grant;
- research that is included in an application submitted to the FDA for approval of a drug, biologic, or certain devices; and
- all research conducted in or by an employee of an institution that has filed a "multiple project assurance" with the Department of Health and Human Services, whether or not a specific project is federally funded.

Thus, research conducted in private clinics or institutions that do not have federal grants or a multiple project assurance appears to fall outside the scope of the Common Rule, as does research conducted by commercial research organizations that will not be used in a regulatory submission, e.g. many epidemiologic and outcomes studies. But since the records of interest in epidemiologic research often are those collected by institutions subject to the Common Rule, the would-be researcher faces a tremendous Catch-22: the research is not subject to the regulation, and under the law, the researcher has no claim on the time or resources of an IRB for obtaining review of the project or waiver of consent. However, each of the multiple academic medical centers from which the researcher wishes to obtain data *is* subject to the rule, and must have the proposal reviewed by its *own* IRB. For example, an epidemiologic researcher who wishes to analyze data from Johns Hopkins, Duke, M.D. Anderson, and Stanford University Medical Centers will have the project

[17] 45 C.F.R. § 46.102.
[18] 45 C.F.R. § 164.508.

reviewed by four separate IRBs each of which must approve the project and waive individual consent in order for it to go forward. In reality, if the researcher is not affiliated with the institution, it may be very difficult to get the IRB to review the proposal without forming a collaborative relationship with someone affiliated with each institution who can get the project on the IRBs' schedules.

STATE LAWS

The informed consent provisions of the Common Rule state: "The informed consent requirements in this policy are not intended to preempt any applicable federal, state, or local laws which require additional information to be disclosed in order for informed consent to be legally effective".[19] Some states, such as Minnesota, have laws that directly regulate research.[20] These state laws are not preempted by the Common Rule, and so long as the federal and state requirements are not inconsistent with one another, the general rule is that one should comply with all applicable laws.

Virtually all states have some form of medical privacy law or law specifying what constitutes informed consent, and the above provision of the Common Rule indicates that IRBs and researchers are obliged to comply with them. In practice, complying with the informed consent requirements of medical privacy laws has not been an extraordinary impediment to epidemiologic research because states typically do not have provisions regarding the waiver of consent; thus the affirmative federal policy has been assumed to govern. In recent years, however, many states have considered legislation that is more restrictive than the Common Rule with respect to waiver of consent.[21] As these laws are implemented, IRBs may find that fewer epidemiologic protocols meet the criteria for waiver of consent.

An even more troubling set of problems for research stems from the increasingly prevalent state laws regulating informed consent and information disclosure when genetic testing or genetic information is involved. As health care interventions increasingly use genetic analyses for diagnostic purposes and for selection of appropriate pharmaceutical interventions, it will be increasingly unlikely that any medical record can be presumed *not* to include genetic information. State genetics laws typically define "genetic information" very broadly, so that carrier status, single gene diseases, multiple gene diseases, and genes that merely indicate a susceptibility for a disease all are encompassed by the definition. As a result, records containing such information generally become subject to state law requirements regarding disclosure of such information. Unless federal regulators and institutions sponsoring IRBs are attentive to the implications for epidemiologic research, the social sensitivity of genetic information (popularly thought of in more narrowly predictive terms than the states' broad definitions), may very well be construed as making any records that include information regarding the results of genetic tests ineligible for expedited review. That is, as discussed above, under the 1998 notice from the FDA and the NIH,[22] research using data that might be used to disadvantage the data subject is not to be deemed "minimal risk" research for purposes of an IRB's expedited review policy. Thus, the breadth of state laws protecting genetic information raises the possibility that routine data-only research will have to be approved and considered by the full IRB—with the potential for fractious "research vs. privacy" debates, as discussed above, that may result in the approval of only a fraction of important protocols.

NEW FEDERAL LAW: MEDICAL PRIVACY UNDER HIPAA

The new federal privacy regulations under the HIPAA establish that "covered entities" may not use or disclose "protected health information"

---

[19] 45 C.F.R. § 46.116(e).
[20] See, for example, Minn. Stat. Ann. § 144.335(3a)(d).
[21] See, for example, 2001 Tex. Sess. Law Serv. ch. 1511 (S.B. 11) (Vernon).

[22] Supra note 12.

except as permitted by the privacy regulation.[23] The regulation defines "covered entities" to include health care providers (e.g. doctors, hospitals, labs, pharmacies, clinics),[24] health plans, and health care clearinghouses.[25] By requiring certain contractual terms in all covered entities' contracts with vendors, suppliers, and anyone else who may process or come into contact with protected health information in performing services for the covered entity, the regulation indirectly applies to business associates of covered entities as well.[26]

Under the privacy regulation, only the following categories of uses and disclosures of protected health information are permitted:

1. for purposes of treatment, payment, and health operations, with an individual's written consent ("Consent");[27]
2. for purposes unrelated to treatment, payment, or health operations (including research), with an individual's written authorization ("Authorization");[28]
3. for certain other purposes enumerated in the regulation, including protecting the public health and conducting research under a waiver of authorization, provided that applicable conditions are met.[29]

Moreover, even with respect to permitted uses and disclosures, a covered entity may use or disclose only the minimum necessary information to accomplish the intended purpose.[30] Unless every use or disclosure of information fits within one of these permitted categories, the provider or health plan would be exposed to potential civil and criminal penalties for supplying information to a researcher. Likewise, the researcher may be exposed to potential criminal penalties for obtaining or disclosing such information if the covered entity did not comply with the regulation in supplying it to the researcher.[31]

DE-IDENTIFIED INFORMATION

Many people have suggested that the regulation should not affect epidemiologic and outcomes research because it generally does not require access to "individually identifiable" information. The statute says that "individually identifiable health information" is

> any information, including demographic information collected from an individual, that (A) is created or received by a health care provider, health plan, employer, or health care clearinghouse; and (B) relates to the past, present, or future physical or mental health or condition of an individual, the provision of health care to an individual, or the past, present, or future payment for the provision of health care to an individual, and (i) identifies the individual, or (ii) with respect to which there is a reasonable basis to believe that the information can be used to identify the individual.[32]

Under the statute, information that does not fall within the category to be considered "individually identifiable" is not subject to the statutory, or regulatory, requirements.

Congress, the US Department of Health and Human Services Regulatory, privacy advocates, the research community, and others have wrestled with the definition of what characteristics of data create a "reasonable basis to believe" that it could be used to identify the individual. What would be a reasonable standard? On one extreme are researchers and public health advocates who may argue that all data should be considered exempt if the key "direct identifiers" are removed. They argue that the importance of research using these data outweighs the low probability that these data might be used (or misused) to re-identify individual patients. On the other end of the spectrum are those who are concerned that any database, even

---

[23] See 65 Fed. Reg. at 82 805 (codified at 45 C.F.R. § 164.502(a)).
[24] Id. at 82 799 (codified at 45 C.F.R. § 160.103).
[25] See id. at 82 798 (codified at 45 C.F.R. § 160.102(a)).
[26] See id. at 82 798, 82 806, 82 808 (codified at 45 C.F.R. §§ 160.103, 164.502(e), 164.504(e)).
[27] See id. at 82 810–11 (codified at 45 C.F.R. § 164.506).
[28] See id. at 82 811–12 (codified at 45 C.F.R. § 164.508).
[29] See id. at 82 813–18 (codified at 45 C.F.R. § 164.512).
[30] See id. at 82 805–06, 82 819 (codified at 45 C.F.R. §§ 164.502(b), –.514(d)). The "minimum necessary" requirement does not apply to disclosures to a health care provider for treatment purposes. See id. at 82 805 (codified at 45 C.F.R. § 164.502(b)(2)(i)).

[31] Social Security Act ("SSA") § 1177, 42 U.S.C. 1320d–2.
[32] SSA § 1171(6), 42 U.S.C. 1320d(6).

with the complete removal of identifiers, could potentially be overlain with other data sources, and through probability matching on certain information fields, *could* be used to re-identify individuals. Many advocates have maintained that even if the researcher has no interest in knowing the patients' identities, no intent to link the files to other files for this purpose, and establishes physical and procedural safeguards to make it difficult or impossible for employees to do so, that the mere possibility that files *could* theoretically be linked to re-identify patients is a privacy risk to society that should be avoided.

For its part, in implementing this definition, the Department of Health and Human Services created an extremely high standard for information to be considered as falling outside the category of individually identifiable health information. It specifically defined such information as "de-identified". It chose to use statistical probability—as determined by a statistician—to establish the permissible practices that can be used to establish a "reasonable basis to believe". The agency's approach is firmly grounded in the art and science of database manipulation. It does *not* ask whether a reasonable person looking at the data fields on an individual record could discern who the person is or how to contact him or her. It does not take into consideration who will use the data, for what purpose, or how the data are protected from being used to identify individuals. Rather, it asks whether the data fields that appear in a data set also appear in databases that are generally available and which therefore *could be used by someone who is **attempting** to identify data subjects*. Examples of such generally available databases include state drivers license data, voter registration lists, the telephone book, birth records, etc.

The regulation offers a "safe harbor" method in which the covered entity must (a) have no actual knowledge that the information could be used alone or in combination with other information to identify participants and (b) *all* of the following must be removed from the data:

- names;
- all geographic subdivisions smaller than a State, including street address, city, county, precinct,

zip code, and their equivalent geocodes (three digit zip codes may be used if the geographical area contains more than 20 000 people or, for areas with less, the three digit zip code is changed to 000);
- all elements of date (except year) for dates directly related to an individual, including birth date, admission date, discharge date, date of death, and all ages over 89 and all elements of dates indicative of such age, unless aggregated into a single category of age 90 or older;
- telephone numbers;
- fax numbers;
- e-mail addresses;
- social security numbers;
- medical record numbers;
- health plan beneficiary numbers;
- account numbers;
- certificate and license numbers;
- vehicle identifiers and serial numbers, including license plate numbers;
- device identifiers and serial numbers;
- web universal resource locators ("URLs");
- Internet Protocol ("IP") address numbers;
- biometric identifiers, including finger and voice prints;
- full face photographic images and any comparable images; and
- any other unique identifying number, characteristic, or code.

Some of the data fields in the list, such as social security number, e-mail address, telephone number and the like, offer a fairly ready way to find out who a data subject is.[33] The other fields chosen for stripping appear to be a list of fields that a statistician would find to be useful for

---

[33] The irony, of course, is that within a set of health care or health benefits data, even the patient's name, address, and telephone number are not necessarily adequate to know that one is looking at the same individual in different records of health encounters. The same household may have many individuals named John Smith, Maria Hernandez, or Sally Wong. As a result, date of birth or social security number—or some other unique code that is known to be associated with a single individual over time—is almost always needed for health information systems to perform at an acceptable level of accuracy in identifying individuals.

triangulating databases in order to zero in on identified cases. Removal of all of the fields listed in the regulation is the only "safe harbor" for any data to be outside the regulation's prohibitions on use or disclosure.

The only alternative to the safe harbor is for a statistician to find that the "risk is very small that the information could be used ... by an anticipated recipient to identify an individual who is the subject of the information" 42 C.F.R. 164.514(a)(1)(i). Under this "statistical" method, a database can be considered "de-identified" if:

> [a] person with appropriate knowledge of and experience with generally accepted statistical and scientific principles and methods for rendering information not individually identifiable: (i) Applying such principles and methods, determines that the risk is very small that the information could be used, alone or in combination with other reasonably available information, by an anticipated recipient to identify an individual who is a subject of the information; and (ii) Documents the methods and results of the analysis that justify such determination.[34]

If the regulation is taken at face value, then it leads to preposterous results. For example, a report of the frequencies stating the total number of admissions to each of ten hospitals on a given day of the year would be "protected health information"—even if that were the only information transmitted about any given patient's case. As the rule is constructed, the inclusion of a patient-related date of any kind in a data set appears automatically to transform the data into protected health information. As a result, unless a statistician made the risk finding, transmission of such tabular data to anyone would be a technical violation of the regulation even if the number of daily admissions for each hospital were in the hundreds. Likewise, a table showing how many of the total number of inpatient admissions in a given county went to each of several hospitals would be a violation of the regulation, as would a table for a given hospital showing how many of its admissions in a year come from which zip

code. "County" and "zip code" are in the list of fields that are automatically considered to be "identifiers" that must be removed in order for data to fit the de-identification "safe harbor". Therefore, unless each patient authorizes the disclosure or unless a statistician renders a risk opinion, the regulation makes disclosure of a table of frequencies that includes any of the suspect fields a disclosure of protected health information. As a result, data that meet the de-identification safe harbor is virtually useless for sound and informative epidemiologic or outcomes research.

AUTHORIZATION FOR THE USE AND RELEASE OF IDENTIFIABLE INFORMATION

The privacy regulation prohibits covered entities from using or disclosing protected health information for research purposes without an individual's written authorization or a waiver of authorization in accord with the regulation. The regulation explicitly provides that using information for research is *not* one of the activities that is permitted under the arrangements for using and disclosing information for treatment, payment and health care operations.

"Authorization" to use information for research is required—*in addition to* the requirements under the Federal Common Rule relating to "Informed Consent" of the subject to participate in the research protocol. Likewise, the criteria for waiver of authorization under the privacy regulation are different from and in addition to the criteria for waiver of informed consent under the Common Rule.

Authorization for Research

The privacy regulation specifies the required element for a valid authorization. To be effective, an authorization must include, among other elements:

- a specific description of the information to be used or disclosed;

---

[34] See *id.* at 82 818 (codified at 45 C.F.R. § 164.514(b)(1)).

- specific identification of the person or entity with whom or to whom the covered entity may make the requested use or disclosure;
- an expiration date;
- a specific description of the purpose of the use or disclosure;
- an explanation of how the individual may revoke the authorization;
- a statement that the information disclosed may be subject to redisclosure by the researcher and no longer protected by the federal regulation; and
- if the covered entity will receive either direct or indirect remuneration from a third party for making the disclosure, a statement to this effect.[35]

The authorization must contain all the elements specified in the privacy regulation, as well as any disclosures or elements required by any applicable state law, unless an IRB or privacy board grants a waiver of authorization or of the *form* of authorization with respect to one or more elements in accord with the regulation's waiver criteria.[36]

Waiver of Authorization Requirement

In lieu of asking individuals to authorize the disclosure of their protected health information, the covered entity may seek waiver of the authorization requirement from an IRB established in accordance with the Common Rule or from a specially constituted privacy board.[37] Either entity may grant a waiver of authorization if the research protocol meets the privacy regulation's waiver criteria. These criteria resemble the Common Rule criteria for waiver of informed consent, although they specify that the reviewing board must determine whether

the *privacy* risks to individuals whose protected health information is to be used or disclosed are reasonable in relation to the anticipated benefits if any to the individuals, and the importance of the

knowledge that may reasonably be expected to result from the research.[38]

Although the question to the Review Board is posed in the same way as under the Common Rule, the Board actually is being asked a very different philosophical question. As discussed above, the Common Rule question stems from our interest in protecting individuals from risks to their autonomy, life, and liberty in the name of science. The IRB identifies the potential risks and considers their probability in approving the research design. In the data context, however, the question as posed assumes that absolute protection of individuals' privacy from theoretical risks is what is desired. The risks to privacy, as discussed above, stem from violations of data security, not from the research itself. However, that is not the specific question before the Board in evaluating the research risk. Separately, the IRB considers whether there is an "adequate" plan to protect identifiers.

The medical privacy regulation became effective as of 14 April 2001. Hospitals, doctors, pharmacies, health plans, labs, and clinics have two years to bring their operations into full compliance. Because the regulation supplements but does not supersede the Common Rule, all data-only research that also is subject to the Common Rule potentially will need to consider *both* a waiver of Informed Consent to

---

[35] See *id.* at 82 811–12 (codified at 45 C.F.R. § 164.508(c), (d)).
[36] See *id.* at 82 816–17 (codified at 45 C.F.R. § 164.512(i)).
[37] See *id.* at 82 816–17 (codified at 45 C.F.R. § 164.512(i)).

[38] To waive the authorization requirement, an IRB or privacy IRB must determine that: (1) the use or disclosure of the protected health information involves no more than minimal risk to the proposed research subjects; (2) waiver of the authorization requirement will not adversely affect the privacy rights and welfare of the subjects; (3) the proposed research could not practicably be conducted without the waiver; (4) the research could not practicably be conducted without access to and use of the health information; (5) the privacy risks to the proposed subjects are reasonable in relation to the anticipated benefits (if any) to those subjects; (6) an adequate plan exists to protect personal identifiers from improper use and disclosure; (7) an adequate plan exists to destroy such identifiers at the earliest opportunity consistent with the conduct of the research (unless there is a health or research justification for retaining the identifiers, or if retention is otherwise required by law); and (8) there are "adequate written assurances" that the identifiable health information will not be reused or disclosed to any third party except as required by law, for oversight of the research project, or for other research for which the use or disclosure would be permitted by the regulation. *Id.* (codified at 45 C.F.R. § 164.512(i)(2)(ii)).

participate in research and a waiver of authorization under the privacy regulation.[39]

Research With Records of Deceased Individuals

Under the Common Rule, deceased individuals are not considered "human subjects".[40] Absent state laws or institutional policies to the contrary, research using the records of deceased persons does not require IRB approval or an IRB waiver of informed consent. The privacy regulation, in contrast, includes deceased persons as "individuals" whose privacy is protected by the regulation. The regulation states that a covered entity can provide access to records of deceased individuals only if it obtains representations from the researcher that the information sought will be used only for research purposes and is in fact necessary for these purposes.[41] In addition, the covered entity, at its discretion, may require the researcher to document the death of the individuals whose protected health information is sought.[42] Of course, an IRB or privacy board could waive authorization with respect to deceased individuals under the regulation's criteria for waiver.[43]

IMPLICATIONS AND NEXT STEP

In our view, there are several key aspects of the existing legal scheme that are cumbersome impediments to the conduct of large-scale epidemiologic studies. In order to make this scheme workable, we will need to:

- Engage in significant education of data sources and IRBs in order to integrate the new privacy

authorization requirements with the existing Common Rule process for waiver of consent. Timely education will be key to avoiding IRB gridlock as the compliance date approaches.

- Engage in significant education of the public regarding the value of epidemiologic research and the protections routinely used to protect individuals' privacy interests. Because the privacy regulation also provides ordinary persons with access to information about all the people who have had access to their records—including researchers who access information under a waiver of authorization—there is a danger of public backlash if individuals are merely given a list of third parties that conduct research programs without an understanding of the purpose and importance of such uses and how the privacy of individual data subjects is protected.[44]

- Assist in developing de-identification strategies that will meet epidemiologists' data needs, and monitor the use of resources invested in building an information infrastructure to ensure that the public interest in research is protected in a cost-effective manner.

At a more basic level, we must return to the more fundamental policy issue that a consent-based regulatory model (with waiver by a Review Board) is little more than an abdication of the government's responsibility for using its power to protect both privacy and the public interest in research. Although this may be an ethically sound model in interventional research where a specific individual is being asked to subject him or herself to risks in the name of scientific curiosity, the ethical issues arguably are entirely different in data studies undertaken for public health and health care quality purposes. The consent model shifts responsibility to the individual: if the individual consents, then the individual assumes the risk of loss. As implemented under the new federal regulation,

---

[39] See id. at 82 817 (codified at 45 C.F.R. § 164.512(i)(2)(iv)(A)).
[40] 45 C.F.R. § 46.102(f) (2000).
[41] See 45 C.F.R. § 164.512(i)(1)(iii).
[42] See id.
[43] Although an IRB might be inclined to grant such a waiver under the Common Rule criteria (particularly since deceased individuals are not "human subjects"), the privacy regulation provides a process for obtaining authorization from the executor of an individual's estate or other personal representative, so it is not clear how these new rights and responsibilities may affect the deliberations of IRBs.

[44] For example, because data that is stripped of "direct identifiers" is nonetheless "protected health information", the covered entity must keep track for each individual of every researcher who has obtained access to a data set. The fact that the data available to the researcher bore no direct identifiers is *not* a fact to which the data subject has access.

government authority is used merely to ensure that each individual is appropriately warned of the risks, and that those who nonetheless attempt to persuade individuals to consent, keep records of those warnings and of the consent, and are accountable for the inappropriateness of their procedures. From a legal perspective, waiver of consent by an IRB may be construed as an indication that the IRB or its institutional sponsor is accepting this responsibility on behalf of the individual. In our litigious society, this is not a legal model that over the long run will make it economically viable for hospitals, doctors, and health plans to provide data to researchers under a waiver.

To bring the discussion full circle, if this approach had been used as the framework for monetary regulation, it would be analogous to forsaking the secure, regulated banking system for one more like venture capital: bankers would have to poll the public for funds, and each would-be investor would bear responsibility for approving the subject matter of each project and, having signed the forms, bear the risk of loss. In our view, the public interests in privacy *and* in the quality of health care that research makes possible argues for a more equitable approach to assuring that the burdens of research are shared by those who benefit, and that government and/or private oversight is used to minimize risks to all by establishing data security standards and holding individuals accountable for violations.

NOTE ADDED IN PROOF

Since the writing of this chapter, the Secretary of Health and Human Services has issued a call for comments regarding the possibility that "facially de-identified data" could be made available for research and public health purposes under a data use agreement in which the researcher promises to protect the privacy of the data subjects and safeguard the data from use or disclosure for impermissible purposes. If the Secretary decides to revise the regulation to permit this option, then many of the untoward effects discussed in this chapter can be avoided. Many in the research community have applauded the possible revisions as achieving a more appropriate balancing of the public interest in research and public health with the public interest in protecting the privacy of data subjects. Some privacy advocates concerned with protecting the data subject's ability to control uses of facts, have expressed concern that even these arrangements for de-personalized, confidential use of facts compromises the privacy interests of the data subjects. Undoubtedly, when the Secretary decides whether and how to modify the regulations, the research and public health communities will need to re-examine yet again the arrangements under which data are made available and analyzed for public health and research purposes.

REFERENCES

Barefoot BL (1998) Comment. Enacting a health information confidentiality law: can Congress beat the deadline? 77 *North Carol Law Rev* **283**: 307–8, 332.
Lowrance WN (1997) *Privacy and Health Research: A Report to the Secretary of Health and Human Services.* Washington, DC: US Department of Health and Human Services, May.

5

Pre-clinical Safety Evaluation

NORMA KELLETT, STUART J. MAIR AND WALTER S. NIMMO

Inveresk Research, Tranent, UK

INTRODUCTION

A unique feature of pre-clinical toxicology studies is the fact that positive and negative results are of equal importance and this is quite different from the work of pharmacologists. Also, an important aspect of toxicology is the search for models that are predictive of adverse effects in humans exposed to chemicals or drugs. The study of laboratory animals is the subject of intense debate in some countries. However, there is currently no adequate alternative to identify the potential toxic effects of new drugs, the target organs of these effects and the relationship to the dose of drug. Toxicology studies are driven by government requirements and historical knowledge and an assumption that toxicity in animals is predictive of human toxicity, that the use of large doses increases the predictability and that there is some relationship between the toxic dose in animals and in humans.

It follows that any failure of the correlation between animal and human toxicity may result in an unnecessary use of animals or the unnecessary limitation or restriction in the use of a valuable drug. Thus, it is necessary to try continuously to relate the predictability of animal studies to the toxicity of drugs in humans.

REGULATORY REQUIREMENTS BEFORE CONDUCTING CLINICAL TRIALS

Historically, the regulatory control of clinical research has been different in Europe, the United States and Japan. Even within Europe there has been no consensus (for example there is no government control of healthy volunteer studies in the United Kingdom but a detailed review process is in place in Scandinavia). Thus, there has been no harmonisation on the precise extent of pre-clinical testing (toxicology and pharmacology) required before conducting the first study of a new drug in man. Various official (FDA, 1968) and unofficial (ABPI, 1985; PMA, 1977) guidelines have provided details of the basic studies that should be conducted in advance of a Phase I study.

Only relatively recently has a (partial) consensus been reached on the pre-clinical testing required with the publishing of the ICH M3 guideline, which came into operation in March 1998 (EMEA, 1998). Even the latest revision of this guideline (November 2000) has areas of non-agreement in the data expectations of the EU, United States and Japan during the various phases of clinical development (e.g. duration of

Pharmacovigilance. Edited by R.D. Mann and E.B. Andrews
© 2002 John Wiley & Sons, Ltd

toxicology testing and timing of reproduction toxicology studies).

Although certain classes of therapeutic agents and drugs for the treatment of certain types of life-threatening or serious disease may warrant a more flexible approach, the general guidance is that, before initiating studies in humans of a pharmaceutical agent, the following studies should be undertaken:

1. Acute toxicity studies in two mammalian species.
2. Repeat-dose toxicity studies in two mammalian species (one non-rodent), the duration of which should equal or exceed the duration of the proposed human clinical study.
3. Safety pharmacology studies to include the assessment of effects on the cardiovascular, central nervous and respiratory systems.
4. *In vitro* evaluation of genotoxicity to include evaluation of mutations and chromosomal damage before Phase I with additional tests required before Phase II.
5. Studies to evaluate the absorption, distribution, metabolism and excretion (ADME) of drugs in animals. Results of these studies should be available by the completion of the Phase I studies and before beginning patient studies.
6. When appropriate, local tolerance studies in animals using the proposed route of administration for human studies. Such evaluations may be included as part of other toxicity studies.
7. Reproduction toxicity studies appropriate for the population to be studied. For example, in the EU embryo–foetal development studies are required before the inclusion of females of childbearing potential in Phase I studies.
8. Carcinogenicity studies are not normally required in advance of the conduct of clinical trials but on occasions may be warranted, e.g. if genotoxicity studies identify a potential risk.

The aim of pre-clinical safety evaluation is to identify potential toxic effects as well as the organs or systems most sensitive to the effects of the drug. The relationship to dose and the potential reversibility of effects are also important. The information generated will give guidance on the selection of a safe starting dose for the first administration-to-man study and will highlight the safety monitoring which is required. Progress through the various stages of drug development will require continued assessment of human safety data with the possibility of further pre-clinical studies being required based on the information generated. However, the basic battery of pre-clinical safety studies is intended to be adequate for the identification and characterisation of potential toxic effects, which may be relevant during the early phase of clinical development.

NUMBERS OF ANIMAL STUDIES IN THE UNITED KINGDOM

In 1999, in the United Kingdom, 2.66 million scientific procedures involving animals began. There has been a downward trend in total numbers since 1976. Species studied were mice (62%), rats (21%), guinea pigs (2%), birds (4%), fish (5%), ungulates (2%), rabbits (1.6%), dogs (0.3%) and non-human primates (0.15%).

Twenty-three percent of the total procedures was for pharmaceutical research and development and consisted mainly of rodents. Toxicology or safety evaluation accounted for 20% of the total number of procedures and this was 4% less than in 1998. Of these procedures, 80% was conducted in rodents. Other species accounted for less than 1% each of all toxicology procedures. Of the toxicology procedures, 86% was for legislative purposes.

HOW PREDICTIVE ARE ANIMAL STUDIES OF HUMAN TOXICITY?

In 1962, Litchfield reviewed six diverse drugs being developed by one company and found that toxicities that occurred in rats only were rarely observed in humans and those that occurred in dogs only slightly more frequently. Toxicities that occurred in rats and dogs showed about a 70% correlation with human toxicity.

In general, cytotoxic anticancer agents cause qualitatively similar toxicity in animals and humans with data from dogs predicting gastrointestinal toxicity well but overpredicting hepatic and renal toxicity.

In a survey of 139 drugs approved in Japan from 1987 to 1991 (Igarashi, 1994), animal toxicity data were drawn from 468 repeated dose studies, mainly in rats and dogs but with a few mice and monkeys. Forty-three percent of clinical toxicities from 69 marketed drugs were not predicted from animal studies. The best predictability was for cardiovascular events and the poorest was for skin and hypersensitivity. In reviews of clinical toxicity resulting in withdrawal from marketing, only 4 of 24 cases and 6 of 114 cases could have been predicted from animals. This is not surprising as late-onset toxic effects are of low incidence, usually idiosyncratic and not related to the drug's pharmacology.

In a review from 12 pharmaceutical companies who supplied data to the International Life Sciences Institute an attempt was made to identify how well toxicities seen in pre-clinical animal studies would predict actual human toxicities for a number of specific target organs (Olson *et al.*, 2000). In addition, the duration of dosing necessary was studied.

A database of 221 human toxicities from 150 compounds was available for study. Over 50% of these became manifest during Phase I trials. Sixty-two cases were seen after single doses and 158 cases were seen after multiple doses. If the human toxicity led to project termination, then 39% were terminated at Phase I, 43% in Phase II and 10% were terminated in Phase III. Only four toxicities were considered to be idiosyncratic.

Overall, the true positive concordance rate was 70% for the pre-clinical animal species to show target organ toxicity in the same organ system as the human toxicity. For the remaining 30% of human toxicities, there was no relationship between toxicities seen in animals and those observed in humans. Concordance was seen in 63% of non-rodent species (particularly the dog) and 43% of rodent species (usually the rat).

The best predictability was for haematological, gastrointestinal and cardiovascular toxicities and the least for skin toxicity. The prediction rate when the human toxicity was observed first

was 75% (Phase I), 58% (Phase II) and 52% (Phase III).

Overall, 94% of animal target organ toxicities which correlated with human toxicity was observed first in studies equal or less than one month in duration.

INCORRECT PREDICTION OR FAILURE TO PREDICT TOXICITY

There are many potential reasons for incorrect predictions from animals to man. These include differences in the way the toxicity is elicited (verbally is not possible in animals), the presence or absence of concomitant medication, pharmacokinetic and metabolic differences, age (animals are young and humans may be old), state of health (animals are free from disease), homogeneity of the animals studied compared with the heterogeneity of the humans, dose differences, housing and nutrition (optimal in animal studies) as well as timing differences.

A significant message from Olson's review is that the human toxicities with the poorest correlation with animal studies (hepatic toxicity and hypersensitivity/skin reactions) were the two toxicities that led most often to termination of clinical development. Further study of mechanisms is required.

It is worthy of note that the pharmacokinetics in any one animal species may be very different from those in other species or in humans (Nimmo and Watson, 1994). This may result in low bioavailability in the animals or a first pass metabolism that results in insufficient target organ concentrations to produce any adverse effects reliably. Toxicokinetic data generated as an integral component of pre-clinical toxicology studies and the use of the data in the interpretation of toxicological findings may improve the predictive value of a particular species. A sensible approach to drug development would be to conduct a single dose tolerability/pharmacokinetic study in humans as soon as possible and to compare concentrations achieved with those observed in the different animal species studied. This would allow interpretation of the findings in the most appropriate animal species with similar concentrations before conducting a multiple dose tolerability or a Phase II study. Toxicokinetic data should contribute to the design of pre-clinical studies after the first human study has been conducted.

WHAT TOXICITY OCCURS IN HEALTHY VOLUNTEER STUDIES?

We have reviewed all adverse events recorded in volunteers during two separate 12-month periods (1993 and 1998) at Inveresk Research's Clinical Unit. All adverse events reported spontaneously, elicited by staff questioning or observed were collected. Two doctors performed the allocation of each event to the trial medication independently with a third arbiter in cases of disagreement. The doctors were blinded to the study medication and allocated causality according to the known pre-clinical pharmacology and toxicology of the drug and the timing of the adverse event.

Of a total of 30 studies (32 drugs) available for review in 1998, 10 were single ascending dose tolerability studies and 5 were multiple-dose toler-ability studies. The remaining studies were phar-macokinetic studies. Several therapeutic classes of drugs were represented. Drug-related adverse events were those considered possibly, probably or definitely related to the medication. Data were compared with those collected in 1993 involving a total of 23 studies (18 drugs). Comparison of the numbers of studies and exposures is made in Table 5.1 and details of the adverse events them-selves are given in Tables 5.2 to 5.4.

Table 5.1. Comparison of number of studies and exposures in 1993 and 1998.

	1998	1993
Studies	30	23
Drugs	32	18
Subjects	704	502
Active exposures	994	627
Placebo exposures	169	120

In the first report in 1993, the frequency of adverse events reported in volunteer studies was much greater than that reported by Orme et al. (1989). However, the incidence we reported in 1993 was confirmed by the 1998 data. Another point of note in 1993 was that there was a similar frequency of adverse events in volunteers receiving an active drug and those receiving a placebo. This was different from the findings of Sibille et al. (1992) who reported a difference in the incidence of adverse events between active drug and placebo treatment, active being significantly higher. Once again, our 1993 results were confirmed in 1998.

Therefore, we conclude that the incidence of adverse event reporting in healthy volunteer studies is 34%–39% with an almost identical incidence in placebo exposures as in active exposures.

Most adverse events were mild and self-limiting and in both 12-month periods the most common event in both active and placebo exposures was headache (19%–30%). It is hard to imagine how this would be predicted from animal studies.

When we look at adverse events considered to be drug related (possibly, probably or definitely) in 1998, the first thing to note is that some placebo

Table 5.2. Comparison of adverse events in healthy volunteer studies in one clinical unit in 1998 and 1993.

	Active 1998	Active 1993	Placebo 1998	Placebo 1993
Total exposures	994	627	169	120
Exposures resulting in at least one adverse event	354 (36%)	246 (39%)	58 (34%)	45 (38%)
Total adverse events	620	468	106	97
Adverse events per subject experiencing one adverse event	1.8	1.9	1.8	2.1

Table 5.3. All adverse events reported in 1998 compared with 1993.

Adverse events	Active		Placebo	
	1998	1993	1998	1993
Total	620 (100%)	468 (100%)	106 (100%)	97 (100%)
Headache	143 (23%)	142 (30%)	21 (20%)	19 (20%)
Rash	56 (9%)	26 (6%)	6 (6%)	13 (13%)
Nausea	41 (7%)	22 (5%)	2 (2%)	0
Dizziness	34 (5%)	24 (5%)	6 (6%)	4 (4%)
Pain (musculo-skeletal)	24 (4%)		9 (8%)	
Pain (other)	22 (4%)		10 (9%)	
Rhinitis	21 (3%)	9 (2%)	6 (6%)	6 (6%)
Pharyngitis	20 (3%)		4 (4%)	
Abdominal pain	19 (3%)		4 (4%)	
Hepatic function abnormal	14 (2%)		0	
Diarrhoea	12 (2%)		0	
Somnolence	11 (2%)	12 (3%)	4 (4%)	2 (2%)
Asthenia	11 (2%)	13 (3%)	0	4 (4%)
Sweating	10 (2%)	9 (2%)	0	1 (1%)
Herpes simplex	9 (2%)		3 (3%)	
Cough	9 (2%)	24 (5%)	0	0
Constipation	9 (2%)		0	
Other	155 (25%)	187 (40%)	31 (29%)	48 (49%)

Table 5.4. Drug-related adverse events in 1998.

Adverse event	Active	Placebo
Total	323 (100%)	29 (100%)
Headache	93 (29%)	12 (41%)
Rash	37 (11%)	1 (3%)
Nausea	30 (9%)	0
Dizziness	26 (8%)	3 (10%)
Hepatic function abnormal	13 (4%)	0
Abdominal pain	12 (4%)	2 (7%)
Diarrhoea	9 (3%)	0
Constipation	9 (3%)	0
Herpes simplex	8 (3%)	2 (7%)
Somnolence	7 (2%)	2 (7%)
Other	79 (24%)	7 (24%)

events were considered related based on the timing of the event in relation to dosing. The events which feature in both the placebo and active groups are those of a more subjective nature, e.g. somnolence, dizziness and headache. These are all events that are not possible to monitor reliably in animal studies. In contrast, those which can be measured in animals, e.g. constipation, diarrhoea and abnormal liver function tests, feature only in the active group. The conclusion is that these are more reliable indicators of drug effect and may differentiate active from placebo. However, in another study in our clinical unit, abnormalities in plasma alanine aminotransferase concentrations (ALT) occurred in subjects in between day 4 and day 10 in multiple-dose studies receiving placebo (Wyld, 1991). The underlying cause was thought to be increased carbohydrate intake but it highlights the need to take all factors into account when assessing the cause of an adverse event.

CONCLUSION

Human toxicity from drugs is predicted in over 70% of cases by pre-clinical studies. Some toxicity is easier to predict than others. It is likely that prediction could be improved by concentrating on developing topics and problem areas, e.g. skin toxicity and hypersensitivity reactions are predicted

poorly. Toxicokinetic data, particularly for highly
metabolised drugs, might identify the most appropriate species to study. At present it appears that
two species—one non-rodent—are necessary to
maximise the predictive value of pre-clinical studies.

REFERENCES

Association of the British Pharmaceutical Industry
(ABPI) (1985) *Guidelines on Data Needed to Support
the Administration of New Chemical Entities to Non-
Patient Volunteers*. London: ABPI.

The European Agency for the Evaluation of Medicinal
Products (EMEA) (1998) *ICH M3 Non-Clinical
Safety Studies For The Conduct of Human Clinical
Trials for Pharmaceuticals*. CPMP/ICH/286/95

Food and Drug Administration (FDA) (1968) *Synopsis
of General Guidelines for Animal Toxicity Studies*.

Igarashi T (1994) The duration of toxicology studies
required to support repeated dosing in clinical
investigation—a toxicologists opinion. *CMR Workshop*.

Litchfield JT (1962) Evaluation of the safety of new
drugs by means of tests in animals. *Clin Pharmacol
Ther* 3: 665–72.

Nimmo WS., Watson N (1994) What a clinical
pharmacologist requires from toxicokinetic studies.
Drug Inf J 28: 185–6.

Olson H, Betton G, Robinson D, Thomas K, Monro A,
et al. (2000) Concordance of the toxicity of pharmaceuticals in humans and in animals. *Regulat Toxicol
Pharmacol* 32: 56–67.

Orme M, Harry J, Routledge P, Hobson S (1989)
Healthy volunteer studies in Great Britain: the results
of a survey into 12 months activity in this field. *Br J
Clin Pharmacol* 27: 125–33.

Parkinson C, McAuslane N, Lumley C, Walker SR
(2000) *The Timing of Toxicological Studies to Support
Clinical Trials*. Boston: Kluwer, pp. 67–74

Pharmaceutical Manufacturers Association (PMA)
(1977) *Pharmaceutical Manufacturers Association
Guidelines for the Assessment of Drug and Medical
Device Safety in Animals*. Washington: PMA.

Sibille M, Deigat N, Olagnier V, Vital Durand D, Levrat
R (1992) Adverse events in phase one studies: a study
in 430 healthy volunteers. *Eur J Clin Pharmacol* 42:
389–93.

Wyld PJ (1991) Clinical pathology measurements: the
detection and significance of what is abnormal. In:
Nimmo WS, Tucker GT, eds, *Clinical Measurement in
Drug Evaluation*. London: Wolfe, pp. 115–25.

6

Metabolic Mechanisms

MUNIR PIRMOHAMED AND B. KEVIN PARK

The Department of Pharmacology and Therapeutics, The University of Liverpool, Liverpool, UK

INTRODUCTION

An *adverse drug reaction* may be defined as "an appreciably harmful or unpleasant reaction, resulting from an intervention related to the use of a medicinal product, which predicts hazard from future administration and warrants prevention or specific treatment, or alteration of the dosage regimen, or withdrawal of the product" (Edwards and Aronson, 2000). This has to be contrasted with the term *adverse drug event*, which refers to untoward occurrences following drug exposure but not necessarily caused by the medicine (Asscher *et al.*, 1995). This chapter focuses on adverse drug reactions rather than adverse events.

While the drug discovery process has been revolutionized by new techniques such as combinatorial chemistry and high-throughput screening, drug safety assessment lags well behind and is still reliant on many of the same technologies that have been used for several decades. By the time a drug is marketed, only about 1500 patients may have been exposed to the drug (Asscher *et al.*, 1995; Rawlins, 1995). Thus, only those adverse reactions occurring at a frequency of greater than 1 in 500 will have been identified at the time of licensing. Assessment of adverse drug reactions therefore is likely to represent an important aspect of drug therapy for

many years to come, and indeed, with the development of new biotechnology compounds, it is likely that the pattern of these reactions will change. Furthermore, through the use of gene and protein screening technologies, many new targets will be discovered. As new drugs are developed to modulate the function of these targets, it is very unlikely that we will fully understand the biology of the new target molecule(s), and this will lead to unforeseen adverse reactions. For example, adverse effects such as exacerbation of multiple sclerosis, systemic lupus erythematosus (SLE) and blood dyscrasias that are being reported with anti-TNF therapies (Sharief and Hentges, 1991; Furst *et al.*, 2000) would not have been expected given that TNF-α is involved in their pathogenesis.

IMPORTANCE OF ADVERSE DRUG REACTIONS

Adverse drug reactions are a major clinical problem, many studies showing that they account for about 2%–6% of all hospital admissions (Einarson, 1993; Bates *et al.*, 1995a, 1995b, 1997; Classen *et al.*, 1997). A recent meta-analysis suggested that adverse drug reactions were between the fourth and sixth commonest cause of

Pharmacovigilance. Edited by R.D. Mann and E.B. Andrews

Table 6.1. The direct and indirect effects of adverse drug reactions.

Cause admission to hospitals, or attendance in primary care

Complicate hospital in-patient stay in 10%–20% of cases

Responsible for deaths, possibly as high as the fourth commonest cause of death

Increase length of hospital stay

Increase cost of patient care

Major economic burden on the pharmaceutical industry

Adversely affect patient quality of life

Cause patients to lose confidence in their doctors

Occurrence of toxicity in a minority of patients will preclude use of the drug in the majority of patients

Mimic disease and result in unnecessary investigations and/or delay treatment

---

death in the United States in 1994 (Lazarou *et al.*, 1998). Recent surveys have also indicated that adverse drug events are associated with an increased length of stay in hospital of 2 days,

and an increased cost of approximately $2500 per patient (Bates *et al.*, 1997; Classen *et al.*, 1997). Besides the above, adverse drug reactions can also have many other indirect effects (Table 6.1), which in total, highlight the overall importance of adverse drug reactions in modern medicine.

CLASSIFICATION OF ADVERSE DRUG REACTIONS

There are many different classifications for adverse drug reactions. For the purpose of this chapter, we will use the original classification proposed by (Rawlins and Thompson, 1991), which divided adverse drugs reactions into two types: type A (pharmacological) and type B (idiosyncratic) (Table 6.2). The type A reactions represent an augmentation of the known pharmacological actions of a drug, are dose-dependent and, perhaps more importantly from the viewpoint of safety, are readily reversible on drug withdrawal, or even simply after dose-reduction

Table 6.2. Characteristics of type A and type B adverse drug reactions.

Characteristic	Type A	Type B
Dose-dependency	Usually shows a good relationship	No simple relationship
Predictable from known pharmacology	Yes	Not usually
Host factors	Genetic factors may be important	Dependent on (usually uncharacterized) host factors
Frequency	Common	Uncommon
Severity	Variable, but usually mild	Variable, proportionately more severe than type A
Morbidity	High	High
Mortality	Low	High
Overall proportion of adverse drug reactions	80%	20%
First detection	Phases I–III	Usually phase IV, occasionally phase III
Mechanism	Usually due to parent drug or stable metabolite	May be due to parent drug or stable metabolite, but chemically reactive metabolites also implicated
Animal models	Usually reproducible in animals	No known animal models

(Table 6.2). In contrast, the type B, or idiosyncratic adverse reactions, are bizarre, cannot be predicted from the known pharmacological actions of the drug, do not show simple dose dependency, and cannot be reproduced in animal models. The type A reactions are more common than the type B reactions (Einarson, 1993) accounting for over 80% of all reactions. Although they cause a great deal of morbidity, in general, type A reactions are proportionately less severe and less likely to result in fatalities than type B reactions.

TYPE A ADVERSE DRUG REACTIONS

Pharmacological (type A) adverse drug reactions are the most common forms of drug toxicity (Pirmohamed *et al.*, 1998). They can be due to the primary and secondary pharmacological characteristics of the drug (Figure 6.1). More emphasis is now placed on the secondary pharmacology of new drugs during pre-clinical evaluation, in order to anticipate, and thus avoid, problems that might arise once the drug is introduced into man.

The recent experience with fialuridine, an experimental drug for hepatitis B, highlights the need for continued development of appropriate *in vivo* and, bridging, *in vitro* test systems for the prediction of secondary pharmacological adverse

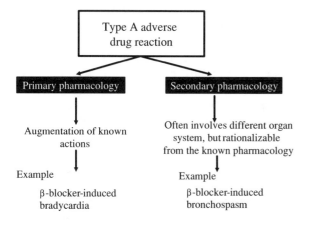

Figure 6.1. Type A adverse drug reactions can be due to the primary and/or secondary pharmacological characteristics of the drug.

effects in man. In June 1993, during phase II trials, 5 out of 15 patients died whilst two others required emergency liver transplants as a result of delayed toxicity which included liver and kidney failure (McKenzie *et al.*, 1995); this had not been observed in four animal species. On the basis of *in vitro* studies in cultured hepatoblasts, the toxicity is thought to be due to inhibition of DNA polymerase γ by fialuridine and its metabolites leading to decreased mtDNA and mitochondrial ultrastructural defects (Lewis *et al.*, 1996).

The development of drugs with greater selectivity should, in theory, lead to improved drug safety. In this respect, there is great expectation for the more selective inhibitors of the cyclo-oxygenase enzymes COX-1 (constitutive form) and COX-2 (inducible form), especially as non-steroidal anti-inflammatory drugs (NSAIDs) represent a therapeutic class of drugs frequently associated with discontinuation for safety reasons, after the product has been granted a licence (Bakke *et al.*, 1995). Data with rofecoxib and celecoxib, selective COX-2 inhibitors, do in fact suggest that they may be associated with a lower incidence of gastrointestinal (GI) toxicity when compared with the non-selective inhibitors such as diclofenac (Bombardier *et al.*, 2000; Silverstein *et al.*, 2000). However, they are not completely devoid of GI adverse effects particularly when they are used in high-risk patients, i.e. those patients who have a history of GI side-effects with the non-selective COX inhibitors.

Factors predisposing to pharmacological adverse reactions include dose, pharmaceutical variation in drug formulation, pharmacokinetic or pharmacodynamic abnormalities, and drug–drug interactions (Pirmohamed *et al.*, 1998) (Table 6.3). In essence, a type A reaction will occur when the drug concentration in plasma or tissue exceeds the perceived therapeutic window. Alternatively, the drug concentration may be within the normal range defined for the population, but because of increased sensitivity of the target in the individual, an adverse reaction results. There are a number of examples of drugs (e.g. captopril) that had been introduced into clinical practice at a dose that was subsequently shown to be associated with an unacceptable frequency of adverse drug reactions,

Table 6.3. Factors predisposing to pharmacological type A adverse drug reactions.

Type	Example	Toxicity	Mechanism
Pharmaceutical	Phenytoin	Phenytoin toxicity (ataxia, nystagmus, etc.)	Increase in bioavailability as a result of a change in formulation
Pharmacokinetic (can involve absorption, distribution, metabolism, and excretion)	Digoxin	Digoxin toxicity (nausea, arrhythmias, etc.)	Decreased elimination if renal function is impaired
Pharmacodynamic	Indomethacin	Left ventricular failure	Water and sodium retention
Genetic	Nortriptyline	Confusion	Reduced hepatic elimination as a result of a deficiency of CYP2D6
Drug–drug interactions (can involve any of the above processes)	Lithium–NSAIDs	Lithium toxicity	Inhibition of excretion of lithium

Adapted from Pirmohamed et al. (1998).

and for which a lower dose was found to be both safe and effective. In general, however, the individual affected by a type A adverse reaction will have impairment of clearance or increased sensitivity as a result of the normal process of ageing, disease, concomitant drugs, or genetic variation, or a combination of these factors (Brodie and Feely, 1991).

GENETIC POLYMORPHISMS AND TYPE A ADVERSE DRUG REACTIONS

A gene can be defined as exhibiting genetic polymorphisms if the variant allele exists in the normal population at a frequency of at least 1%. Genetic polymorphisms are a source of variation to drug response in the human body. In relation to type A adverse drug reactions, polymorphisms in both pharmacokinetic and pharmacodynamic parameters can act as predisposing factors (Table 6.4).

To date, most attention has focused on genetically mediated deficiencies of the P450 enzymes, in particular on CYP2D6 (Park, 1986; Pirmohamed and Park, 1996). A drug metabolized by this pathway will show reduced elimination from the body with a consequent increase in half-life. This will lead to dose-dependent toxicity; a typical example is bradycardia with metoprolol in CYP2D6-poor metabolizers (Lennard et al., 1982).

The role of genetic variation in the metabolism of warfarin by CYP2C9 has attracted a great deal of attention recently. Warfarin is the oral anticoagulant of choice in the United Kingdom (Hart et al., 1998). The number of patients attending anticoagulant clinics has doubled in the last 5 years, largely because of its use in atrial fibrillation. The major risk of warfarin treatment is haemorrhage with an incidence of 8–26 per 100 patient-years (Petty et al., 1999); this is related to the intensity of anticoagulation. Minimization of the risk of bleeding depends on accurate clinical prediction of dosage requirements during warfarin therapy. However, this is difficult since there is wide inter-individual variability in the dose necessary to maintain the international normalized ratio (INR) within a target range.

The S-enantiomer of warfarin, which is predominantly responsible for the anticoagulant effect, is metabolized by CYP2C9 (Rettie et al., 1992). Polymorphisms in the CYP2C9 gene result in at least two allelic variants, CYP2C9*2 ($Arg_{144} \rightarrow Cys$) and CYP2C9*3 ($Ile_{359} \rightarrow Leu$) (Furuya et al., 1995), both of which have been shown to decrease warfarin clearance in vitro (Haining et al., 1996; Takahashi et al., 1998) and in vivo (Takahashi et al., 1998). Clinically, these variants have been shown to be associated with a reduced warfarin dose requirement, greater difficulty in

Table 6.4. Genetic polymorphisms and dose-dependent adverse drug reactions.

Area affected	Polymorphic gene	Example of drug affected	Adverse reaction
Phase I metabolizing enzyme	Cytochrome P450 2D6 (CYP2D6)	Metoprolol	Bradycardia
Phase II metabolizing enzyme	Thiopurine methyl transferase	6-mercaptopurine	Bone marrow suppression
Drug transporter	P-glycoprotein (MDR1)	Digoxin	Digoxin toxicity
Target enzyme	Acetylcholinesterase	Pyridostigmine	Neurotoxicity
Receptor	Dopamine D_3 receptor	Chlorpromazine	Tardive dyskinesia
Ion channel	Delayed rectifier potassium channel (I_{Kr})	Clarithromycin	Prolonged QT interval and torsades de pointe

Adapted from Pirmohamed and Park (2001a).

initiating warfarin treatment, and an increased risk of bleeding (Aithal *et al.*, 1999). Although the relationship between CYP2C9 genotype and dose requirement has been confirmed in two other studies (Freeman *et al.*, 2000; Taube *et al.*, 2000), one of which was much larger ($n = 561$) (Taube *et al.*, 2000), the relationship with severe over-anticoagulation and hence bleeding was not.

On the basis of these studies, should all patients starting warfarin be genotyped? This is probably premature since a number of confounding factors need to be studied (Pirmohamed and Park, 2001a). First, the anticoagulant response is partly dependent on R-warfarin, which is metabolized by CYP1A2 and CYP3A4 (Kaminsky and Zhang, 1997). Second, there are a number of pharmacodynamic factors, such as vitamin K status and thyroid disease, which alter sensitivity to anticoagulants (Scott, 1989). Third, there are mutations in the clotting factors such as prothrombin that may alter sensitivity to warfarin (Taube *et al.*, 2000). Fourth, there are other methods of dose titration and dose maintenance with warfarin, for example prescribing by computer program (Poller *et al.*, 1998) or home monitoring (Cromheecke *et al.*, 2000), which have been shown to be more effective than conventional prescribing. Finally, the clinical use of warfarin dictates that the genotype of the patient would be required within 24 hours of admission. Thus, before genotyping prior to warfarin treatment can become a routine part of clinical practice, there is a need for a prospective randomized clinical trial, which not only incorporates into its trial design the different methods for monitoring and altering warfarin dosage, but also the confounding factors mentioned above.

DRUG INTERACTIONS AND ADVERSE DRUG REACTIONS

Patients on polytherapy are more likely to have type A reactions. The likelihood of developing an adverse interaction increases with the number of drugs prescribed (D'Arcy, 1986). To date, this has largely been a problem in the elderly where polypharmacy is prevalent (Williamson and Chopin, 1980), but is becoming increasingly frequent in younger patients with chronic diseases such as AIDS, where patients may be on 6–10 different drugs (Bayard *et al.*, 1992). An Australian study showed that 4.4% of all adverse drug reactions resulting in hospital admission were due to drug interactions (Stanton *et al.*, 1994).

Drug interactions due to effects on metabolic pathways may either be due to enzyme induction or enzyme inhibition (Brodie and Feely, 1991). Enzyme induction usually leads to increased metabolism of the drug and thus increases drug clearance. This will lead to reduced drug efficacy rather than drug toxicity (unless the adverse reaction is due to a metabolite rather than to the parent drug). Enzyme inhibition, on the other hand, is more likely to lead to type A adverse drug reactions since the clearance of the affected drug is reduced; this is particularly likely when the affected drug has a narrow therapeutic index (Brodie and Feely, 1991). Indeed, enzyme inhibitory drug interactions have resulted in regulatory action in a number of instances. An important recent example was the interaction between the CYP3A4 inhibitors ketoconazole and erythromycin and the non-sedating antihistamine terfenadine (Konig *et al.*, 1992; Woosley *et al.*, 1993). This resulted in decreased conversion of terfenadine to its active metabolite (now marketed as fexofenadine). Terfenadine has been shown to affect the delayed rectifier potassium current (Chen *et al.*, 1991), which results in prolongation of the QT interval, torsades de pointe, and sudden death. A similar interaction with cisapride and CYP3A4 inhibitors (Michalets and Williams, 2000) has also resulted in regulatory action against cisapride.

A new mechanism of adverse interaction has recently been described following the identification of the role of drug transporters in the disposition of drugs. Many drug transport proteins are present on membranes, some of which are responsible for drug influx, some are responsible for drug efflux, while others can transport in both directions. Most of the focus to date has been on P-glycoprotein (Pgp), which is encoded by the MDR1 gene. Over-expression of Pgp is one of the mechanisms responsible for resistance of tumours to chemotherapy (Germann, 1996). However, Pgp is also responsible for the transport of a number of other drugs including digoxin. Digoxin does not undergo any significant degree of metabolism, but is known to interact with drugs such as quinidine, verapamil, and amiodarone, all of which can precipitate digoxin toxicity. A recent study has shown that the mechanism of this interaction involves inhibition of Pgp, thereby reducing the efflux of digoxin from the gut and kidney (Fromm *et al.*, 1999). As knowledge of the transporters and their drug substrates increases, it is likely that this will be identified as the mechanism underlying many adverse drug interactions.

TYPE B OR IDIOSYNCRATIC ADVERSE DRUG REACTIONS

Idiosyncratic adverse reactions are less common than the pharmacological adverse reactions, but are as important, if not more so, because they are often more serious, and account for many drug-induced deaths. The possible mechanisms of idiosyncratic adverse effects (Park *et al.*, 1992) are listed in Table 6.5. The toxic reactions may affect many organ systems either in isolation or in combination (Table 6.6).

Type B adverse drug reations have been characterized as being dose-independent (Table 6.2), or rather, there is no simple relationship between dose and the occurrence of toxicity (Park *et al.*, 1998). Certainly, evaluation of patients with and without hypersensitivity to a particular compound shows very little difference in doses received, and indeed in the patients with hypersensitivity, the doses may have been lower since the drug had to be withdrawn. Furthermore, even within the hypersensitive group, there is little relationship to the occurrence and severity of toxicity and the dose administered.

Table 6.5. The mechanisms of type B or idiosyncratic adverse drug reactions.

Mechanism	Example
Pharmaceutical variation	Eosinophilia-myalgia syndrome with L-tryptophan
Receptor abnormality	Malignant hyperthermia with general anaesthetics
Abnormal biological system unmasked by drug	Primaquine-induced haemolysis in patients with G6PD deficiency
Abnormalities of drug metabolism	Isoniazid-induced peripheral neuropathy in slow acetylators
Immunological	Penicillin-induced anaphylaxis
Drug–drug interactions	Increased incidence of isoniazid hepatitis with concomitant administration of rifampicin
Multifactorial	Halothane hepatitis

Adapted from Park *et al.* (1992).

Table 6.6 Examples of organs affected by type B or idiosyncratic adverse drug reactions.

Organ system	Type of reaction	Drug examples
Generalized reaction	Anaphylaxis	Penicillins
Generalized reaction	Hypersensitivity	Temafloxacin
Skin	Toxic epidermal necrolysis	NSAIDs
Liver	Hepatitis	Halothane
Haematological system	Aplastic anaemia	Remoxipride
	Agranulocytosis	Clozapine
	Haemolysis	Nomifensine
Central nervous system	Guillain–Barré syndrome	Zimeldine
Kidney	Interstitial nephritis	Penicillins
Lung	Pneumonitis	Dapsone
Heart	Cardiomyopathy	Tacrolimus
Reproductive toxicity	Etretinate	Various foetal abnormalities

However, intuitively there must be some kind of dose–response relationship since if the patient had not received the drug they would not have developed the hypersensitivity reaction. Since many type B adverse drug reations are thought to be mediated by the formation of chemically reactive metabolites through metabolism by P450 enzymes (a process termed bioactivation) (Park *et al.*, 1998), perhaps a relationship exists with the "internal dose", i.e. the concentration of the toxic metabolite formed in the body. However, since these metabolites by definition are unstable, it has not been possible with the currently available technologies to evaluate the dose–response relationship. The situation is further compounded by the fact that the different sources of variation in the human body may all have a different dose–response relationship. Nevertheless, evidence for the existence of such a dose–response relationship can be gleaned from clinical situations where different doses have to be given to the same group of patients in different circumstances. For example, in HIV-positive patients, the anti-infective agent co-trimoxazole has to be given at low doses for prophylaxis against *Pneumocystis carinii* pneumonia (PCP) (960 mg once daily), while for acute treatment of PCP, much higher doses (up to 8 g/day) may be administered. The frequency of hypersensitivity reactions is lower with the prophy-lactic dose (30%) than with the acute dose, where rates as high 80% have been reported (Carr and Cooper, 1995; Pirmohamed and Park, 1995).

THE ROLE OF DRUG METABOLISM IN TYPE B ADVERSE DRUG REACTIONS

In general, drug metabolism can be considered to be a detoxication process in that it converts therapeutically active compounds to inactive metabolites, which can then be excreted harmlessly from the body. This process may require one or more than one drug metabolizing an enzyme which may be a phase I and/or phase II enzyme (Woolf and Jordan, 1987) (Figure 6.2). A drug may undergo sequential phase I and phase II metabolism, or alternatively, it may only undergo either phase I or phase II metabolism (Tephly and Burchell, 1990).

In certain circumstances, the drug-metabolizing enzymes can convert a drug to a toxic, chemically reactive metabolite (CRM), a process termed bioactivation (Pirmohamed *et al.*, 1994, 1996) (Figure 6.2). Bioactivation may represent less than 1% of the overall metabolism of a drug. The body is equipped with formidable defence mechanisms, and in most cases the CRM will be detoxified (a process which can be termed bioinactivation)

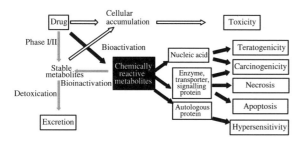

Figure 6.2. The role of metabolism in drug toxicity. A decrease in metabolism can lead to increased drug concentration and dose-dependent toxicity (which may also be due to cellular accumulation). The drug may undergo bioactivation to form chemically reactive metabolites, which if not adequately bioinactivated may bind to various cellular macromolecules, and lead to different forms of toxicity.

before it can initiate tissue damage. Indeed, it is possible that most therapeutically used drugs undergo some degree of bioactivation, but do not cause toxicity because the amount of toxic metabolite formed is below a "toxic" threshold or it is promptly detoxified. Both phase I and phase II enzymes can cause drug bioactivation, but in most cases it is the former, i.e. the cytochrome P450 enzymes, which are responsible (Pirmohamed *et al.*, 1994).

Inadequate detoxication of a CRM is often the first step in the initiation of idiosyncratic drug toxicity (Park *et al.*, 1992; Pirmohamed *et al.*, 1994). This may occur if there is an imbalance between drug bioactivation and bioinactivation pathways. Tissue-specific expression of enzymes involved in drug bioactivation and drug detoxication may lead to a selective imbalance in that tissue resulting in tissue-selective toxicity (Park *et al.*, 1995). An imbalance may be the consequence of a genetically determined deficiency of an enzyme, or alternatively it may be acquired as a result of environmental factors such as infection, diet, or concomitant drug intake. It is important to note that inadequate detoxication of a CRM, although an important first step in the occurrence of toxicity, is not necessarily the ultimate step (Pirmohamed *et al.*, 1996). Other factors, such as tissue repair enzymes, immune responsiveness and the biochemical processes that modulate tissue

injury, may all serve as factors determining not only whether idiosyncratic toxicity occurs but also its severity.

An inadequately detoxified CRM can combine with or damage cellular macromolecules such as proteins and nucleic acids and result in various forms of toxicity, including teratogenicity, carcinogenicity, cellular necrosis, and hypersensitivity (Park *et al.*, 1995) (Figure 6.2). Binding of a CRM to nucleic acid may result in teratogenicity or carcinogenicity (Figure 6.2).

Binding to cellular macromolecules may result in either direct or immune-mediated toxicity (Pirmohamed *et al.*, 1994) (Figure 6.2). With direct toxicity, binding of the CRM to a protein will interfere with its normal physiological function leading to cellular necrosis. Alternatively, the CRM can act as a hapten and initiate an immune reaction which may be due to a specific humoral (antibody) response, a cellular response (T lymphocytes), or a combination of both (Park *et al.*, 1987, 1998, 2001; Pohl *et al.*, 1988; Naisbitt *et al.*, 2000a). The immune response can be directed against the drug (haptenic epitopes), the carrier protein (autoantigenic determinants), or the neoantigen created by the combination of the drug and the protein (new antigenic determinants). The factors that determine what type of toxicity is mediated by a CRM are poorly understood, but are likely to include the following (Gillette *et al.*, 1984; Park *et al.*, 1987; Boelsterli, 1993):

- the relative stability of the CRM, and thus its reactivity;
- the half-life of any drug–protein adducts which are formed and their concentration within the cell;
- the epitope density, i.e. the number of groups of the CRM which are covalently bound to a protein molecule; and
- the nature, physiological function, and subcellular site of the carrier protein to which the CRM binds.

In most cases, the differentiation between these two forms of idiosyncratic toxicity is largely empirical being based on symptomatology; for example, the occurrence of manifestations such as rash, fever, lymphadenopathy, and eosinophilia all suggest drug hypersensitivity (Pessayre and Larrey, 1988; Pirmohamed *et al.*, 1998). The lack of laboratory methodology by which to make a definitive diagnosis largely reflects our ignorance of the mechanism of toxicity in most cases of idiosyncratic toxiity.

PARACETAMOL: AN EXAMPLE OF A DRUG THAT CAUSES TOXICITY THROUGH THE FORMATION OF A CHEMICALLY REACTIVE INTERMEDIATE

For a number of drugs that undergo metabolism, CRM will be formed irrespective of the dose of the drug (Pirmohamed *et al.*, 1996). When a drug is taken in therapeutic dosage, any toxic metabolite formed will be detoxified by normal enzymatic or non-enzymatic cellular defence mechanisms. An imbalance between bioactivation and bioinactivation leading to toxicity may however be created by taking a drug overdose. This will lead to the formation of large amounts of chemically reactive metabolites, overwhelming the cellular detoxication capacity, and leading to cell damage. The clearest example of this is paracetamol, which causes hepatotoxicity when taken in overdosage, and still causes about 160 deaths per year in the United Kingdom (Bray, 1993). According to the conventional definition of adverse drug reactions, paracetamol hepatotoxicity should not be classified as an adverse drug reaction, since the hepatic injury occurs when the drug is used inappropriately. However, it is important to note that the occurrence of liver damage with paracetamol and its severity is a function not only of the dose but also of various host factors (Pirmohamed *et al.*, 1994). Indeed, paracetamol hepatotoxicity has been reported with therapeutic drug use. For example, a recent study in 67 alcoholics who had sustained liver injury after paracetamol ingestion showed that 40% had taken less than 4 g/day (the maximum recommended therapeutic dose) while another 20% had taken between 4 and 6 g/day (which is also regarded as a non-toxic dose) (Zimmerman and Maddrey, 1995).

In therapeutic dosage, paracetamol is largely metabolized by phase II processes (glucuronida-tion and sulphation) to stable metabolites, but between 5% and 10% also undergoes P450 metabolism to the toxic N-acetyl p-benzoquino-neimine (NAPQI) metabolite (Nelson, 1990) (Figure 6.3). This is detoxified by cellular glutathione. In overdosage, saturation of the phase II metabolic pathways results in a greater proportion of the drug undergoing bioactivation. This ultimately leads to depletion of cellular glutathione, and allows the toxic metabolite to bind to hepatic proteins resulting in hepatocellular damage (Nelson, 1990). The use of N-acetylcysteine in the treatment of paracetamol overdosage illustrates the important point that elucidation of the mechanism of drug toxicity can lead to the development of rational therapies that will prevent the toxicity. Alcoholics show increased susceptibility to paracetamol overdosage because excess alcohol consumption results in depletion of glutathione (Lauterburg and Velez, 1988) and induction of the P450 isoform CYP2E1 (Raucy *et al.*, 1989). Recent studies in knockout mice have shown that CYP2E1 is the primary isoform involved in the bioactivation of paracetamol (Lee *et al.*, 1996).

Although experiments with transgenic mice have shown that in the absence of phase I oxidative pathways and therefore NAPQI formation, hepatotoxicity does not occur, the precise pathway

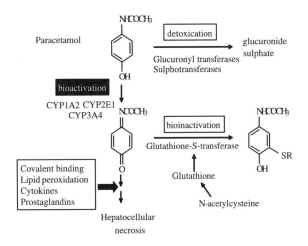

Figure 6.3. The role of metabolism in the hepatotoxicity associated with paracetamol.

leading to liver damage is still unclear (Gibson *et al.*, 1996). Several mechanisms have been proposed, including effects on plasma membrane Ca^{2+} pumps (Tsokos-Kuhn, 1989), which can lead to Ca^{2+}-induced DNA damage (Ray *et al.*, 1990), mitochondrial damage (Meyers *et al.*, 1988) resulting in glutathione depletion and oxidative stress (Jaeschke, 1990), and apoptosis (Ray *et al.*, 1996). Recently, it has been shown that Fas antisense oligonucleotide protects mice from paracetamol toxicity, suggesting that the ultimate cytotoxic event involves more than simply necrosis, and that cells of the immune system may be recruited in the inflammatory response (Zhang *et al.*, 2000). Interestingly, several studies have revealed that cells exposed to chemical or oxidant stress will respond with an orchestrated and robust transcriptional response aimed at detoxifying the offending chemical and preventing or repairing cellular damage (Hayes *et al.*, 1999; Moinova and Mulcahy, 1998, 1999). If unsuccessful, the culmination of this response, known as the antioxidant response, is to commit the cell to suicide through apoptosis. The target genes for the antioxidant response encode a set of enzymes and other proteins that scavenge free radicals, neutralize electrophiles, or up-regulate the critical cellular thiol, glutathione. Glutathione depletion caused by a range of chemicals leads to up-regulation of c-jun and c-fos mRNA, and enhances AP-1 DNA binding activity (Kitteringham *et al.*, 2000). This response was also accompanied by induction of γ-glutamyl cysteine synthetase (GCS). What was surprising for paracetamol, in contrast to the other compounds, was that despite the increased GCS protein levels, catalytic activity was in fact reduced. This finding, which presumably involves a post-translational modification of the protein, may contribute to the inability of hepatocytes to defend themselves against paracetamol, whilst recovery from other compounds that deplete glutathione to the same extent can be achieved through enhanced synthetic activity.

Paradoxically, studies performed with transgenic mice aimed at clarifying events subsequent to NAPQI formation have only served to confound rather than to clarify. For example, deletion of components of the glutathione detoxication system such as glutathione peroxidase (Mirochnitchenko *et al.*, 1999) and glutathione transferase pi (Henderson *et al.*, 2000) both afforded partial protection against paracetamol hepatotoxicity. The loss of a major hepatic form of GST, which represents over 3% of total soluble protein (Fountoulakis *et al.*, 2000), would have been expected to predispose the animals to hepatotoxicity through a reduction in the glutathione conjugation of NAPQI (Coles *et al.*, 1988). This suggests that GST-pi may be involved in a novel mechanism that determines susceptibility to paracetamol hepatotoxicity. Indeed, a recent study has shown that GST-pi may have a role in cell signalling; it has been shown to be an efficient inhibitor of Jun kinase (also known as stress-activated kinase), the enzyme that activates c-jun and several other transcription factors (Adler *et al.*, 1999). Future studies using other transgenic mice models will be useful in determining the exact pathway by which paracetamol causes liver damage, and may therefore provide novel therapeutic strategies by which to reverse liver damage in patients who present late after paracetamol overdosage.

THE ROLE OF THE IMMUNE SYSTEM IN TYPE B ADVERSE DRUG REACTIONS

On the basis of clinical criteria, it has been postulated that many idiosyncratic adverse drug reactions are immune-mediated (Park *et al.*, 1998; Pirmohamed *et al.*, 1998). Research into this area is now providing some direct evidence to support the clinical impression. The mechanism by which a drug leads to an immune-mediated adverse reaction is explained by the hapten hypothesis (Park *et al.*, 1998) (Figure 6.2). Central to the hapten hypothesis is the assumption that small molecules such as drugs (< 1000 Da) can be recognized as immunogens (i.e. a substance capable of eliciting a specific immune response) only when they become covalently bound to an autologous high molecular weight (> 50 000 Da) macromolecular carrier such as a protein (Park *et al.*, 1987). The term hapten has been coined to describe such substances that are not immunogenic *per se* but become immunogenic when conjugated to a macromolecular carrier (this has been termed signal 1). The type of hypersensitive reaction will be partly determined by the nature of the immune response and the site of antigen formation. The best understood reactions are the type I hypersensitivity reactions induced by penicillins and cephalosporins and mediated by IgE antibodies directed against a drug hapten conjugated to protein (Weiss and Adkinson, 1988; Pirmohamed et al., 1994). Severe anaphylactic reactions occur in only a minority of patients (1 in 2000); atopic patients are at increased risk, although the genetic basis of this and of the IgE response to penicillins remains to be elucidated.

Less well understood are the immunological mechanisms that underlie severe skin reactions such as Stevens–Johnson syndrome and immunoallergic hepatitis. There is clear chemical evidence from in vitro studies that the drugs associated with these reactions can undergo oxidative metabolism to chemically reactive metabolites that can haptenate proteins (Park et al., 1995). In addition, both humoral and cell-mediated responses directed against drug-induced antigen have been detected in patients, for example in halothane hepatitis (Pohl et al., 1990). With some compounds the immune response seems to be directed predominantly towards an autoantigen. For example, in tienilic acid-induced hepatitis, patients have circulating autoantibodies directed against the P450 isoform (CYP2C9), which is responsible for the bioactivation of tienilic acid (Beaune and Bourdi, 1993).

The fundamental concept that protein-conjugation is an obligatory step in the process of immune recognition of drugs has however recently been challenged by the observation that T-cell clones from patients hypersensitive to a number of drugs undergo proliferation in an antigen-processing independent [but major histocompatibility complex (MHC) restricted] manner (Schnyder et al., 1997; Zanni et al., 1998). This requires labile, reversible binding of a drug to the MHCs on antigen-presenting cells. The presence of T-cell clones that proliferate only in response to the parent drug rather than the metabolite, and the rapid down-regulation in expression of the T-cell receptor upon stimulation are consistent with this mechanism. It is of course possible that both mechanisms may be important in the overall

pathogenesis. For example, the hapten-dependent pathway may be more important for primary immune stimulation (sensitization), while the metabolism-independent pathway may be all that is necessary for secondary stimulation and elicitation of tissue damage (Pirmohamed and Park, 2001b). Further studies are needed to define the roles of the two pathways of drug (antigen) presentation in the pathogenesis of immune-mediated adverse drug reactions.

Irrespective of the mechanism of antigen presentation, T cells are of fundamental importance in the immune response against a drug (Naisbitt et al., 2000a). The interaction between the T cell and the drug (antigen) in the groove of the MHC governs the immune response. MHC class I molecules bind the peptides of 8–10 amino acids and present to the CD8 + T cells (Pamer and Creswell, 1998). MHC class II molecules present longer peptide molecules (13–17 amino acids) to CD4 + cells (Jensen, 1997). While class I molecules are found on all cell surfaces, class II molecules are only expressed on specialized antigen-presenting cells such as macrophages, but can become expressed on other cells such as keratinocytes in the presence of pro-inflammatory cytokines such as interferon gamma (Pichler and Yawalkar, 2000). The nature of the immune response is governed by differentiation of T cells into T helper-1 (T_H1), T helper-2 (T_H2), T cytotoxic-1 (T_C1) or T cytotoxic-2 (T_C2) subsets. T_H1 and T_C1 cells mediate cytotoxicity and local inflammatory reactions, while T_H2 and T_C2 cells stimulate B-cell dependent antibody production (Romagnani, 1999; Singh et al., 1999).

It is important to note that the presence of an antigen (i.e. signal 1) in the absence of co-stimulatory molecules will lead to tolerance and T-cell apoptosis (Naisbitt et al., 2000a). Although the role of surface molecules such as B7.1 and B7.2 as co-stimulatory molecules has long been known, the importance of cytokines has only been recognized recently. In addition to signal 1, two other signals are required to stimulate a full immune response (Curtsinger et al., 1999). Signal 2 is represented by a series of pro-inflammatory cytokines such as IL-2, TNF-α, and IFN-gamma that act indirectly on antigen presenting cells to up-regulate the expression of co-stimulatory molecules. Signal 3 represents polarizing cytokines that act directly on T cells. It is known that T_H1 cells produce IL-12 and IFN-gamma, which promote the activation of macrophages and cell-mediated immunity. By contrast, T_H2 cells produce IL-4 and IL-13; these provide help for the humoral immune response by promoting IgG to IgE class switching.

An interesting hypothesis, termed the danger hypothesis, has recently been proposed in the field of immunology to explain the basis of self-tolerace (Matzinger, 1994; Anderson and Matzinger, 2000; Gallucci and Matzinger, 2001). This can also be applied to the mechanism of drug hypersensitivity (Park et al., 1998; Uetrecht, 1999). This hypothesis states that the immune system responds to most antigens with tolerance, and only in the presence of a danger signal will presentation of an antigen result in an immune response. The nature of the danger signals has not been accurately defined, but pro-inflammatory and polarizing cytokines, intracellular contents resulting from cell necrosis and exogenous proteins including those derived from viruses, are all potential candidates (Gallucci and Matzinger, 2001). With respect to drug hypersensitivity, it can be hypothesized that the chemically reactive metabolite may not only provide signal 1 (by conjugating with a protein), but it could also provide the co-stimulatory signals 2 and 3 by activation of signalling pathways linked to oxidative stress and protein damage, including the secretion of cytokines (Park et al., 2001). Furthermore, the hypothesis also allows the possibility that the co-stimulatory molecules are completely independent of the drug, and could, for example, be concomitant viral infections (see below).

THE ROLE OF VIRUSES IN TYPE B ADVERSE DRUG REACTIONS

There is increasing evidence that concomitant virus infections can predispose to the development of idiosyncratic adverse drug reactions, particularly those reactions that are thought to be immune-mediated. The mechanism of this is unclear, but as postulated above, the viruses may be acting as a source of danger signal.

Evidence for the role of viruses first came from the observation that the use of ampicillin in patients with active EBV infection (i.e. infectious mononucleosis) results in a rash in 95% of patients (Sullivan and Shear, 2001). Another member of the herpes virus family, human herpes virus 6 (HHV6) has recently been implicated in hypersensitivity reactions associated with a number of drugs, including sulphasalazine (Suzuki et al., 1998; Descamps et al., 2001). However, whether this is a true predisposition or merely a coincidental factor needs further study. Perhaps the most striking association between viral infection and drug hypersensitivity has been observed in HIV-infected individuals. These patients have a higher frequency of hypersensitivity reactions with numerous anti-infective drugs including co-trimoxazole, sulphadiazine, dapsone, clindamycin, primaquine, and thioacetazone (Koopmans et al., 1995; Pirmohamed and Park, 2001b). This has been best shown with co-trimoxazole that is used for the treatment of Pneumocystis carinii pneumonia (PCP). Approximately 50% of patients being treated acutely for PCP will develop skin rashes, whereas when used for prophylaxis the figure is 30% (van der Ven et al., 1991). This contrasts with a frequency of 3% in HIV-negative individuals (van der Ven et al., 1991). A deficiency of thiols such as glutathione and cysteine has been suggested to be responsible for the increase in susceptibility of HIV-positive patients (van der Ven et al., 1991; Koopmans et al., 1995). A recent study has demonstrated that in the presence of plasma cysteine deficiency, HIV-positive patients have a lower capacity to detoxify the toxic nitroso metabolite of sulphamethoxazole (Naisbitt et al., 2000b). However, the fact that prophylactic N-acetylcysteine does not prevent co-trimoxazole hypersensitivity (Walmsley et al., 1998) suggests that the reasons for the higher frequency are likely to be more complex and multifactorial, and include the dose of the drug, changes in drug metabolizing capacity (both in bioactivation and bioinactivation), and immune dysregulation (Pirmohamed and Park, 2001b). In addition, HIV itself may act as a source of a danger signal (Park et al., 1998; Uetrecht, 1999; Pirmohamed and Park, 2001b; Sullivan and Shear, 2001).

Interestingly, the peculiar predisposition of HIV patients to hypersensitivity reactions is now being witnessed with the new antiretrovirals such as abacavir (severe hypersensitivity is seen in 3% of patients) and non-nucleoside reverse transcriptase inhibitors such as nevirapine, efavirenz, and delavirdine, all of which produce skin rashes at a frequency of between 18% and 40% (Pirmohamed and Park, 2001b).

GENETIC PREDISPOSITION TO TYPE B ADVERSE DRUG REACTIONS

Type B adverse drug reactions have typically been defined to be host-dependent (Rawlins and Thompson, 1991). However, the nature of this host-dependency has not been defined for most drugs, although genetic factors have long been suspected. Indeed, genetic factors are also important for type A reactions; however, while type A reactions may conform to a monogenic or oligogenic model, it is likely that type B adverse drug reactions will be polygenic in nature (Pirmohamed and Park, 2001a), and will be as difficult to unravel as polygenic diseases such as ischaemic heart disease, with the added complication that they are not as common, and therefore it will be more difficult to recruit adequate numbers of patients.

The nature of the polygenic predisposition is unclear, but in general could be divided into several areas (Figure 6.4), as follows (Pirmohamed *et al.*, 1998; Park and Pirmohamed, 2001; Pirmohamed and Park, 2001a):

- *Activation*: This involves activation of a drug to chemically reactive metabolites. Bioactivation of drugs is largely mediated by cytochrome P450 enzymes, many of which have now been shown to be polymorphically expressed (Park *et al.*, 1995). Importantly, a deficiency of an enzyme will lead to reduced bioactivation of a drug and will act as a protective factor. No good examples have been identified to date. By contrast, amplification of a P450 isoform, as seen with CYP2D6 (CYP2D6*2xN) (Ingelman-Sundberg *et al.*, 1999), would increase bioactivation, but again no good example has yet been identified.

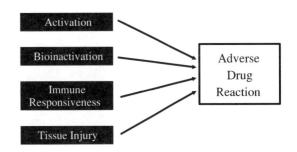

Figure 6.4. Type B or idiosyncratic drug reactions have a multi-factorial aetiology. Variation, which may be genetically determined, in drug *bioactivation* and *bioinactivation*, can lead to persistence of a chemically reactive metabolite. If the adverse reaction is immune-mediated, the binding of the chemically reactive metabolite will lead to the formation of an antigen, which will be recognized by the body's immune system resulting in an *immune response* and *tissue injury*.

- *Detoxification*: The absence or reduced activity of a detoxification enzyme would lead to a decrease in bioinactivation of the reactive metabolite (Pirmohamed and Park, 1999), and hence increase the possibility of the reactive metabolite interacting with important cellular macromolecules resulting in different forms of toxicity. The best characterized example of this is the slow acetylator phenotype predisposing to hypersensitivity with co-trimoxazole in HIV-negative patients (Rieder *et al.*, 1991), and SLE with hydralazine and procainamide (Park *et al.*, 1992). There has also been interest in the role of the glutathione-S-transferase genes, many of which have been shown to be polymorphically expressed. However, although these gene polymorphisms may be important with respect to certain cancers, studies to date have not shown any association of the glutathione transferase gene polymorphisms with idiosyncratic drug reactions observed with co-trimoxazole (Pirmohamed *et al.*, 2000), carbamazepine (Leeder, 1998), and tacrine (Green *et al.*, 1995b; De-Sousa *et al.*, 1998).
- *Immune response genes*: Most importantly this includes the major histocompatibility complex of genes, including those encoding the human leukocyte antigen (HLA) molecules. HLA associations have been shown with numerous idiosyncratic drug reactions including clozapine

agranulcoytosis and hydralazine-induced SLE (Park *et al.*, 1992). However, research in this area has been by the lack of reproducibility in results between different populations. This may be a reflection of the high degree of linkage disequilibrium in this area of the MHC, which is located on the short arm of chromosome 6. This has recently been sequenced, and initial findings suggest that over 60% of the genes on this area are of unknown function (The MHC Sequencing Consortium, 1999), and may serve as a fruitful area of research in the search for predisposing genes.

- *Tissue injury genes*: There are many molecules that are important in mediating the tissue injury resulting from a drug insult. Of particular importance may be cytokines such as IL-1, IFN-gamma and TNF-α. We have recently investigated the role of TNF-α gene locus in carbamazepine hypersensitivity (Pirmohamed *et al.*, 2001). This syndrome is characterized by skin rash, fever, eosinophilia, lymphadenopathy, and extra-cutaneous manifestations. Skin biopsy data have shown the involvement of cytotoxic T cells and pro-inflammatory cytokines such as TNF-α (Friedmann *et al.*, 1994). There is both clinical and biochemical data that suggest that this form of idiosyncratic toxicity has a genetic basis (Strickler *et al.*, 1985; Edwards *et al.*, 1999). *Ex vivo* studies have shown that cells from hypersensitive patients are more susceptible to the toxic effects of drug metabolite(s) generated *in situ* (Shear *et al.*, 1988; Pirmohamed *et al.*, 1991). However, analysis of genes coding for enzymes responsible for drug bioinactivation, including microsomal epoxide hydrolase, glutathione transferases, catechol-O-methyl transferase, and quinone reductase, failed to reveal an association with carbamazepine hypersensitivity (Gaedigk *et al.*, 1994; Green *et al.* 1995a). Analysis of the promoter region polymorphisms in the TNF-α gene that may be functionally active has shown that serious, but interestingly not non-serious, hypersensitivity reactions to CBZ showed an association with the—308, but not the—238, polymorphism (Pirmohamed *et al.*, 2001). Demonstration in

an independent sample population is required to confirm this association.

For the future, it may be possible to use a comprehensive, densely spaced, genome-wide single nucleotide polymorphism (SNP) map which may allow conduction of screens for pharmacogenetically active genes as whole-genome, unbiased searches (Roses, 2000). SNPs are single-base differences in the DNA sequence, observed between individuals, which occur throughout the human genome. The International SNP Map Working Group has recently published a map of 1.42 million SNPs throughout the genome, occurring at an average density of one SNP every 1.9 kilobases (The International SNP Map Working Group, 2001). At least 60 000 SNPs are within coding regions (coding SNPs) and are therefore more likely to be functionally active. This high density SNP map provides an opportunity to perform SNP profiling in order to identify genetic factors predisposing to adverse drug reactions. However, before this can become a reality many obstacles need to be overcome including the development of both the technologies to perform SNP profiling and less expensive genotyping strategies (Pirmohamed and Park, 2001a). Furthermore, given the need to test for multiple markers simultaneously, an issue that needs to be considered is the sample size and the level of statistical significance required to prevent detection of false-positive associations. A recent study has reported that for testing 100 000 loci in a genome-wide screen will require a three-fold greater sample size at a significance level of 2.5×10^{-7} (Cardon *et al.*, 2000). This does suggest that for pharmacogenomic detection of rare adverse events, testing in phases I–III is not likely be practicable, and will require prospective storage of samples and evaluation in phase IV when a problem has been identified.

CONCLUSION

The importance of adverse drug reactions is often underestimated. They are common, can be life threatening, and unnecessarily expensive. Because of the wide range of drugs available, the manifestations of toxicity can be variable and affect any organ system. In fact, adverse drug reactions have taken over from syphilis and tuberculosis as the great mimics of other diseases. It is also likely that the pattern of toxicity is going to change with the introduction of new biotechnology products. It is therefore important for the prescribing clinician to be aware of the toxic profile of drugs they prescribe and to be ever vigilant for the occurrence of unexpected adverse reactions.

Both type A and type B adverse reactions are complex, and their prevention for future populations will depend on an understanding of their pathogenesis, and exactly how a foreign chemical, i.e. a drug, interacts with macromolecules within the body. Pharmacogenomic strategies have been proposed for the prevention of these reactions in the future by prediction of susceptible individuals (Roses, 2000). However, despite the hype surrounding the area, this is likely to be a long-term goal and will crucially depend on (a) the availability of accurately phenotyped patients, which for the rare reactions will necessitate multi-centre international collaborations, (b) the demonstration that genotyping is clinically- and cost-effective, (c) an understanding of the mechanisms of the adverse reactions so that more targeted SNP profiling can be undertaken, and (d) most crucially, education of the end-users, i.e. clinicians, so that they understand the rationale for performing the tests, and how to interpret the results.

ACKNOWLEDGEMENTS

The authors wish to thank the Wellcome Trust, MRC, NHS Executive North West, Sir Jules Thorn Charitable Trust, and GSK, Pfizer and Astra-Zeneca Pharmaceuticals for their support.

REFERENCES

Adler V, Yin Z, Fuchs SY, Benezra M, Rosario L, Tew KD, Pincus MR, Sardana M, Henderson CJ, Wolf CR, Davis RJ, Ronai Z (1999) Regulation of JNK signaling by GSTp. *Embo J* **18**: 1321–34.

Aithal GP, Day CP, Kesteven PJL, Daly AK (1999) Association of polymorphisms in the cytochrome P450 CYP2C9 with warfarin dose requirement and risk of bleeding complications. *Lancet* **353**: 717–9.

Anderson CC, Matzinger P (2000) Danger: The view from the bottom of the cliff. *Semin Immunol* **12**: 231–8; discussion 257–344.

Asscher AW, Parr GD, Whitmarsh VB (1995) Towards the safer use of medicines. *Br Med J* **311**: 1003–5.

Bakke OM, Manocchia M, de-Abajo F, Kaitin KI, Lasagna L (1995) Drug safety discontinuations in the United Kingdom, the United States, and Spain from 1974 through 1993: a regulatory perspective. *Clin Pharmacol Ther* **58**: 108–17.

Bates DW, Boyle DL, Vliet MVV, Schneider J, Leape L (1995a) Relationship between medication errors and adverse drug events. *J Gen Intern Med* **10**: 199–205.

Bates DW, Cullen DJ, Laird N, Petersen LA, Small SD, Servi D, Laffel G, Sweitzer BJ, Shea BF, Hallisey R, Vandervliet M, Nemeskal R, Leape LL (1995b) Incidence of adverse drug events and potential adverse drug events—implications for prevention. *Am Med Assoc* **274**: 29–34.

Bates DW, Spell N, Cullen DJ, Burdick E, Laird N, Petersen LA, Small SD, Sweitzer BJ, Leape LL (1997) The costs of adverse drug events in hospitalized patients. *J Am Med Assoc* **277**: 307–11.

Bayard PJ, Berger TG, Jacobson MA (1992) Drug hypersensitivity reactions and human immunodeficiency virus disease. *J AIDS* **5**: 1237–57.

Beaune PH, Bourdi M (1993) Autoantibodies against cytochrome P-450 in drug-induced autoimmune hepatitis. *Ann NY Acad Sci* **685**: 641–5.

Boelsterli UA (1993) Specific targets of covalent drug-protein interactions in hepatocytes and their toxicological significance in drug-induced liver injury. *Drug Metab Rev* **25**: 395–451.

Bombardier C, Laine L, Reicin A, Shapiro D, Burgos-Vargas R, Davis B, Day R, Ferraz MB, Hawkey CJ, Hochberg MC, Kvien TK, Schnitzer TJ (2000) Comparison of upper gastrointestinal toxicity of rofecoxib and naproxen in patients with rheumatoid arthritis. VIGOR Study Group. *N Engl J Med* **343**: 1520–8.

Bray GP (1993) Liver failure induced by paracetamol. *Br Med J* **306**: 157–8.

Brodie M, Feely J (1991) Adverse drug interactions. In: Feely J, ed., *New Drugs*. London: BMJ, pp. 29–39.

Cardon LR, Idury RM, Harris TJ, Witte JS, Elston RC (2000) Testing drug response in the presence of genetic information: sampling issues for clinical trials [In Process Citation]. *Pharmacogenetics* **10**: 503–10.

Carr A, Cooper DA (1995) Pathogenesis and management of HIV-associated drug hypersensitivity. *AIDS Clin Rev* **96**: 65–97.

Chen Y, Gillis RA, Woosley RL (1991) Block of delayed rectifier potassium current, Ik, by terfenadine in cat ventricular myocytes. *J Am Coll Cardiol* **17**: 140A.

Classen DC, Pestotnik SL, Evans RS, Lloyd JF, Burke JP (1997) Adverse drug events in hospitalized patients. Excess length of stay, extra costs, and attributable mortality. *J Am Med Assoc* **277**: 301–6.

Coles B, Wilson I, Wardman P, Hinson JA, Nelson SD, Ketterer B (1988) The spontaneous and enzymatic reaction of N-acetyl-p-benzoquinonimine with glutathione: a stopped-flow kinetic study. *Arch Biochem Biophys* **264**: 253–60.

Cromheecke ME, Levi M, Colly LP, de Mol BJ, Prins MH, Hutten BA, Mak R, Keyzers KC, Buller HR (2000) Oral anticoagulation self-management and management by a specialist anticoagulation clinic: a randomised cross-over comparison. *Lancet* **356**: 97–102.

Curtsinger JM, Schmidt CS, Mondino A, Lins DC, Kedl RM, Jenkins MK, Mescher MF (1999) Inflammatory cytokines provide a third signal for activation of naive CD4 + and CD8 + T cells. *J Immunol* **162**: 3256–62.

D'Arcy PF (1986) Epidemiological aspects of iatrogenic disease. In: D'Arcy PF, Griffin JP, eds, *Iatrogenic Diseases*. Oxford: Oxford University Press, pp. 29–58.

Descamps V, Valance A, Edlinger C, Fillet AM, Grossin M, Lebrun-Vignes B, Belaich S, Crickx B (2001) Association of human herpesvirus 6 infection with drug reaction with eosinophilia and systemic symptoms. *Arch Dermatol* **137**: 301–4.

DeSousa M, Pirmohamed M, Kitteringham NR, Woolf T, Park BK (1998) No association between tacrine transaminitis and the glutathione transferase theta genotype in patients with Alzheimer's disease. *Pharmacogenetics* **8**: 353–5.

Edwards IR, Aronson JK (2000) Adverse drug reactions: definitions, diagnosis, and management. *Lancet* **356**: 1255–59.

Edwards SG, Hubbard V, Aylett S, Wren D (1999) Concordance of primary generalised epilepsy and carbamazepine hypersensitivity in monozygotic twins. *Postgrad Med J* **75**: 680–1.

Einarson TR (1993) Drug-related hospital admissions. *Ann Pharmacother* **27**: 832–40.

Fountoulakis M, Berndt P, Boelsterli UA, Crameri F, Winter M, Albertini S, Suter L (2000) Two-dimensional database of mouse liver proteins: changes in hepatic protein levels following treatment with acetaminophen or its nontoxic regioisomer 3-acetamidophenol. *Electrophoresis* **21**: 2148–61.

Freeman BD, Zehnbauer BA, McGrath S, Borecki I, Buchman TG (2000) Cytochrome P450 polymorphisms are associated with reduced warfarin dose. *Surgery* **128**: 281–5.

Friedmann PS, Strickland I, Pirmohamed M, Park BK (1994) Investigation of mechanisms in toxic epidermal necrolysis induced by carbamazepine. *Arch Dermatol* **130**: 598–604.

Fromm MF, Kim RB, Stein CM, Wilkinson GR, Roden DM (1999) Inhibition of P-glycoprotein-mediated drug transport: a unifying mechanism to explain the interaction between digoxin and quinidine. *Circulation* **99**: 552–7.

Furst DE, Breedveld FC, Burmester GR, Crofford JJ, Emery P, Feldmann M, Kalden JR, Kavanaugh AF, Keystone EC, Klareskog LG, Lipsky PE, Maini RN, Russell AS, Scott DL, Smolen JS, Van de Putte LB, Visher TL, Weisman MH (2000) Updated consensus statement on tumour necrosis factor blocking agents for the treatment of rheumatoid arthritis (May 2000). *Ann Rheum Dis* **59** (Suppl 1): i1–2.

Furuya H, Fernandez-Salguero P, Gregory W, Taber H, Steward A, Gonzalez FJ, Idle JR (1995) Genetic polymorphism of CYP2C9 and its effect on warfarin maintenance dose requirement in patients undergoing anticoagualtion therapy. *Pharmacogenetics* **5**: 389–92.

Gaedigk A, Spielberg SP, Grant DM (1994) Characterization of the microsomal epoxide hydrolase gene in patients with anticonvulsant adverse drug reactions. *Pharmacogenetics* **4**: 142–53.

Gallucci S, Matzinger P (2001) Danger signals: SOS to the immune system. *Curr Opin Immunol* **13**: 114–9.

Germann UA (1996) P-glycoprotein—a mediator of multidrug-resistance in tumor-cells. *Eur J Cancer* **32A**, 927–44.

Gibson JD, Pumford NR, Samokyszyn VM, Hinson JA (1996) Mechanism of acetaminophen-induced hepatotoxicity: covalent binding versus oxidative stress. *Chem Res Toxicol* **9**: 580–5.

Gillette JR, Lau SS, Monks TJ (1984) Intra- and extracellular formation of metabolites from chemically reactive species. *Biochem Soc Trans* **12**: 4–7.

Green VJ, Pirmohamed M, Kitteringham NR, Gaedigk A, Grant DM, Boxer M, Burchell B, Park BK (1995a) Genetic analysis of microsomal epoxide hydrolase in patients with carbamazepine hypersensitivity. *Biochem Pharmacol* **50**: 1353–9.

Green VJ, Pirmohamed M, Kitteringham NR, Knapp MJ, Park BK (1995b) Glutathione S-transferase u genotype (GSTM1*O) in Alzheimer's patients with tacrine transaminitis. *Br J Clin Pharmacol* **39**: 411–15.

Haining RL, Hunter AP, Veronese ME, Trager WF, Rettie AE (1996) Allelic variants of human cytochrome P450 2C9: baculovirus-mediated expression, purification, structural characterization, substrate stereoselectivity, and prochiral selectivity of the wild-type and I359L mutant forms. *Arch Biochem Biophys* **333**: 447–58.

Hart RG, Sherman DG, Easton JD, Cairns JA (1998) Prevention of stroke in patients with nonvalvular atrial fibrillation. *Neurology* **51**: 674–81.

Hayes JD, Ellis EM, Neal GE, Harrison DJ, Manson MM (1999) Cellular response to cancer chemopreventive agents: contribution of the antioxidant responsive element to the adaptive response to oxidative and chemical stress. *Biochem Soc Symp* **64**: 141–68.

Henderson CJ, Wolf CR, Kitteringham N, Powell H, Otto D, Park BK (2000) Increased resistance to acetaminophen hepatotoxicity in mice lacking glutathione S-transferase Pi. *Proc Natl Acad Sci USA* **97**: 12741–5.

Ingelman-Sundberg M, Oscarson M, McLellan RA (1999) Polymorphic human cytochrome P450 enzymes: an opportunity for individualized drug treatment. *Trends Pharmacol Sci* **20**: 342–9.

Jaeschke H (1990) Glutathione disulfide formation and oxidant stress during acetaminophen-induced hepatotoxicity in mice in vivo: the protective effect of allopurinol. *J Pharmacol Exp Ther* **255**: 935–41.

Jensen PE (1997) Peptide binding and antigen presentation by class I I histocompatibility glycoproteins. *Biopolymers* **43**: 303–22.

Kaminsky LS, Zhang ZY (1997) Human P450 metabolism of warfarin. *Pharmacol Ther* **73**: 67–74.

Kitteringham NR, Powell H, Clement YN, Dodd CC, Tettey JN, Pirmohamed M, Smith DA, McLellan LI, Park BK (2000) Hepatocellular response to chemical stress in CD-1 mice: induction of early genes and gamma-glutamylcysteine synthetase. *Hepatology* **32**: 321–33.

Konig PK, Woosley RL, Zamani K, Conner DP, Cantilena LR (1992) Changes in the pharmacokinetics and electrocardiographic pharmacodynamics of terfenadine with concomitant administration of erythromycin. *Clin Pharmacol Ther* **52**: 231–38.

Koopmans PP, van der Ven AJAM, Vree TB, van der Meer JWM (1995) Pathogenesis of hypersensitivity reactions to drugs in patients with HIV-infection—allergic or toxic? *AIDS* **9**: 217–22.

Lauterburg BH, Velez ME (1988) Glutathione deficiency in alcoholics: risk factor for paracetamol hepatotoxicity. *Gut* **29**: 1153–7.

Lazarou J, Pomeranz BH, Corey PN (1998) Incidence of adverse drug reactions in hospitalized patients—a meta-analysis of prospective studies. *J Am Med Assoc* **279**: 1200–5.

Lee SST, Buters JTM, Pineau T, Fernandezsalguero P, Gonzalez FJ (1996) Role of cyp2e1 in the hepatotoxicity of acetaminophen. *J Biol Chem* **271**: 12063–7.

Leeder JS (1998) Mechanisms of idiosyncratic hypersensitivity reactions to antiepileptic drugs. *Epilepsia* **39** (Suppl. 7): S8–S16.

Lennard MS, Silas JH, Freestone S, Ramsey LE, Tucker GT, Woods HF (1982) Oxidation phenotype—a minor determinant of metoprolol metabolism and response. *New Engl J Med* **303**: 1558–60.

Lewis W, Levine ES, Griniuviene B, Tankersley KO, Colacino JM, Sommadossi J-P, Watanabe KA, Perrino FW (1996) Fialuridine and its metabolites inhibit DNA polymerase gamma at sites of multiple adjacent analog incorporation, decrease mtDNA abundance, and cause mitochondrial structural defects in cultured hepatoblasts. *Proc Natl Acad Sci (USA)* **93**: 3592–7.

Matzinger P (1994) Tolerance, danger, and the extended family. *Ann Rev Immunol* **12**: 991–1045.

McKenzie R, Fried MW, Sallie R, Conjeevaram H, Dibisceglie AM, Park Y, Savarese B, Kleiner D, Tsokos M, Luciano C, Pruett T, Stotka JL, Straus SE, Hoofnagle JH (1995) Hepatic-failure and lactic-acidosis due to fialuridine (fiau), an investigational nucleoside analog for chronic hepatitis-b. *New Engl J Med* **333**: 1099–1105.

Meyers LL, Beierschmitt WP, Khairallah EA, Cohen SD (1988) Acetaminophen-induced inhibition of hepatic mitochondrial respiration in mice. *Toxicol Appl Pharmacol* **93**: 378–87.

Michalets EL, Williams CR (2000) Drug interactions with cisapride: clinical implications. *Clin Pharmacokinet* **39**: 49–75.

Mirochnitchenko O, Weisbrot-Lefkowitz M, Reuhl K, Chen L, Yang C, Inouye M (1999) Acetaminophen toxicity. Opposite effects of two forms of glutathione peroxidase. *J Biol Chem* **274**: 10349–55.

Moinova HR, Mulcahy RT (1998) An electrophile responsive element (EpRE) regulates beta-naphthoflavone induction of the human gamma-glutamylcysteine synthetase regulatory subunit gene. Constitutive expression is mediated by an adjacent AP-1 site. *J Biol Chem* **273**: 14683–9.

Moinova HR, Mulcahy RT (1999) Up-regulation of the human gamma-glutamylcysteine synthetase regulatory subunit gene involves binding of Nrf-2 to an electrophile responsive element. *Biochem Biophys Res Commun* **261**: 661–8.

Naisbitt DJ, Gordon SF, Pirmohamed M, Park BK (2000a) Immunological principles of adverse drug reactions: the initiation and propagation of immune responses elicited by drug treatment. *Drug Safety* **23**: 483–507.

Naisbitt DJ, Vilar J, Stalford A, Wilkins EGL, Pirmohamed M, Park BK (2000b) Plasma cysteine and decreased reduction of nitroso sulphamethoxazole with HIV infection. *AIDS Res Hum Retrov* **16**: 1929–38.

Nelson SD (1990) Molecular mechanisms of the hepatotoxicity caused by acetaminophen. *Semin Liver Dis* **10**: 267–78.

Pamer E, Creswell P (1998) Mechanisms of MHC class-I restricted antigen processing. *Ann Rev Immunol* **16**: 323–58.

Park BK (1986) Metabolic basis of adverse drug reactions. *J R Coll Phys* **20**: 195–200.

Park BK, Coleman JW, Kitteringham NR (1987) Drug disposition and drug hypersensitivity. *Biochem Pharmacol* **36**: 581–90.

Park BK, Naisbitt DJ, Gordon SF, Kitteringham NR, Pirmohamed M (2001) Metabolic activation in drug allergies. *Toxicology* **158**: 11–23.

Park BK, Pirmohamed M (2001) Toxicogenetics in drug development. *Toxicol Lett* **120** (1–3): 281–91.

Park BK, Pirmohamed M, Kitteringham NR (1992) Idiosyncratic drug reactions: a mechanistic evaluation of risk factors. *Br J Clin Pharmacol* **34**: 377–95.

Park BK, Pirmohamed M, Kitteringham NR (1995) The role of cytochrome P450 enzymes in hepatic and extrahepatic human drug toxicity. *Pharmacol Ther* **68**: 385–424.

Park BK, Pirmohamed M, Kitteringham NR (1998) The role of drug disposition in drug hypersensitivity: a chemical, molecular and clinical perspective. *Chem Res Toxicol* **11**: 969–88.

Pessayre D, Larrey D (1988) Acute and chronic drug-induced hepatitis. *Bailliere's Clin Gastroenterol* **2**: 385–423.

Petty GW, Brown RD, Whisnant JP, Sicks JD, OFallon WM, Wiebers DO (1999) Frequency of major complications of aspirin, warfarin, and intravenous heparin for secondary stroke prevention—a population-based study. *Ann Intern Med* **130**: 14–22.

Pichler WJ, Yawalkar N (2000) Allergic reactions to drugs: involvement of T cells. *Thorax* **55** (Suppl 2): S61–S65.

Pirmohamed M, Alfirevic A, Vilar J, Stalford A, Wilkins EG, Sim E, Park BK (2000) Association analysis of drug metabolizing enzyme gene polymorphisms in HIV-positive patients with co-trimoxazole hypersensitivity. *Pharmacogenetics* **10**: 705–13.

Pirmohamed M, Breckenridge AM, Kitteringham NR, Park BK (1998) Adverse drug reactions. *Br Med J* **316**: 1295–8.

Pirmohamed M, Graham A, Roberts P, Smith D, Chadwick D, Breckenridge AM, Park BK (1991) Carbamazepine hypersensitivity: assessment of clinical and in vitro chemical cross-reactivity with phenytoin and oxcarbazepine. *Br J Clin Pharmacol*, **32**: 741–9.

Pirmohamed M, Kitteringham NR, Park BK (1994) The role of active metabolites in drug toxicity. *Drug Safety* **11**: 114–44.

Pirmohamed M, Lin K, Chadwick D, Park BK (2001) TNF-alpha promoter region gene polymorphisms in carbamazepine-hypersensitive patients. *Neurology* **56** (7): 890–6.

Pirmohamed M, Madden S, Park BK (1996) Idiosyncratic drug reactions: metabolic bioactivation as a pathogenic mechanism. *Clin Pharmacokinet* **31**: 215–30.

Pirmohamed M, Park BK (1995) Drug reactions in HIV infected patients. *Postgrad Doctor* **18**: 438–44.

Pirmohamed M, Park BK (1996) Adverse drug reactions. In: Kaufman L, Taberner PV, eds, *Pharmacology in the Practice of Anaesthesia*. London: Edward Arnold, pp. 641–60.

Pirmohamed M, Park BK (1999) Adverse drug reactions: role of enzyme inhibition and induction. In: Erill S, ed., *Proceedings of the Esteve Foundation Symposium VIII: Variability in Human Drug Response*. Amsterdam: Elsevier, pp. 41–51.

Pirmohamed M, Park BK (2001a) Genetic susceptibility to adverse drug reactions. *Trends Pharmacol Sci* **22**(6): 298–305.

Pirmohamed M, Park BK (2001b) HIV and drug allergy. *Curr Opin Allergy Clini Immunol* **1**: 311–16.

Pohl LR, Satoh H, Christ DD, Kenna JG (1988) Immunologic and metabolic basis of drug hypersensitivities. *Ann Rev Pharmacol* **28**: 367–87.

Pohl LR, Thomassen D, Pumford NR, Butler LE, Satoh H, Ferrans VJ, Perrone A, Martin BM, Martin JL (1990) Hapten carrier conjugates associated with halothane hepatitis. In: Witmer CM, *et al.*, eds, *Biological Reactive Intermediates*, Vol. IV. New York: Plenum, pp. 111–20.

Poller L, Shiach CR, MacCallum PK, Johansen AM, Munster AM, Magalhaes A, Jespersen J, European Concerted Action on Anticoagulation (1998) Multicentre randomised study of computerised anticoagulant dosage. *Lancet* **352**: 1505–9.

Raucy JL, Lasker JM, Lieber CS, Black M (1989) Acetaminophen activation by human liver cytochromes P-450IIE1 and P-450IA2. *Arch Biochem Biophys* **271**: 270–83.

Rawlins MD (1995) Pharmacovigilance: paradise lost, regained or postponed? *J R Coll Phys Lond*, **29**: 41–9.

Rawlins MD, Thompson JW (1991) Mechanisms of adverse drug reactions. In: Davies DM, ed., *Textbook of Adverse Drug Reactions*. Oxford: Oxford University Press, pp. 18–45.

Ray SD, Mumaw VR, Raje RR, Fariss MW (1996) Protection of acetaminophen-induced hepatocellular apoptosis and necrosis by cholesteryl hemisuccinate pretreatment. *J Pharmacol Exp Ther* **279**: 1470–83.

Ray SD, Sorge CL, Raucy JL, Corcoran GB (1990) Early loss of large genomic DNA in vivo with accumulation of $Ca2+$ in the nucleus during acetaminophen-induced liver injury. *Toxicol Appl Pharmacol* **106**: 346–51.

Rettie AE, Korzekwa KR, Kunze KL, Lawrence RF, Eddy AC, Aoyama T, Gelboin HV, Gonzalez FJ, Trager WF (1992) Hydroxylation of warfarin by human cdna-expressed cytochrome-p-450—a role for p-4502C9 in the etiology of (s)-warfarin drug-interactions. *Chem Res Toxicol* **5**: 54–9.

Rieder MJ, Shear NH, Kanee A, Tang BK, Spielberg SP (1991) Prominence of slow acetylator phenotype among patients with sulfonamide hypersensitivity reactions. *Clin Pharmacol Ther* **49**: 13–7.

Romagnani S (1999) Th1/Th2 cells. *Inflamm Bowel Dis* **5**: 285–94.

Roses AD (2000) Pharmacogenetics and the practice of medicine. *Nature* **405**: 857–65.

Schnyder B, Mauri-Hellweg D, Zanni M, Bettens F, Pichler WJ (1997) Direct, MHC-dependent presentation of the drug sulfamethoxazole to human alpha/beta T cell clones. *J Clin Invest* **100**: 136–41.

Scott AK (1989) Warfarin usage: can safety be improved? *Pharmacol Ther*, **42**, 429–57.

Sharief MK, Hentges R (1991) Association between tumor necrosis factor-alpha and disease progression in patients with multiple sclerosis. *New Engl J Med* **325**: 467–72.

Shear NH, Spielberg SP, Cannon M, Miller M (1988) Anticonvulsant hypersensitivity syndrome: in vitro risk assessment. *J Clin Invest* **82**: 1826–32.

Silverstein FE, Faich G, Goldstein JL, Simon LS, Pincus T, Whelton A, Makuch R, Eisen G, Agrawal NM, Stenson WF, Burr AM, Zhao WW, Kent JD, Lefkowith JB, Verburg KM, Geis GS (2000) Gastrointestinal toxicity with celecoxib vs nonsteroidal anti-inflammatory drugs for osteoarthritis and rheumatoid arthritis: the CLASS study. A randomized controlled trial. *J Am Med Assoc* **284**: 1247–55.

Singh VK, Mehrotra S, Agarwal SS (1999) The paradigm of Th1 and Th2 cytokines: its relevance to autoimmunity and allergy. *Immunol Res* **20**: 147–61.

Stanton LA, Peterson GM, Rumble RH, Cooper GM, Polack AE (1994) Drug-related admissions to an Australian hospital. *J Clin Pharm Therapeut* **19**: 341–7.

Strickler SM, Miller MA, Andermann E, Dansky LV, Seni M-H, Spielberg SP (1985) Genetic predisposition to phenytoin-induced birth defects. *Lancet* **ii**, 746–9.

Sullivan JR, Shear NH (2001) The drug hypersensitivity syndrome: what is the pathogenesis? *Arch Dermatol* **137**: 357–64.

Suzuki Y, Inagi R, Aono T, Yamanishi K, Shiohara T (1998) Human herpesvirus 6 infection as a risk factor for the development of severe drug-induced hypersensitivity syndrome. *Arch Dermatol* **134**: 1108–12.

Takahashi H, Kashima T, Nomoto S, Iwade K, Tainaka H, Shimizu T, Nomizo Y, Muramoto N, Kimura S, Echizen H (1998) Comparisons between in-vitro and in-vivo metabolism of (S)-warfarin: catalytic activities of cDNA-expressed CYP2C9, its Leu359 variant and their mixture versus unbound clearance in patients with the corresponding CYP2C9 genotypes. *Pharmacogenetics* **8**: 365–73.

Taube J, Halsall D, Baglin T (2000) Influence of cytochrome P-450 CYP2C9 polymorphisms on warfarin sensitivity and risk of over-anticoagulation in patients on long-term treatment. *Blood* **96**: 1816–19.

Tephly TR, Burchell B (1990) UDP-glucuronyl transferases: a family of detoxifying enzymes. *Trends Pharmac Sci* **11**: 276–229.

The International SNP Map Working Group (2001) A map of human genome sequence variation containing 1.42 million single nucleotide polymorphisms. *Nature* **409**: 928–33.

The MHC Sequencing Consortium (1999) Complete sequence and gene map of a human major histocompatibility complex. *Nature* **401**: 921–23.

Tsokos-Kuhn JO (1989) Evidence in vivo for elevation of intracellular free Ca2+ in the liver after diquat, acetaminophen, and CCl4. *Biochem Pharmacol* **38**: 3061–65.

Uetrecht JP (1999) New concepts in immunology relevant to idiosyncratic drug reactions: the "danger hypothesis" and innate immune system. *Chem Res Toxicol* **12**: 387–95.

van der Ven AJAM, Koopmans PP, Vree TB, van der Meer JW (1991) Adverse reactions to co-trimoxazole in HIV-infection. *Lancet* **ii**, 431–33.

Walmsley SL, Khorasheh S, Singer J, Djurdjev O (1998) A randomized trial of N-acetylcysteine for prevention of trimethoprim-sulfamethoxazole hypersensitivity reactions in Pneumocystis carinii pneumonia prophylaxis (CTN 057). Canadian HIV Trials Network 057 Study Group. *J AIDS Hum Retrovirol* **19**: 498–505.

Weiss ME, Adkinson MF (1988) Immediate hypersensitivity reactions to penicillin and related antibiotics. *Clin Allergy* **18**: 515–40.

Williamson J, Chopin JM (1980) Adverse reactions to prescribed drugs in the elderly: a multicentre investigation. *Age Ageing* **9**: 73–80.

Woolf TF, Jordan RA (1987) Basic concepts in drug metabolism: Part 1. *J Clin Pharmacol* **27**: 15–17.

Woosley RL, Chen YW, Freiman JP, Gillis RA (1993) Mechanism of the cardiotoxic actions of terfenadine. *J Am Med Assoc* **269**: 1532–36.

Zanni MP, vonGreyerz S, Schnyder B, Brander KA, Frutig K, Hari Y, Valitutti S, Pichler WJ (1998) HLA-restricted, processing- and metabolism-independent pathway of drug recognition by human alpha beta T lymphocytes. *J Clin Invest* **102**: 1591–98.

Zhang H, Cook J, Nickel J, Yu R, Stecker K, Myers K, Dean NM (2000) Reduction of liver Fas expression by an antisense oligonucleotide protects mice from fulminant hepatitis. *Nat Biotechnol* **18**: 862–67.

Zimmerman HJ, Maddrey WC (1995) Acetaminophen (paracetamol) hepatotoxicity with regular intake of alcohol: analysis of instances of therapeutic misadventure. *Hepatology* **22**: 767–73.

7

Drugs and the Elderly

UNA MARTIN

The University of Birmingham, Queen Elizabeth Hospital, Edgbaston, Birmingham, UK

CHARLES GEORGE

British Heart Foundation, London, UK

THE AGEING POPULATION AND CHANGING DEMOGRAPHY

The past century has seen major changes in the age structure of Western countries. For example, Americans and UK citizens live far longer than previously. Thus, a person born in the United States at the beginning of the twentieth century could expect to live to around 49 years, while the life expectancy at the end of the century was 76.5 years, a gain of over 27 years (Olshansky *et al.*, 2001).

These changes have been brought about by an improved standard of living with better housing, clean water and immunisation programmes, together with better medical treatments, especially drugs. The past 50 years have also seen a major change in the age structure of the population. In 1951 the population of England and Wales contained 4.83 million persons aged 65 or over but by 30 years later the figure had risen to 7.57 million and now exceeds 8 million elderly people. More important is the number of old elderly persons (over 75 years), the number of whom has roughly doubled in the same time period. These trends over time are set to continue and it is forecast that there will be continued expansion of the elderly population over the next 30 years (Figure 7.1).

DISEASE PREVALENCE IN THE ELDERLY

The prevalence of many diseases is age-related and several may co-exist in the same patient. These include hypertension (Hawthorne *et al.*, 1974) osteoarthrosis (Lawrence, 1977) and prostatic hypertrophy (Berry *et al.*, 1984). Age-specific mortality rates are shown for cardiovascular and cerebrovascular diseases, together with data for cancers, in Table 7.1 (British Heart Foundation, 2000) and morbidity data in Table 7.2 (British Heart Foundation, 2001).

Cardiovascular and cerebrovascular problems related to atheroma are the most common cause of death in the elderly but are also a major source of suffering. Nevertheless, a huge majority of old people have osteoarthrosis of the joints and the lower limbs (Blackburn *et al.*, 1994) causing pain and disability without threatening life

Pharmacovigilance. Edited by R.D. Mann and E.B. Andrews

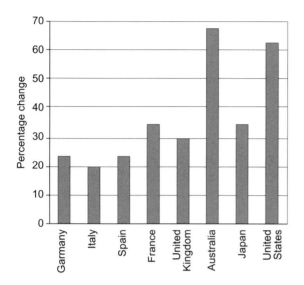

Figure 7.1. Percentage growth in number of 60 and over, 2000–2020. *Source*: UK Govt. Actuaries Dept. 1998 based projections, UN Census Bureau 2000. Reproduced with permission from Dept. of Trade & Industry. Foresight, Ageing Population Panel (2000) *The Age Shift*. DTI.

directly. By contrast, treatments for osteoarthrosis can give rise to severe adverse reactions and to fatalities (Castleden and Pickles, 1988; see below).

MEDICINE-TAKING BY THE ELDERLY

Several studies have examined the nature and prevalence of medicines prescribed for old people living in the community. One of the best known is that by Cartwright and Smith (1988) which was based on a random sample of people aged 65 and over drawn from the electoral registers of 10 parliamentary constituencies in England. Information was obtained from 78% (805 patients) of the 1032 included in the original sample. Of these 805 patients, 60% had taken one or more prescribed medicines within the preceding 24 hours. Drugs for diseases of the heart and circulation were widely prescribed and diuretics formed a therapeutic category in most widespread use. Diuretics were followed by analgesics, hypnotics, sedatives and anxiolytics; drugs for rheumatism and gout and then β-adrenoceptor antagonists. Similar findings were recorded in two studies from Southampton (Ridout *et al.*, 1986; Sullivan and George, 1996). A more recent review by Jones and Poole (1998) has confirmed the rising use of cardiovascular drugs amongst elderly people; and widespread use of agents with an effect on the central nervous system. There was, however, some geographic variation in the use of medicines for musculo-skeletal and joint disease. By contrast, the use of

Table 7.1. Deaths by cause, sex and age 1998, United Kingdom.

		Age under 35	Age 35–44	Age 45–54	Age 55–64	Age 65–74	Age 75 and over
All disease of the circulatory system (390–459)	MEN	575	1600	5 575	13 616	32 751	68 101
	WOMEN	392	634	1 923	5 632	20 244	105 667
	TOTAL	967	2234	7 498	19 248	52 995	173 768
Coronary Heart Disease	MEN	148	1004	3 971	8 795	21 622	38 002
	WOMEN	40	180	837	3 080	11 167	47 307
	TOTAL	188	1184	4 808	12 875	32 789	85 309
Stroke	MEN	134	246	730	1 775	5 269	16 338
	WOMEN	120	255	611	1 323	4 708	34 299
	TOTAL	254	501	1 341	3 098	9 777	50 637
Cancer	MEN	883	1280	5 034	12 675	26 048	35 447
	WOMEN	781	1949	5 613	10 206	19 695	37 004
	TOTAL	1664	3229	10 647	22 881	45 743	72 451

Adapted from *Coronary Heart Disease Statistics*, BHF (2000).

Table 7.2. Prevalence of treated CHD by sex and age 1994/98, England and Wales.

	No. of cases	Age 0–34 (%)	Age 35–44 (%)	Age 45–54 (%)	Age 55–64 (%)	Age 65–74 (%)	Age 75–84 (%)	Age 85 and over (%)
Men	107 777	0.015	0.50	2.90	9.34	17.51	21.68	20.53
Women	87 289	0.010	0.18	1.26	4.83	10.81	16.16	17.17

Adapted from *Coronary Heart Disease Statistics: Morbidity Supplement*, BHF (2001).

drugs with an action on the central nervous system varies according to individual circumstances: psychotropic agents are used particularly in patients in residential nursing homes and in long-term care (McGrath and Jackson, 1996).

Besides prescribed medicines, elderly people as a group are high consumers of non-prescription medication. Indeed, it has been estimated that over 50% of elderly people take one or more over the counter (OTC) preparations every day (Chrischilles *et al.*, 1992b). Those OTCs most commonly taken are oral analgesics and vitamins and tonics, but recently the popularity of herbal medicines has increased (Barnett *et al.*, 2000). Women are particularly likely to consume medicines and some of these can interact with prescription medicines (see below) to cause adverse events.

There are two other features which are characteristic of drug therapy in the elderly: long duration and polypharmacy. Drug treatment for older people is often for chronic conditions, which means that once started, medicines tend to be continued for six months or longer (Ridout *et al.*, 1986). This may account for the increased rates of gastrointestinal bleeding in patients taking non-steroidal anti-inflammatory drugs (NSAIDs) (Langman *et al.*, 1994). This latter problem highlights the need for improvements in repeat prescribing and for regular review of medication in the elderly.

There are several legitimate reasons for polypharmacy in the elderly. First, as indicated previously, the prevalence of many diseases is age-related and several may co-exist in the same patient. Secondly, it may not be possible to achieve an adequate therapeutic response from the use of a single drug. Examples include the patient who has

sustained an acute myocardial infarction and will normally be offered treatment with a beta adreno-ceptor antagonist and aspirin to reduce the risks of further infarction, as well as a statin to lower cholesterol and stabilise atheromatous plaques in the arterial circulation. Many will also be treated with an inhibitor of the angiotensin converting enzyme (ACE). Thirdly, patients with heart failure will normally be offered treatment with an ACE inhibitor and diuretic. Digoxin may also be prescribed as may spironolactone and, for those with atrial fibrillation, consideration given to the use of warfarin to prevent a stroke from thrombo-embolism.

A third reason for giving more than one drug simultaneously is to counteract or minimise the risk of a side effect (type A adverse reaction) occurring. For example, potassium loss can be corrected with spironolactone or amiloride in patients who are receiving either a benzothiadiazine or loop-type diuretic. However, one of the most important predictors of adverse drug reactions is the total numbers of drugs given simultaneously (Leach and Roy, 1986; Bax *et al.*, 1987). In the study by Cartwright and Smith (1988), the average number of medicines prescribed for the patient was 2.8, but many patients living in the community received more than this. Additionally, polypharmacy can cause confusion leading to errors in medicine taking, particularly amongst those over the age of 85 (Parkin *et al.*, 1976; Vestal, 1978).

INTERACTIONS IN RELATION TO MULTIPLE DRUG PRESCRIBING

Adverse drug reactions (see below) are common in the elderly. This is frequently a consequence of multiple drug prescribing which leads to the occurrence of drug–drug interactions. Drug interactions represent a change in either the magnitude or duration of action of one drug caused by the presence of a second. This may enhance or reduce the efficacy of one or both of the drugs or a new effect may appear which is not seen with either of the drugs alone. Interactions may be pharmacokinetic or pharmacodynamic. The most important adverse interactions occur with drugs that have easily recognisable toxicity and a low therapeutic index (i.e. the dose or plasma concentration of drug which is effective lies close to that which causes toxicity) (Lin and Lu, 1998).

PHARMACOKINETIC INTERACTIONS

Drug interactions may result in impaired drug absorption from the gastrointestinal tract. The rate at which a drug is absorbed may be decreased by drugs such as anticholinergics, which inhibit gastric motility; conversely, drugs such as metoclopramide (which increase gastric motility) may enhance the absorption rate. Certain drugs form chelates and complexes with other drugs, altering their solubility and absorption. For example, agents that bind to digoxin in the gut (such as antacids and cholestyramine) reduce the extent of its absorption by 20%–35% (Brown and Juhl, 1976). However, despite these potential interactions few drug–drug interactions affect drug absorption to a clinically significant extent (May et al., 1987; McInnes and Brodie, 1988). Drugs that undergo extensive first-pass metabolism may be affected by other drugs, which alter liver blood flow or compete for metabolism. For example, the non-selective monoamine oxidase inhibitors (MAOIs), such as phenelzine, reduce the first-pass metabolism of tyramine (found in cheese, tomatoes and chocolate) and pseudoephedrine (in cough mixtures) and many other direct and indirect sympathomimetic agents (Tollefson, 1983). As a result, large amounts of these amines reach the sympathetic nervous system, where they stimulate the interneuronal release of noradrenaline. MAO inhibition prevents noradrenaline breakdown, producing a syndrome of sympathetic over-activity characterised by headache,

hypertension, excitement and delirium (Tollefson, 1983).

Drugs may also affect the distribution of others within the body. When two or more highly protein-bound drugs are administered concurrently, competitive binding by one may increase the free fraction or unbound portion of the other. The importance of this interaction has probably been overstated. For example, the NSAIDs may displace warfarin from its binding site and increase its anticoagulant effect, but this effect is negligible in vivo (O'Callaghan et al., 1984); it is much more likely that the NSAIDs inhibit warfarin metabolism (O'Reilly et al., 1980). Similarly, tolbutamide-induced hypoglycaemia with the addition of azapropazone has been reported (Waller and Waller, 1984). Although the interaction may have been due to displacement of the oral hypoglycaemic agent from albumin leading to enhanced hypoglycaemia, inhibition of tolbutamide metabolism by the NSAID was probably more important (Andreasen et al., 1981).

Inhibition or induction of drug metabolism is one of the most important mechanisms for drug–drug interactions. Interactions involving a loss of action of one of the drugs are at least as frequent as those involving an increased effect (Seymour and Routledge, 1998). There are many examples of one drug interfering with the metabolism of another by inhibition of the cytochrome P450 (CYP) enzymes in the liver (Tanaka, 1998). The enzymes responsible for transforming drugs in humans belong to 6 CYP subfamilies, i.e. CYP1A, 2A, 2C, 2D, 2E and 3A. Each subfamily contains a number of different isoforms. It has been estimated that about 90% of human drug oxidation can be attributed to six of these, i.e. CYP1A2, CYP2C9, CYP2C19, CYP2D6, CYP2E1, CYP3A, and enzyme inhibition interactions have been reported with all (Kinirons and Crome, 1997; Seymour and Routledge, 1998). Each CYP isoenzyme may metabolise many drugs, so the potential for drug–drug interactions is high in patients taking several medications (Lin and Lu, 1998). For example, in a group of elderly male patients, cimetidine inhibited the metabolism of procainamide, giving rise to toxic plasma concentrations of the antiarrhythmic (Bauer et al., 1990).

Other drugs which are similarly affected by cimetidine are benzodiazepines, β-adrenoceptor blockers, tricyclic antidepressants, theophylline, phenytoin and oral anticoagulants. Although few of these drug–drug interactions are of clinical significance (Sax, 1987), caution is indicated when cimetidine is given concomitantly with drugs that have a narrow range of therapeutic concentration such as warfarin, theophylline and phenytoin: in one study, two days of cimetidine therapy decreased theophylline clearance by 39% (Jackson et al., 1981). Other common inhibitors of one or more CYP isoenzymes include amiodarone, fluconazole, erythromycin, clarithromycin, sulphonamides, ciprofloxacin, omeprazole and paroxetine. Occasionally, clinically severe interactions occur as has been shown recently with combined administration of terfenadine and ketoconazole (Honig et al., 1993; Monaghan et al., 1993), erythromycin (Honig et al., 1992) and itraconazole (Pohjola-Sintonen et al., 1993) resulting in prolongation of the QT interval and torsades de pointes. At present there is no evidence that CYP inhibition by these agents is affected by age (Kinirons and Crome, 1997).

Liver enzyme induction by one drug may lead to inactivation of a second drug. Well-recognised examples include the decreased efficacy of warfarin seen with barbiturate therapy and the reduced efficacy of dihydropyridine calcium-channel blocking drugs with carbamazepine therapy (Capewell et al., 1988). The delay between the commencement of the enzyme-inducing agent and its full effect can take 7 to 10 days, making recognition of the interaction more difficult (Seymour and Routledge, 1998). However, in general terms, elderly individuals appear to be less sensitive to drug induction than younger individuals (Lin and Lu, 1998). For example, the distribution of hexobarbitol before and after treatment with rifampicin was studied in young and elderly volunteers. Rifampicin produced differential increases in hexobarbitol metabolism with 90- and 19-fold increases in the young and elderly volunteers, respectively (Smith et al., 1991).

Finally, drug–drug interactions may occur in the kidney resulting in altered drug elimination. This subject has been recently been reviewed by Bonate et al. (1998), who concluded that clinically significant drug interactions due to a renal mechanism are relatively rare. Five potential mechanisms exist for drug interactions in the kidney (Table 7.3) and the best recognised is competitive inhibition of tubular secretion leading to an increase in drug concentration. An example of this interaction is the co-administration of probenecid with penicillin. Non-competitive interference with drug secretion may also occur, e.g. prolonged treatment with thiazide diuretics causes a compensatory increase in proximal tubule reabsorption of sodium, resulting in increased lithium reabsorption (Peterson et al., 1974). This interaction has resulted in serious lithium toxicity due to lithium accumulation (Mehta and Robinson, 1980). NSAIDs also decrease the renal elimination of lithium by up to 60%, but the mechanism is uncertain (Amdisen, 1982; Jefferson et al., 1986). Similarly, the administration of quinidine results in an increase in the plasma concentration of digoxin in over 90% of patients (Bigger, 1982). Although this is partly due to displacement of digoxin from its binding sites in tissues, its renal clearance is reduced by 40%–50% with regular administration of quinidine. Similar interactions have been reported with amiodarone (Moysey et al., 1981; Oetgen et al., 1984) and verapamil (Pederson et al., 1983), leading to 70%–100% increases in serum digoxin concentrations. Although the precise mechanisms have not been elucidated, recent reports suggest that inhibition of ATP-dependent P-glycoprotein-mediated drug transport in renal tubular cells (Inui et al., 2001) by verapamil and quinidine may lead to decreased renal tubular elimination of digoxin (Fromm et al., 1999; Verschraagen et al., 1999).

Table 7.3. Mechanisms for drug–drug interactions at the renal level.

1. Displacement of bound drug results in an increase in drug excretion by glomerular filtration
2. Competition at the tubular secretion site resulting in a decrease in drug excretion
3. Competition at the tubular reabsorption site resulting in an increase in drug excretion
4. Change in urinary pH and/or flow rate that may increase or decrease the drug excretion depending on the pKa of the drug
5. Inhibition of renal drug metabolism

PHARMACODYNAMIC INTERACTIONS

An antagonistic pharmacological interaction between two drugs may counteract the intended therapeutic effects. For example, the non-specific β-adrenoceptor-blocking drug propranolol may induce bronchoconstriction in a patient taking theophylline for asthma. Co-administration of NSAIDs and antihypertensives may lead to a reduced hypotensive effect due to sodium retention by the analgesics. One Australian study found that 12% of almost 3000 non-institutionalised elderly

Table 7.4. Drug interactions that may lead to an enhanced effect.

Drug A	May interact with drug B	Effect of interaction	Mechanism of interaction
ACE inhibitors	NSAIDs	Hyperkalaemia, reduced renal function	Additive nephrotoxic effects
Antidepressants (tricyclic)	Enzyme Inhibitors	Increased effect of A	Reduced clearance of A
Antihypertensive agents	Vasodilators (e.g. nitrates for angina) antipsychotics and some antidepressants	Postural hypotension	Combined hypotensive effects
Aspirin (acetylsallcylic acid) (low dose)	NSAIDs	Peptic ulceration	Additional risk of peptic ulceration
Carbamazepine	Enzyme inhibitors, verapamil	Increased effect of A	Reduced clearance of A
Corticosteroids (oral)	NSAIDs (including aspirin)	Peptic ulceration	Corticosteroid prevents healing
Ciclosporin	Enzyme inhibitors	Increased effect of A	Reduced clearance of A
Digoxin	Amiodarone, diltiazem, verapamil	Increased effect of A	Reduced clearance of A
Digoxin	Diuretics (loop and thiazides)	Increased effect of A (e.g. arrhythmias)	Diuretic induced hypokalaemia
Diuretics (potassium sparing)	ACE inhibitors, potassium supplements	Hyperkalaemia, impaired renal function	Combined potassium elevating effects
Lithium	NSAIDs, thiazide diuretics	Increased effect of A	Reduced clearance of A
Phenothiazines and butyrophenones	Anticholinergic drugs (e.g. some antihistamines and tricyclic antidepressants)	Excessive anticholinergic effects (e.g. constipation, urinary hesitancy, dry mouth, confusion)	Combined anticholinergic effects
Phenytoin	Enzyme inhibitors	Increased effect of A	Reduced clearance of A
Quinolones	NSAIDs	Seizures	Pharmacodynamic interaction at CNS effector site
Theophylline	Enzyme inhibitors Quinolones	Increased effect of A	Reduced clearance of A

Reproduced from Seymour RM, Routledge PA (1998). Important drug–drug interactions in the elderly. *Drugs & Ageing* **12**, 485–94 by permission of Adis International Ltd, Auckland, New Zealand.

patients studied were taking NSAIDs and anti-hypertensive medication simultaneously. Furthermore, NSAID usage was an independent risk factor for hypertension in this age group (Johnson et al., 1993).

Finally, indirect pharmacodynamic effects may occur when one drug's pharmacological effect influences another drug's action. For example, the toxicity of digoxin is increased by hypokalaemia, which may occur with the co administration of a diuretic. Similarly, enhanced myocardial depression, hypotension and atrioventricular block may occur when β-adrenoceptor blockers are administered with verapamil or diltiazem (Krikler and Spurrell, 1974; Edoute et al., 2000).

Despite the many ways in which drug–drug interactions may occur, it is likely that only about 10% of potential interactions result in clinically significant events. However, while death or serious clinical consequences are rare, low grade, clinical morbidity in the elderly may be much more common (Seymour and Routledge, 1998). Non-specific complaints such as confusion, lethargy, weakness, dizziness, incontinence, depression and falling may indicate an underlying drug–drug interaction. The drug interactions of clinical importance in the elderly have recently been reviewed by Seymour and Routledge (1998) and are listed in Tables 7.4 and 7.5. In some cases the cause of the interaction is complex, involving both pharmacokinetic and pharmacodynamic mechanisms. For example, epileptic patients with psychiatric co-morbidity may be particularly vulnerable due to combined use of psychotropic and antiepileptic drugs. In particular, antidepressants and antipsychotic drugs are believed to lower the seizure threshold (Alldredge, 1999). In general, the potential for drug–drug interactions in psychiatric patients is high because of the need for combined therapy to treat co-morbid psychiatric disorders, to treat the adverse effect of a medication or to treat concomitant medical conditions. In particular, the selective serotonin uptake inhibitors fluoxetine and paroxetine are potent inhibitors of CYP2D6 and have the potential to increase the plasma concentrations of many of the major tranquilisers, including haloperidol and thioridazine; fluvoxamine inhibits the metabolism of many of the benzodiazepines (Sproule et al., 1997).

Table 7.5. Drug interactions that may lead to a reduced effect.

Drug A	May Interact with Drug B	Effect of Interaction	Mechanism of Interaction
Antidepressants	Enzyme inducers	Reduced effect of A	Increased clearance of A
Antihypertensives (e.g. ACE inhibitors, thiazides and β-adrenoceptor antagonists (β-blockers))	NSAIDs	Reduced effect of A	Pharmacodynamic antagonism of antihypertensive effect of A
Calcium antagonists	Enzyme inducers	Reduced effect of A	Increased clearance of A
Corticosteroids	Enzyme inducers	Reduced effect of A	Increased clearance of A
Ciclosporin	Enzyme inducers	Reduced effect of A	Increased clearance of A
Digoxin	Cholestyramine, colestipol	Reduced effect of A	Reduced absorption of A
Quinolones	Cholestyramine, colestipol	Reduced effect of A	Reduced absorption of A
Theophylline	Enzyme inducers	Reduced effect of A	Increased clearance of A
Thyroxine	Enzyme inducers	Reduced effect of A	Increased clearance of A

Reproduced from Seymour RM, Routledge PA (1998). Important drug–drug interactions in the elderly. Drugs & Ageing 12, 485–94 by permission of Adis International Ltd, Auckland, New Zealand.

ALTERED PHARMACOKINETICS IN THE ELDERLY

Elderly patients may also develop drug-related problems even when their medication is confined to a single agent or non-interacting multiple agents. This may relate to pharmacokinetic and pharmacodynamic changes associated with ageing. Such age-related physiological changes may alter the way in which the body handles medication, leading to changes in drug disposition in the elderly patient.

ABSORPTION

Following oral administration, most drugs dissolve in the stomach. Little absorption takes place here due to the small surface area and low pH, which means that drugs which are weak bases are in an ionized state. Absorption primarily takes place in the small intestine because of the large surface area and high pH, which favours the unionised state of most drugs. With increasing age a number of changes occur in the gastrointestinal tract which should make the rate of absorption less predictable, including a reduction in acid secretion in the stomach, decreased gastric emptying, diminished splanchnic blood flow and decreased gastrointestinal mobility (Geokas and Haverback, 1969; Evans et al., 1981; Greenblatt et al., 1982; Goldberg and Roberts, 1983; Montamat et al., 1989; Woodhouse, 1994). However, in practice few drugs have significantly delayed rates of absorption (Greenblatt et al., 1982; Woodhouse, 1994). This is probably because potentially rate-limiting factors in the small intestine (such as surface area and lumenal pH) are not altered to a critical degree.

Once drugs are absorbed from the gut, they enter the portal circulation and must pass through the liver before entering the systemic circulation. The bioavailability of most polar or water-soluble drugs is not affected by age because they are not highly extracted by the liver. For many lipophilic drugs, this first pass through the liver is accompanied by pronounced (sometimes over 90%) extraction with only 5%–10% of the dose reaching the systemic circulation. It is clear that a small change in hepatic function may result in a large increase in bioavailability in those drugs which undergo a high presystemic first-pass metabolism (Montamat et al., 1989; Woodhouse, 1994). For example, decreased presystemic extraction in the elderly may lead to increases in the bioavailability of propranolol (Castleden and George, 1979) and nifedipine (Robertson et al., 1988), but usually not to a clinically significant extent. The changes may be more marked, however, in the frail and hospitalised elderly (Woodhouse, 1994).

DISTRIBUTION

Following absorption of a drug, the extent to which it is distributed within the body depends on body composition, plasma protein binding and blood flow.

Body Composition

With age there is a decrease in lean body mass and body water and a corresponding increase in adipose tissue in relation to total body weight (Edelman and Leibman, 1959; Forbes and Reina, 1970; Novak, 1972). Adipose tissue increases from about 18% to 36% in men and from 33% to 45% in women (Novak, 1972). Therefore the distribution of lipid-insoluble drugs such as paracetamol (Divoll et al., 1982) or ethanol (Vestal et al., 1977) may decrease in the elderly. This means that plasma concentrations per unit dose are higher. Lipid-soluble drugs such as diazepam are more widely distributed in the elderly and may have prolonged action and a "hangover" effect because of the longer elimination half-life (Macklon et al., 1980).

Protein Binding

Serum albumin levels decline with age but in healthy elderly people this change is minimal. More marked reductions appear to relate to disease, immobility and poor nutrition rather than age itself (MacLennan et al., 1977; Campion et al., 1988). This reduction may result in a decrease in the binding capacity of weakly acidic drugs such as salicylates and phenytoin (Wallace and Verbeeck, 1987). Measurement of the plasma free-drug concentration (which will be increased under these circumstances) may be a better guide to the dose requirements than the total plasma concentration, particularly if the therapeutic ratio is low (Grandison and Boudinot, 2000). However, a raised free fraction will also result in an increased clearance allowing a new steady state to be achieved with regular dosing. Total plasma drug concentrations may then be lower but free-drug concentrations will remain the same since these are determined by hepatic or renal clearance of free drug. On the other hand, α-1-acid glycoprotein increases with age and basic drugs such as lignocaine display increased protein binding in elderly patients (Cusack et al., 1980).

Metabolism

Although some drugs are eliminated directly by the kidneys, many undergo metabolism in the liver first. Clearance of drugs by the liver depends on the activity of the enzymes responsible for biotransformation and on blood flow, which determines the rate of delivery of the drug to the liver. For drugs that are metabolised relatively slowly by the liver (those with low intrinsic clearance), clearance is proportional to the rate of hepatic metabolism (Woodhouse, 1994). Hepatic mass decreases with age by 25%–35%, so the metabolism of such drugs may be reduced (Woodhouse and James, 1990).

The metabolic pathways involved in the biotransformation of drugs may be divided into two phases (Williams, 1967). Phase 1 reactions comprise oxidative, reductive or hydrolytic processes which render the compound less lipophilic but can be fully or partly active. Products of phase 1 may then undergo phase 2 reactions which involve glucuronidation, sulphation or acetylation. The resulting conjugates are much more polar than the parent compound, usually have little or no pharmacological activity and are generally excreted in the urine. Phase 1 oxidative drug metabolism may be reduced in the elderly (O'Malley et al., 1971), but phase 2 reactions are generally thought not to be altered, at least in fit elderly patients. However, in the frail elderly, in those who have suffered injury or have undergone surgery, enzyme activity may be significantly depressed, resulting in higher blood concentrations and an increased risk of adverse reactions (Woodhouse, 1994). In particular, a reduction in plasma aspirin esterase activity, paracetamol conjugation and metabolism of metoclopromide and theophylline have been reported in frail elderly patients (Wynne et al., 1990; Groen et al., 1993; Israel et al., 1993; Wynne et al., 1993).

Metabolism of a number of drugs, such as the benzodiazepines, may involve phase 1 followed by phase 2 reactions. Diazepam undergoes oxidative (phase 1) metabolism and its elimination is prolonged in the elderly (Belantuono et al., 1980). It is also partly converted to an active metabolite, desmethyldiazepam, which has a half-life of up to 220 hours in elderly people. However, other benzodiazepines, such as lorazepam, undergo conjugation reactions in the liver and their metabolism is unaltered by age. These compounds which do not give rise to active compounds, may therefore be safer for elderly people to use than the other benzodiazepines (Williams and Lowenthal, 1992).

Age may be only one factor that affects drug metabolism. Cigarette smoking, alcohol intake, dietary considerations, drugs, illnesses and caffeine intake may be equally important (Vestal et al., 1975; Montamat et al., 1989). In addition, hepatic blood flow rather than microsomal enzyme activity is the major determinant of total clearance of many drugs which have a very rapid rate of metabolism and consequently high extraction rates across the liver. Hepatic blood flow is 35% lower in healthy people over 65 years of age than in young people (Wynne et al., 1989). Reductions in systemic clearance of drugs with high hepatic extraction ratios (including presystemic clearance) have been reported in elderly people. Such drugs include propranolol (Castleden and George, 1979), chloromethiazole (Nation et al., 1976) and morphine (Baillie et al., 1989) and the reduced clearance is compatible with a decline in liver blood flow.

RENAL EXCRETION

Most polar drugs or polar drug metabolites are eliminated by the kidney after filtration at the glomerulus. In addition, drugs such as the β-lactam antibiotics are actively secreted in the proximal tubules. As part of normal ageing, both renal functional capacity and renal reserve diminish. The structural changes include a decrease in renal weight, thickening of the intrarenal vascular intima, a reduction in the number of glomeruli with increased sclerogenous changes within those remaining and infiltration by chronic inflammatory cells and fibrosis in the stroma (Muhlberg and Platt, 1999). Altered renal tubular function may also lead to impaired handling of water, sodium and glucose in old age. There is a steady decline in the glomerular filtration rate by approximately 8 ml/minute per decade (Rowe *et al.*, 1976). By the age of 70, therefore, a person may have a 40%–50% reduction in renal function (even in the absence of overt renal disease).

Drug elimination may be reduced even in patients with normal serum creatinine concentrations because creatinine production decreases with age. Many drugs which are dependent on the kidney for elimination will accumulate to toxic levels if given in the usual doses to elderly people. Examples include digoxin (Smith, 1973), atenolol (McAinsh, 1977) and amiloride (George, 1980). Furthermore, many drugs themselves adversely affect renal function in the elderly, e.g. aminoglycosides, diuretics, NSAIDs and angiotensin-converting enzyme (ACE) inhibitors. In this way age-dependent changes in renal function are responsible for altered pharmacokinetics in the elderly but in many cases the kidneys are the target for the adverse drug reactions produced by these changes (Muhlberg and Platt, 1999).

As drug elimination is correlated to creatinine clearance, estimating the creatinine clearance may be helpful in deciding whether a dose reduction is necessary. A useful method that may be used at the bedside is the Cockcroft formula (Cockcroft and Gault, 1976):

Creatinine clearance (male)

$$= \frac{1.23 \times (140 - \text{age}) \times \text{body weight (kg)}}{\text{Plasma creatinine } (\mu\text{mol } l^{-1})}$$

Creatinine clearance (female)

$$= \frac{1.04 \times (140 - \text{age}) \times \text{body weight (kg)}}{\text{Plasma creatinine } (\mu\text{mol } l^{-1})}$$

The diagnostic value of age and creatinine clearance (calculated by the Cockcroft formula) for the prediction of potentially toxic drug plasma levels has recently been reviewed by Muhlberg and Platt (1999). They found that 256 geriatric patients with many different illnesses have been studied in 17 pharmacokinetic studies with 17 different drugs, including angiotensin-converting enzyme inhibitors, NSAIDs, antibiotics, beta-blockers, bronchodilators and benzodiazepines. Mathematical simulation and pharmacokinetic methods were used to determine whether a dose reduction was necessary in elderly patients with a reduced creatinine clearance determined by the Cockcroft formula. For most drugs studied elevated plasma levels at steady state could be correctly predicted when the creatinine clearance was < 40 ml/min, particularly when age was taken into account, suggesting that a dose reduction was necessary. This confirms the usefulness of the Cockcroft formula for clinical use in elderly patients taking drugs which are eliminated in the kidney and which are toxic at higher plasma concentrations.

ALTERED PHARMACODYNAMICS IN THE ELDERLY

Age-related changes in pharmacodynamics may also be relevant. The most important concept in regard to pharmacodynamics is sensitivity, i.e. the measurement of a response to a given dose of drug. Sensitivity is independent of dose- and age-related changes in the pharmacokinetics (Jackson, 1994). It may be difficult to quantify in elderly patients, who may show both increased and decreased responsiveness to medication. The mechanisms include changes to organ systems such as age-related impairment of homeostatic mechanisms, as well as changes at receptor and cellular level (Jackson, 1994).

Warfain acts by inhibiting the synthesis of clotting factors II, VII, IX and X by inhibiting regeneration of vitamin K oxide. Early studies suggested that responsiveness to warfarin increases with age (O'Malley *et al.*, 1977), possibly due to greater inhibition of vitamin K-dependent clotting factors per plasma concentration of warfarin in this age group (Shepherd *et al.*, 1977). However, two retrospective studies have failed to show any association of increased age and bleeding complications (Gurwitz *et al.*, 1988) or deviation from target international normalised ratio (Britt *et al.*, 1992). None the less, elderly patients were found to require, on average, a lower dose of warfarin than younger patients to maintain the same degree of anticoagulation (Redwood *et al.*, 1991). Although there is uncertainty as to the precise mechanism of the increased sensitivity to warfarin amongst elderly people, one possibility is an increased sensitivity to enzyme inhibition rather than differences in substrate availability (Jackson, 1994). Warfarin is a racemate of R and S stereoisomers and is subject to interindividual variability in stereospecific metabolism, which may be exaggerated in the elderly.

Elderly people also show increased sensitivity to the effects of the benzodiazepines; this may be due to altered tissue sensitivity or different rates of entry of the drug into the central nervous system, as well as the alteration in pharmacokinetics already mentioned. For example, the extent and duration of action of nitrazepam on psychomotor function was more marked in elderly subjects despite the plasma concentrations being similar in young and old, suggesting increased sensitivity of the ageing brain to this benzodiazepine (Castleden *et al.*, 1977). Similarly, the plasma concentration of diazepam required to induce a predetermined level of sedation for dental and endoscopic procedures fell progressively between the ages of 20 and 80 years (Cook *et al.*, 1984). Although there is some evidence of pharmacodynamic tolerance developing to the sedative effects of benzodiazepines with long-term use (Swift *et al.*, 1984), dizziness, fainting, blackouts and falls are more common in elderly people taking these drugs regularly (Hale *et al.*, 1985). Furthermore, benzodiazepines appear to adversely affect the safety of the older driver, particularly when compounds with long half-lives or very high doses are used (Ray *et al.*, 1993).

In many cases the increased response to a drug in an elderly patient can be explained by pharmacokinetic changes. For example, the administration of nifedipine to elderly people is associated with a reduction in first-pass metabolism and

clearance compared with young volunteers. This results in higher and more prolonged plasma concentrations and explains the increased hypotensive effect in this age group (Robertson *et al.*, 1988). However, altered homeostatic mechanisms due to impaired baroreceptor function in the elderly may also contribute (Gribbin *et al.*, 1971). In younger patients a fall in blood pressure leads to a compensatory tachycardia partly offsetting the fall in cardiac output, but with increasing age this effect is reduced. This means that the heart-rate response to standing is diminished and may cause orthostatic hypotension, which is defined as a reduction in systolic blood pressure of at least 20 mmHg occurring in response to a change from a supine to an upright position (Mets, 1995). The prevalence of orthostatic hypotension has been reported to be between 10% and 30% for elderly people and is particularly associated with the use of antihypertensive medication (Mets, 1995).

On the other hand, β-adrenoceptors may show a reduction both in numbers (Schocken and Roth, 1977) and in responsiveness to agonists and antagonists with age (Dillon *et al.*, 1980; Ullah *et al.*, 1981; Kendall *et al.*, 1982; Feldman *et al.*, 1984; Pan *et al.*, 1986; Scarpace, 1986). Despite this, elderly patients with hypertension appear to respond well to β-adrenoceptor blockers, but they may be more troubled by postural hypotension due to the impaired homeostatic mechanisms already mentioned. Similarly, although there is a decline in function in the renin-angiotensin system with age (Skott and Giese, 1984) the ACE inhibitors cause a greater reduction in blood pressure in elderly people (Ajayi *et al.*, 1986), particularly after the first dose (Cleland *et al.*, 1985). This may relate to higher baseline blood pressure in the elderly.

ADVERSE DRUG REACTIONS IN THE ELDERLY

DEFINITION OF AN ADVERSE DRUG REACTION

These age-related changes in pharmacokinetics and pharmacodynamics in addition to increased prescribing rates and multiple drug therapy leave the elderly patient vulnerable to drug-related adverse events. An adverse drug reaction (ADR) can be described as any undesirable effect produced by a drug, and the World Health Organisation (WHO) has suggested that it is any response to a drug which is noxious and unintended and which occurs at doses used in humans for prophylaxis, diagnosis or therapy (WHO, 1970). This definition does not include intentional or accidental poisoning or drug abuse and it has been suggested that it should also exclude therapeutic failures (Karch and Lasagna, 1975).

ADRs have been divided into two classes: type A and type B (Rawlins and Thompson, 1977). Type A reactions are pharmacologically predictable for the known activity of the drug—e.g. the dry mouth associated with the use of the tricyclic antidepressants due to anticholinergic effects—and are common, dose-related and usually not serious. Conversely, type B reactions are unpredictable and usually more serious (e.g. anaphylactic shock with penicillin). They may be caused by hypersensitivity to the drug or by an "idiosyncratic" reaction.

Unfortunately, it is often difficult to establish a clear cause-and-effect relationship between the drug and the reaction. To try to overcome this difficulty, ADRs have been classified as definite, probable, possible, conditional or doubtful (Karch and Lasagna, 1975). However, this classification relies on clinical judgement. Difficulties *may arise* when the patient is taking several medications or when the symptoms attributed to the drug, such as headache or nausea, are non-specific and subjective. Attempts have been made to improve precision in the diagnosis of ADRs by developing algorithms to standardise assessments of presumed ADRs (Karch and Lasagna, 1977; Leventhal *et al.*, 1979; Naranjo *et al.*, 1981). These algorithms ask a series of questions in sequence, and the answers are scored to measure the probability that a given clinical event was an ADR. Questions include the timing of the event relative to exposure to the drug, whether the event represents a known reaction to the drug, the possible role of the patient's condition at the time and the effects of drug withdrawal and, where appropriate, rechallenge.

INCIDENCE OF ADRS IN THE ELDERLY

Many studies have suggested that ADRs are a common problem in elderly patients and are the cause of 3%–12% of hospital admissions in this age group (Williamson and Chopin, 1980; Smucker and Kontak, 1990; Lindley *et al.*, 1992; Moore *et al.*, 1998; Mannesse *et al.*, 2000). Various risk factors have been identified. These include prescription of unnecessary or interacting drugs or drugs with relative or absolute contraindications (Lindley *et al.*, 1992). It has also been demonstrated that ADRs are particularly likely in patients who have had a fall before admission, or in those presenting with gastrointestinal bleeding or haematuria (Mannesse *et al.*, 2000).

Fewer studies have been done to determine the incidence of ADRs during hospital admission, but the incidence is about 5% with a range from 1.5% to over 20% (Seidl *et al.*, 1966; Hurwitz, 1969; Skott and Geise, 1984; Leach and Roy, 1986; Lindley *et al.*, 1992). The incidence is higher in the elderly. For example, in a prospective study of 1160 inpatients who were prescribed medication during admission, 10.2% experienced an ADR—and in patients over 60 years the incidence was higher, at 15.4% (Hurwitz, 1969). Seidl *et al.* (1966) found that while 13.6% of a resident hospital population in the United States acquired an ADR during hospitalisation, the incidence was as high as 24% in patients in their eighties. In addition, ADRs have been shown to be risk factors for delayed discharge from hospital (Skott and Geise, 1984) as well as early hospital readmission (Chu and Pei, 1999). Finally, in the out-patient population, about 5%–10% of patients have ADRs and slightly less than 1% of all patients are sent to hospital because of these (Skott and Geise, 1984; Chrischilles *et al.*, 1992b).

DRUGS THAT FREQUENTLY CAUSE ADRS IN ELDERLY PEOPLE

Some medicines are much more likely than others to cause problems when prescribed to elderly people. Three groups of drugs consistently cause problems in this age group: cardiovascular, NSAIDs and drugs acting on the central nervous system.

CARDIOVASCULAR DRUGS

Antihypertensives

Several studies have confirmed the high incidence of ADRs in elderly patients taking antihypertensives. For example, on a geriatric ward de V Mering noted severe cough induced by captopril, enalapril-induced angioedema and bronchospasm, peripheral vascular symptoms caused by β-adrenoceptor blockers and gout precipitated by thiazides (de V Mering, 1991). In the community, 3.1% of respondents reported an ADR with propranolol, 2.5% with methyldopa and 2.2% with nifedipine (Chrischilles et al., 1992a). For patients admitted to geriatric wards, antihypertensive drugs were a frequent cause of ADRs leading to hospital admissions (Hallas et al., 1992). The β-adrenoceptor blockers were a particularly common cause, and in some patients had been prescribed despite contraindications (Gosney and Tallis, 1984; Lindley et al., 1992).

Diuretics

Diuretics are one of the most common group of drugs being used by elderly patients before entering hospital. They are often stopped following admission, without causing any deterioration in clinical status (Burr et al., 1977; Abrams and Andrews, 1984). They are also a common cause of ADRs in this age group. Williamson and Chopin (1980) found that the largest number of ADRs in elderly patients admitted to hospital were due to diuretics, which were the most commonly prescribed group of drugs.

When elderly patients were observed during hospital admissions it was found that diuretics and antibiotics caused the most ADRs and were by far the most commonly prescribed drugs (Leach and Roy, 1986). In support of this, 50% of elderly in-patients in a teaching hospital were found to be receiving diuretics (Burr et al., 1977). In the community, patients complained of adverse side-effects with antihypertensives, diuretics and β-adrenoceptor blockers; these together accounted for 55% of reported ADRs (Chrischilles et al., 1992a).

Digoxin

Digoxin is frequently prescribed in the elderly but may cause problems in this age group, particularly in the presence of impaired renal function and low body weight. One study investigated 1433 in-patients who had digoxin assays performed and found that 8% had elevated levels (Marik and Fromm, 1998). This was most likely in older patients with higher serum creatinine levels. Of those patients who had elevated digoxin levels on admission, almost 50% were on a recommended maintenance dose suggesting that clinical vigilance and use of therapeutic monitoring is essential to minimise toxicity in this age group.

NON-STEROIDAL ANTI-INFLAMMATORY DRUGS

Elderly patients are among those who appear predisposed to NSAID-induced gastrointestinal bleeding (Carson et al., 1987). A case–controlled study by Collier and Pain (1985) found a twofold increase in risk of perforated peptic ulcer in patients over 65 years, whereas the risk was not increased in those under 65. Although all NSAIDs may be implicated, ibuprofen and diclofenac carry the lowest risk and azapropazone and ketoprofen the highest (Langman et al., 1994). Elderly people are also at increased risk of other ADRs from NSAIDs including hyperkalaemia, fluid retention and nephrotoxicity (Blackshear et al., 1983). A prospective study of elderly residents in a large nursing home who were started on NSAIDs demonstrated a deterioration in renal function in 13% over a short course of therapy (Gurwitz et al., 1990). This adverse effect was associated with higher NSAID doses and concomitant use of loop diuretics. The elderly are also at risk from central nervous system effects such as headaches and giddiness (O'Brien and Bagby, 1985).

DRUGS ACTING ON THE CENTRAL NERVOUS SYSTEM

In general, elderly people are more sensitive to medications that affect central nervous system function. Drugs of particular relevance in this regard are benzodiazepines, major tranquillisers and antidepressants, which are all frequently used by elderly patients. In a study of medicine use in general practice, psychotropic drugs were prescribed more commonly than any other group and accounted for up to one-fifth of all prescriptions (Skegg *et al.*, 1977). The proportion of patients receiving such medicines increased steadily with age: 21.4% of men and 29.9% of women over 75 years of age were receiving a sedative or hypnotic. Adverse reactions due to psychotropic drugs are known to be a frequent cause of hospital admission in the elderly (Williamson and Chopin, 1980; Hallas *et al.*, 1992).

IMPLICATIONS FOR DRUG DEVELOPMENT

The need for research in elderly persons has been addressed by Williams and Denham (1998). It should be clear from the studies referred to in this chapter that the effects of drugs can alter significantly with age as a consequence of changes in body composition and physiology and the effectiveness of various detoxifying mechanisms. Additional factors include the presence of disease, polypharmacy and possible differences in patient behaviour. Consequently, doses of drugs required to achieve desired results in elderly people may be substantially different from those used in younger persons. Furthermore, the risk of ADRs and interactions is enhanced by the presence of concomitant diseases and remedies for them.

The need for clinical trials to involve elderly people is obvious if treatments are to be used safely and effectively in this age group. Yet, the major part of the so-called "therapeutic explosion" which occurred during the twentieth century relied on research carried out in younger patients and there were casualties. These included the development of a hepato-renal syndrome associated with the use of benoxaprofen (Hamdy *et al.*, 1982) and problems with other NSAIDs (Castleden and Pickles, 1988). The need for dose modification for agents such as triazolam (Greenblatt *et al.*, 1991) was identified, as was the need for attention to labelling and modification of package inserts. However, by the time that a new medicine has been marketed, experience with its use remains confined to a relatively small number of people, of whom only a proportion will be elderly. There is, therefore, a need for careful pharmacovigilance to identify unexpected adverse effects such as those produced by terodiline. This agent, which was introduced for use in urinary incontinence due to detrusor muscle instability, was subject to prescription event monitoring by the Drug Safety Research Unit in Southampton (Freemantle *et al.*, 1997). The latter system relies on reporting of significant events "such as a broken leg" which may be due to hypotension, ataxia or metabolic bone disease. In the case of terodiline, an excess of fractures was identified, many of which were the result of falls. Further investigations revealed that the cause was syncope due to torsades de pointes which can be identified by means of Holter Monitoring (Committee on Safety of Medicines, 1991).

Although prescription event monitoring is likely to identify important adverse reactions occurring at a low frequency, we rely on other systems to identify those which occur more rarely. Most of these are so-called type B adverse effects. Examples include agranulocytosis caused by co-trimoxazole and by oxyphenbutazone, eventually shown by voluntary reporting systems, e.g. the Yellow Card system operated by the Committee on Safety of Medicines, to occur predominantly in old people (Inman, 1977). This led to the advice to avoid using co-trimoxazole in the elderly and the revocation of the licence for oxyphenbutazone. Fortunately, the need for clinical studies and trials in the elderly is now recognised by all major drug regulatory bodies. Thus, in Europe, official recognition by the European Commission occurred in the 1970s and a regulatory requirement (Directive 78 of the 318 of the EC) and similar regulations were introduced by the Food and

Drugs Administration in the United States (Food and Drug Administration Center, 1989; International Conference on Harmonisation, 1993).

REFERENCES

Abrams J, Andrews K (1984) The influence of hospital admission on long-term medication of elderly patients. *J R Coll Phys Lond* **18**: 225–7.

Adreasen PB, Simonsen D, Brocks K, Dimo B, Bouchelouche P (1981) Hypoglycaemia induced by azapropazone–tolbutamide interaction. *Br J Clin Pharmacol* **12**: 581–3.

Ajayi AA, Hocking N, Reid JL (1986) Age and the pharmacodynamics of angiotensin converting enzyme inhibitors enalapril and enalaprilat. *Br J Clin Pharmacol* **21**: 349–57.

Alldredge BK (1999) Seizure risk associated with psychotropic drugs: clinical and pharmacokinetic considerations. *Neurology* **53** (Suppl 2): S68–S75.

Amdisen A (1982) Lithium and drug interactions. *Drugs* **24**: 133–9.

Baillie SR, Bateman DN, Coates DE, Woodhouse KW (1989) Age and the pharmacokinetics of morphine. *Age Ageing* **18**: 258–62.

Barnett NL, Denham MJ, Francis S-A (2000) Over-the-counter medicines and the elderly. *J R Coll Phys Lond* **34**: 445–6.

Bauer LA, Black D, Gensler A (1990) Procainamide cimetidine drug interaction in elderly male patients. *J Am Geriatr Soc* **38**: 467–9.

Bax DE, Woods HS, Christie J, Bearn M, Woods HF, Bax NDS (1987) Therapeutic audit on a general medical ward. *Clin Sci* **72**: 29P.

Belantuono C, Reggi V, Tognoni G, Garattini S (1980) Benzodiazepines: clinical pharmacology and therapeutic use. *Drugs* **19**: 195–219.

Berry SJ, Coffey DS, Walsh PC, Ewing LL (1984) The development of human benign prostatic hyperplasia with age. *J Urol* **132**: 474–9.

Bigger JT (1982) The quinidine–digoxin interaction. *Mod Concepts Cardiovasc Dis* **51**: 73–8.

Blackburn SCF, Ellis R, George CF, Kirwan JR (1994) The impact and treatment of arthritis in general practice. *Pharmacoepidemiology and Drug Safety* **3**: 123–38.

Blackshear JL, Davidman M, Stillman MT (1983) Identification of risk for renal insufficiency from non-steroidal anti-inflammatory drugs. *Arch Intern Med* **143**: 1130–4.

Bonate PL, Kelly R, Weir S (1998) Drug interactions at the renal level. Implications for drug development. *Clin Pharmacokinet* **34**: 375–405.

British Heart Foundation (2000) *Coronary Heart Disease Statistics*. London: BHF.

British Heart Foundation (2001) *Coronary Heart Disease Statistics: Morbidity Supplement*. London: BHF.

Britt RP, James AH, Raskino CL, Thompson SG (1992) Factors affecting the precision of warfarin treatment. *J Clin Pathol* **45**: 1003–6.

Brown DD, Juhl RP (1976) Decreased bioavailability of digoxin due to antacids and kaolin-pectin. *New Engl J Med* **295**: 1034–7.

Burr ML, King S, Davies HEF, Pathy MS (1977) The effects of discontinuing long-term diuretic therapy in the elderly. *Age Ageing* **6**: 38–45.

Campion EW, de Labrey LO, Glynn RJ (1988) The effect of age on serum albumin in healthy males: report from the normative ageing study. *J Gerontol* **43**: M18–M20.

Capewell S, Freestone S, Critchley JAJH, Pottage A, Prescott LF (1988) Reduced felodipine bioavailability in patients taking anticonvulsants. *Lancet* **2**: 480–2.

Carson JL, Strom BL, Morse ML, West SL, Soper KA, Stolley PD, Jones JK (1987) The relative gastrointestinal toxicity of the non-steroidal anti-inflammatory drugs. *Arch Intern Med* **147**: 1054–9.

Cartwright A, Smith CRW (1988) *Elderly People, Their Medicines and Their Doctors*. London: Routledge.

Castleden CM, Pickles H (1988) Suspected adverse drug reactions in elderly patients reported to the CSM. *Br J Clin Pharmacol* **26**: 347–53.

Castleden CM, George CF, Marcer D, Hallett C (1977) Increased sensitivity to nitrazepam in old age. *Br Med J* **1**: 10–12.

Castleden CM, George CF (1979) The effect of ageing on the hepatic clearance of propranolol. *Br J Clin Pharmacol* **7**: 49–54.

Chrischilles EA, Foley DJ, Wallace RB, Lemke JH, Semla TP, Hanlon JT, Glynn RJ, Ostfeld AM, Guralnik JM (1992a) Use of medications by persons 65 and over: data from the established populations for epidemiologic studies of the elderly. *J Gerontol* **47**: M137–M144.

Chrischilles EA, Segar ET, Wallace RB (1992b) Self-reported adverse drug reactions and related resource use. *Ann Intern Med* **117**: 634–40.

Chu LW, Pei CK (1999) Risk factors for early emergency hospital readmission in elderly medical patients. *Gerontology* **45**: 220–6.

Cleland JGF, Dargie JH, McAlpine H, Ball SG, Morton JJ, Robertson JIS, Ford I (1985) Severe hypotension after first dose of enalapril in the elderly. *Br Med J* **291**: 1309–12.

Cockroft DW, Gault MH (1976) Prediction of creatinine clearance from serum creatinine. *Nephron* **16**: 31–41.

Collier DSTJ, Pain JA (1985) Non-steroidal anti-inflammatory drugs and peptic ulcer perforation. *Gut* **26**: 359–63.

Committee on Safety of Medicines (1991) *Withdrawal of Terodiline (Micturin, Kabi Pharmacia Limited)*. Current problems 32.

Cook PJ, Flanagan R, James IM (1984) Diazepam tolerance: effect of age, regular sedation and alcohol. *Br Med J* **289**: 351–3.

Cusack B, Kelly JG, Lavan J, Noel J, O'Malley K (1980) Pharmacokinetics of lignocaine in the elderly. *Br J Clin Pharmacol* **9**: 293P–294P.

de V Mering P (1991) Prescribing for the elderly—a new perspective required. *S Afr Med J* **79**: 293–4.

Dillon N, Chung S, Kelly J, O'Malley K (1980) Age and beta adrenergic receptor mediated function. *Clin Pharmacol Ther* **27**: 769–72.

Divoll M, Ameer B, Abernathy DR, Greenblatt DJ (1982) Age does not alter acetaminophen absorption. *J Am Geriatr Soc* **30**: 240–4.

Edelman IS, Leibman J (1959) Anatomy of body water and electrolytes. *Am J Med* **27**: 256.

Edoute Y, Nagachandran P, Svirski B, Ben-Ami H (2000) Cardiovascular adverse drug reaction associated with combined beta-adrenergic and calcium entry-blocking agents. *J Cardiovasc Pharmacol* **35**: 556–9.

Evans MA, Triggs EJ, Cheung M, Broe GA, Creasey H (1981) Gastric emptying in the elderly: implications for drug therapy. *J Am Geriatr Soc* **29**: 201–5.

Feldman RD, Limbird LE, Nadeau J, Robertson D, Wood AJ (1984) Alterations in leukocyte beta-receptor affinity with ageing: a potential explanation for alatered beta adrenergic sensitivity in the elderly. *New Engl J Med* **310**: 815–9.

Food and Drug Administration Center (1989) Guidelines for the study of drugs likely to be used in the elderly. Food and Drug Administration Center for Drug Evaluation and Research, Rockville, Maryland, USA 16.

Forbes GB, Reina JC (1970) Adult lean body mass declines with age: some longitudinal observations. *Metabolism* **9**: 653–63.

Freemantle SN, Pearce GL, Wilton LV, Mackay FJ, Mann RD (1997) The incidence of the most commonly reported events with 40 new marketed drugs—a study by Prescription-Event and Monitoring. *Pharmacoepidemiology and Drug Safety* **6** (Suppl 1): 1–8.

Fromm MF, Kim RB, Stein CM, Wilkinson GR, Roden DM (1999) Inhibition of P-glycoprotein-mediated drug transport: a unifying mechanism to explain the interaction between digoxin and quinidine. *Circulation* **99**: 552–7.

Geokas M, Haverback BJ (1969) The ageing gastrointestinal tract. *Am J Surg* **117**: 881–92.

George CF (1980) Amiloride handling in renal failure. *Br J Clin Pharmacol* **9**: 94–5.

Goldberg PB, Roberts J (1983) Pharmacological basis for developing rational drug regimes for elderly patients. *Med Clin North Am* **67**: 315–31.

Gosney M, Tallis R (1984) Prescription of contraindicated and interacting drugs in elderly patients admitted to hospital. *Lancet* **2**: 564–7.

Grandison MK, Boudinot FD (2000) Age-related changes in protein binding of drugs: implications for therapy. *Clin Pharmacokinet* **38**(3): 271–90.

Greenblatt DJ, Haematz JS, Shapiro L, Englehardt N, Gouthro TA, Shader RI (1991) Sensitivity to triazolam in the elderly. *New Engl J Med* **324**: 1691–8.

Greenblatt DJ, Sellers EM, Shader RI (1982) Drug disposition in old age. *New Engl J Med* **306**: 1081–8.

Gribbin B, Pickering TG, Sleight P, Peto R (1971) Effect of age and high blood pressure on baroreceptor sensitivity in man. *Circ Res* **29**: 424–31.

Groen H, Horan MA, Roberts NA (1993) The relationship between phenazone (antipyrine) metabolite formation and theophylline metabolism in healthy and frail elderly women. *Clin Pharmacokinet* **25**: 136–44.

Gurwitz JH, Avorn J, Ross-Degnan D, Lipsitz LA (1990) Nonsteroidal anti-inflammatory drug-associated azotemia in the very old. *J Am Med Assoc* **264**: 471–5.

Gurwitz JH, Goldberg RJ, Holden A, Knapie N, Ansell J (1988) Age-related risks of long-term oral anticoagulant therapy. *Arch Intern Med* **148**: 1733–6.

Hale WE, Stewart RB, Marks RG (1985) Antianxiety drugs and central nervous system symptoms in an ambulatory elderly population. *Drug Intell Clin Pharm* **19**: 37–40.

Hallas J, Gram LF, Grodum E, Demsbo N, Brosen K, Haghflet T (1992) Drug related admissions to medical wards: a population based survey. *Br J Clin Pharmacol* **33**: 61–8.

Hamdy RC, Murnane B, Perera N (1982) Pharmacokinetics of benoxaprofen in elderly subjects. *Eur J Rheumatol Inflamm* **5**: 69–76.

Hawthorne VM, Greaves DA, Beevers DG (1974) Blood pressure in a Scottish town. *Br Med J* **3**: 600–3.

Honig PK, Woosley RL, Zamani K, Conner DP, Cantilena LR Jr (1992) Changes in the pharmacokinetics and electrocardiographic pharmacodynamics of terfenadine with concomitant administration of erythromycin. *Clin Pharmacol Ther* **52**: 231–8.

Honig PK, Wortham DC, Zamani K, Conner DP, Mullin JC, Cantilena LR (1993) Terfenadine–ketoconazole interaction: pharmacokinetic and electrocardiographic consequences. *J Am Med Assoc* **269**: 513–8.

Hurwitz N (1969) Predisposing factors in adverse reactions to drugs. *Br Med J* **1**: 536–9.

Inman WHW (1977) Study of fatal bone marrow depression with special reference to phenylbutazone and oxyphenbutazone. *Br Med J* **1**: 1500–5.

International Conference on Harmonisation (ICH) Expert Working Group E7 (1993) Studies in support of Special Populations; Geriatrics III/3388/93.

Inui KI, Masuda S, Saito H (2000) Cellular and molecular aspects of drug transport in the kidney. *Kidney International* **58**: 944–58.

Israel BC, Blouin RA, McIntyre W, Shedlofsky ST

(1993) Effects of interferon-alphamonotherapy on hepatic drug metabolism in cancer patients. *Br J Clin Pharmacol* **36**: 229–35.

Jackson JE, Powell JR, Wandell M, Bentley J, Dorr R (1981) Cimetidine decreases theophylline clearance. *Am Rev Respir Dis* **123**: 615–7.

Jackson SHD (1994) Pharmacodynamics in the elderly. *J R Soc Med* **23**: 5–7.

Jefferson JW, Greist JH, Carroll J, Baudhuin M (1986) Drug–drug and drug–disease interactions with non-steroidal anti-inflammatory drugs. *Am J Med* **81**: 948.

Johnson AG, Simons LA, Simons J, Friedlander Y, McCallum J (1993) Non-steroidal anti-inflammatory drugs and hypertension in the elderly: a community based cross-sectional study. *Br J Clin Pharmacol* **35**: 455–9.

Jones D, Poole C (1998) Medicine taking by elderly people: an overview. In: George CF, Woodhouse KW, Denham MJ, MacLennan WJ, eds, *Drug Therapy in Old Age*. Chichester: Wiley, pp. 111–22.

Karch FE, Lasagna L (1975) Adverse drug reactions. *J Am Med Assoc* **234**: 1236–41.

Karch FE, Lasagna L (1977) Toward the operational identification of adverse drug reactions. *Clin Pharmacol Ther* **21**: 247–54.

Kendall MJ, Woods KL, Wilkins MR, Worthington DJ (1982) Responsiveness to β-adrenergic receptor stimulation: the effects of age are cardioselective. *Br J Clin Pharmacol* **14**: 821–6.

Kinirons MT, Crome P (1997) Clinical pharmacokinetic considerations in the elderly. An update. *Clin Pharmacokinet* **33**: 302–12.

Krikler DM, Spurrell RAJ (1974) Verapamil in the treatment of paroxysmal supraventricular tachycardia. *Postgrad Med J* **50**: 447–53.

Langman MJS, Weil J, Wainwright R, Lawson DH, Rawlins MD, Logan RFA, Murpy M, Vessey MP, Colin-Jones DG (1994) Risks of bleeding peptic ulcer associated with individual non-steroidal anti-inflammatory drugs. *Lancet* **343**: 1075–8.

Lawrence JS (1977) *Rheumatism in Populations*. London: Heinemann.

Leach S, Roy SS (1986) Adverse drug reactions: an investigation on an acute geriatric ward. *Age Ageing* **15**: 241–6.

Leventhal JM, Hutchinson TA, Kramer MS, Feinstein AR (1979) An algorithm for the operational assessment of adverse drug reactions. *J Am Med Assoc* **242**: 1991–4.

Lin JH, Lu AY (1998) Inhibition and induction of cytochrome P450 and the clinical implications. *Clinical Pharmacokinet* **35**: 361–90.

Lindley CM, Tully MP, Paramsothy P, Tallis RC (1992) Inappropriate medication is a major cause of adverse drug reactions in elderly patients. *Age Ageing* **21**: 294–300.

Macklon AF, Barton M, James O, Rawlins MD (1980) The effect of age on the pharmacokinetics of diazepam. *Clin Sci* **59**: 479–83.

MacLennan WJ, Martin P, Mason BJ (1977) Protein intake and serum albumin levels in the elderly. *Gerontology* **23**: 360–7.

Mannesse CK, Derkx FH, De Ridder MA, Man in't Veld AJ, Van der Cammen TJ (2000) Contribution of adverse drug reactions to hospital admission of older patients. *Age Ageing* **29**: 35–9.

Marik PE, Fromm L (1998) A case series of hospitalized patients with elevated digoxin levels. *Am J Med* **105**: 110–5.

May JR, Dipiro JT, Sisley JF (1987) Drug interactions in surgical patients. *Am J Surg* **153**: 327–35.

McAinsh J (1977) Clinical pharmacokinetics of atenolol. *Postgraduate Med J* **53** (Suppl 3): 74–8.

McGrath AM, Jackson GA (1996) Survey of neuroleptic prescribing in residents of nursing homes in Glasgow. *Br Med J* **312**: 611–2.

McInnes GT, Brodie MJ (1988) Drug interactions that matter. A critical appraisal. *Drugs* **36**: 83–110.

Mehta BR, Robinson BHB (1980) Lithium toxicity induced by triamterene-hydrochlorothiazide. *Postgrad Med J* **56**: 783–4.

Mets TF (1995) Drug-induced orthostatic hypotension in older patients. *Drugs Ageing* **6**: 219–28.

Monaghan BP, Ferguson CL, Killeavy ES, Lloyd BK, Troy J, Cantilena LR (1993) Torsades de pointes occurring in association with terfenadine use. *J Am Med Assoc* **264**: 2788–90.

Montamat SC, Cusack BJ, Vestal RE (1989) Management of drug therapy in the elderly. *New Engl J Med* **321**: 303–9.

Moore N, Lecointre D, Noblet C, Mabille M (1998) Frequency and cost of serious adverse drug reactions in a department of general medicine. *Br J Clin Pharmacol* **45**: 301–8.

Moysey JO, Jaggarao NSV, Grunoy EN, Chamberlain DA (1981) Amiodarone increases plasma digoxin concentrations. *Br Med J* **282**: 272.

Muhlberg W, Platt D (1999) Age-dependent changes of the kidneys: pharmacological implications. *Gerontology* **45**: 243–53.

Naranjo CA, Busto U, Sellers EM, Sandor P, Ruiz I, Roberts EA, Janeck E, Domecq C, Greenblatt DJ (1981) A method for estimating the probability of adverse drug reactions. *Clin Pharmacol Ther* **30**: 239–45.

Nation RL, Learoyd B, Barber J, Triggs EJ (1976) The pharmacokinetics of chlormethiazole following intravenous administration in the aged. *Eur J Clin Pharmacol* **10**: 407–15.

Novak LP (1972) Ageing, total body potassium, fat-free mass, and cell mass in males and females between ages 18 and 85 years. *J Gerontol* **27**: 438–43.

O'Brien W, Bagby GF (1985) Rare adverse reactions to

non-steroidal-antiinflammatory drugs. Part IV. *J Rheumatol* 12: 785–90.

O'Callaghan JW, Thompson RN, Russell AS (1984) Combining NSAIDs with anticoagulants: yes and no. *Can Med Assoc J* 131: 857–8.

O'Malley K, Crooks J, Duke E, Stevenson IH (1971) Effect of age and sex on human drug metabolism. *Br Med J* 3: 607–9.

O'Malley K, Stevenson IH, Ward CA, Wood AJJ, Crooks J (1977) Determinants of anticoagulant control in patients receiving warfarin. *Br J Clin Pharmacol* 4: 309–14.

O'Reilly RA, Trager WF, Motley CH, Howald W (1980) Stereoselective interaction of phenylbutazone with (12C/13C) warfarin pseudo racemates in man. *J Clin Invest* 65: 746–53.

Oetgen WJ, Sobol SM, Tri TB, Heydorn WH, Rakita L (1984) Amiodarone–digoxin interaction: clinical and experimental observations. *Chest* 84: 75–9.

Olshansky SJ, Carnes BA, Désesquelles A (2001) Prospects for human longevity. *Science* 291: 1491–2

Pan HY, Hoffman BB, Pershe RA, Blaschke TF (1986) Decline in beta-adrenergic-receptor-mediated vascular relaxation with ageing in man. *J Pharmacol Exp Ther* 239: 802–7.

Parkin DM, Henney CR, Quirk J, Crooks J (1976) Deviation from prescribed drug treatment after discharge from hospital. *Br Med J* 2: 686–8.

Pederson KE, Tayssem P, Klitgaard NA, Christiansen BD, Nielsen-Kudski F (1983) Influence of verapamil on the inotropism and pharmacokinetics of digoxin. *Eur J Clin Pharmacol* 25: 199–206.

Peterson V, Hvidts S, Thomsen K, Shou M (1974) Effect of prolonged thiazide treatment on enal lithium clearance. *Br Med J* 2: 143–5.

Pohjola-Sintonen S, Viitasalo M, Toivonen L, Neuvonen P (1993) Ketoconazole prevents terfenadine metabolism and increases risk of torsades de pointes' ventricular tachycardia. *Eur J Clin Pharmacol* 45: 191–193.

Rawlins MD, Thompson JW (1977) Pathogensis of adverse drug reactions. In: Davies DM, ed., *Textbook of Adverse Drug Reactions*. Oxford: Oxford University Press, p. 44.

Ray WA, Thapa PB, Shorr RI (1993) Medications and the older driver. *Clin Geriatr Med* 9: 412–38.

Redwood M, Taylor C, Bain BJ, Matthews JH (1991) The association of age with dose requirement for warfarin. *Age Ageing* 20: 217–20.

Ridout S, Waters WE, George CF (1986) Knowledge of and attitudes to medicines in the Southampton community. *Br J Clin Pharmacol* 21: 701–12.

Robertson D, Waller DG, Renwick AG, George CF (1988) Age-related changes in the pharmacokinetics and pharmacodynamics of nifedipine. *Br J Clin Pharmacol* 25: 297–305.

Rowe JW, Adres R, Tobin JD, Norris AH, Shock NW (1976) The effect of age on creatinine clearance in men: a cross-sectional and longitudinal study. *J Gerontol* 31: 155–63.

Sax MJ (1987) Clinically important adverse effects and drug interactions with H_2-receptor antagonists: an update. *Pharmacotherapy* 7: 1105–55.

Scarpace PJ (1986) Decreased β-adrenoceptor responsiveness during senescence. *Fed Proc* 45: 51–4.

Schocken D, Roth G (1977) Reduced beta-adrenergic receptor concentration in ageing man. *Nature* 267: 856–8.

Seidl LG, Thorton GF, Smith JE, Cluff LE (1966) Studies on the epidemiology of adverse drug reaction III. Reactions in patients on a general medical service. *Bull Johns Hopkins Hosp* 119: 299–315.

Seymour RM, Routledge PA (1998) Important drug–drug interactions in the elderly. *Drugs Ageing* 12: 485–94.

Shepherd AMM, Hewick DS, Moreland TA, Stevenson IH (1977) Age as a determinant of sensitivity to warfarin. *Br J Clin Pharmacol* 4: 315–20.

Skegg DCG, Doll R, Perry J (1977) Use of medicines in general practice. *Br Med J* 1: 1561–3.

Skott P, Giese J (1984) Age and the renin angiotensin system. *Acta Med Scand* (Suppl) 676: 45–51.

Smith DA, Chandler MHH, Shedlofsky SI, Wedland PJ, Blouin RA (1991) Age-dependent stereoselective increase in the oral clearance of hexobarbitone isomers caused by rifampicin. *Br J Clin Pharmacol* 32: 735–9.

Smith TW (1973) Digitalis glycosides. *New Engl J Med* 288: 942–6.

Smucker WD, Kontak JR (1990) Adverse drug reactions causing hospital admission in an elderly population: experience with a decision algorithm. *J Am Board Fam Pract* 3: 105–9.

Sproule BA, Naranjo CA, Brenmer KE, Hassan PC (1997) Selective serotonin reuptake inhibitors and CNS drug interactions. A critical review of the evidence. *Clinical Pharmacokinet* 33: 454–71.

Sullivan MJ, George CF (1996) Medicine taking in Southampton: a second look. *Brit J Clin Pharmacol* 42: 567–71.

Swift CG, Swift MR, Hamley J, Stevenson IH (1984) Side-effect "tolerance" in elderly long-term recipients of benzodiazepines hypnotics. *Age Ageing* 13: 335–43.

Tanaka E (1998) clinically important pharmacokinetic drug–drug interactions: role of cytochrome P450 enzymes. *J Clin Pharmacol Ther* 23: 403–16.

Tollefson GD (1983) Monoamine oxidase inhibitors: a review. *J Clin Psychiatry* 44: 280–6.

Ullah MI, Newman GB, Saunders KB (1981) Influence of age on response to ipratropium and salbutamol in man. *Thorax* 36: 523–9.

Verschraagen M, Koks CH, Schellens JH, Beijnen JH (1999) P-glycoprotein system as a determinant of drug interactions: the case of digoxin–verapamil. *Pharmacol Res* 40: 301–6.

Vestal RE (1978) Drug use in the elderly: a review of problems and special considerations. *Drug* **16**: 358–82.

Vestal RE, McGuire EA, Tobin JD, Andres R, Norris AH, Mezey E (1977) Ageing and ethanol metabolism. *Clin Pharmacol Ther* **21**: 343–54.

Vestal RE, Norris AH, Tobin JD, Cohen BH, Shock NW, Andres R (1975) Antipyrine metabolism in man: influence of age, alcohol, caffeine and smoking. *Clin Pharmacol Ther* **18**: 425–32.

Wallace SM, Verbeeck RK (1987) Plasma protein binding of drugs in the elderly. *Clin Pharmacokinet* **12**: 41–72.

Waller DG, Waller D (1984) Hypoglycaemia due to azapropazone–tolbutamide interaction. *Br J Clin Rheumatol* **23**: 24–5.

World Health Organisation (1970) International Drug Monitoring—the role of hospital. *Drug Intell Clin Pharm* **4**: 101.

Williams A, Denham MJ (1998) The ethics of biomedical research in the elderly. In: George CF, Woodhouse KW, Denham MJ, MacLennan WJ, eds, *Drug Therapy in Old Age*. Chichester: Wiley.

Williams L, Lowenthal DT (1992) Drug therapy in the elderly. *South Med J* **85**: 127–31.

Williams RT (1967) Comparative patterns of drug metabolism. *Fed Proc* **26**: 1029–39.

Williamson J, Chopin JM (1980) Adverse reactions to prescribed drugs in the elderly: a multicentre investigation. *Age Ageing* **9**: 73–80.

Woodhouse KW, James OFW (1990) Hepatic drug metabolism and ageing. *Br Med Bull* **46**: 22–35.

Woodhouse KW (1994) Pharmacokinetics of drugs in the elderly. *J R Soc Med* **87** (Suppl 23): 2–4.

Wynne H, Cope LH, Herd MD, Rawlins MD, James OFD, Woodhouse KW (1990) The association of age and frailty with paracetamol conjugation in man. *Age Ageing* **19**: 419–24.

Wynne H, Yelland C, Cope LH, Boddy A, Woodhouse KW, Bateman DN (1993) The association of age and frailty in the phamacokinetics and pharmacodynamics of metoclopromide. *Age Ageing* **22**: 354–9.

Wynne HA, Cope E, Mutch E, Rawlins MD, Woodhouse KW, James OFW (1989) The effect of age upon liver volume and apparent liver blood flow in healthy man. *Hepatology* **9**: 297–301.

8

Natural History

PAUL E. STANG

Galt Associates, Inc., Blue Bell, PA, USA, and University of North Carolina School of Public Health at Chapel Hill, NC, USA

INTRODUCTION

Disease natural history is a broad term that reflects the events and outcomes that characterize the course of illness. It has been referred to as "background rate", "background noise", or expected rate in the pharmacovigilance world. For acute disease such as many infections, the natural history may be relatively simple and uncomplicated as in the case of wound infections or acute otitis media. For chronic disease, the picture can be drastically different as over time, different events may present themselves and the passage of time itself increases the likelihood that other illnesses or exposures may exert an influence. The natural course of disease is a dynamic process with variations in severity, comorbidities and exacerbations over time. Knowledge of the disease natural history provides the context against which the risk and benefit of any therapy can be judged. One need only look at the CIOMS IV recommendations to see the integral role of these data in providing the context for risk tolerance and assessment of the risk–benefit profile of a product (CIOMS IV, 1998). This chapter will outline the relevant concepts of disease natural history and how they are applicable to pharmacovigilance.

WHAT CONSTITUTES DISEASE NATURAL HISTORY

A chief goal of natural history research is to understand the spectrum of the disease, the different manifestations, patterns of recognition and care. It is critical for differentiating self-limiting illnesses (e.g. acute infection) from chronic states (e.g. heart disease, cancer, diabetes, chronic respiratory illness) and distinguishing underlying disease from the exacerbations of chronic illness (e.g. multiple sclerosis, pain syndromes). There is often talk of "confounding by indication" where our concern is determining events that may be attributable to the "indication" or disorder for which the therapy is prescribed rather than the therapy itself: disease natural history is the indication side of this dilemma.

The first rule of good epidemiology is to clearly define case and exposure criteria that enable us to designate subjects as being in one state of illness or another (pre-symptomatic, symptomatic, with disease or not with disease). Although it is easiest to consider "disease" as present or absent, most diseases change over time. Over the course of a lifetime a subject may move in and out of disease states across many

---

Pharmacovigilance. Edited by R.D. Mann and E.B. Andrews

diseases at any given point in time. The natural history of disease and interventions are consistent with the public health model of prevention and reflects the changes in an individual over time. It includes the following stages, which coincide with the public health model of prevention (Figure 8.1):

● Primary prevention—intervention during the stage of susceptibilty; intended to reduce new occurrences of disease.
● Secondary prevention—intervention during the pre-symptomatic phase; intended to delay the onset of disease or reduce its duration or severity.
● Tertiary prevention—intervention during the clinical stage; intended to reduce complications and disabilities.

The manifestations of the disease are not always stable over time and may be sporadic. These are often referred to as exacerbations, flares, or episodes, as seen with epilepsy, migraine, asthma, irritable bowel syndrome, depression, multiple sclerosis, or anxiety or when the symptoms themselves are unstable over time (Stang and Von Korff, 1995). This may also connote sporadic therapy, whether prescribed "as needed" or self-medicated as such. To address this complexity, some authors distinguish between clinical course

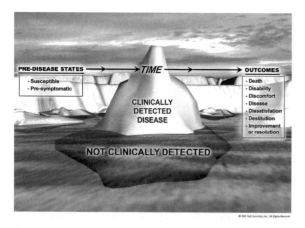

Figure 8.1. A model of disease natural history showing the phases of disease, passage of time, clinical detection, and outcomes.

and disease natural history (Fletcher *et al.*, 1996). The distinction made is that clinical course describes the evolution of disease that has come under medical care with its consequent interventions that may impact the course of events. The course of an illness not under medical care is then referred to as "disease natural history." There are any number of reasons why a disorder may go untreated, including lack of symptoms, lack of detection, or failure to seek medical attention. The examples are plentiful in the literature, most prominent among which are found in the cardiovascular field and in mental illnesses.

The pattern of utilization of services itself may be a clue to the natural course of disease or help identify those who may otherwise go undetected. In addition, those under treatment with the therapy of interest bring with them the combined risks and benefits of this treatment, concomitant illness and their treatments, as well as the risks associated directly with the illness. Under these circumstances, the attribution of risk to the medication of interest in combination with treatments for concomitant illness can become quite difficult if we do not have information about the events that occur with each level or combination of therapy.

There are many who seek medical attention for their symptoms who fail to receive the proper diagnosis or treatment (for example, Stang and Von Korff, 1994). In many circumstances, they are still "cases" who may be contrasted with those who clearly do not suffer the target indication but receive treatment anyway. This reality makes pharmacovigilance more difficult. Patients receiving therapy who do not suffer the target indication may not carry with them the biological or clinical "burden" of that disease. If extensive medication use falls into this category, additional information may need to be provided to patients and physicians to place the potential risks and benefits in a context that differs from the intended target population. Nonetheless, the capture of information on the spectrum of illnesses, their associated demographics and illness are the foundation used for the interpretation of adverse event signals within a spectrum of uses.

For studies that depend on clinical detection of disease or events, the researcher should be wary of any potential distortion in the identification of disease or events (detection bias) as it may be that only those who undergo "screening" or have the opportunity to present with symptoms will likely be detected which leaves one to speculate about the status of those who were not screened. This may be particularly true for symptoms, rather than illnesses, as the natural history of symptoms of a particular illness are even more difficult to ascertain since those with the target disorder may report a symptom more frequently. This is the case in pain syndromes. An interesting example of this was seen in a study of the systematic assessment of chest pain among migraine sufferers (Sternfeld *et al.*, 1995).

COMORBIDITY

Comorbid disease or illness refers to other diseases that coexist with the disease of interest, and on a population level, usually more frequently than by chance alone. The term is exacting and even enjoys a position as a Medical Subject Heading (MeSH) used in the indexing of the medical literature. Comorbidities may arise by chance, selection bias, shared environmental or genetic factors, or as part of the causal path of another condition. These associated factors are extremely important as they are often markers of disease severity (as evidenced by their judicious use in the health services research literature in chronic disease scores), can modify the risk of a given outcome, and are often undetected or ignored when attempting to understand potential adverse consequences of pharmacotherapy. A comorbid condition may imply differential risk attributable to the disorder itself (e.g. risk of suicide with comorbid depression) or suggest effects from self-treatment or pharmacotherapy that may not have otherwise come to the attention of the treating clinician or researcher. Principal to be considered among these disorders are those that may not be easily shared with a clinician including substance abuse (including alcohol) or smoking.

It is a prudent approach for the safety professional to "backtrack" by starting with the adverse event of interest and determining the possible disease and therapy mechanisms that are known

to be associated with the given type of event (clinically, a differential diagnosis that enumerates the possible etiologies). Once identified, they can query what is known about the comorbidities and natural history of the disease to determine if they can explain any or all of the events under scrutiny and the degree to which they are known in the given case. This approach is more focused and can be inefficient across a number of events; however, it does provide the necessary clear direction in the search of the literature, data and follow-up often necessary with cases of interest.

Comorbidity can also be a modifier of effect: in the presence of a comorbidity, the effect of the drug of interest may be magnified or attenuated which consequently would impact the risk of a given outcome. Depression itself, whether a consequence or a contributing factor, is highly comorbid with a number of chronic medical conditions and often affects compliance, outcome and may affect the potential risk–benefit of a given therapy. Cardiovascular disease has long had a history of identifying comorbid factors as a means of determining risk of outcome (Figure 8.2). One only need look at the various risk scoring schemes that include body mass index, hypertension, cholesterol level, and family history to see how important comorbidities are in the assessment of risk.

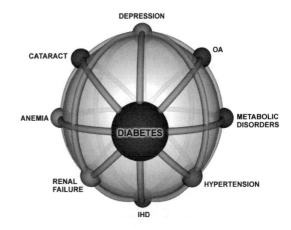

Figure 8.2. A representation of the comorbidity of illnesses related to diabetes.

Comorbidity is of such importance in some fields that entire studies have been undertaken to examine them. Most prominent among these is the National Comorbidity Survey (Kessler, 1994), a systematic interview and screening for mental illness in a representative sample of the US population. From this study, an incredible wealth of information has emerged about the impact and natural history of mental illness and comorbid mental illness on patient outcomes.

So what does all this have to do with drug safety? Aside from its potential impact on risk, comorbidities and their treatments may modify the risk of adverse events either directly or by increasing the probability of a drug interaction or exacerbation of one illness due to the treatment for another. Comorbidities may suggest product exposures that may not be captured by pharmacy claims data because they are over-the-counter (OTC) products, nutraceuticals, vitamins or substances like alcohol, tobacco or street drugs. However, detection of comorbidities, like the index diseases themselves, is dependent on the source of information. In studies using claims data, there are the obvious issues relating to coding, ascertainment, eligibility of patients for insurance coverage for certain services; in clinical data, as in claims data, detection is dependent on the patient presenting with symptoms, the physician making the diagnosis, and the coding reflecting the encounter. This is very similar to the issues in spontaneous reporting where capture of the potential event depends on the patient presenting to the doctor with the complaint, the physician recognizing it as potentially an adverse event, and reporting it to the proper system. The precision of that coding is of interest as well, and has been shown to vary depending on the disease and the source of the data where the method of ascertainment may result in substantial differences in estimates of prevalence (Sanders, 1962). Relying on coded diagnoses in an existing database requires that the scientist have a keen understanding of the coding scheme, any restrictions on the number of codes allowed for any given site of service, in addition to how disease (or symptom), medication, procedure, hospitalization and social data are captured and recorded, and whether there are potential weaknesses given the study design. These limitations are particularly important when considering comorbidities and attempting to assess their impact.

SOURCES OF DATA AND TOOLS

Now that we recognize the role and the need for information about the natural course of illness and treatment, where can we find the information that we need? A reasonable place to begin any scientific inquiry is the literature and it is important to examine the standard clinical, epidemiological and social science literatures. Although not prominent in the mind of many pharmacovigilance professionals, we are often given hints from disparate sources that suggest additional details that might be relevant to the issue under study. The literature may also help guide the researcher to other articles, data sources or experts for further work. Beware however, that although "comorbidity" is a MeSH term, there is no equivalent for "disease natural history".

Population-based studies are perhaps the most difficult but useful of all samples. These studies are undertaken in a population usually defined by geographic boundaries and has reasonable certainty for capturing any critical data of interest for that population. Perhaps the most well-known population-based resource is the Rochester Epidemiology Project, housed at the Mayo Clinic (Melton, 1996). The Rochester Epidemiology Project has a unique medical records linkage system that provides comprehensive capture of all care delivered to residents of Rochester and Olmsted County, Minnesota. Any medical care delivered to a resident of the county is reflected in their unique medical dossier and is available for research, which has produced over 900 publications since its organization in 1966. Olmsted County is one of the few places in the world where the occurrence and natural history of diseases can be accurately described and analyzed in a defined population for a half century or more.

Longitudinal study data are the key source of information to any researcher, particularly in pharmacovigilance. Virtually impossible to obtain, they do exist, mostly as longitudinal records of the subjects' interactions with the medical care system as in medical claims data or clinical databases. Some are population-based (i.e. the Rochester Epidemiology Project, Scandinavian registries), others represent stable clinical populations (i.e. the General Practice Research Database (GPRD)), while others are only as longitudinal as the subject's fiscal coverage of a particular reimbursement (i.e. a particular Health Maintenance Organization, Medicaid). Many longitudinal studies have been undertaken with a principal disease target (i.e. Atherosclerosis Risk in Communities, MONICA) or a general group under study (e.g. the Nurse's Health Study); however, in the course of the conduct of the study, other disorders are captured. Framingham stands as an example of a population-based longitudinal cohort that regularly screens their subjects for signs, symptoms and social factors to help us assemble a picture of disease natural history although it does not capture medical care interactions throughout the follow-up period. The popularity of the disease registry as a method for collecting natural history data is a testament to the power and utility of these data.

Such studies provide a rich resource of information in this field either through extant publications or through additional exploration of the data. The US government, as well as other governments, routinely undertake population studies and make the data available to the public for further analyses. One need only visit any country's center for health or population statistics website to see the extent of the data available. One of the more interesting and valuable of these is the National Health and Nutrition Examination Survey (NHANES) which every decade in the United States provides us with rich data on disease prevalence (incidence if you use the follow-up data), comorbidity, test results which allow the researcher to identify clinically detected and undetected cases of disease because of its capture of signs and symptoms as well as diagnoses (Mannino *et al.*, 2000). Data on hospitalizations, outpatient visits, surgical procedures and more are often available. The Food and Drug Administration uses these data to generate the "expected rates" of illness (La Grenade *et al.*, 2000). Even

long-term simplified trials that have become the mainstay of cardiovascular disease, can offer insight into the natural history of disease.

With the computerization of medical care, enormous aggregates of patient-level data have become available. Whether based on clinical encounters with a general practitioner (i.e. GPRD, MediPlus) or the claims from the encounter used in billing (most managed care databases, Medicare, Medicaid), much about practitioner recognized and treated disease can be understood. Analysis is also facilitated by the computerized nature of the data. The reader is referred to Chapters 30–32 in this same volume for more discussion about these resources.

CLINICAL TRIALS AND OBSERVATIONAL DATA

Clinical trials themselves provide some opportunity to effectively screen at baseline and follow any number of comorbid conditions and gain a brief snapshot of the history of the disease. However, clinical trials by design seek relatively uncomplicated patients, randomize them to a medication, and capture information from the beginning of their medication "trial". If we really want to be able to compare the impact of an intervention based on clinical trials and observational data, we must identify an incident or inception cohort, i.e. a cohort of patients at a definitive point in the course of their illness that can be reliably identified across all patients or at the point of their initial intervention.

Observational data can produce a sense of the real spectrum of disease and provide a clinical context for the "clean" patients normally enrolled in a clinical trial program. This will aid in the anticipation of adverse event issues and may help direct product labeling. However, it does put additional demands on any observational data source but is consonant with the goal of true characterization of the users of the medication. It is not uncommon for the initial users of a new therapy to be those who have failed on a currently available therapy. This is especially true when a new therapy is initially promoted as "safer": clinicians are then motivated to place all their more problematic treatment failures, or those who have suffered side-effects, on the new therapy. These patients invariably have more complicated clinical histories and by capturing information from the true beginning of therapy, one is able to better ascertain earlier periods of risk that may be associated with the medication (including other risk factors that may be modified by the new medication) that may not be obvious in a cross-sectional approach.

Longitudinal data are critical to the planning and interpretation of clinical trials as it would be foolhardy to design a trial whose length is too short to detect the events of interest or is under-powered for lack of information about the frequency of an outcome. It would be difficult to design a clinical trial in asthma with the intent of reducing Emergency Department (ER) admissions if the trialists had little insight into how frequently ER visits occur or how to at least identify the characteristics of the patients who do use the ER most frequently for their asthma. Disease natural history is critical to determine the appropriateness and effectiveness of clinical interventions, especially for those illnesses whose measures of treatment effect are unclear. Research from the Rochester Epidemiology Project illustrates this point well in work on benign prostatic hypertrophy (Guess et al., 1995), again pointing to the relative value of the data and the data source.

For all of the advantages offered by longitudinal data, there are some issues to be aware of especially when using clinical data. The issues are well described elsewhere (Stang, 1998; Strom, 2000); however, they bear brief mention here. Paramount among the concerns of the scientist using longitudinal or any data for that matter, is to understand why and how these data were collected. Data that derive from clinical practice or billing will only represent detected clinical illness and may not contain other factors that are useful in assessing risk (e.g. non-prescription drug use (OTC, street drugs, alcohol, smoking) or other medical disorders that may not be clearly or consistently captured in the data). The lack of capture may be due to how data are captured for a segment of care (hospitalizations for example) which may lack the necessary detail (as in the

aggregates of claims data) or rely on the practitioner to make a separate entry based on a referral letter (as in GPRD).

For many databases, it is also important to understand the reason why people are in the database and if that confers its own special risk. For instance, government entitlement programs (e.g. Medicaid) capture information on a population of relatively low socio-economic status which, as a comorbidity, confers its own risks. Eligibility is determined on a monthly basis so that one often finds an interrupted series of information about a given patient. Clinical databases, such as the GPRD and the Rochester Epidemiology Project, are based on the medical care provided to a relatively well-defined population, but again reflects their medical care and may capture some additional information about social and psychological risk factors. The reader is encouraged to explore the amassing literature on databases and their applications in this area.

An important feature that often eludes adequate study, in large part because of the paucity of longitudinal data, is the relevance and station of time in both the onset and progression of disease. Cancer and environmental epidemiologists have long studied the lag time between putative exposures and detection of disease. However, it is a difficult study when faced with charting the natural history of disease whose outcomes may take 15 or 20 years to present themselves. However, the importance of this information is critical as we strive to understand the risk, benefit and costs of treating the asymptomatic patient prior to the onset of any serious outcomes. In these instances we may rely on other study designs or case series to obtain information that may otherwise be difficult to find.

With longitudinal data come more complicated methodologies as time introduces a very complicated covariate. New techniques, such as data mining, are also being introduced more and more into the signal detection effort, which is expanding our knowledge in one respect while generating the need for more "context" in our effort to determine statistical from clinically meaningful patterns. Data mining is able to find relationships between factors that may have escaped our detection but these findings will still require a basis for evaluation.

THE APPLICATION OF LONGITUDINAL DISEASE NATURAL HISTORY DATA

The application of this information in the hands of a safety professional varies from the generation of expected rates of and time to events, development of risk prediction models based on the natural history, comorbidities and current therapy. The basis for the assessment of causality and strength of association is determining the expected rate of events in some referent population. Signal detection routines that depend on chi-square, Bayesian methods, or any number of suggested approaches depend largely on one's ability to detect a departure from the "expected" rate (Figure 8.3). Clinical trials and sample size calculations depend, to a large extent, on much the same information.

One only need look at the cardiovascular risk prediction models based on the Framingham data to see how powerful this information can be when properly applied. Not every safety professional needs to consider launching a Framingham study; however, accessing and integrating these data are time-consuming but very worthwhile endeavors.

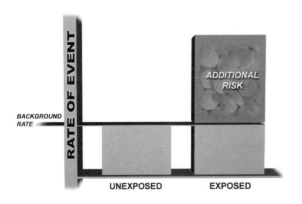

Figure 8.3. The role of "disease natural history" in determining background or expected rates so that proper determinations can be made for the risk attributable to a particular intervention.

But be warned that natural history data is a general representation of the course of an illness that can at best provide the user with probabilities of events that must be considered as a portion of the information necessary to determine the relationship between a potential adverse event and the intervention under scrutiny. It may provide some insight into the predisposition of some patients for an event or guide the pharmacovigilance professional in determining what additional data need to be aggressively sought to determine the role of a particular comorbidity or other risk factor for a given event.

Mapping of the natural history of disease can also be helpful in the interpretation and planning of clinical trials. As surrogate markers are used more frequently, it is important to understand the various pathways of illness and which path is reflected by a given surrogate (Fleming and DeMets, 1996) as regulators and scientists alike are becoming more and more skeptical of surrogates that are employed without full understanding of all the different pathways.

There are difficulties in ascribing causality in the face of reasonable doubt. Disease natural history information is intended to assure the scientist that she has considered the role and contribution of the disease context when evaluating cases or a series of cases. It is not intended to substitute or overwhelm other evidence for a given case. One cannot readily ascribe an event to the natural history of the illness in the face of a positive rechallenge, for instance, but can question whether the biological mechanism responsible for an event is explained more readily by the disease than by the pharmacology of the intervention.

How is it best to capture all of this information and present it in a useful format? We have worked on several ways, most of them graphical and in some ways dependent on the magic of the internet and hypertext linkage. Figure 8.2, for example, is one way that we display the relationship between disorders which can be annotated with actual data. We have found that graphical representations often make data accessible to more users. One can also use a decision-analytic modeling framework with branches and nodes that represent the different probabilities of treatment and outcome.

Finally, we have developed disease "maps" with a longitudinal pathway, comorbidities, probabilities of outcomes and hypertext linkage of data that allows the map to continue to be refined as new data become available. These "maps" look much like Figure 8.1. This approach has provided the most flexibility since any number of users with different perspectives can access the data and apply it to their need. For those who produce formal safety surveillance plans and risk assessment documents, it also facilitates storage and capture of the relevant information over repeated reviews of spontaneous and clinical data.

CONCLUSION

A keen understanding of the natural course of illness should be considered a critical component of any assessment of drug risk or benefit. Although a daunting task that does not lend itself to the rapid assessments that are often necessary, these data provide the critical context against which all events should be evaluated. The acquisition, integration and application of these data into the safety surveillance process require an ongoing commitment; however, the data can be continually referred to and elaborations made on different parts as the need arises or as data become available. These data can also be applied to other areas in the drug development and safety assessment areas.

Its important for the pharmacovigilance professional to have a good understanding of the natural course of an illness; otherwise he or she may well be blinded to the indication for therapy. It will take an investment in time and resource, but it will help you to understand what you don't know. By the same token, it is important to know what you don't know, but could.

REFERENCES

CIOMS Working Group IV (1998) *Benefit–Risk Balance for New Drugs: Evaluating Safety Signals.* Geneva: CIOMS.

Fleming TR, DeMets DL (1996) Surrogate end points in clinical trials: are we being misled? *Ann Intern Med* **125**: 605–13.

Fletcher RH, Fletcher SW, Wagner EH, eds (1996) *Clinical Epidemiology: The Essentials*, 3rd edn. Baltimore: Williams and Wilkins, Inc., pp. 112–13.

Guess HA, Jacobsen SJ, Girman CJ, *et al.* (1995) The role of community-based longitudinal studies in evaluating treatment effects. Example: benign prostatic hyperplasia. *Med Care* **33**: AS26–AS35.

Kessler RC (1994) The National Comorbidity Survey of the United States. *Int Rev Psychiatry* **6**: 365–76.

La Grenade LA, Kornegay C, Graham DJ (2000) Using publicly-available data to derive background rates when evaluating adverse drug reaction reports. *Pharmacoepidemiology and Drug Safety* **9**: S70–S71 (abstract).

Mannino DM, Gagnon RC, Petty TL, Lydick E (2000) Obstructive lung disease and low lung function in adults in the United States: data from the National Health and Nutrition Examination Survey, 1988–1994. *Arch Intern Med* **160**(11): 1683–9.

Melton LJ (1996) History of the Rochester Epidemiology Project. *Mayo Clin Proc* **71**: 266–74.

Sanders BS (1962) Have morbidity surveys been oversold? *Am J Publ Health* **52**: 1648–59.

Stang PE (1998) I hear the data singing: considerations when the siren calls. *New Med* **2**: 233–8.

Stang PE, Von Korff M (1994) The diagnosis of headache in primary care: factors in the agreement of clinical and standardized diagnosis. *Headache* **34**: 138–42.

Stang P, Von Korff M (1995) The stability of reported headache symptoms over time. In: Oleson J, ed., *Headache Classification and Epidemiology*. New York: Raven Press, pp. 45–9.

Sternfeld B, Stang P, Sidney S (1995) Relationship of migraine headaches to experience of chest pain and subsequent risk of myocardial infarction. *Neurology* **45**: 2135–42.

Strom BL, ed (2000) *Pharmacoepidemiology*, 3rd edn. New York: Wiley.

9

Responding to Signals

PATRICK C. WALLER AND PETER ARLETT

Post-Licensing Division, Medicines Control Agency, London, UK

INTRODUCTION

In this chapter we take a practical look at the handling of post-marketing drug safety issues. The process of handling such issues is shown in Figure 9.1 and this forms the basis on which this chapter is structured.

There may be differences in the way issues are handled, and in perceptions, depending on whether one is coming from a regulatory or industry perspective. However, in both cases the goal is to protect patients and the means of achieving this should coincide from both directions. The broad aims of pharmacovigilance personnel are that any medicine should be used as safely as possible and that, where necessary, steps should be taken to improve its safety and users informed promptly (Waller et al., 1996).

In order to meet the above aims, both regulatory authorities and companies need to identify safety issues proactively. With proper use of the systems available, many potential issues will be identified but only some of them will turn out to be real and/or important. Judgements will need to be made, sometimes based on limited information, as to whether there is an issue in need of attention. When this is considered to be the case, it will be necessary to investigate it by assembling all the

relevant evidence available and, sometimes, by designing specific new studies. Consideration will need to be given at an early stage to the possible outcomes and specifically as to how safety might be improved. The output of the process will usually be a risk–benefit analysis with proposals for changes in the recommendations for use of a medicine, withdrawal on safety grounds being relatively unusual (Jefferys et al., 1998). Communicating any necessary changes is a key issue in determining the effectiveness of the measures that are ultimately taken.

The first stage is the identification of a possible hazard. What you find depends on where and how

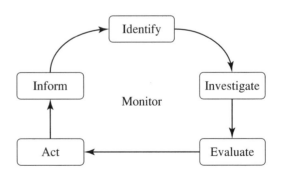

Figure 9.1. Process of handling a drug safety issue.

Pharmacovigilance. Edited by R.D. Mann and E.B. Andrews

you look, and this is our starting point for considering how to respond to a drug safety issue.

IDENTIFYING DRUG SAFETY ISSUES

Assessment of drug safety involves bringing together all the available information from multiple sources (Figure 9.2). It begins with the basic pharmacological and pre-clinical studies and should continue until the end of potential sequelae of marketing exposure, a period which may span many decades. Potentially important drug safety issues can be identified at any stage of drug development. In the post-marketing phase they are particularly likely to be identified in the first few years after marketing, although new issues also arise with long-established drugs. There are several reasons why important drug safety issues may not be detected until after marketing, and these are listed in Table 9.1.

In order to ensure that safety problems that have not been recognised or fully characterised pre-marketing are handled promptly, proactive processes are required for screening emerging data for potential issues. At the stage of initial identification, it is unusual for it to be clearcut that the hazard is drug-related and this has led to the concept of "signalling". Alternative terms that may be regarded as synonymous in this context are "alerting", "early warning" and "hypothesis-

Table 9.1. Reasons why drug safety issues may not be identified until the post-marketing period.

1. The adverse reaction is rare and therefore undetectable until a large number of patients have been exposed to the drug
2. There is a long latency between starting the drug and development of the adverse reaction
3. The drug has not been studied in normal clinical practice:
   - patients treated in clinical practice are likely to have different characteristics to trial patients (e.g. demography, other diseases, other medication);
   - in clinical practice a drug is less likely to be used strictly in accordance with the recommendations by both doctors and patients, and with less monitoring

generation". A signal is simply an alert from any available source that a drug may be associated with a previously unrecognised hazard or that a known hazard may be quantitatively (e.g. more frequent) or qualitatively (e.g. more serious) different from existing knowledge. Spontaneous adverse drug reaction (ADR) reporting is the classic signalling system and its major purpose is to provide early warnings of possible hazards. Indeed, a signal could be defined on the basis of single case reporting, although we prefer the broader concept indicated above. Other than spontaneous adverse reaction reporting, signals may come from studies of various types. The subsequent processes for assessment, investigation and possible action (see below) are required regardless of the type of data leading to identification of an issue.

SIGNALS: WHERE TO LOOK

Effective monitoring of drug safety requires a systematic approach in order to identify and use information from many sources, both published and unpublished, as it becomes available. The most important sources from which drug safety hazards may be identified post-marketing are summarised in Figure 9.2. These are the principal sources of information on adverse drug effects which need to be regularly monitored for new evidence which may contribute to knowledge of drug risks. Information from all these sources

- Pre-clinical studies
- Clinical trials
  – pre-and post-marketing
- Spontaneous adverse reaction reporting
  – national
  – international
- Epidemiological studies
  – case–control
  – cohort
- Data collected for other purposes
  – routine statistics
  – databases of prescriptions and outcomes

Figure 9.2. Principal sources of information on drug safety.

needs to be evaluated and used to build a picture of the safety profile of drugs on a continuous basis. There are now many drug safety bulletins published, for example by regulatory authorities and the World Health Organisation. These and other published sources need to be screened systematically and as carefully as any other data source by those involved in drug safety monitoring.

Whilst the utility of spontaneous ADR reporting schemes and formal studies in the identification of drug safety issues is well-established, the use of databases containing prescriptions and outcomes, and disease registries for generating signals have been under-utilised. Such databases can be screened for single cases of disorders likely to be drug-induced. Alternatively, when adequate usage data are available, the frequencies of associations between drugs and medical events can be examined for differences from expected values. These methods might be able to detect signals missed by other approaches, and are likely to be developed and used more in the future.

SIGNALS: WHAT TO LOOK FOR

Identifying signals is a selective process based on the apparent strength of the evidence and the potential importance of association. In practice, a signal is something that, if found to be drug-related, would be considered clinically important and might impact on patient management or the balance of benefits and risks. What to look for depends on the type of data being used, which can be broadly divided into data from spontaneous reporting or from formal studies. Both types of data may be published or unpublished.

Spontaneous ADR reporting data

The commonest source for identification of significant drug safety concerns arising with marketed medicines is spontaneous suspected adverse reaction reporting. These are individual case reports from health professionals (and, in some countries, consumers) of adverse events which the reporter considers *may* be related to the drug or drugs being taken. Reporters are not asked to provide all adverse events that follow drug administration but to selectively report those that they suspect were adverse reactions. There may be several reasons why a reporter suspects a drug may have caused an adverse reaction, and these are summarised in Table 9.2. None of these factors on their own (apart from the need for drug administration to precede the suspected adverse reaction) is essential in leading to suspicion of a causal association, but the more that apply, the greater suspicion is likely to be. Greater suspicion does not invariably lead to greater likelihood of reporting since knowledge of a mechanism and the effects of similar drugs may deter reporting.

One common feature to all spontaneous ADR reporting systems is under-reporting. The possible reasons why an adverse reaction may not be reported are well-recognised : the "seven deadly sins" (Inman and Weber, 1986). It is less clear which factors are, in practice, the most important, and this may vary between countries and over time. A figure of 10% of ADRs being reported has often been quoted but the reality is likely to be that

Table 9.2. Reasons for suspecting a relationship between a drug and an adverse event.

Reason	Requirement
Temporal association	Plausible temporal relationship between taking the drug and development of the possible adverse effect
Dechallenge	Relationship between discontinuation of the drug and abatement of the possible adverse effect
Dose–response	Relationship between dose and severity of the possible adverse effect
Rechallenge	Recurrence of the possible adverse effect with re-introduction of the drug
Mechanism	Pharmacological or toxicological basis for an adverse effect
Class effect	Knowledge that a similar drug or class of drugs produces this adverse effect
Absence of alternatives	Lack of another explanation (e.g. other drugs and diseases) for the possible adverse effect

the level of under-reporting is probably highly variable according to many factors, the most well-recognised being as follows: (1) seriousness of the reaction, (2) novelty of the drug, and (3) whether or not the effect is recognised and has been publicised. It is clear that appropriate feedback to reporters and specific measures to encourage reporting are an essential element of an effective scheme. The latter comes into three categories as follows: (1) promotion of the scheme, (2) facilitation of reporting, and (3) education about drug safety and the benefits of ADR reporting.

Inherent in any spontaneous adverse reaction reporting system is a monitoring process that recognises the dynamic nature of data. A prerequisite for an effective system is a database from which data can be retrieved in a format useful for screening. Regular and systematic review of what is new on the database in the context of what was there previously is needed. Usually this is done by reviewing all the data for individual drugs or products looking for reactions of potential concern. However, an alternative approach is to bring together all the data for a particular ADR and review the drugs that have been suspected of producing the reaction and the numbers of cases. This approach is likely to be more useful to regulatory authorities than companies because they can cover all marketed medicines.

Spontaneous reporting systems exist throughout the developed world and in some developing countries. The World Health Organisation maintains a database of worldwide spontaneous reports in Sweden (Uppsala Monitoring Centre, 1998). Screening of spontaneous ADR data needs to be performed on both a national and an international basis, and there should be a worldwide perspective to this function. Companies have to collate worldwide data for their products in order to meet statutory obligations for ADR reporting and periodic safety updates.

Utilising Spontaneous Reporting Data

In the context of spontaneous reporting, a signal is normally a series of cases of similar suspected adverse reactions reported by health professionals associated with a particular drug. A single case is not usually sufficient (Edwards *et al.*, 1990). When the ADR is a disease which is rare in the general population (e.g. aplastic anaemia, toxic epidermal necrolysis), a small number of cases associated with a single drug is unlikely to be a chance phenomenon (Bégaud *et al.*, 1994), even if the drug has been used quite widely. In this situation three cases may be considered a signal and five cases a strong signal. An illustration of this point based on conditions that might apply for aplastic anaemia is given in Figure 9.3. Even if all the cases occurring in users were reported, the maximum number of cases that could be accepted as coincidental under the conditions shown is two.

The level of drug usage is important in assessing the likely order of magnitude of frequency. However, as illustrated in Figure 9.3, it is not necessarily critical in determining whether or not there is a signal that needs to be evaluated. Likewise, the strength of evidence for the individual cases will be important to consider later but, initially, the key issue is whether or not there is an "unexpected" number of cases. If the event is common in the general population, then a large number of cases would be needed to raise a signal but calculations of the type shown in Figure 9.3 cannot be applied. A judgement has to be made from all the information available which depends more on the apparent strength of the evidence than the number of reported cases.

A number of comparative methods are available for using spontaneous reporting data to generate signals. Calculating reporting rates based on usage

---

Assumptions (based on aplastic anaemia)

- Background frequency 6 per million per year
- 100% of cases reported
- 300 000 users for 3 months
- significance level cut-off 5%

Maximum number of reported cases that could be accepted as coincidental = 2

▶ 3 reported cases is a signal if the background frequency is rare

---

Figure 9.3. Numbers of cases needed to generate a signal.

denominator data (Speirs, 1986), either as pre-scriptions dispensed or defined daily doses, may enable a signal of an increased frequency of a particular ADR in comparison with alternative treatments to be derived. All spontaneous ADR reporting schemes are subject to a variable and unknown degree of under-reporting, which means that such comparisons are crude. They need to be interpreted carefully, particularly if the drugs being compared have been marketed for different indications or durations, or if there has been significant publicity about the adverse effects of one of the drugs.

The other principal approach for making comparisons between drugs is to use the propor-tions of all ADRs for a particular drug that are within a particular organ system class of reactions (e.g. gastrointestinal or cutaneous). This is known as profiling (Inman and Weber, 1986), a method that has an advantage over reporting rates in that it is independent of the level of usage. The data may easily be displayed graphically as adverse reaction profiles (Figure 9.4).

Related mathematical approaches have also been developed, involving calculation of odds ratios and confidence intervals from 2×2 tables which compare the proportion of all ADRs for a particular drug that are the ADR of interest against the analogous proportion across all drugs

in the database (Egberts *et al.*, 1997). These may be termed proportional reporting ratios (PRRs) (Evans *et al.*, 2001) and used as one indication of the strength of a signal. The associated statistical significance is calculated by the chi-squared test and criteria may be set for automatic signal generation, for example a PRR greater than 3, chi-squared greater than 5 and at least three cases (Figure 9.5). An alternative approach which uses Bayesian methods in a "neural network" has been developed by the World Health Organisation (Bate *et al.*, 1998). The mathematical nature of these approaches should not be used to obscure the inherent nature of the data and limitations in respect of determining causality.

Drugs are authorised and used differently across the world and even in neighbouring countries there are often major differences in clinical practice and labelling which may impact on ADR reporting. Whilst it reasonable to review, for example, the number of cases of a possible reaction reported worldwide in the context of worldwide sales data, it should be recognised that the above differences and varying patterns of reporting across countries limit this approach. One approach to dealing with this is to focus particularly on the source of the greatest number of cases and to attempt to identify why it may have emerged from that source.

Formal Studies

Although formal studies of drug safety have a particular place in the investigation of signals generated by methods such as spontaneous ADR reporting (i.e. hypothesis-testing), they may also

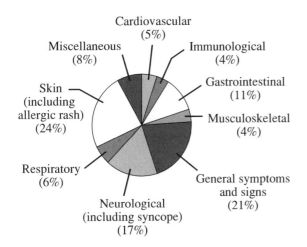

Figure 9.4. Adverse reaction reporting profile for Measles/Rubella vaccine.

	Rifabutin	All other drugs
Uveitis	41	754
All other ADRs	14	591 958

Proportion of rifabutin uveitis ADRs = 0.75
Proportion for all other drugs = 0.0013
PRR = 586 ; chi-squared = 22 740

Figure 9.5. Use of proportional reporting ratios (PRRs) for signal generation.

provide the initial evidence producing a drug safety concern. Such studies often start with efficacy rather than safety as the primary objective but, if they have the potential to provide new safety data, it is important that the emerging evidence is kept under regular review. In particular, it is vital to maximise the potential of studies to identify adverse effects, particularly if they are to expose large numbers of patients relative to exposure in previous studies. This should be achieved by ensuring that the design, methods and analyses facilitate safety assessment (e.g. by including comparator groups and measuring important outcomes) and by monitoring the data using a sequential approach which is specified in advance. In a randomised double-blind study, a safety monitoring group with access to the codes but no direct contact with investigators or other study personnel is essential. An analogous group is also desirable in open studies. It is important to define in advance the criteria that would lead to actions such as stopping the trial. If unexpected cases of an adverse outcome occur, these need to be evaluated both individually and in the context of the frequencies in the different exposure groups. The advantages of the trial design (e.g. control groups, known denominators) and a statistical analysis should be fully utilised in judging whether or not a signal is present, and in assessing the likelihood of a causal association.

PROCESSES FOR IDENTIFYING DRUG SAFETY HAZARDS

In order to undertake the systematic approach to drug safety monitoring described above, systems and processes must be established to ensure that all the necessary information is brought together at a single point. For pharmaceutical companies this is recognised in European legislation through the establishment of a requirement for a qualified person for pharmacovigilance. Likewise, regulatory authorities now have clear obligations to transmit data to companies and other authorities. Within a pharmaceutical company or regulatory authority there may be several groups dealing with data that are relevant to drug safety. Links between groups handling pre-clinical studies, clinical trials and

pharmacovigilance data are needed, and effective communication between such groups is essential. Functional drug safety groups that review all safety data generated internally or externally are required to avoid issues being overlooked. Drugs or groups of drugs should have individuals assigned (physicians, pharmacists, scientists) who have a particular interest in the field and who take prime responsibility for reviewing emerging information and undertaking initial assessments.

Any group involved in drug safety should aim to identify an emerging signal rapidly. Once an issue has been identified, information about it may be disseminated in many ways. It is important for both regulatory authorities and companies to be prepared to evaluate and manage issues regardless of the original source. Once a signal has been identified from any source the next step is to perform an initial assessment. This process is described in the next section.

INITIAL ASSESSMENT

The main purpose of the initial assessment is to make a decision regarding whether or not the possible hazard requires further investigation. The key principles of the initial assessment are to review the strength of the evidence which indicates a possible drug-related hazard, consider how that evidence can be extended (e.g. by further analyses) and to consider the other evidence that is immediately available which may help to support or refute the hypothesis. There are four key issues that will determine whether or not a signal should be investigated further, as signified by the acronym "SNIP":

1. the *strength* of the signal;
2. whether or not the issue or some aspect of it is *new*;
3. the clinical *importance* as judged by the seriousness of the reaction and severity of the cases; and
4. the *potential* for preventive measures.

The main factors influencing the assessment vary depending on the source of the signal and, in particular, whether it derives from spontaneous reporting or from a formal study.

SIGNALS DERIVED FROM SPONTANEOUS REPORTING

In many cases the initial signal will consist of a case series of similar adverse reactions occurring with a particular medicine. The principal factors that need to be taken into account in the assessment of such signals are given in Table 9.3. Broadly this consists of the details of the cases themselves and other evidence which may provide insights into the issue.

The cases producing the signal need to be reviewed individually. Evidence for causality in individual cases can be assessed by a number of methods (Meyboom *et al.*, 1997; Edwards and Aronson, 2000). At this stage further information

Table 9.3. Factors influencing the initial assessment of a possible hazard arising from a case series.

Evidence to be considered	Underlying issue
1. The cases producing the signal Individual case assessment: temporality, effect of dechallenge/rechallenge, alternative causes (see Table 9.2)	Causality
Quality of the information regarding cases	Documentation
Number of cases in relation to usage of the medicine	Frequency/reporting rate
Severity of the reactions	Implications for patients
Seriousness of the hazard	and public health
2. Other evidence Pharmacological or toxicological effects of the drug	Mechanism
Known effects of other drugs in the class	Possible class effect
Pre-clinical studies	Existence of other evidence which may
Clinical trials	support or refute the
Epidemiological studies	signal

on the cases may need to be obtained but may take some time to gather. This does not, however, preclude an initial view as to whether the problem warrants further evaluation. A large number of poorly documented cases of an adverse reaction which has important consequences for users (e.g. because they are serious and/or potentially preventable) will at least warrant consideration of other evidence whilst further information is being obtained. However, the greater the number of cases in relation to usage and the better documented they are, the greater will be the need to investigate the problem fully. It is important to establish a case definition and to clearly identify those cases which may provide reasonable evidence of a drug-related hazard (the cardinal cases). A view of the case series as a whole should be formed in addition to assessments of the individual cases. Depending on the quality of data, the same number of spontaneous reports and the same level of usage may provide good or poor evidence of a hazard. The key difference is often whether or not there are frequent alternative causes (these are often called "confounding factors").

Consideration of Alternative Causes

Table 9.4 lists the explanations other than a causal relation between suspect drug and event which need to be considered. The most common alternative causes are concomitant medication and co-existing disease. In the first case, the adverse event is a reaction to a drug and the issue is which drug is implicated, or sometimes whether there might be an interaction between two drugs. A common

Table 9.4. Possible explanations for a reported ADR other than a causal relationship between suspect drug and the adverse event.

1. Related to medication
   (a) Single other drug—recognised cause
   (b) Single other drug—unrecognised cause
   (c) Combination of drugs (may include suspect drug)

2. Not an ADR
   (a) Coexisting disease unrelated to indication for suspect drug
   (b) Complication of indication for suspect drug

situation is that there is an alternative explanation because the patient was concomitantly exposed to a drug which is recognised to cause the adverse reaction in question. An example might be a patient with schizophrenia taking chlorpromazine who is also given a new antipsychotic drug and develops hepatitis. The reporter may suspect either drug or both, but is much more likely to report it if the new drug is suspected. Clearly, such a case of suspected hepatitis due to the new drug may not have been caused by it but there are several reasons why it might have been reported. In some cases the reporter will have been unaware of the recognised adverse reaction or the reporter may have had good reasons (perhaps relating to the temporal relationships of drug administration and the reaction, or response to dechallenge) for suspecting that the new drug is implicated.

The situation where the patient has been taking two or more medicines, none of which is recognised to produce the suspected adverse reaction, is also common. Only one drug may be suspect— often because the event occurred shortly after its initial administration or because the drug is new— but sometimes all the drugs are listed as suspect. In these circumstances it may be possible to form a view of the most likely cause or combination of causes, based on pharmacology, temporality and dechallenge. However, often no clear judgement can be made and formal studies are needed. This is particularly likely when patients start taking multiple drugs simultaneously as in highly-active anti-retroviral therapy.

Possible interactions are often particularly difficult to interpret when the signal arises from spontaneous reporting. The number of cases is usually very small and a watching brief would usually be an appropriate initial response in the absence of one or more of the following circumstances: (1) there are several plausible cases; (2) the reported cases provide objective evidence of interaction (e.g. repeated laboratory measurements during periods of single and dual drug exposure); (3) there is a plausible mechanism based on the known pharmacokinetics and pharmacodynamics of the drugs which has not yet been investigated in formal interaction studies (in which case such studies should be initiated); or (4) the

drug has a narrow therapeutic index and the suspected adverse reactions reported are serious.

Often the major alternative explanation for one or more suspected ADR reports is that the event was not an ADR but was a naturally occurring disease which may or may not be related to the indication for the suspected drug. Since most ADRs are similar to diseases that occur naturally (a notable exception is fibrosing colonopathy with high-strength pancreatic enzymes (Smyth *et al.*, 1995)), this explanation almost always requires consideration. A recent example for which the possible roles of drugs and underlying diseases is still not resolved is the occurrence of lipodystrophy and various metabolic abnormalities in patients treated for HIV infection.

Two important factors to take into account are the rarity of the disease in the population and whether or not the disease is related to any intercurrent illness, including the indication for the suspect drug. A series of cases of a rare disease occurring in relation to exposure to a particular drug is much stronger evidence of an association than a similar series of cases of a common disease. This does not mean that drugs are less likely to cause common diseases but that such associations are harder to detect. When the suspected adverse drug reaction is a complication of the underlying disease for which that drug was given, spontaneous reporting is likely to be unhelpful. Whilst it is possible that a drug may increase the risk of the complication developing (e.g. re-perfusion arrhythmias with streptokinase), data from a formal study measuring risk are almost invariably required in order make a satisfactory judgement about the issue.

In some of the circumstances described above, information derived from a series of cases is, by its nature, unsuited for making the necessary judgements. In this situation the possible implications for public health and the other evidence listed in section 2 of Table 9.3 are the key factors in determining whether and how to progress the issue. If the cases are scanty and most are associated with reasonable alternative explanations, a watching brief is likely to be the most appropriate course. At the other extreme, a well-documented series of cases of a particular suspected ADR without obvious alternative explanation and/or with evidence of a possible mechanism should rapidly lead to consideration of both what further investigation may be warranted, and what action is needed to minimise the risks. Many issues come between these extremes and require careful consideration of evidence from various sources and of the possible ways in which the issue might be investigated further.

SIGNALS DERIVED FROM FORMAL STUDIES

There are many possible sources from which drug safety issues may arise (see above). Those that do not come from reporting of individual case reports derive from formal studies, usually either a clinical trial or an epidemiological study. However, occasionally new safety issues may arise with a marketed medicine as a result of pre-clinical (i.e. animal) data, examples being the possible carcinogenicity of carbaryl (Calman *et al.*, 1995) and danthron (Committee on Safety of Medicines/Medicines Control Agency, 2000), or human volunteer work (e.g. interaction studies).

Signals derived from studies have the potential to be stronger than those derived from spontaneous reporting. This is because the design and analysis of the study may enable much better judgements about causality and frequency to be made (e.g. in the case of randomised, double-blind trials). However, at the stage of initial assessment there is often only one study available and, even if this has a strong design and apparently clear findings there is no certainty that it is providing the correct answer. Examples of formal studies with findings that seem likely to be false positives include those associating selegiline with increased mortality (Lees, 1995), and neonatal vitamin K with childhood cancer (von Kries, 1998).

The underlying issues listed in Table 9.3 are also pertinent to the assessment of signals derived from a formal study. The frequency of the relevant event is likely to be a triggering factor in that a greater frequency of the event relative to a comparator (either an alternative treatment or no active treatment) usually constitutes the signal. The assessment of increased risk depends on the quality of the study design and the statistical power of the analysis. Causality may be established by exclusion of three major causes of false positive findings—chance, bias and confounding. The strength of the evidence for causality is a key consideration for an initial assessment. The assessment of causality based on data from formal studies is summarised in Table 9.5. Finally, consideration must be given to the implications for patients and public health, taking particular account of the severity, seriousness and frequency of the outcome in the context of the disease for which the study is used to treat.

Bias and Confounding

There are many types of bias which may affect the results of clinical trials and epidemiological studies. Bias is a systematic distortion of the

Table 9.5. Assessment of causality based on formal studies.

Possible explanation	Key evidence to be considered
Chance	Levels of statistical significance and power of study Whether or not there was a prior hypothesis How many tests were performed?
Bias	Study design—how were patients allocated to treatments? How were the data on outcomes collected?
Confounding	What factors other than drug treatments could explain differences between groups? What steps have been taken to control for confounding in the design or analysis?
Causal	Extent to which chance, bias and confounding have been excluded as alternative explanations Availability of evidence from other sources which may support an association or explain it (e.g. a mechanism)

findings by a specific factor and does not imply deliberate manipulation by the investigator (i.e. fraud). An example of bias is recall bias in case–control studies. Cases with a disease are often much more likely to recall exposures which may have led to their illness than controls who are not ill. Such a bias could be overcome by using an objective record of whether or not the patients were exposed, if available.

In general, clinical trials are less prone to bias because they tend to incorporate particular design features (e.g. prospective random allocation to treatments and double-blinding) for this purpose. Epidemiological studies observe patients treated in the "real world" and the possibility of bias is ever present (Collet and Boivin, 2000). Nevertheless such studies are important because (a) some issues cannot, in practice, be studied by controlled trials; (b) bias can often be eliminated or minimised; and (c) "real world" data are more generally applicable than those derived from clinical trials.

A confounder in an epidemiological study is a factor that is related to both the outcome and exposure of interest. An example of a confounder is smoking, which is related to both use of the oral contraceptive (OC) pill (smokers are more likely to use the pill than non-smokers) and an adverse outcome for which OCs may increase the risk (myocardial infarction). In a study of myocardial infarction and oral contraceptive use it is essential to measure smoking status and to attempt to control for it. A study that did not do this could provide only weak evidence of a causal association between OC use and myocardial infarction since an increased risk in OC users could simply be a consequence of smoking. Confounding can be controlled for in two broad ways—in the design by matching (ensuring through selection that cases and controls are similar for specified variables) or in the analysis by statistical adjustment of the data to account for any imbalances between groups which could impact on the results. When data have been adjusted for confounders it is important to take into account both the crude (i.e. unadjusted data) and the adjusted risks, but usually greater weight should be placed on the latter.

Overall Assessment

The overall assessment of causality depends on the extent to which alternative explanations have been excluded and also on the availability of other supporting evidence. Formal criteria for causality assessment such as those described by Hill (1965) are often hard to apply at the stage of the initial assessment. However, it may be possible to bring all the evidence from clinical trials or epidemiological studies together in a formal meta-analysis (Berlin, 2000). This will indicate the overall strength of the evidence for or against a causal association and the likely magnitude of the risk. Meta-analysis is an increasingly used and valuable technique that is well-established in the field of randomised clinical trials but more controversial for epidemiological studies. When evaluating any meta-analysis, it is important to consider whether all the available evidence has been included, the quality of that evidence, and whether there is significant heterogeneity between study populations which may limit the overall conclusions that can be drawn.

Signals arising from studies can sometimes be supported by data from spontaneous ADR reporting. Although the primary purpose is to provide signals, spontaneous reporting data can also be used for hypothesis-strengthening and, in particular, for identifying risk factors in ordinary practice. If there are already a substantial number of cases, then the issue should have already been signalled, but sometimes signals are missed or considered unassessable. Most signals derived from studies lead to a review of the available spontaneous reporting data although absence, or near absence, of cases cannot be considered to strongly refute a signal. This is because spontaneous reporting systems may fail to signal some drug safety hazards.

The final step in the initial assessment is to consider the way forward. The key decision is whether to simply keep a watching brief or to proactively gather further evidence. The overall strength of the evidence for a hazard and its potential implications for the balance of risks and benefits are the principal factors that should underpin this decision. The process of further investigation is described in the next section.

FURTHER INVESTIGATION

When the initial assessment has indicated that there is sufficient evidence of concern to warrant further investigation, detailed consideration should be given to the most appropriate means of resolving the outstanding issues. There is no standard recipe for this process because every issue is different. The factors that are most likely to require clarification relate to causality, mechanism, frequency and preventability. Assessment of these issues may require new formal studies, but the hypothesis may be strengthened or weakened using immediately available sources of retrospective information such as epidemiological databases (Wood and Waller, 1996) (see below).

The principal epidemiological databases that are used for drug safety purposes are shown in Table 9.6. These databases have the potential to provide rapid answers to important questions, facilitating immediate risk management and the design process of definitive studies. Their individual strengths, limitations and overall utility have been well summarised by Strom (2000).

To address the key factors listed above may require laboratory, clinical or epidemiological studies. Detailed consideration of the first two are beyond the scope of this chapter, but we will consider the principles underlying the epidemiological approach in some detail.

Table 9.6. Principal databases used for drug safety studies.

Country	Database
United Kingdom	General Practice Research Database
	Medicines Monitoring Unit—Tayside
	Prescription–Event Monitoring (DSRU)
	MediPlus (formerly AAH Meditel)
Netherlands	Pharmo
Italy	Friuli-Venezia Giulia
Germany	MediPlus
United States	Puget Sound
	Medicare
	Medicaid
Canada	Saskatchewan

EPIDEMIOLOGICAL STUDIES OF DRUG SAFETY

The basic elements necessary for an epidemiological study of drug safety are: (1) a record of drug exposure; (2) a record of outcomes; and (3) access to detailed medical information about individual cases. The first two elements may be held in the same database (as in the UK General Practice Research Database) or in separate databases which are "record-linked". The key element of record linkage is the cross-identification of individuals in both databases so that exposures and outcomes are linked for individual patients (Figure 9.6). This is exemplified in the Medicines Monitoring Unit (MEMO) system based in Tayside, UK, where completely separate databases of encashed prescriptions and hospital discharge records are linked through a unique identifier known as the Community Health Index number (Evans and MacDonald, 2000).

Even though no source of data is perfect, the quality and accuracy of the data are important considerations when setting up an investigation. The effect of random inaccuracies in the data will be a tendency to underestimate a true association. Inaccuracies in the data would generally have to be very marked to cause a true association to be completely missed, but the practical problem is that they might produce sufficient dilution of the association to lead to an uncertain result. Data inaccuracies will only explain an apparent positive

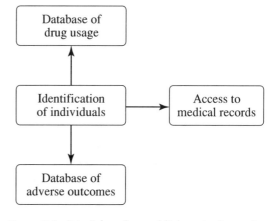

Figure 9.6. Principles of record linkage in drug safety.

association if they are gross or if systematic bias is present. A modest degree of inaccuracy in the data is unlikely to produce a positive finding when no such association exists.

Drug Exposure Data

The record of drug exposure in epidemiological studies is invariably imperfect. In the General Practice Research Database (GPRD) it is a record that a prescription was issued by a doctor. In the MEMO scheme it is a record that the prescription was encashed, which is likely to be substantially preferable. In a study in Tayside, UK, up to 15% of patients did not cash the prescription issued (Beardon *et al.*, 1993). However, in neither case is their any certainty that the patient consumed the prescribed medicine as intended (Sackett *et al.*, 1986)—this can only be assessed by interviewing subjects or by monitoring compliance. The interview approach has some advantages (for example, it can be applied to non-prescription medicines), but because patients are generally not precise observers of their own behaviour, it is not necessarily more accurate than a prescription record. Furthermore, such data are potentially subject to systematic biases, notably recall bias (see above for explanation).

Outcome Data

Similar issues arise regarding the quality and accuracy of the outcome data. It is usually considered necessary to verify outcomes held on a computer record by reviewing the medical records. This will eliminate basic data entry errors and, to an extent depending on the outcome being studied and the diagnostic criteria used, improve the accuracy of the outcome data. It may also allow the time of onset of the disease to be clarified (it is important to know whether or not cases are "incident", i.e. new) and better measurement of potential confounders. However, it should be recognised that there is also a disadvantage inherent in this process, which is that selection of the best-documented cases is being practised. There is therefore potential for selection bias and the incidence of the outcome is

likely to be underestimated. It has been argued that these disadvantages may outweigh the benefits of case validation (Evans and Mac-Donald, 1997) and this is an issue that needs further research.

Selective Use

A particular issue that arises in the design and interpretation of many epidemiological studies of drug safety relates to whether or not the drug of interest is being used selectively in patients who have different characteristics to those using comparators. It is well-recognised that this is a common occurrence and that it may in part relate to marketing strategies. For example, claims that a non-steroidal anti-inflammatory drug has less gastrointestinal toxicity than others may lead to it being selectively used in patients with a history of such problems, a phenomenon known as channelling (Petri and Urquhart, 1991). The result in an observational study is that such a drug will apparently be associated with a higher risk of gastrointestinal toxicity than comparators. This is called "confounding by indication". It is analogous to an imbalance at baseline in a randomised trial. The most satisfactory way to deal with this problem is by adjustment for the relevant risk factors, but this is not always feasible, leading to difficulties in data interpretation.

Use of Computerised Databases

For reasons of cost and speed, epidemiological studies of drug safety are increasingly being based on data from computerised databases that have primarily been collected for another purpose (Jick *et al.*, 1991). Use of the databases listed in Table 9.6 has demonstrated the potential of this approach in the investigation of a wide range of drug safety issues. Both major types of epidemiological study design have been used, i.e. cohort and case–control designs.

In a cohort design, a defined population is followed forwards in time and the incidence of the outcome in question is measured and compared in individuals exposed or not-exposed to the drug of interest. Both absolute and relative risks can be measured using this approach.

In a case–control design, cases of the outcome of interest are identified along with a group of controls drawn from the same population who do not have the outcome. Prior exposure to the drug(s) of interest is then compared in cases and controls. These studies provide measures of relative risk in the form of odds ratios but they do not directly measure absolute risks. A further approach is for a case–control study to be "nested" within a cohort design. This method has the advantages of both approaches, particularly if it used used to facilitate more detailed control of potential confounding than can be achieved in a complete cohort.

INITIATING NEW STUDIES

Study design is a key issue when initiating a new study for the specific purpose of further investigating a drug safety issue (i.e. hypothesis-testing). Important specific issues which should be addressed are: (1) clear specification of the hypothesis to be tested; (2) achieving adequate statistical power to detect as significant clinically important risks compared with those attributable to therapeutic alternatives (a power calculation should always be performed); (3) minimisation of bias (primarily through processes for selecting subjects and collecting exposure and outcome data); and (4) control of confounding in the design (by matching) or analysis (by adjustment, normally using multivariate statistical techniques).

In addition to study design there are many logistic issues to be addressed regarding the processes for assuring the quality of the data and the validity of the study. Particular consideration should be given to potential ethical issues and to how the data are going to be monitored if the study is prospective. The guidelines cited above encourage pharmaceutical companies to set up independent advisory boards to oversee such studies. Advisory boards are now becoming the norm for most studies that are relevant to drug safety.

UTILISING THE DATA

When new data become available from purpose-designed studies it is important that they are reviewed in the context of the existing data. An assessment should be made as to whether and how the new evidence changes the previous evaluation, focusing particularly on the strength of the evidence for a drug-related association and possible approaches to prevention. In the latter respect, detailed analysis of the data to identify possible risk factors for the hazard is important. Suppose that a rare hazard has been identified along with several risk factors. It may well be that the benefits of the medicine are clearly sufficient to outweigh the hazard overall but not in particular individuals with risk factors for the outcome. An example of this would be venous thromboembolism (VTE) with hormone replacement therapy (HRT). The risk of VTE is two to three times greater in users than non-users of HRT (Castellsague et al., 1998), i.e. there is an increased relative risk. However, the probability of VTE occurring in a healthy middle-aged women is small (the background absolute risk is about 1 in 10 000 per year) and the benefits of HRT to an individual may be considerable. Patients with a high baseline risk of VTE, perhaps because they have previously had a deep venous thrombosis, will be subjected to the same increase in relative risk if they use HRT, but this represents a much higher absolute risk of VTE. Unless the benefits of the treatment are substantial, such a risk could outweigh the benefits to that individual.

The role of those involved in drug safety is to make recommendations that are justified by the scientific evidence and allow users to make informed decisions. A detailed approach to balancing risks and benefits of marketed medicines has been put forward by CIOMS (CIOMS Working Group IV, 1998). Sometimes the balance of risks and benefits will be sufficiently clear-cut to allow firm recommendations (such as contraindications), whilst in other situations less directive advice will be warranted. The next section deals with how we can use the evidence gathered in the processes described above to take action that improves the safe use of medicines.

IMPROVING THE SAFETY OF MEDICINES

When a drug safety hazard has been identified and sufficient information is available on which to base a judgement about the implications for users, the overall aim of promoting the safest possible use of the agent becomes foremost. A plan is required for providing appropriate information to health professionals and patients, so as to minimise the risk of the hazard. The urgency of implementation of this plan will vary depending upon the frequency and seriousness of the adverse reaction and the place of the drug in clinical practice. An important principle is that whenever the actions proposed may significantly alter prescribing, the necessary information needs to be made available rapidly. Rarely, there is a need to withdraw the drug from the market on safety grounds. This invariably requires immediate actions by both company and regulatory authority in order to ensure users are informed and to recall distributed supplies of the drug.

The nature of the action taken in reaction to a drug safety issue will depend on several factors, which are listed in Table 9.7. In terms of the hazard, the influencing factors here are much the same as the underlying issues in the initial assessment phase (see Table 9.3) but also included here should be consideration of the benefits of the drug in relation to alternatives and the nature of the disease being treated (CIOMS Working Group IV, 1998).

An important aim is the provision of clear product information. Several sections of the

Table 9.7. Factors influencing the type of action taken and timing in relation to a drug safety issue.

Seriousness of the hazard (i.e. its potential for a fatal outcome, or to lead to hospitalisation or disability)

Frequency

Preventability

Nature of the disease being treated

Benefits of treatment with the drug

Availability of alternative treatments

---

product information may include vital information for safe use. These are listed in Table 9.8, with examples. Changes to product information need to be tailored to specific issues and placed in the context of the existing information. Key safety information should come first within a particular section and may need to be highlighted. The amount of information added should be proportionate to the importance of the issue and care must be taken to avoid duplication (cross-referencing between sections is preferable to repetition) or adding excessive information which does not aid the prescriber. Non-contributory information dilutes important messages and may increase the likelihood of the key facts being missed. The principles of how to address safety aspects of product information have been reviewed in detail by the CIOMS Working Group III (1995).

ACTIONS TO PREVENT ADRS AND PROMOTE SAFER USE OF MEDICINES

The types of the action that may be taken vary according to potential means of preventing the adverse reaction. In particular, hazards may be minimised by targeting the drug at patients least likely to be at risk of the ADR and by specifically contraindicating it in patients with identifiable risk factors. Many factors impact on the potential for preventing ADRs. These relate to both patient and drug characteristics and are summarised in Table 9.9.

Dose and duration of treatment are often important issues in resolving drug safety issues since the risk of many hazards is related to one or both of these parameters. It is quite common for dosage regimens to change during the post-marketing period in response to safety concerns and many drugs have been initially recommended at doses higher than necessary (e.g. thiazide, diuretics, prazosin, captopril). In re-evaluating dose in response to a safety concern, it is important that consideration is also given to the evidence of efficacy at lower doses. It is conceivable that reducing dose could lessen efficacy whilst having only a limited effect on safety. In theory, therefore, the balance of benefits and risks could be made less favourable and empirical

Table 9.8. Sections of product information which may require amendment in response to a drug safety issue.

Section	Examples
Indications/uses	Limiting the indications to particular conditions with the greatest benefits by removal of indications (a) for which the benefits are insufficient to justify use and (b) for which use is associated with a greater risk of the ADR
Dosing instructions	Reductions in dose (may be applied to specific groups, e.g. the elderly); limitations on duration or frequency of treatment (especially for ADRs related to cumulative dose); provision of information on safer administration
Contraindications	Addition of concomitant diseases and/or medications for which the risks of use are expected to outweigh the benefits
Interactions	Addition of concomitant medications or foods which may interact; advice on co-prescription and monitoring
Pregnancy/lactation	Addition of new information relating to effects on fetus or neonate; revised advice about use in these circumstances based on accumulating experience
Warnings/precautions	Addition of concomitant diseases and/or medications for which the risks of use need to be weighed carefully against the benefits; additional or modified recommendations for monitoring patients
Undesirable effects	Addition of newly recognised adverse reactions; improving information about the nature, frequency and severity of effects already listed
Overdosage	Adverse effects of overdosage; management including the need for monitoring

Table 9.9. Factors which may impact on the potential for prevention of ADRs.

1. User characteristics
   Demographics: age, sex, race
   Genetic factors: polymorphisms (e.g. acetylator status)
   Concomitant diseases (e.g. impaired hepatic or renal failure)
   Compliance

2. Drug characteristics
   Route of administration
   Formulation (e.g. sustained vs. immediate release, excipients)
   Dosage regimen
   Therapeutic index
   Mechanisms of drug metabolism and route of excretion
   Potential for drug interactions

reductions of dose to levels that have not been shown to be efficacious should be avoided. Proposing limiting the duration of treatment also requires consideration of the benefit side and must be coherent with the therapeutic objective. For

example, it may be entirely rational for antibiotic-related hepatitis if the risk is associated with longer courses of therapy but it would be a pointless move where chronic therapy is needed such as with an antihypertensive or antidiabetic drugs.

TIMING

An important consideration is how quickly information needs to be made available to users. A new life-threatening adverse reaction, such as cardiac arrhythmias with terodiline (Rawlins, 1997), requires immediate communication, whereas the addition of a symptom which does not appear to be associated with serious consequences (e.g. nausea) to the undesirable effects section of the product information could be actioned at the next routine revision. Further-more, in the latter case there may be no particular need to draw attention to the problem. Most issues come between these two extremes and a judgement needs to be made about the speed of action and the most appropriate method of communication.

CHANGING PRODUCT INFORMATION

Product information is both a potential tool for communicating with users of medicines and a regulatory document with legal implications (for example, in the EU advertising must be consistent with the authorised Summary of Product Characteristics). The identification of a new adverse drug reaction or the accumulation of important new evidence about a recognised reaction leads to a need to make changes to the product information, and hence to vary the marketing authorisation(s). Variations to marketing authorisations on safety grounds may be initiated by the regulatory authority or pharmaceutical company. Regardless of who proposes the changes, it is essential that there is exchange of information and discussion between the parties before a proposed variation is submitted, since this is likely to promote agreement on the actions proposed and facilitate rapid implementation.

Decisions about the actions needed to respond to a specific drug safety issue require consultation between the regulatory authorities and the relevant marketing authorisation holder(s). When the regulatory authorities and companies are in broad agreement about the nature and impact of a drug safety issue, it is likely that negotiations regarding the necessary action will be successful and changes can be made on a voluntary basis. If the parties do not agree about the actions required, then authorities may exercise compulsory powers to remove a drug from the market or change the conditions of the authorisation. These are usually accompanied by rights of appeal for the company. Both companies and authorities normally try to avoid such procedures for safety issues since they may involve unsatisfactory delay and limit the actions that can be taken until the outcome is known. When the issue has urgent public health implications the authority may act rapidly without a right of appeal by the company. In such situations, the usual action taken is immediate withdrawal of the product(s) from the market.

Any change to the marketing authorisation and product information that has significant safety implications should be actively drawn to the attention of the relevant health professionals, usually by circulating the new product information under cover of a "Dear Doctor/Pharmacist" letter. Invariably such changes also require production of a new patient information leaflet and may require revision of the information on the packaging. When the changes being made are vital for ensuring patient safety they need to be implemented very quickly and it may be necessary to recall all stock.

The distribution of revised safety information may be targeted at specialists or generalists. However, even for drugs used primarily by specialists there may be a need to ensure that generalists are made aware. This is because the generalist may supervise long-term patient care and be in a position to prevent, identify or manage adverse reactions. If there is doubt about how widely information should be distributed it is therefore wise to distribute the information more rather than less widely. Consultation with the relevant experts, professional bodies and patient groups is important before making such a decision.

SAFETY ISSUES AFFECTING DRUG CLASSES

Drug safety issues affecting a large class of drugs (an example is the increased risk of VTE associated with the use of HRT) provide particular difficulties. In such cases it is important for information provided about the issue to be consistent unless there is clear evidence of a difference between products. Thus there is less likely to be a place for individual companies informing users. In such circumstances communication may be best achieved via a regulatory authority safety bulletin (such as *Current Problems in Pharmacovigilance* in the United Kingdom) or, if the matter is urgent, a "Dear Doctor/Pharmacist" letter may be sent directly by the regulatory authority.

In summary, minimising the risks of ADRs usually requires a variety of measures, and effective communication to professional and lay audiences. The latter issue is dealt with in the next section.

COMMUNICATING ABOUT DRUG SAFETY

INTRODUCTION

Communicating information to users is a vital step in the process of handling a safety issue with a marketed medicine. Ultimately, the successful handling of a specific problem does not only depend on making the right decisions but also on presenting the proposed action in a way that leads users to react appropriately. In this section we review the principles underlying successful communication in drug safety in terms of getting the messages right for health professionals, patients and the media, and distributing and timing them effectively.

GETTING STARTED

Once a decision has been taken on the appropriate action to reduce the risk from a drug safety issue, it is essential that planning is undertaken. Planning will include how and when action is taken and the optimisation of communications to ensure all those that need to know about the action are informed in a clear and timely manner. If the safety issue represents a major hazard to the public and significant action, such as a product withdrawal is planned, then it is essential to act quickly. A project team should be formed made up of a leader to oversee the planning and execution of communications and members with the necessary knowledge and experience of drug safety, communication and distribution networks. A communication plan will be drafted which makes clear the key messages, the audiences to be targeted (and how to reach them), who is responsible for drafting documents, who should review them and who will sign them off. The plan should include dates and times for production of drafts, for initiating distribution and for communications being received. The plan should be reviewed regularly and may need to be changed in light of emerging events. The plan should also include contingency for a major change in events, such as a leak of information to the media.

GETTING THE MESSAGE RIGHT

The key requirements for a successful drug safety communication are summarised in Table 9.10, i.e. targeted, understandable, open, informative and balanced. These are the factors around which the formulation process should be built. Any proposed communication should be tested against these requirements by a review process that includes both individuals who are experts in the field and those who are generalists. Communications intended for patients should be written in plain English and reviewed by lay people. In urgent situations it is vital to spend the time that is available ensuring that these requirements are met.

It is particularly important in any communication about drug safety to ensure that essential information is clearly conveyed and not obscured by other less important information. The key facts and recommendations must be worded unambiguously and should be placed in a prominent early position, if necessary with use of highlighting.

Table 9.10. Key requirements for a successful drug safety communication.

Requirement	Comments
Targeted	First, consider your audience and their specific information needs
Understandable	Keep it as straightforward as possible—the reader is more likely to respond appropriately if the message is simple and clear
Open	Be honest about the hazard—don't hide or minimise it; make it clear what has led you to communicate now
Informative	Make sure you include all the information which the reader needs to know; what should they do if they are concerned or require further information?
Balanced	The final test—is it clear that you have considered both risks and benefits; is the overall message right?

Healthcare Professionals

A model for a written communication to health-care professionals is shown in Figure 9.7. The numbered paragraphs are intended to describe the content of the particular section rather than to be used as headings. The model should aid making the letter open and informative, and can be tailored to the specific issue. It is important for credibility that communications to health professionals are signed by a senior professional, such as the company Medical Director. One of the key aspects is to inform healthcare professionals of any action that they need to take. Simple instructions will help prevent unnesessary consultations and minimise further enquiries. Contact points should be given for the provision of further information. This is particularly important as some individuals will not have understood the messages, some will want more information on the data leading to the action, others will want detailed advice on patient management, and some will want to complain. Contact points might include a website address, the number of a telephone helpline and an address for written correspondence.

Patients and the Public

The key principles with patient information are that it should, in substance, be the same as the information provided to healthcare professionals and it should be presented in language that they can understand. Good patient information adds to and reinforces the main issues which should be

---

IMPORTANT SAFETY INFORMATION
(also on envelope)

Dear Health Professional,
PRODUCT (Approved name) : HAZARD DESCRIPTION
1. The problem
2. The evidence
3. Conclusions drawn from the evidence
4. Practical recommendations
Mention enclosures (if any)
Contact(s) for further information (phone, fax, e-mail)
Signed : Senior Professional

Figure 9.7. Model letter to health professionals.

---

discussed between health professionals and patients, and does not make statements that could interfere with that relationship.

The Media

Most important drug safety issues will receive attention in the media. Often this will originate in medical journals with a scientific paper or news item forming the basis of subsequent television and newspaper coverage. The lay media have great potential influence on the perceptions of large numbers of users of medicines. Furthermore, healthcare professionals may first hear about a drug safety issue through the media. Therefore the media need to be handled with considerable care. It should be recognised that the immediate need of journalists is for a story that will interest their customers. The aim should be to provide them with the necessary facts and interpretation so as to give them maximum opportunity for balanced reporting. Unfortunately, a balanced perspective of risks and benefits may not lead to a newsworthy item, and journalists often tend to over-rate anecdotal evidence (e.g. in putting emphasis on the problems experienced by a particular individual). Journalists' expectations may also be unrealistic in relation to the level of safety of medicines or the quality of the evidence suggesting harm. They can be expected to highlight disagreement amongst experts in the field or any other factor that increases the newsworthiness of the item. With these considerations in mind, a basic model for providing the media with information is proposed in Table 9.11.

Professional Organisations and Patient Representative Groups

Professional organisations and patient representative groups offer both potential benefits and potential threats to a communication plan. Such organisations may be willing to input into the drafting of communication documents and in so doing improve them by offering perspectives which regulatory or company personnel do not have. They may be willing to give quotes relating to the action being taken which can then be used in

Table 9.11. Model for providing information to the media.

---

1. Nature of the problem: drug, hazard, precipitating factor(s)

2. Evidence for the hazard: strengths, weaknesses

3. What is being done: e.g. reviewing, investigating, new studies, changing labelling, etc.

4. What are the implications for (a) health professionals and (b) patients?

5. Overall balanced view of risks and benefits

---

media briefing and in response to complaints. These organisations may be willing to help with the distribution of communications and, if they are adequately briefed (for example with a detailed "question and answer" document), may be able to handle some of the enquiries that inevitably follow communication about a major safety issue. However, if the relationship with the organisation is poor prior to the safety issue emerging, then consultation can significantly complicate the communications plan and may lead to a leak to the media. Ideally, contacts with these organisations should be built proactively rather than making first contact at the time of an urgent drug safety issue.

DISTRIBUTING THE MESSAGES

Healthcare Professionals

It is essential to be clear which healthcare professionals need to know about the safety issue. It is also important to ensure that relevant health authority staff are informed about major drug safety issues. They may be willing to help with the dissemination of information. Usually all general practitioners will need to be informed, with hospital medical staff, hospital and community pharmacists, and nursing staff being informed depending on the drug in question. Occasionally, when the safety issue relates to a drug only used by a small number of hospital specialists, it may be acceptable to target this specialist group, together with those pharmacists and nursing staff working in the relevant speciality. However, if there is any

doubt as to whether generalists may be providing healthcare to those receiving the specialist treatment, then a letter distributed widely is necessary.

Distribution lists can be accessed via commercial and professional organisations. Which to choose will depend on how the drug is used. Some commercial organisations also offer faxing services, which can be very useful when a leak has occurred, or is likely to occur.

Information being distributed should also be added to the regulatory authority and company websites. This also provides an opportunity to provide more detailed information such as a summary of the data leading to the action and a "question and answer" document.

Patients and the Public

In certain situations, particularly if the hazard is potentially life-threatening, it may be appropriate to include "boxed warnings" on patient information leaflets and/or the packaging. An example of such a case is the contraindication to use of beta-blockers in patients with a history of asthma or bronchospasm, where it is vital that the patient does not use the product. Here, good patient information adds an extra safeguard in the event of a prescription being dispensed which would have potentially lethal consequences for the patient.

When information is provided to health professionals regarding an urgent drug safety issue which is likely to attract media attention, an information sheet, which can be copied and given to patients, may be of considerable value to practitioners. An example of such a leaflet is given in Figure 9.8.

It is increasingly likely that patients will first learn of a drug safety issue via the media. This reinforces the need to ensure that media briefing is clear, balanced, explains any action that patients need to take, and provides contact points for further information. Telephone helplines are essential for major safety issues. They should be staffed by appropriately trained personnel who have access to comprehensive "question and answer" documents. The internet is a further medium for patients to access information and for some patients will be their first port of call.

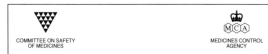

COMMITTEE ON SAFETY OF MEDICINES

MEDICINES CONTROL AGENCY

INFORMATION ON THE RISK OF BLOOD CLOTS FOR WOMEN TAKING HORMONE REPLACEMENT THERAPY (HRT)

You may have read in the press or heard people discuss that women taking hormone replacement therapy (HRT) are prone to blood clots in their veins. The purpose of this leaflet is to explain the benefits and risks, and what this means for you.

The benefits of HRT

HRT relieves symptoms of the menopause and when taken for several years prevents fractures by reducing thinning of the bones (osteoporosis). It has also been suggested that it may reduce heart disease.

The risk of a blood clot

New information was published in a medical journal in October 1996 which suggests that blood clots in the veins are more common in women who take HRT, whatever the type. However, the chance of getting a blood clot is low regardless of whether or not you take HRT.

Chances of getting a blood clot:

Not taking HRT — 1 in 10,000 per year
While taking HRT — 3 in 10,000 per year

What are the consequences of a blood clot?

Blood clots can occur in any vein but are most common in the legs (deep vein thrombosis or DVT) where they may cause pain, swelling or redness. If this occurs patients may require certain tests and a few days treatment in hospital. Occasionally blood clots pass to the lungs, this is more serious but usually responds to treatment.

How serious can a blood clot be?

Most people who get a blood clot in a vein make a complete recovery after treatment so the chance of dying from a blood clot is very low indeed. If you are not taking HRT your chance of dying from a blood clot is 1 in a million per year while if you are taking HRT your chance is 3 in a million per year.

What to do if you are concerned

The risk of blood clots is low and needs to be balanced against the benefits that HRT may have for you. If you are already on HRT, you do not need to stop it. If you are concerned about what you have heard or read and would like to discuss these concerns further, make a routine appointment to see your doctor who can talk through the pros and cons of HRT with you.

Figure 9.8. Example of a drug safety communication targeted at patients.

Therefore, adding clear information to the regulatory authority or company website is essential.

The Media

Providing written information to newspapers and the makers of television programmes through a spokesperson should be the usual method of interaction, with informal conversations being best avoided. Interviews for television or radio may be requested and careful consideration should be given to their potential benefits and harm in the context of the specific situation in question. Such interviews invariably have the potential to inflame an issue but refusal to appear can also be damaging. If it is decided that the interview should be accepted, then

it is important that the individual to be interviewed has both undertaken media training and is fully briefed about the issue, the key messages and the pitfalls likely to be encountered.

When it is predicted that a drug safety issue is likely to attract media attention and where there is considerable potential for unbalanced reporting to lead to patient alarm and possibly harm, it is usually best to adopt a proactive approach. One model is to issue a press briefing rather than awaiting enquiries from the press, so allowing the opportunity to present the facts in a balanced way. An alternative is to hold a press conference backed up with written briefing for journalists. A press conference requires considerable planning but will allow the facts to be clearly presented and journalists an opportunity to clarify issues they do not understand. When successful, a press conference can lead to journalists printing the exact messages you want the public and health professionals to receive. This may be achieved by using experienced staff to explain the facts and required action and backing it up through providing journalists with written briefing.

Professional Organisations and Patient Representative Groups

At an early stage in the communications planning a list of relevent professional and patient representative groups, together with named contacts and telephone and fax numbers, should be drawn up. If it is intended that these groups input into draft communications, help with distribution or take enquiries, then the first contact will need to be made many days before communications "go live". If their input is not required, then such organisations should at least be faxed, in confidence and for information, the letter being sent to healthcare professionals.

TIMING THE MESSAGES

As a major safety issue is being evaluated, it is good practice to begin considering communication issues and to form a communications project team. This should minimise the amount of crisis management required. Ideally, professional and patient organisations will be informed prior to all relevant healthcare professionals. In turn relevant healthcare professionals will be informed prior to any media briefing. Although the media will inevitably hear about a major safety issue before all relevant healthcare professionals have been informed, timing the communications in this way will minimise the chances of major media coverage with no mechanism in place for getting communications to healthcare professionals.

AUDIT

To ensure an efficient and effective system for handling drug safety issues, audit should be performed of all the steps in the process. Audit will include measuring performance against targets for data collection and processing, signal generation and evaluation, decision-making, regulatory action and communication.

ENSURING ACTION TO PROTECT PATIENTS IS EFFECTIVE

Perhaps the most important aspect of audit is ensuring that any action taken to protect the public from a drug risk is effective. With the exception of when a drug is withdrawn from the market, all action on drug safety will aim to reduce rather than eliminate risk. If the drug in question is of proven therapeutic benefit, then this is entirely appropriate. However, simply adding warnings to product information, recommending monitoring or contraindicating an at-risk patient group may not adequately protect public health. It is therefore important to monitor that the action has been effective and to continue to monitor the safety issue on an ongoing basis. A list of possible methods of evaluation is given in Table 9.12. In the past, the number and nature of spontaneous reports received has been used as the main method of evaluating the effectiveness of action. However, for the reasons discussed above, this approach has significant limitations. Ideally, adverse reactions following use of the drug would be prospectively monitored. This might be done using a formal observational study or by monitoring prescribing

Table 9.12. Possible methods of evaluating the effectiveness of actions taken.

1. Communications—have they been received and understood (using market research techniques)?

2. Prescribing—extent to which it is consistent with revised recommendations in product information (using longitudinal patient databases)

3. Spontaneous reporting—do serious cases continue to be reported? Do reported cases reflect contraindicated use?

4. Observation/formal study of prescribing and events—has the action resulted in reduced morbidity/mortality from the ADR in practice (using longitudinal patient databases or epidemiological study)?

events in a longitudinal patient database such as the GPRD. If there is evidence that the action taken has not reduced the morbidity or mortality associated with the drug, then further action and communications will usually be necessary.

CONCLUSIONS

The data resources and processes for identifying and responding effectively to drug safety issues have been reviewed above. Pharmaceutical companies and regulatory authorities have clear obligations to use them in order to recognise and address safety concerns promptly so that marketed medicines can be used as safely as possible. To achieve this objective organisations must be proactive in identifying and investigating issues, and responsive to a moving target. Most important, drug safety issues are unpredictable and an open-minded approach is necessary to ensure that significant changes in the evidence lead to appropriate actions. Once action has been taken there is invariably a need for continued monitoring.

The methodologies underpinning pharmacovigilance have been developed over the last 30 years to a level that affords patients a reasonable degree of protection against the unwanted effects of medicines. However, these still need to become more sophisticated to meet the challenges of the changing world of therapeutics. Innovative methodologies are also needed in order to enhance the capabilities of drug safety personnel to respond quickly to important issues. Technological advances, and the increasingly availability of computerised databases which can be used to research drug safety issues, are providing new opportunities for better investigation and communication about drug safety.

Consumer expectations of drug safety have recently increased and are likely to continue to do so (Asscher *et al.*, 1995). The primary consideration in this field must always be the patients using the medicine. When making decisions based on risk–benefit analysis, a fine line often has to be drawn between restricting availability and choice, and minimising the risks that inevitably accompany the use of any pharmacological agent. Improving the quality of the evidence on which such judgements are based is a clear priority for all working in the field of drug safety.

ACKNOWLEDGEMENTS

This chapter is based on an article by Patrick Waller and Ennis Lee published in *Pharmacoepidemiology and Drug Safety* in 1999 (Volume 8, pp. 535–552). We would like to thank Dr Iain Cockburn for helpful comments. The views expressed in this chapter are those of the authors and should not be taken to represent the official view of the Medicines Control Agency.

REFERENCES

Asscher AW, Parr GD, Whitmarsh VB (1995) Towards safer use of medicines. *Br Med J* 311 1003–5.

Bate A, Lindquist, Edwards IR, Olsson S, Orre R, Lasner A, De Freitas RM (1998) A Bayesian neural network for adverse drug reaction signal generation. *Eur J Clin Pharmacol* 54: 315–21.

Beardon PHG, McGilchrist MM, McKendrick AD, McDevitt DG, MacDonald TM (1993) Primary non-compliance with prescribed medication in primary care. *Br Med J* 307: 846–8.

Bégaud B, Moride Y, Tubert-Bitter P, Chaslerie A, Haramburu F (1994) False-positives in spontaneous reporting: should we worry about them? *Br J Clin Pharmacol* 38: 401–4.

Berlin JA (2000) The use of meta-analysis in pharmacoepidemiology. In: Strom BL, ed., *Pharmacoepidemiology*, 3rd edn. Chichester: Wiley, pp. 633–59.

Calman K., Moores Y, Hartley BH (1995) Carbaryl. Department of Health PL CMO(95)4.

Castellsague J, Perez Gutthann S, Garcia Rodriguez LA (1998) Recent epidemiological studies of the association between Hormone Replacement Therapy and venous thromboembolism. *Drug Safety* 18: 117–23.

CIOMS Working Group III (1995) *Guidelines for Preparing Core Clinical Safety Information on Drugs.* Geneva: CIOMS.

CIOMS Working Group IV (1998) *Benefit–Risk Balance for Marketed Drugs: Evaluating Safety Signals.* Geneva: CIOMS.

Collet JP, Boivin JF (2000) Bias and confounding in pharmacoepidemiology. In: Strom BL, ed., *Pharmacoepidemiology*, 3rd edn. Chichester: Wiley, pp. 765–84.

Committee on Safety of Medicines/Medicines Control Agency (2000) Danthron restricted to constipation in the terminally ill. *Current Problems in Pharmacovigilance* 26: 4.

Edwards IR, Aronson JK (2000) Adverse drug reactions: definitions, diagnosis and management. *Lancet* 356: 1255–59.

Edwards IR, Lindquist M, Wiholm B-E, Napke E (1990) Quality criteria for early signals of possible adverse drug reactions. *Lancet* 336: 156–8.

Egberts ACG, Meyboom RHB, de Koning FHP, Bakker A, Leufkens HGM (1997) Non-puerperal lactation associated with antidepressant drug use. *Br J Clin Pharmacol* 44: 277–81.

Evans JMM, MacDonald TM (1997) Misclassification and selection bias in case–control studies using an automated database. *Pharmacoepidemiology and Drug Safety* 6: 313–8.

Evans JMM, MacDonald TM (2000) The Tayside Medicines Monitoring Unit (MEMO). In: Strom BL, ed., *Pharmacoepidemiology*, 3rd edn., Chichester: Wiley, pp. 361–74.

Evans SJW, Waller PC, Davis S (2001) Use of proportional reporting ratios for signal generation from spontaneous adverse drug reaction reports. *Pharmacoepidemiology and Drug Safety* 10: 483–6.

Hill AB (1965) The environment and disease: association or causation? *Proc Roy Soc Med* 58: 295–300.

Inman WHW, Weber JCP (1986) The United Kingdom. In: Inman WHW, ed., *Monitoring for Drug Safety*, 2nd edn. Lancaster: MTP Press, pp. 13–47.

Jefferys DB, Leakey D, Lewis J, Payne S, Rawlins MD (1998) New active substances authorized in the United Kingdom between 1972 and 1994. *Br J Clin Pharmacol* 45: 151–6.

Jick H, Jick SS, Derby LE (1991) Validation of information recorded on general practitioner based computerised data resource in the United Kingdom. *Br Med J* 302: 766–8.

Lees AJ on behalf of the Parkinson's Disease Research Group in the United Kingdom (1995) Comparison of therapeutic effects and mortality data of levodopa and levodopa combined with selegiline in patients with early, mild Parkinson's disease. *Br Med J* **311**: 1602–7.

Meyboom RHB, Hekster YA, Egberts AC.G, Gribnau FWJ, Edwards IR (1997) Causal or casual? The role of causality assessment in pharmacovigilance. *Drug Safety* **17**: 374–89.

Petri H, Urquhart J (1991) Channeling bias in the interpretation of drug effects. *Stat Med* **10**: 577–81.

Rawlins MD (1997) Predicting the future from lessons of the past. *Int J Pharmaceut Med* **11**: 37–40.

Sackett DL, Haynes RB, Gent M, Taylor DW (1986) Compliance. In: Inman WHW, ed., *Monitoring for Drug Safety*, 2nd edn. Lancaster: MTP Press, pp. 471–83.

Smyth RL, Ashby D, O'Hea U, Burrows E, Lewis P, van Velzen D, Dodge JA (1995) Fibrosing colonopathy in cystic fibrosis: results of a case–control study. *Lancet* **346**: 1247–51.

Speirs CJ (1986) Prescription-related adverse reaction profiles and their use in risk–benefit analysis. In: D'Arcy PF, Griffin JP, eds., *Iatrogenic Diseases*, 3rd edn. Oxford: Oxford University Press, pp. 93–101.

Strom BL (2000) How should one perform pharmacoepidemiology studies? Choosing among the available alternatives. In: Strom BL, ed., *Pharmacoepidemiology*, 3rd edn. Chichester: Wiley, pp. 401–13.

Uppsala Monitoring Centre (1998) *A Network for Safety*. Uppsala: WHO Collaborating Centre for International Drug Monitoring.

von Kries R (1998) Neonatal Vitamin K prophylaxis: the Gordian knot still awaits untying. *Br Med J* **316**: 161–2.

Waller PC, Coulson RA, Wood SM (1996) Regulatory pharmacovigilance in the United Kingdom: current principles and practice. *Pharmacoepidemiology and Drug Safety* **5**: 363–75.

Wood SM, Waller PC (1996) Record linkage databases for pharmacovigilance: a UK perspective. In: Walker SR, ed., *Databases for Pharmacovigilance*. Carshalton: Centre for Medicines Research, pp. 47–54.

10

Micturin and Torsades de Pointes

RICHARD N. WILD*

Arakis Ltd, Saffron Walden, UK

RESPONDING TO SIGNALS

MICTURIN AND TORSADES DE POINTES

Micturin® (Mictrol®, terodiline hydrochloride) was withdrawn from sale in 1991 after the discovery of an association with serious cardiac arrhythmias, most notably a rare form of ventricular tachycardia known as torsades de pointes (TP) (Wild, 1992). In most patients, TP occurs in short, self-limiting bursts that lead to temporary interruption of the circulation, causing symptoms of cerebral impairment such as dizziness, acute confusion, syncope or epileptiform fits. Occasionally, it may convert into ventricular fibrillation from which death may result. TP may co-exist with sinoatrial depression, bradycardia and heart block in some patients, which may require temporary or permanent cardiac pace-making. TP is always associated with prior QT interval lengthening in the electrocardiograph (ECG) (Ben-David and Zipes, 1993). Micturin caused prolongation of the QT interval (Stewart et al.; 1992, Thomas et al., 1995; Hartigan-Go et al., 1996; Shuba et al., 1999).

Micturin had been licensed in the United Kingdom in 1986, indicated for the management of detrusor instability (urge incontinence). Pharmacologically, it was a tertiary amine with dominant anti-muscarinic activity, but it also had modest calcium antagonist properties (Husted et al., 1980). Importantly, as will become clear, prior to launch as Micturin, terodiline had been licensed since the mid-1960s in Sweden as an anti-anginal drug (Bicor®). It was side effects on the urinary bladder that led to its re-development as Micturin (Andersson et al., 1988; Langtry and McTavish, 1990).

Micturin had been successfully marketed for two years before the first report of TP. A second report was received almost exactly a year later, quickly followed by a third. A full review of the corporate safety database, and of the pre-clinical data, yielded no information that pointed to a causal relationship. Terodiline's early use as a cardiac drug historically preceded the first published descriptions of TP (Desertenne, 1966), so it is highly likely that any cases of TP were simply not recognised, any emergent arrhythmias being attributed to the disease state. Emphasis had been put on the review because of a serious event

---

* Formerly Medical Director, Pharmacia, UK.

Pharmacovigilance. Edited by R.D. Mann and E.B. Andrews
© 2002 John Wiley & Sons, Ltd

that, according to the literature, had virtually no spontaneous incidence; it was usually associated with drugs or metabolic derangement (Stratman and Kennedy, 1987). (There is also a rare congenital lengthening of QT interval.) All these early cases (and most of the subsequent cases) were complicated by histories of ischaemic heart disease (IHD) and polypharmacy.

Early in 1991 the fourth report of TP was received (McCleod *et al.*, 1991) and, most significantly, a UK cardiac centre notified the company of an impending publication (Connolly *et al.*, 1991) involving five cases of TP, three of which were the first reports received by the company back in 1988 and 1989. The other two were, until then, not known to the company. Six cases of a very rare disorder, apparently associated with Micturin treatment, could not be ignored. It constituted a potential safety issue and required sharing with the regulators. (Each case had, of course, been reported individually to the regulators according to prevailing serious adverse drug event (ADE) requirements. These had provoked no comments from the Medicines Control Agency (MCA) at the time.)

At this stage, it was far from certain that Micturin might have a direct causal relationship with TP:

- Experts would not entirely rule out an association of the TP with IHD, or its drug treatment, a feature in many of the reported cases.
- Despite the launch of Micturin in other countries, the United Kingdom remained alone in reporting the ADE.
- Index patients had been safely on the drug for a mean of 13 months (the longest was two years) before the onset of the symptoms (usually blackouts) associated with TP.

Despite these doubts, the MCA was informed of our concerns. The MCA did not share any prior concern they themselves may have had, and added no more cases to the company database. The MCA saw no need for immediate action on their part, and accepted the company plan of action that included:

- Full validation of each case received with on-site due diligence

- Quantifying the level of risk through sales data
- Reviewing prescribing experience with key prescribers for unreported cases (none was discovered)
- Re-analysis of the Prescription Event Monitoring database (PEM, Drug Safety Research Unit, University of Southampton), as the original study had not identified an arrhythmia hazard
- Commissioning a search and case–control study of the GP research database (VAMP).
- Studying the effects of Micturin on QT interval lengthening

By July 1991, 13 cases of TP (plus three other ventricular tachycardias) had been reported from the United Kingdom, and Micturin was reviewed at a routine meeting of the Committee on Safety of Medicines (CSM). Unexpectedly, CSM decided immediate restriction in the use of the drug was required, despite no new information from any of the research actions the company had agreed with the MCA. A "Dear Doctor" letter with revised prescribing information was issued on 25 July 1991 (Asscher, 1991). Not unexpectedly, this had immediate effects. Patient and prescriber confidence was immediately lost, and prescriptions dwindled to less than 10% of peak levels in just six weeks. Reporting rates for not only TP, but also other arrhythmias, and sudden, unexplained deaths, increased rapidly. Many of these reports were retrospective once the association was recognised. On Friday, 13 September 1991, the company decided, voluntarily, to withdraw the drug worldwide.

At this point of withdrawal, some 69 cases of cardiac arrhythmia and sudden, unexplained death (14 of the 69) had been reported in the United Kingdom. Only three cases had been reported from outside the United Kingdom. Reports included 13 cases of other ventricular arrhythmias and 18 brady-dysrhythmias, in addition to the TP (24 cases). Prior to this point, it was estimated that approximately 450 000 UK patients (and a further 550 000 elsewhere) had been prescribed Micturin. The risk for TP (based only on UK data) was calculated at around 1 in 18 750, but this risk increased to 1 in 6500 for any of the cited events.

Preliminary analysis results became available from the PEM and VAMP databases. In the original PEM study of 1986–1987, no case of TP was discovered amongst 12 457 patients. In 1991 these data were revisited (Inman *et al.*, 1993). As it was quite possible that cases of TP could have missed diagnosis (owing to its transient and self-limiting nature in most cases), re-analysis included all incidents that could have been attributable to cardiac or vascular events. A comparison of the incidence of these events, and deaths, was also made with another drug (nabumetone) that had also undergone a PEM study in a similar age-range of patients. There were no pertinent differences between the two groups of patients.

In the VAMP analysis of 9716 Micturin-treated patients, one case of TP was found (Hall *et al.*, 1993). A subsequent retrospective cohort study, taken from this group of patients, showed no differences in the overall incidence of diagnosed cardiac arrhythmias between Micturin-treated patients and controls matched for age, sex and urinary consultations. Admittedly, the power provided by the VAMP and PEM databases was not high (covering only 22 000+ patients) but, at least, they provided reassurance that there was not a larger, unrecognised problem. Most relevant cases appeared to be being reported.

Studies of QT interval lengthening on ECG have shown an undoubted correlation with Micturin treatment (Stewart *et al.*, 1992; Thomas *et al.*, 1995; Hartigan-Go *et al.*, 1996; Shuba *et al.*, 1999). As QT interval lengthening is pre-requisite for TP, it must be accepted that Micturin probably played a role in the development of TP. However, it is not the purpose of this chapter to examine QT interval lengthening and its association with TP. It is important to note that since the withdrawal of Micturin, effects on QT interval have been recorded in a much wider range of drugs than the anti-arrhythmics and psychotropic drugs that dominated the early publications (Stratman and Kennedy, 1987; Yap and Camm, 2000). Perhaps the most notable of the drugs affected have been two humble, and very widely used, over-the-counter (OTC) anti-histamines, astemizole and terfenadine. (Both are available now only on prescription.) Owing to the prevalence of QT interval lengthening with so

many classes of drugs now, and the ease with which the effect can be detected and measured, it is important to rule it out early in clinical development.

There are important lessons to be learned from managing the Micturin alert:

1. Never to take false comfort from the fact that a drug has had an apparently long history of safe use. The development for the earlier use will probably have pre-dated modern standards of development and adverse event reporting.
2. A change of use or indication may be exposing a new profile of the patient, more susceptible to the ADE.
3. Because an event is rare, or even previously undescribed (as TP was until 1966), do not dismiss a possible association. Thalidomide teratogenicity and practolol-associated fibrosing peritonitis caused much morbidity before anyone dared to make the association.
4. We could have reacted more to the early signals. It would have been very easy, and quick, to conduct a case–control study in patients for effects on QT interval lengthening. Unfortunately, thought processes, then, did not immediately encompass the notion that patients without TP might have QT prolongation.

In these sorts of circumstances, it is always easier to find excuses to absolve than reasons to blame.

Would earlier action have actually made any difference to the outcome? This can, perhaps, be answered by examining the reasons that lead to the withdrawal. The drug was not life saving but had potentially lethal side effects. The side effects (taken as a whole) were not all that rare, at about 1 in 6500 patients exposed (between 1 in 10 000 and 1 in 20 000 for TP alone). The risk was probably doubled in the over 75s, a large patient group for the drug (Inman *et al.*, 1993). ECGs were not helpful, as anyone exposed to terodiline will lengthen their QT interval (but, at the time, defining when it became a pathological increase was controversial).

Terodiline had been recognised as being metabolised and excreted more slowly in the elderly during clinical development (Hallén *et al.*, 1989), and appropriate prescribing information resulted. Whilst some patients with TP had been on inappropriately high doses for their age, most were not. Unfortunately, a serum level of terodiline had been measured in only one of the reported cases (Connolly *et al.*, 1991). It is noteworthy that the level in this case was in fact around six times the accepted therapeutic level, and this was from, apparently, recommended dosage. Thus, there was the suspicion that QT prolongation might be related to blood levels. (This was subsequently proven—Thomas *et al.*, 1995.)

Why did many of the index patients apparently live happily with their (presumed) prolonged QT for up to two years, and then develop TP? Were there co-factors that combined with the QT prolongation and precipitated the TP? Hypokalaemia increases the risk of TP, also through QT lengthening. Co-prescription of other drugs also known to prolong QT interval would have been another risk factor.

Finally, it had to be accepted that there were safer, alternative treatments available. All these reasons left the company with little choice but to withdraw the drug. Some patients thought otherwise, saying they were quite prepared to risk death in order to enjoy the freedom the drug had given back to them. Most patients, and their doctors, however, had already decided the risk was not worth taking.

The irony in this recount will not have escaped the alert reader. Terodiline had owed its renaissance, as Micturin, to the discovery of side effects on the urinary bladder in cardiac patients. Cardiac side effects in urological patients proved to be its undoing.

POSTSCRIPT

Terodiline has since been superceded by another molecule, tolterodine. This new molecule does *not* prolong the QT interval. The risk was peculiar to terodiline and is not a class effect. Oxybutinin, for instance, has been shown not to affect the QT interval (Hussain *et al.*, 1996).

REFERENCES

Andersson K-E, Ekström B, Mattiasson A (1988) Actions of terodiline, its isomers and main metabolite on isolated detrusor muscle from rabbit and man. *Acta Pharmacol Toxicol* **63**: 390–5.

Asscher AW (1991) Terodiline (Micturin) and adverse cardiac events. *Committee on Safety of Medicines* (letter).

Ben-David J, Zipes DP (1993) Torsades de pointes and proarrhythmia. *Lancet* **341**: 1578–82.

Connolly MJ, Astridge PS, White EG, Morley CA, Campbell Cowan J (1991) Torsades de pointes ventricular tachycardia and terodiline. *Lancet* **338**: 344–5.

Desertenne F (1966) La tachycardie ventriculaire á deux foyers opposés variable. *Archives des Maladies du Coeur et des Vaisseaux* **59**: 263–72.

Hall GC, Chukwujindu J, Richardson J, Lis Y, Wild RN (1993) Micturin (terodiline hydrochloride), torsades de pointe and other arrhythmias—a study using the VAMP database. *Pharmacoepidemiology and Drug Safety* **2**: 127–32.

Hallén B, Bogentoft S, Sandquist S, Stromberg S, Setterberg G, Ryd-Kjellen E (1989) Tolerability and steady state pharmacokinetics of terodiline and its main metabolites in elderly patients with urinary incontinence. *Eur J Clin Pharmacol* **36**: 487–93.

Hartigan-Go K, Bateman N, Daly AK, Thomas SHL (1996) Stereoselective cardiotoxic effects of terodiline. *Clin Pharmacol Ther* **60**: 89–98.

Hussain RM, Hartigan-Go K, Thomas SHL, Ford GA (1996) Effect of oxybutinin on the QTc interval in elderly patients with urinary incontinence. *Br J Clin Pharmacol* **41**: 73–5.

Husted S, Andersson K-E, Sommer L, Ostergaard JR (1980) Anticholinergic and calcium antagonistic effects of terodiline in rabbit urinary bladder. *Acta Pharmacologica et Toxicologica (Copenhagen)* (Suppl 1), **46**: 20–30.

Inman W, Clarke J, Wilton L, Pearce G, Veldhuis GJ (1993) PEM Report Number 2. Terodiline. *Pharmacoepidemiology and Drug Safety* **2**: 287–319.

Langtry HD, McTavish D (1990) Terodiline: a review of its pharmacological properties and therapeutic use in the treatment of urinary incontinence. *Drugs* **40**: 748–61.

McCleod AA, Thorogood S, Barnett S (1991) Torsades de pointes complicating treatment with terodiline. *Br Med J* **302**: 1469.

Shuba LM, Kasamaki Y, Jones SE, Ogura T, McCullough JR, McDonald TF (1999) Action potentials, contraction, and membrane currents in guinea pig ventricular preparations treated with the antispasmodic agent terodiline. *J Pharmacol Exp Ther* **290**: 1417–26.

Stewart DA, Taylor J, Ghosh S, Macphee GJA, Abdullah I, McLenachan, Stott DJ (1992) Terodiline causes polymorphic ventricular tachycardia due to reduced heart rate and prolongation of QT interval. *Eur J Clin Pharmacol* **42**: 577–580.

Stratman HS, Kennedy HL (1987) Torsades de pointes associated with drugs and toxins: recognition and management. *Am Heart J* **113**: 1470–82.

Thomas SHL, Higham PD, Hartigan-Go K, Kamali F, Wood P, Campbell RWF, Ford GA (1995) Concentration dependent cardiotoxicity of terodiline in patients treated for urinary incontinence. *Br Heart J* **74**: 53–6.

Wild RN (1992) Micturin and torsades de pointe—experience of a post-marketing alert. *Pharmacoepidemiology and Drug Safety* **1**: 147–150.

Yap YG, Camm J (2000) Risk of torsades de pointes with non-cardiac drugs. *Br Med J* **320**: 1158–9.

11

Withdrawal of Terodiline: A Tale of Two Toxicities

RASHMI R. SHAH

Medicines Control Agency, London, UK

INTRODUCTION

It is difficult to think of a type A pharmacological adverse drug reaction other than drug-induced prolongation of the QT interval, and its subsequent degeneration into torsade de pointes, which has been responsible for the withdrawal in recent times of so many drugs from the market over a short period. Withdrawal of prenylamine in 1988, followed by that of terodiline in 1991, was to herald a similar misfortune for many other drugs such as terfenadine, astemizole, cisapride, sertindole, grepafloxacin, droperidol and levoacetylmethadol. Many other drugs, such as pimozide, halofantrine and thioridazine, to name just three, had severe prescribing restrictions placed on their clinical use for the same reason. In addition, a significant number of drugs have had their clinical development, some at a fairly advanced stage, curtailed resulting from early identification of their potential to prolong the QT interval while others such as moxifloxacin, gatifloxacin and ziprasidone have been deemed unapprovable in some Member States of the European Union (EU) because their potential to prolong the QT interval was determined to adversely affect their risk–benefit ratio.

In essence, withdrawal of terodiline represents the perils of failure to learn from precedents and to apply all available techniques to characterise the safety of a drug. This is particularly unfortunate since drug-induced torsade de pointes is a concentration-dependent, and therefore a predictable, type A adverse drug reaction.

From a regulatory perspective, terodiline is almost too perfect an example of drugs whose more potent secondary pharmacological effects, observed as an adverse drug reaction during the originally intended clinical use, led to its clinical re-development for a completely different indication. It further highlights how such a strategy can be eclipsed by the virulent appearance of additional, not fully explored, secondary pharmacological effects. It illustrates, therefore, the limitations of drug development programmes in characterising a relatively rare but potentially fatal clinical hazard. In addition, the post-marketing identifica-

The views expressed in this chapter are those of the author and do not necessarily represent the views or the opinions of Medicines Control Agency, other regulatory authorities or any of their advisory committees.

tion of its proarrhythmic potential through a spontaneous reporting system emphasises the strengths of systems such as the UK Yellow Card System in comparison with formal post-marketing surveillance studies.

RE-BIRTH OF TERODILINE

Terodiline (Figure 11.1) was first marketed in 1965 as an antianginal agent ("Bicor") in Scandinavia (Wibell, 1968), a relatively small market. This period of original marketing of terodiline is worthy of note for three reasons: (a) it antedates any serious regulatory or clinical interest in drug-induced prolongation of the QT interval, (b) it antedates the first description of torsade de pointes, a unique proarrhythmia associated with prolonged QT interval (Dessertenne, 1966) and (c) the drug probably co-existed with prenylamine, also an antianginal agent. Because of its potent anticholinergic properties, urinary retention proved to be a frequent and troublesome side-effect during its use as an antianginal agent and terodiline was therefore re-developed in early 1980s for clinical use in urinary incontinence due to detrusor instability.

In the period intervening between these two indications, it was also being investigated by some workers for use in chronic obstructive airways disease (Castenfors et al., 1975), presumably in an attempt to harness the same, otherwise unwanted, pharmacological property. In isolated airways preparations from rats, terodiline had been shown to block the bronchoconstrictor effect of acetylcholine but was ineffective against that caused by serotonin and bradykinin. The shift in the dose–response curves of acetylcholine by terodiline indicated that this property may explain the cilio-

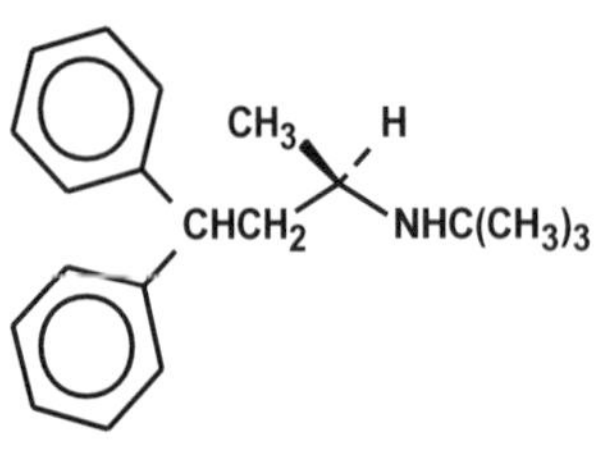

Figure 11.1. (+)-(R)-terodiline.

stimulatory effect of this drug (Iravani and Melville, 1975).

It was first introduced in the United Kingdom as "Terolin" (later changed to "Micturin") in July 1986 for use in urinary frequency, urgency and incontinence in patients with detrusor instability and neuogenic bladder disorders. In the EU, it was approved at that time in Denmark, Ireland, Luxembourg, Belgium, the Netherlands, Spain and West Germany, but not in France, Greece, Italy or Portugal. Overall, the drug was approved in 20 countries worldwide and marketed in a number of these but the major markets were the United Kingdom, Sweden and Japan. The recommended dose of the drug was 12.5–25 mg twice daily in young adults and otherwise healthy elderly but 12.5 mg twice daily in frail elderly patients. In general, the doses used in Sweden were lower than those used in the United Kingdom while the dose approved in Japan was half the UK recommended dose.

TERODILINE-INDUCED PROARRHYTHMIAS

One of the fist indications of proarrhythmic activity of terodiline was a sudden unexpected death following an overdose in 1987 reported by Cattini et al. (1989). Forensic toxicological analysis on this 20-year-old previously healthy man with fatal overdose of terodiline revealed the presence of a potentially fatal blood level of terodiline. His blood and urine levels were greater than 10 µg/mL, whereas therapeutic concentrations in serum are usually not more than 1 µg/mL. No other drugs were detected. At post-mortem, his organs did not reveal any natural diseases. Although death was suspected to have followed inhalation of vomitus, the probability of a proarrhythmic event preceding aspiration cannot be excluded. Boyd (1990) has attempted to provide a clarification on the probable dose ingested. The first proarrhythmic reactions to clinical doses of terodiline were reported to have actually occurred in 1987 when there was one case of ventricular tachycardia and one of bradycardia. These reports were followed by an additional one report each of the two reactions in 1988.

The first three reports of torsade de pointes in association with the use of terodiline, following its post-approval routine clinical use, were notified to the licence holder during 1988 and 1989 and the fourth report in 1990 (Wild, 1992). Beginning early 1991, additional reports of QT interval prolongation and torsades de pointes began to appear (Andrews and Bevan, 1991; Connolly *et al.*, 1991; Davis *et al.*, 1991; Mcleod *et al.*, 1991). These events, reported individually to the Medicines Control Agency (MCA), did not raise any immediate concern at first because of the associated confounding factors. However, by May 1991 the marketing authorisation holder was aware of 10 cases of torsades de pointes when the MCA was alerted of the potential hazard collectively signalled by these reports.

Additional reports followed and by 21 July 1991, there were 14 reports of ventricular tachycardias (including 13 of torsades de pointes) and 7 of bradyarrhythmias. None had a fatal outcome. Therefore, the Chairman of the UK Committee on Safety of Medicines (CSM) wrote to all doctors in the United Kingdom warning them of this potentially fatal adverse reaction and summarising the risk factors (Anon, 1991a). On the basis of the reports received, the prescribers were advised of the risk factors such as age greater than 75 years, ischaemic heart disease, co-prescription with cardioactive drugs, diuretics, antidepressants and antipsychotics, hypokalaemia and patients with any cardiac arrhythmias including ECG evidence of prolonged QT interval. Age *per se* was not regarded as an absolute contraindication.

Following this warning, many additional reports were received and by September 1991 there were 69 reports of serious cardiac arrhythmias. These consisted of 50 reports of tachyarrhythmias and 19 reports of bradyarrhythmias and heart blocks. Amongst these 69 cases were 14 cases of sudden or unexplained deaths (13 in the tachyarrhythmia group). Fifty-one cases had recovered and there was no information on outcome in 4 reports. Of the 55 non-fatal cases, 24 were ventricular tachycardia of the torsades de pointes variety, 5 ventricular fibrillation, 7 unspecified

ventricular tachycardia, one of multifocal ventricular ectopics and 18 of bradyarrhythmias including all degrees of heart blocks.

Patient demography and pattern of drug usage was essentially similar in the tachyarrhythmias and bradyarrhythmias groups. Of the 50 patients with tachyarrhythmias, 40 were females and 43 were aged 61 years or more. A dose of 25 mg daily or less was taken by 25 (56%) of the 45 patients with tachyarrhythmias in whom the dose was stated. Information on duration of treatment was available in 40 of these 50 patients. It was less than 1 month in 8 cases, up to 2 months in 10 cases, up to 6 months in 8 cases and more than 6 months in the remaining 14 cases. A dose of 25 mg or less was taken by 11 (65%) of the 17 patients with bradyarrhythmias and heart blocks in whom the information on dose was available.

An analysis of predisposing factors in the 69 reports of cardiotoxicity due to terodiline confirmed previous conclusions on potential risk factors: (a) an age greater than 75 years, (b) concurrent use of cardioactive medication ($n = 33$), (c) concurrent use of diuretics ($n = 27$), (d) concurrent use of antidepressants or antipsychotic agents, and (e) hypokalaemia ($n = 8$). Ischaemic heart disease was present in 13 and other cardiovascular pathology in 39 patients. In 12 cases (18%), there were no clinically identifiable risk factors at all.

Of the 69 cases, 21 had been reported at the time of the warning from the Chairman of CSM and an additional 48 cases were reported within 2 months following this warning. Clearly, there were cases of cardiac effects of terodiline but were simply not reported—the association may have appeared too implausible to the prescribing community. However, once alerted, the real magnitude of the potential risk began to become clearer. While the regulatory action was under consideration, the drug was withdrawn voluntarily by the licence holder from the market worldwide on 13 September 1991 (Anon, 1991b).

Interestingly enough, at the time of its withdrawal, only 3 reports had come from Sweden (daily doses were 37.5 mg, 50 mg and 50 mg), 1 from the Netherlands (dose unknown) and none from Japan. There were no reports of cardiac arrhythmias from Denmark, Germany or Ireland. There was no information from Luxembourg. The drug was not marketed in Belgium, France, Greece, Italy, Spain, or Portugal. Following its withdrawal, there were isolated reports of terodiline-induced torsades de pointes published from Denmark and Norway and additional ones from the Netherlands and one report of sudden expected death from Germany.

At the time of its withdrawal, about one million patients had been treated with terodiline worldwide, including about 450 000 in the United Kingdom. Even assuming a generous spontaneous reporting rate of 20%, the incidence of the risk is estimated at 1 in 1300 patients exposed. This remarkably high cardiotoxic potential of terodiline, uncovered through a spontaneous reporting system, is in sharp contrast to the generally reassuring safety profile that was being asserted on the basis of observations from post-marketing surveillance studies.

LIMITATIONS OF FORMAL POST-MARKETING SURVEILLANCE STUDIES

A general practice based Prescription Event Monitoring (PEM) study (Inman *et al.*, 1993) profiled the safety of terodiline in 12 457 patients treated between November 1986 and September 1987. Of these patients, 72.5% were females. The mean age was 65.6 (range 5–98) years in males and 63.3 (range 5–102) years in females. Incontinence (47.8%), frequency (16.9%), bladder irritability (7.7%) and urgency (6.6%) accounted for the majority of the indications for use of terodiline in females. In clinical practice, 62.2% of the patients were receiving a maximum daily dose of 25 mg, 18.2% were receiving 50 mg and a minority used other regimes up to a maximum of 100 mg per day. Terodiline was reported to have been effective in 56% of the patients. Cardiovascular events reported during the first 6 months and at any time during and after treatment with terodiline but *not* considered to be adverse reactions to it included dizziness ($n = 135$ and 255, respectively), syncope (41 and 105), hypotension (15 and 30), atrial

fibrillation (8 and 30), tachycardia (8 and 17), bradycardia (2 and 10), arrhythmias (2 and 8), ventricular fibrillation (0 and 3), heart block (0 and 2) and cardiac arrest (0 and 2). Even in a subsequent survey (initiated in 1990) of co-prescribing of various cardioactive medications, it could not be established whether the excess of syncope, arrhythmias, bradycardia, hypotension and other cardiovascular events was due to drug combinations or to the presence of co-existing cardiovascular disease. Of all the events reported in the cohort, only 51 events were noted to have been suspected adverse reactions to terodiline and these included 2 cases of dizziness. No case of cardiovascular collapse attributable to torsade de pointes could be found.

Even a retrospective study, undertaken in the aftermath of this powerful signal from spontaneous reports and withdrawal of the drug from the market, failed to better quantify the risk of cardiotoxicity of terodiline. In this study (Hall *et al.*, 1993), using the VAMP database, a preliminary open study identified a total of 9176 terodiline-treated patients. Altogether, a total of 59 patients were found to have had a cardiac arrhythmia during the follow-up period and a total of 77 (0.8%) of the patients had an ECG investigation during the study period. There was only one confirmed case of torsades de pointes in a 41-year-old female who had hypokalaemia at the time of the event. Apart from 50 mg terodiline, she was concurrently receiving a tricyclic antidepressant. This open study estimated the risk of terodiline-induced torsades de pointes to be 1.1 per 10 000 patients. In a retrospective cohort extension of this study, 5705 terodiline-treated patients were compared with 9604 controls. It concluded that there was no significant difference in the risk of developing an arrhythmia in the terodiline-treated patients compared with that of their controls. The risk compared with controls was estimated at 1.1 (95% CI: 0.64–1.90). Even the patients reporting symptoms suggestive of cardiac arrhythmias (syncope, collapse, blackouts) were not overly represented in the terodiline-treated cohort. Only dizziness and falls were reported significantly more frequently in the terodiline-treated patients (5.13% vs. 3.35%). A retrospective but limited inquiry into the nature of arrhythmias in the 59 patients elicited information in 19 patients. These included 6 bradycardia, 4 heart blocks, 3 ventricular tachycardias, 2 ventricular conduction defects, 2 extrasystoles, 1 tachy-brady syndrome and 1 cardiac arrest! None had previously been reported to the CSM through the yellow cards and 16 of the 19 practitioners concerned agreed to complete a yellow card.

Both of these studies had failed spectacularly if it was intended that they would test or strengthen a "hypothesis" signalled through the spontaneous reporting system.

ELECTROPHYSIOLOGICAL BASIS OF TORSADES DE POINTES

The QT interval on the surface electrocardiogram, measured from the beginning of the Q wave to the end of the T wave, represents the period from the beginning of depolarisation to the end of repolarisation of the ventricular myocardium. Prolongation of this interval is most frequently and necessarily associated with class III (potassium channel blocking) antiarrhythmic activity. This class of antiarrhythmic drugs produces, by definition, the desired therapeutic benefit by a controlled prolongation in ventricular repolarisation, and therefore the myocardial refractory period. Unfortunately, however, excessive prolongation of the QT interval can be proarrhythmic and degenerates into a potentially fatal ventricular tachyarrhythmia known as torsades de pointes. Clinical manifestations of this usually transient tachyarrhythmia include palpitation, syncope, blackouts, dizziness and/or seizures. Torsades de pointes subsequently degenerates into ventricular fibrillation in about 20% of cases (Salle et al., 1985) and, not uncommonly, cardiac arrest and sudden death may be the outcome. The overall mortality is of the order of 17% (Salle et al., 1985). It is plainly evident that the balance between the therapeutic antiarrhythmic effect and the potentially fatal proarrhythmic activity of QT interval prolongation is a very delicate one, depending not only on the drug concerned and its plasma concentration but also on a number of host

factors. These include electrolyte imbalance (especially hypokalaemia), bradycardia, cardiac disease, cirrhosis, autonomic failure and pre-existing prolongation of QT interval. Females are at greater risk.

At a molecular level, QT interval prolongation reflects prolongation of the ventricular action potential duration due to delayed repolarisation resulting from blockade of the outward current responsible for repolarisation during phases 2 and 3 of the action potential. Exceptionally, it could result from enhanced inward sodium current. Against a background of prolonged QT interval, the presence of slow heart rates gives rise to early after-depolarisations (EADs), mediated by slow inward calcium current during the late phase 2 of the action potential, that trigger torsades de pointes. Although a number of currents, predominantly mediated by potassium ions, are involved during repolarisation, the one almost universally affected by all the drugs—non-cardiovascular and non-antiarrhythmics alike—prolonging the QT interval is the rapid component of the delayed rectifier potassium channel and known as the I_{Kr} current.

The expression of this and other potassium channels is under the control of genes that are known to carry mutations responsible for channels with diminished or absent functional capacity—the so-called "diminished cardiac repolarisation reserve". The clinical phenotypes of these patients are the congenital long QT syndromes such as Romano–Ward and Jervell Lange–Neilsen syndromes. Evidence is now also accumulating that in view of the low penetration of many of these mutations, the size of population with mutations of potassium channels may be substantially larger than those diagnosed by ECG recording alone. Relatively large numbers of individuals who carry these "silent" mutations of long QT syndrome genes have been identified. Despite a diminished repolarisation reserve, they have a normal ECG phenotype. It has been postulated that drug-induced long QT syndrome might represent a genetically-mediated "forme fruste" of the long QT syndrome.

Unicellular recordings of action potential could be conducted in ventricular tissues or in Purkinje fibres in order to evaluate the effect of drugs on QT interval. In general, higher concentrations are necessary to induce EADs in ventricular cell preparations than in Purkinje preparations, thus introducing an added complexity in interpretation of the findings. A ventricular cell subtype, designated the M cells, which are found in the deep subepicardial to midmyocardial layers, has been identified as a very sensitive preparation for testing the drugs for their potential to prolong the QT interval and induce EADs. These cells, also found in human ventricles, have electrophysiological properties that are different from those of epicardial or endocardial ventricular cells and intermediate between those of the ventricular muscle or the Purkinje fibres. The hallmark of these M cells is the ability of their action potential to prolong markedly with decreasing stimulation rate. The presence of a smaller potassium current in the M cells is thought to be largely responsible for their unique pharmacologic responsiveness. Arising from the qualitative and quantitative distribution of various ion channels, these cells seem to have a better predictive value than do other tissues. From one set of investigations, it is possible to obtain a broad range of clinically useful results. The species used for these experiments could be guinea pig, rabbit or dog, depending on laboratory skills and database. The relevance of the selected species and the tissue to man is perhaps the most important determinant of how useful the information obtained will be with regard to whether a drug will pose a liability following exposure of humans to the drug.

In vitro studies using unicellular preparations have many advantages over *in vivo* or perfused organ studies. Preparations that have been used most frequently include ventricular myocytes including the use of M cells, papillary muscle and Purkinje fibres. Inclusion of a positive control, preferably from the same therapeutic, pharmacologic or chemical class, will further increase the reliability of the results.

If electrophysiological studies with unicellular preparations confirm an effect of the drug on cardiac action potential duration, it is then appropriate to proceed to define the channels and ionic currents involved. As stated earlier, the vast majority of the drugs known to adversely (or intentionally for class III antiarrhythmic drugs) prolong ventricular repolarisation do so by blocking the rapid component of the delayed rectifier potassium current, I_{Kr}. At the molecular level, the channel for the I_{Kr} current is expressed by proteins encoded by the HERG (human ether-a-go-go) gene on chromosome 7. The α-subunit forming the HERG K^+ channel carries the I_{Kr} current. *In vitro* tests could be conducted to evaluate a potential blocking effect of a new chemical entity (NCE) on endogenous cardiac I_{Kr} current or on recombinant HERG (human ether-a-go-go gene, responsible for encoding for delayed rectifier potassium channel 1) channels in heterologous expression systems. The use of HERG channels as a screening test is a relatively new *in vitro* tool but its track record to date has been impressive in being highly predictive of a drug's potential to prolong the QT interval and probably induce torsades de pointes. False positives may result if, for example, there is defective protein trafficking of the HERG potassium channel. In addition, channels with α-subunits or accessory β-subunits encoded by HERG gene mutations conduct a current of smaller amplitude. In consequence, the repolarisation process is delayed when these mutations are present.

Of the drugs listed earlier in the Introduction, studies with HERG channels would have successfully predicted the proarrhythmic activities of pimozide, sertindole, astemizole, terfenadine and cisapride. Studies using HERG channels have not been performed to date with the others. Even these drugs have, however, been shown in unicellular preparations to prolong the action potential and hence the QT interval.

Recent *in vitro* studies have confirmed that terodiline blocks the rapid component of the delayed rectifier potassium current—the molecular substrate for prolongation of the QT interval (Jones *et al.*, 1998). In guinea pig papillary muscles and ventricular myocytes, clinically relevant concentrations of terodiline lengthened the action potential duration by up to 12% while higher concentrations shortened the duration in a concentration-dependent manner. Voltage-clamp studies indicated that terodiline inhibits three membrane currents that govern repolarisation—an E4031-sensitive, rapidly activating K^+ current (IC_{50} near 0.7 μM), a slowly activating, delayed-rectifier K^+ current (IC_{50} value of 26 μM), and an L-type Ca^{2+} current (IC_{50} value of 12 μM) (Shuba et al., 1999).

INITIAL REGULATORY DELIBERATIONS

Questions arise, inevitably in retrospect, as to whether terodiline should have been approved at all and whether its proarrhythmic potential could have been anticipated. While it may be easy to answer these in retrospect, the commentary that follows is not based entirely on the benefit of hindsight because the nature of the problem had become apparent at the regulatory authority immediately on receipt of the first two to three reports of cardiotoxicity.

There is little doubt that urinary incontinence, although relatively benign in terms of morbidity, is a highly prevalent condition that has a serious adverse effect on the quality of life. No other drug with a comparably satisfactory and favourable risk–benefit ratio was available at the time of the approval of terodiline in 1986. Clinical trials had shown terodiline to be effective and, by all accounts, relatively safe. The efficacy of terodiline had been demonstrated in a number of studies (Yoshihara et al., 1992; Anon, 1993; Norton et al., 1994). The majority of the reactions reported were mild and anticholinergic. The safety of terodiline 50 mg daily was evaluated in a 6-month study in 100 women with urgency/urge incontinence by recording of adverse reactions and measurements of haematology, liver function, creatinine, ESR, heart rate and blood pressure (Fischer-Rasmussen, 1984). Mean levels of all variables on clinical chemistry were well within the normal range. Ninety-one patients were evaluated after 3 months and 70 after both 3 and 6 months. No significant changes were seen except for a small increase in platelet, serum creatinine and ESR. No significant changes in heart rate or blood pressure occurred except for a small but statistically significant increase (about 2 mmHg) in resting diastolic blood pressure after 6 months. Adverse reactions, usually those to be expected from the anticholinergic pharmacological effects of the drug, caused withdrawals in 12 patients. In a randomised, double-blind, two-period cross-over (3-week period) trial in 89 women with motor urge incontinence without other neurological symptoms, no statistically significant difference in incidence of side-effects could be demonstrated between 37.5 mg daily of terodiline and placebo (Peters, 1984).

Given the therapeutic options available at the time, there is no question that its approval was a highly justified decision. Even during the few months immediately following its withdrawal, many patients and urologists continued to write to the Agency, testifying to its benefits, how the lives of many patients had been transformed and complaining about the abrupt loss of a highly valuable drug. An option to make the drug available on a named patient basis was considered but never followed through. The withdrawal of terodiline was an equally less difficult decision since its risk–benefit was found to be clearly unfavourable and another drug, oxybutynin, had already been approved in January 1991.

However, four vital pieces of information that might have heralded the potential proarrhythmic hazard of terodiline were already available at the time of its redevelopment. The analogy between terodiline and prenylamine extends well beyond their structures into their pharmacology and toxicity profiles. Firstly, the association between prenylamine, also an antianginal agent, and its propensity to prolong the QT interval and induce torsades de pointes; secondly, the stereoselectivity in the proarrhythmic potential of prenylamine; thirdly, the stereoselectivity in the pharmacodynamic activities of the two enantiomers of terodiline and the unexpectedly high frequency of anticholinergic effect observed during its use as an antianginal agent should have suggested an unusual behaviour of one of the enantiomers, and lastly, the wide inter-individual variability in the metabolism of terodiline with aberrant pharmacokinetic behaviour of one of the enantiomers.

To illustrate the regulatory thinking at the time, frequent references will be made to prenylamine in this commentary. This will highlight the striking similarity between these two drugs and, hence, the logic that should have supported the re-development of the drug. Importantly, this comparison emphasises the strengths of a scientific synthesis of all the available information when evaluating the significance of the first two to three reports and determining the best regulatory options.

STRUCTURAL ALERT

Structurally, terodiline (Figure 11.1) and prenylamine (Figure 11.2) are both closely related. Introduced in the United Kingdom in the early 1960s, prenylamine is a diphenylpropyl derivative of phenylethylamine while terodiline is a diphenylpropyl derivative of butylamine. The presence of a chiral centre in each drug gives rise to a pair of enantiomers. It is acknowledged that even a minor modification in the structure of a molecule can dramatically alter the activity of a drug, and indeed this is the basis of metabolic inactivation of most drugs. However, notwithstanding the minor structural differences between terodiline and prenylamine, it is intuitive that terodiline must have some cardiac effects since it was marketed originally as a cardioactive antianginal agent.

PRENYLAMINE-INDUCED PROARRHYTHMIAS

Prenylamine was also withdrawn from the market worldwide in 1988 because of its high potential to prolong the QT interval and induce torsade de pointes, often with a fatal outcome (Anon, 1988).

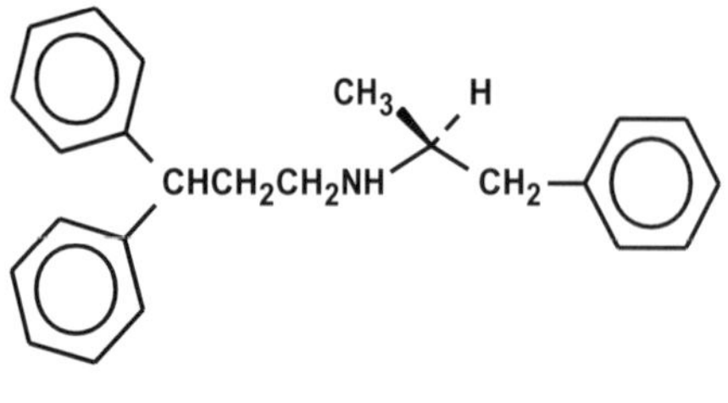

Figure 11.2. (+)-(S)-prenylamine.

When first marketed, the standard recommended dose of prenylamine for the majority of patients was 60 mg three times daily, which could be increased to 60 mg four or five times daily in those patients who did not respond within 7 days of starting treatment. It was not until 1971 that reports (mostly from France and the United Kingdom) linking prenylamine with prolongation of the QT interval, ventricular tachycardia, ventricular fibrillation and torsades de pointes began to appear (Picard *et al.*, 1971). Despite changes in dose schedules and warnings, prenylamine-induced proarrhythmias continued to be reported and by 1988, 158 cases of polymorphous ventricular tachycardia were reported in association with prenylamine and the drug was withdrawn worldwide soon after its removal from the UK market. About 80% of patients were female. The mean age was 68 ± 11 years and 30 of the 109 patients had received prenylamine as the only medication. The vast majority of the patients were taking 180 mg daily. Hypokalaemia was present in 34 of the 82 patients for whom this information was available.

Strikingly, neither drug had declared its proarrhythmic potential during their development. Cardiotoxicity following their routine clinical use did not become evident for at least 2–3 years after marketing. A number of prospective studies with prenylamine were conducted to study its effect on QT interval but none could demonstrate a significant difference before and after treatment with the drug. A review of the clinical trials data on terodiline proved unhelpful for evaluation of its effect on ECG. However, in one study in 12 patients in sinus rhythm, undertaken after its withdrawal from the market (Thomas *et al.*, 1995), mean QTc interval and QT dispersion were significantly prolonged to 491 and 84 ms during racemic terodiline treatment compared with measurements of 443 and 42 ms, respectively, made off therapy. The mean drug-induced increases were 48 ms for the QTc interval and 42 ms for QT dispersion. QT interval prolongation was shown to correlate closely with steady state plasma concentrations of (+)-(R)- and (−)-(S)-terodiline.

Both drugs further illustrate a more general difficulty in successfully containing a clinical risk by amending the prescribing information. These changes may include new dose schedules, contra-indications, precautions for use, risks of drug interactions and monitoring requirements. Unfortunately, this strategy has proved to be highly disappointing in risk management, as evidenced recently by a number of high profile drugs such as terfenadine, astemizole, cisapride (all associated with proarrhythmias), troglitazone and bromfenac (both associated with hepatotoxicity) (Shah, 1999). All these drugs have been withdrawn from the market. Most recent casualty was cerivastatin which continued to be inappropriately prescribed concurrently with gemfibrozil (resulting in rhabdomyolysis) despite a contraindication.

PHARMACOKINETIC SIMILARITY TO PRENYLAMINE AND RECOMMENDED DOSE SCHEDULES

Both terodiline and prenylamine bear an uncanny resemblance in their pharmacokinetics and the dose schedules of the two drugs should be scrutinised in the context of their elimination half-lives.

Prenylamine is extensively metabolised in man by ring hydroxylation and further methylation of the phenolic metabolites—its absolute bioavailability is estimated to be 15%. This metabolism displays wide inter-individual variation. The pharmacokinetics are enantioselective, favouring the elimination of the (+)-(S)-enantiomer (Geitl et al., 1990; Paar et al., 1990). The mean plasma half-lives after a single dose were 8.2 hours for the (−)-(R)-enantiomer and 24 hours for the (+)-(S)-enantiomer. With chronic dosing, however, the mean half-lives for the (−)-(R)- and (+)-(S)-prenylamine in 8 volunteers were 13.7 and 17.4 hours respectively. The maximum plasma concentration and AUC (area under curve of plasma concentration vs. time) of the (−)-(R)-enantiomer were shown to exceed those of the (+)-(S)-enantiomer by 4- to 5-fold—the apparent oral clearance of the (+)-(S)-form was 4.6-fold and the renal clearance 2.4-fold higher than that of the (−)-(R)-form.

Thus, another area of concern in the re-development of terodiline should have been its metabolic

disposition. Terodiline is also extensively (85%) metabolised to a phenol, p-hydroxy-terodiline, which is as active as the parent compound. There is wide inter-individual variation in its metabolism (Karlén et al., 1982; Hallén et al., 1994).

The effects of racemic terodiline on isolated detrusor preparations from rabbit and man were compared with those of its (+)-(R)- and (−)-(S)-isomers, and with those of its main metabolite, p-hydroxy-terodiline (Andersson et al., 1988). It was concluded that (+)-(R)-terodiline is the main contributor of the detrusor effects of the racemate, and that a component of this activity is anticholinergic in nature. p-Hydroxy-terodiline had a profile of pharmacological activity similar to that of racemic terodiline, but its potency was low. Since this metabolite is present in the plasma in low concentrations even at steady state (about 0.05 µg/mL), its contribution to the clinical effects of terodiline is probably small. The estimated potencies of the parent drug and the main metabolite and the fact that p-hydroxyterodiline constitutes only 10%–20% of the terodiline steady-state plasma level in man indicate that the contribution of this metabolite to the chronotropic effect observed in clinical studies is minor (Hallén et al., 1990).

In studies using human liver microsomes, the metabolism of terodiline at high concentrations has been shown to be stereoselective for the (+)-(R)-enantiomer (Norén et al., 1989) although, at steady state, the ratio of the concentrations of the two enantiomers at clinical doses is close to unity (Hallén et al., 1995).

The average steady-state serum concentrations on a 12.5 mg twice daily dose are 0.518 µg/mL in geriatric patients and 0.238 µg/mL in healthy volunteers. The mean half-lives of the drug are 57 (range 35–72) hours in young adults and 131 (range 63–237) hours in the elderly (Hallén et al., 1989). Therefore, the corresponding times to steady-state plasma levels would be 7–15 days in young adults and 2–7 weeks in the elderly.

Following their studies on the pharmacokinetics of terodiline in 9 healthy volunteers who were given (i) 12.5 mg intravenously and orally and (ii) 20 mg intravenously and 25 mg orally on two different occasions, Karlén et al. (1982) had concluded that the long serum half-life of terodiline should permit its once daily administration. Side-effects were often encountered at concentrations exceeding 0.6 μg/mL (Andersson, 1984).

When announcing its withdrawal, the marketing authorisation holder of terodiline advised prescribers to identify immediately all their patients being treated with it and stop the drug as soon as practicable. They also cautioned the prescribers to bear in mind the long half-life of terodiline if alternative anticholinergic treatment was considered and recommended a washout period, which on average would be 2–3 weeks but in some cases as long as 6 weeks.

ROLE OF PHARMACOGENETICS AS A RISK FACTOR

It appears probable that the metabolism of both terodiline and prenylamine may be controlled by the P450 cytochrome CYP2D6, the isoform responsible for debrisoquine hydroxylation. This major drug metabolising isozyme is expressed polymorphically in a population, resulting in two major phenotypes: extensive (EM) and poor (PM) metabolisers. The latter are unable to effect the metabolic elimination of many CYP2D6 substrates which include antiarrhythmics, β-blockers, antihypertensives, neuroleptics and antidepressants.

On chronic dosing, the half-lives for the (−)-(R)- and (+)-(S)-prenylamine were 13.7 and 17.4, hours respectively (Geitl et al., 1990). Generally, the steady-state plasma level was reached after 5–7 days indicating that the terminal half-lives of both the enantiomers of prenylamine were in the region of 24 hours. The high average value for the (+)-(S)-enantiomer following a single dose was mainly a consequence of the extremely long plasma half-life of 82 and 83 hours in 2 of the 8 volunteers. The remaining 6 subjects showed an average half-life of 11 hours. Although none of these subjects had been phenotyped for their metabolic capacity, prenylamine fulfils all the structural requirements of a CYP2D6 substrate and it is worth speculating whether the two individuals were poor metabolisers of CYP2D6 with an impaired ability to eliminate (+)-(S)-prenylamine.

Studies with rat liver microsomes suggest that more than one CYP isoform may be involved in the metabolism of terodiline, with different isoforms involved for the two enantiomers (Lindeke et al., 1987). Although much of the data in man are incomplete, puzzling or often difficult to reconcile, there is a fairly persuasive body of evidence to suggest that the major isozyme involved in the metabolism of (+)-(R)-terodiline is CYP2D6 and hence subject to genetic polymorphism. The formation of p-hydroxy-terodiline from (+)-(R)-terodiline was found to be impaired in one poor metaboliser of debrisoquine (Hallén et al., 1993). In this study of the pharmacokinetics of 25 mg oral dose of (+)-(R)-terodiline in healthy volunteers, the mean half-life of the isomer in 4 EMs of debrisoquine was 42 (range 35–50) hours and in the only PM, it was 117 hours. In another study (Thomas and Hartigan-Go, 1996) in healthy volunteers, which included 7 EMs and 2 PMs administered a single oral dose of 200 mg racemic terodiline, the maximum plasma concentrations and AUC of (+)-(R)-terodiline were significantly higher compared with (−)-(S)-terodiline and their half-lives were similar. The PM/EM clearance ratios for (+)-(R)-terodiline and (−)-(S)-terodiline were 45% and 56%, respectively.

Oxidative hydroxylation of the R-enantiomer of tolterodine, a new structural analogue of terodiline with antimuscarinic properties and marketed for the treatment of urinary incontinence, has also been shown in vitro and in vivo studies to be mediated principally by CYP2D6 (Brynne et al., 1998; Postlind et al., 1998), with CYP3A4-mediated dealkylation providing the main route of elimination in those who are the PMs of CYP2D6 (Brynne et al., 1999).

However, in a study investigating the stereoselective cardiotoxicity of terodiline in healthy volunteers given high doses, elimination of terodiline enantiomers was not significantly delayed in two genotypic PMs of CYP2D6 (Hartigan-Go et al., 1996). Another study of the CYP2D6 and CYP2C19 genotypes of 8 patients who survived terodiline-induced proarrhythmias, 6 with torsades de pointes and 2 with ventricular tachycardia, concluded that the CYP2D6 alleles were no more frequent in these 8 individuals than in the normal population (Ford *et al.*, 2000). This study also found a statistically higher frequency of mutant CYP2C19*2 allele in this population and it was suggested that CYP2D6 poor metaboliser status was not primarily responsible for terodiline cardiotoxicity and that possession of the CYP2C19*2 allele appeared to contribute to adverse cardiac reactions to terodiline. This study has serious limitations that have been acknowledged by its authors, and among others include the lack of ECG evidence of QT interval prolongation or torsade de pointes, lack of information on co-medications in 2 patients and co-administration of diuretics in another 2 patients.

The susceptibility role of CYP2C19*2 suggested by Ford *et al.* (2000), however, does not explain either the absence of terodiline cardiotoxicity among the Japanese in whom the frequency of the CYP2C19*2 allele is much higher at 0.29–0.35 or the high frequency of anticholinergic effects of (+)-(R)-terodiline in Scandinavia, where the frequency of the CYP2C19*2 allele is far lower at no more than 0.08. Neither is there any evidence that the frequency of this allele is any higher among the elderly. Neither can the closely related CYP2C9 isoform be implicated. Terodiline 50 mg daily did not influence the anticoagulant effect of continuous daily administration of a mean dose of 5.3 mg warfarin or the plasma levels of the warfarin enantiomers (Hoglund *et al.*, 1989).

It is worth recalling that, among the 69 cases of terodiline-induced proarrhythmias reported to the CSM, there were 12 in whom there were no identifiable risk factors. Connolly *et al.* (1991) and Andrews and Bevan (1991) have also reported one case each of torsades de pointes in patients without any risk factors and in whom plasma terodiline levels were markedly elevated. Information on the genotypes of such patients would have been helpful in elucidating the role of genetic susceptibility to terodiline-induced proarrhythmias.

The consequence of this stereosensitive polymorphic metabolism is that the calcium antagonistic (−)-(S)-terodiline would accumulate in all patients over time, but in addition there will also be an accumulation of (+)-(R)-terodiline in the poor and intermediate CYP2D6 metabolisers.

Thus, genetically determined accumulation of (+)-(R)-terodiline could constitute another risk factor. While it is true that the doses used in Sweden and Japan were generally lower, this CYP2D6-mediated metabolism of (+)-(R)-terodiline might also explain the striking inter-ethnic differences in the incidence of ventricular arrhythmias associated with its use. Whereas 9% of the UK population are PMs, the corresponding figures for Sweden and Japan are only 2.5% and less than 1%, respectively. Such a metabolic pattern would indicate a high potential for drug–drug interaction in the United Kingdom between terodiline and other QT interval prolonging substrates of CYP2D6, such as neuroleptics, antidepressants and other antiarrhythmic drugs.

Mutations of potassium channels, resulting in diminished repolarisation reserve and increased pharmacodynamic susceptibility to prolongation of the QT interval, are common. Female gender is a particularly striking example of genetically conferred susceptibility. Furthermore, any cardiac disease-induced down-regulation of potassium channels will also increase this susceptibility to proarrhythmias. Genetic factors may also operate remotely through other mechanisms. For example, cardiac failure is the end result of many genetically (and non-genetically) determined cardiac diseases. Cardiac failure is typically associated with such a down-regulation. It is interesting to note that despite urinary incontinence, 27 of the 69 patients with terodiline-induced proarrhythmias analysed above were receiving diuretics and 33 were in receipt of other cardioactive medications. Hypokalaemia induced by these diuretics or electrophysiological activities of these cardioactive medications further potentiate pharmacodynamic susceptibility. In addition, there is increased susceptibility to QT prolonging drugs in patients with autonomic failure or neuropathy.

PHARMACODYNAMIC SIMILARITY TO PRENYLAMINE

Pharmacologically, too, terodiline resembles prenylamine. Although prenylamine has been labelled as a calcium antagonist, it is not a true antagonist since it does not act selectively at the membrane-associated, voltage-dependent calcium channels. However, it is a potent inhibitor of calmodulin-dependent enzymes, relaxes smooth muscle and reduces slow inward current. It has been shown to depress peak sodium conductance (Hashimoto *et al.*, 1978; Bayer *et al.*, 1988). Hashimoto *et al.* (1978) have also shown that prenylamine increased the duration of action potential, indicating that the drug may interfere with the late outward current. Thus, prenylamine has potassium channels blocking activity in addition to its negative inotropic and sodium channel blocking effects.

Terodiline not only blocks the uptake of calcium but, in addition, it blocks the utilistion of some intracellular stores of calcium. Some data suggest that the drug also has local anaesthetic activity comparable to that of lignocaine. Additional recent studies have confirmed that terodiline ($\geqslant$1–2 µM) leads to the blockade of the sodium and calcium channels as well as muscarinic receptors in canine cardiac tissues. Terodiline ($\geqslant$2 µM) also depressed the action potential plateau but did not significantly alter the action potential duration at concentrations $\leqslant$10 µM (Pressler *et al.*, 1995). In another study in anaesthetised dogs, terodiline (10 mg/kg given intravenously) significantly prolonged the QTc interval by 6%–8%, an effect thought to be associated with torsades de pointes (Natsukawa *et al.*, 1998). The primary pharmacological activities of terodiline are potent calcium antagonistic and non-selective antimuscarinic effects within the same concentration range. Although both activities probably contribute to the therapeutic effect to a variable extent, the anticholinergic effect predominates at low concentrations and the calcium entry blocking action at high concentrations (Andersson, 1984), suggesting the dominance of (+)-(R)-terodiline at low daily doses of 25–50 mg.

As with prenylamine, the pharmacological activities of terodiline are enantioselective. (−)-(S)-terodiline is almost ten times more potent than its antipode as a calcium antagonist, while (+)-(R)-terodiline is almost ten times more potent than (−)-(S)-terodiline in its anticholinergic activity (Larsson-Backström *et al.*, 1985; Andersson

et al., 1988). In a later study, the affinity and selectivity of racemic terodiline for muscarinic receptor subtypes was determined from functional responses of rabbit vas deferens (M1), guinea pig atria (M2) and bladder detrusor muscle (M3). The results suggest that the *in vivo* actions of racemic terodiline at (M3) receptors mediating bladder contraction may not be separable from its actions at receptors mediating mydriasis and salivation. Moreover, its effects on the pupil and salivary glands are apparently not mediated through M1 receptors (Noronha-Blob *et al.*, 1991).

STEREOSELECTIVITY IN PROARRHYTHMIC POTENTIAL

Stereoselectivity in the activity of β-blockers and dihydropyridine calcium channel blockers at receptors and ion channels is well known. Stereoselectivity in activity at potassium channels has also been described more recently for enantiomers of other drugs such as (+)-(R)-bupivacaine, (+)-(R)-halofantrine and (−)-(4S,6S)-acetylmethadol (levoacetylmethadol).

As regards their adverse secondary cardiac pharmacodynamics, both prenylamine and terodiline display stereoselectivity (Rodenkirchen *et al.*, 1980; Bayer *et al.*, 1988; Hartigan-Go *et al.*, 1996).

In cat papillary muscle preparations (Bayer *et al.*, 1988), (+)-(S)-prenylamine exhibited a positive inotropic action over a wide concentration range, while the (−)-(R)-isomer had a negative inotropic effect. The positive inotropic effect of the (+)-(S)-isomer was particularly evident at low concentrations and at low stimulation rates. The maximum velocity of depolarisation was decreased by the (−)-(R)-isomer and somewhat increased by the (+)-(S)-isomer and the racemic mixture at low concentrations. (+)-(S)-prenylamine prolonged the action potential plateau and the duration of total action potential and dysrrhythmia occurred in 4 of 12 isolated papillary muscle preparations. In contrast, (−)-(R)-isomer shortened the action potential duration to a minor extent. This effect was independent of stimulation rates but evident at low concentrations. Therefore, overall, the data suggest that the proarrhythmic effect of prenylamine in man may have been mediated by (+)-(S)-prenylamine. This finding must be seen in the context of the finding that although the maximum plasma concentration and AUC of the (−)-(R)-enantiomer exceed those of the (+)-(S)-enantiomer by 4- to 5-fold normally, the reverse may be the case in PMs of CYP2D6. This difference between the EMs and the PMs would be more evident at low doses. Not surprisingly, most patients with prenylamine-induced proarrhythmias were receiving doses in the lower range of the recommended schedule.

As far as the author is aware, no *in vitro* study investigating the activity of individual enantiomers of terodilene on action potential duration has been reported to date. *In vivo*, however, the proarrhythmic potential of terodiline has been shown to reside exclusively in (+)-(R)-terodiline. A double-blind, placebo-controlled, randomised, crossover study in 9 healthy volunteers, given single oral doses of 200 mg racemic terodiline, 100 mg (+)-(R)-terodiline, 100 mg (−)-(S)-terodiline or placebo, revealed that both racemic and (+)-(R)-terodiline significantly increased the QT interval and the corrected QT interval (QTc). (−)-(S)-terodiline did not affect the QTc interval (Hartigan-Go *et al.*, 1996). Peak effects occurred 8 hours after dosing when mean increases in the QTc from baseline were −3 ms for the placebo, 23 ms for racemic terodiline, 19 ms for (+)-(R)-terodiline and 0 ms for (−)-(S)-terodiline. Although differences were observed between the pharmacokinetics of the two enantiomers, these were not sufficient to account for the differences in ECG effects, and their elimination half-lives (at these high doses) were similar. It will be recalled that (+)-(R)-terodiline predominates at low concentration, is normally preferentially eliminated and could accumulate in PMs of CYP2D6.

LESSONS TO BE LEARNT

The most important lessons to be learnt from re-development and withdrawal of terodiline are the necessity to draw on experiences with other drugs of the same class and the perils of exploiting adverse secondary pharmacological effects to re-target any drug. An analysis, even in hindsight, of the problems associated with previous drugs, especially of the same chemical and pharmacotherapeutic class, is the cornerstone of a strategic drug development of new drugs in future.

Additionally, there is still a more compelling need to appreciate the limitations of clinical trials and the weaknesses of the more formal studies in identifying post-marketing risks. Since QT interval prolongation and/or torsades de pointes are ECG-based diagnoses, the negative findings from PEM and VAMP studies are not surprising. It is the author's view that the databases used for these studies (general practice based) are not appropriate for the identification or quantification of risks that require ECG diagnosis and may not be sensitive enough to sample hospital-based diagnoses. It is inconceivable that the risk of QT interval prolongation can be characterised when only 0.8% of the cohort under investigation had an ECG investigation (Hall *et al.*, 1993). Inman *et al.* (1993) acknowledge that

> In what is likely to be the largest study ever conducted on this drug, we can find no case of cardiovascular collapse which was attributed to the so-called torsade de pointes arrhythmia …. It is very unlikely, however, that this abnormality would be encountered in general practice since it would only be identified by ECG.

Following the alert by McLeod *et al.* (1991) associating terodiline with torsade de pointes, Veldhuis and Inman (1991) therefore re-examined the PEM database for several possible clinical manifestations of these abnormalities and compared their incidence in terodiline-treated patients with that in a broadly matched nabumetone-treated patients. Confusion, syncope, cerebrovascular accidents, transient ischaemic attacks and falls and fractures were appreciably more frequent in the terodiline group. Although this *post hoc* analysis was not considered conclusive, these investigators recommended that an ECG should be performed on patients who develop confusion, syncope or cerebrovascular accidents while taking terodiline. From a regulatory perspective, such a *post hoc* analysis of clinical manifestations does not confirm the risk of potentially fatal proarrhythmias and cannot form the basis of any regulatory actions, particularly when, of all the events reported in the cohort, only 51 were noted to have been suspected adverse reactions to terodiline and these included only 2 cases of dizziness.

The problem was further compounded by the fact that neither the PEM nor VAMP study had included a large enough sample of patients. Even when the drug is known to possess the property to prolong the QT interval, it requires large prospectively designed hospital-based studies to uncover the real risk. A particularly good example of such a study is the SWORD study, which had to be terminated prematurely following recruitment of as many as 3121 of the planned 6400 patients (Waldo *et al.*, 1996). The mortality (presumed to be due to arrhythmias) was 5% in the (+)-(S)-sotalol group and 3.1% in the placebo group—an increase of 65% in mortality following the active treatment. Even in this study, patients were closely monitored during the first few weeks for excessive (and therefore, proarrhythmic) prolongation of their QTc interval and those with a QTc interval in excess of 560 ms during this period were excluded. For a potentially fatal reaction such as pro-arrhythmias, even a risk as low as 1 in say 3000 recipients is unlikely to be acceptable for relatively benign indications. Even if the background frequency of torsades de pointes is zero, it would require approximately 15 000 patients to identify a risk of 0.03% at 99% confidence level, even assuming that the database is sensitive enough in terms of the population and the adverse reaction to be studied. The strength of spontaneous reporting systems in identifying a serious clinical risk that requires hospital-based resources has been repeatedly demonstrated and almost all major regulatory actions in managing the clinical safety of drugs or averting major risks to public health have followed signals from spontaneous reports.

Furthermore, it is obvious that the pharmacokinetics and pharmacodynamics of each individual enantiomer of chirally active drugs should be fully investigated. Unfortunately, even today, the cytochrome P450 (CYP) isoform(s) responsible for the metabolism of terodiline has not been adequately identified and the role of genetic factors remains

a matter of informed and inferred speculation. Despite the known stereoselectivity in primary pharmacodynamics of terodiline enantiomers, little was investigated with respect to their cardiac effects, most particularly the electrophysiological effects at ion channels, and yet the techniques were available at the outset. In the absence of these vital data, it is impossible to predict any special patient populations at risk and the hazards from potential drug interactions. It is an unfortunate coincidence that terodiline should have been withdrawn from the market in the year in which the CPMP adopted a guideline on "Clinical Investigation of Chiral Active Substances" (Anon, 1998a; Shah *et al.*, 1998).

Above all, the most important lesson is the need to consider and thoroughly explore the potential of the candidate drug for the hazards associated with other drugs of the same chemical, pharmacological and/or therapeutic classes. In this context, the International Conference on Harmonisation (ICH) guideline on "The Extent of Population Exposure to Assess Clinical Safety for Medicines Intended for Long-term Treatment of Non-life threatening Conditions" is helpful (Anon, 1998b). For the most usual case, i.e. frequent and early onset events, the guideline provides for 1500 patients studied over 3 months and it is estimated that this database will characterise a cumulative 3-month incidence of about 1% or more.

The clinical and public health concerns on the potential of non-cardiac drugs to cause QT interval prolongation and potentially fatal torsades de pointes have been eloquently summarised in a recent editorial (Priori, 1998) Concerns have legitimately been expressed that:

> Almost every week a new agent is added to the list of drugs associated with acquired long QT syndrome (LQTS) and torsades de pointes (TdP). Despite this impressive number of reports, the awareness of this subject is still limited among medical professionals and ...

> It is likely that prevention of drug-induced TdP will never be fully successful, because it is a moving target. A patient may not be at risk when therapy is initiated, and may become at risk 5 days later because ...

> It is intuitive that when two or more agents sharing potassium-channel-blocking activity are

simultaneously administered, the risk of excessive prolongation of repolarisation is substantially increased.

... The exclusion of potassium-channel-blocking properties might be considered in the future as a requirement before new molecules are approved for marketing, and more strict warnings in the package insert of drugs with known repolarisation prolonging activity could be enforced.

The ICH guideline recognises that a longer period of observation than usual may also be required and provides for exceptional situations when the harmonised general standards for clinical safety evaluation may not be applicable. These exceptions cover a diverse range of circumstances when they may become applicable and can be best discussed by using drug-induced QT interval prolongation/torsade de pointes as an example. Five major exceptional circumstances are described which would require expanding the safety database in terms of numbers or duration of exposure. The scenario is equally applicable to other rare but serious adverse effects such as cholestatic jaundice, gastro-intestinal haemorrhage, neutropenia, etc.

EXCEPTIONAL CIRCUMSTANCES REQUIRING EXTENDED DATABASE

One can now examine how a very detailed evaluation of the safety of terodiline would have been required under the exceptions listed in the above ICH guideline. Although there are a number of exceptional circumstances specified in the guideline, five are of the greatest relevance to most new chemical entities.

CHEMICAL STRUCTURE

Arguably, any drug that shares a structural similarity with prenylamine is a candidate for a thorough preclinical and clinical evaluation of its potential to prolong the QT interval. Not surprisingly, terfenadine, terodiline, cisapride and pimozide all bear an obvious structural similarity to prenylamine and have all been associated with QT interval prolongation and torsades de pointes.

Apart from the study by Thomas *et al.* (1995), other studies have shown that adequate ECG monitoring of the patients during clinical trials ought to have identified the proarrhythmic risk. In the study by Yoshihara *et al.* (1992) in 109 Japanese patients receiving 24 mg daily of terodiline for 4 weeks, side-effects such as orthostatic hypotension and arrhythmia were observed but these symptoms disappeared following discontinuation of the treatment. Of note is the prospective study of Stewart *et al.* (1992) in 8 elderly in-patients treated with terodiline for urinary incontinence. They found a significant increase in the QT interval by a mean of 29 ms, the QTc interval by 15 ms and a decrease in the resting heart rate by a mean of 6.7 beats per minute after 7 days treatment with terodiline 12.5 mg twice daily.

PHARMACODYNAMIC/ PHARMACOKINETIC PROPERTIES KNOWN TO BE ASSOCIATED WITH SUCH ADVERSE EVENTS

In an effort to further characterise the pharmacodynamics of the drug, *in vitro* studies with isolated tissue preparations are undertaken. *In vitro* electrophysiological studies should form part of this programme. Interestingly, when investigated in retrospect for their effect on potassium channels, prenylamine, terodiline, terfenadine, astemizole, pimozide and cisapride were all found to block these channels. As far as their metabolites are concerned, those of halofantrine and terfenadine are devoid of this activity. However, the desmethyl metabolite of astemizole blocks potassium channels with the same potency as the parent compound but it has a much longer elimination half-life, thereby increasing the risk from accumulation of this metabolite, especially following an overdose. Findings such as these during preclinical studies would require a detailed ECG evaluation of the drug during its clinical development. Among non-cardiovascular agents, such drugs would include all neuroleptics, antidepressants, H1-antihistamines, antimalarials and quinolone antibacterials.

DATA FROM ANIMAL STUDIES

Information on the findings from animal studies with prenylamine is now difficult to obtain but the requirements for preclinical investigations at the time of developing prenylamine were rudimentary. Terodiline had no effect on the QT interval in conscious dog or rat. However, ECG effects (including prolongation of the QT interval) were reported in studies on anaesthetised cats. Arising from this observation, subsequent electrophysiological studies and more rigorous ECG monitoring in clinical trials could have been undertaken to evaluate its potential for proarrhythmias.

OTHER AGENTS OF THE SAME PHARMACOLOGICAL CLASS

This particular scenario requires that the safety database be expanded to exclude any class-related risks. A number of antianginal drugs have been shown to prolong the QT interval and induce proarrhythmias. These include prenylamine, bepridil, lidoflazine, tedisamil, perhexiline, fendiline and aprindine. Therefore, terodiline as well as other antianginal drugs should be evaluated routinely during their preclinical and clinical development for their potential to prolong the QT interval just as all non-steroidal anti-inflammatory drugs (NSAIDs) are evaluated for gastrointestinal toxicity.

As it was, the clinical trials database on terodiline was comparable with those for other drugs intended for urinary incontinence. In retrospect, however, it was not large enough for a drug with its chemical and antianginal pedigree. It had included 8 controlled ($n = 229$) and 6 uncontrolled ($n = 147$) studies with a total patient population of 376 exposed to terodiline. Of these, 241 had received the drug for up to 1 month and a further 39 for 2–3 months. Seventy-five patients had been treated for 4–12 months.

Following structural modifications of a lead compound, drugs are often discovered to have more potent activity at pharmacological targets other than originally intended. Therefore, drugs cross "therapeutic boundaries". A number of important QT-prolonging drugs belong to a specific chemical class usually associated with one therapeutic area but have later been developed or used clinically in an entirely different therapeutic area. Terfenadine is another typical example. It was discovered through a central nervous system programme aimed at synthesising new neuroleptic agents but because of its potent secondary pharmacological effects at the H_1-antihistamine receptor, it was developed as the first non-sedating H_1-antihistamine. It was a highly successful and popular drug until withdrawn due to reports of torsade de pointes resulting from drug interactions. Like all neuroleptics, it attracted considerable regulatory attention because of its effect on the QT interval. Sildenafil, originally intended for development as an antianginal drug, was developed instead for male erectile dysfunction and it is not surprising that at high concentrations, it has been shown to prolong cardiac repolarisation by blocking the rapid component of the delayed rectifier potassium current (Geelen et al., 2000). At clinical doses, a significant effect on QT interval is most unlikely (Sofowora et al., 2001), especially since the drug is used intermittently.

ALERTS/SIGNALS DURING CLINICAL TRIALS

When the risk of QT interval prolongation is high, signals are often present in the clinical trials database. Pimozide, for example, was found to prolong the QT interval in about 10% of the patients in one study in 1989. Similarly, halofantrine was also found during early clinical trials to produce an effect on the QT interval.

As a result of experiences with some of the established as well as newly introduced drugs, clinical trials programmes now usually include electrocardiographic monitoring in at least one or two large studies, particularly those investigating high doses or use of metabolic inhibitors. Depending on the findings from these "exploratory" studies, the database may require expansion to address the risk more fully.

In view of the many high profile drugs, which had attracted considerable regulatory attention in the years 1990–1996 due to their potential to prolong the QT interval and induce torsades de pointes, the CPMP adopted two significant documents in December 1997.

One of these was the CPMP document "Points to Consider: The Assessment of the Potential for QT Interval Prolongation by Non-cardiovascular Medicinal Products" (Anon, 1997a). The recommendations contained within this document are not mandatory but they do represent a strategy by which EU regulators would like to see an NCE investigated for its potential to induce proarrhythmic prolongation of the QT interval.

Following the regulatory concerns and the CPMP document, the European Society of Cardiology (ESC) organised a Policy Conference on drug-induced QT interval prolongation under the auspices of the ESC Committee for Scientific and Clinical Initiatives. A Report from this conference has now been published, endorsing a more rigorous investigation of the preclinical electrophysiological and clinical electrocardiographic effects of new drugs (Haverkamp *et al.*, 2000).

The other significant document was the CPMP "Note for Guidance on the Investigation of Drug Interactions" (Anon, 1997b). A number of drugs such as terfenadine, astemizole, pimozide, and cisapride have the propensity to induce torsade de pointes and other proarrhythmias as a result of drug interactions.

DEVELOPMENT OF SINGLE ENANTIOMERS OF MARKETED RACEMIC DRUGS

The marketing authorisation holder of terodiline is to be commended for the speed and the willingness with which it withdraw the drug as soon as it became evident that the risk is unlikely to be immediately manageable. Unfortunately, it did not follow up the recommendation from the regulatory assessor to investigate separately the two enantiomers systematically for their pharmacology, and possibly develop one of these if it can be shown to be devoid of potassium channel blocking activity while retaining a beneficial therapeutic effect. In light of the subsequent investigations, it seems possible that (−)-(S)-terodiline may have a favourable risk–benefit ratio. At the time of its

withdrawal in 1991, the development of a single enantiomer may have appeared a tedious and potentially unrewarding activity but this, paradoxically, has been one of the striking features of new drug development in the period 1994–2001. This trend has resulted in the development of (S)-ketoprofen, (S)-ofloxacin, (S)-omeprazole, (R)-salbutamol, (S)-citalopram and (S)-ketamine among many others that are still in the pipeline (Shah, 2000). The other notable trend is the development of active but safer metabolites, such as fexofenadine, norcisapride, norastemizole and desmethyl-loratadine, all virtually devoid of the unwanted secondary cardiotoxic pharmacology or unwanted metabolic profile and drug interaction potential.

REFERENCES

Andersson KE (1984) Clinical pharmacology of terodiline. *Scand J Urol Nephrol Suppl* **87**: 13–20.

Andersson K-E, Ekström B, Mattiasson A (1988) Actions of terodiline, its isomers and main metabolite on isolated detrusor muscle from rabbit and man. *Pharmacol Toxicol* **63**: 390–5.

Andrews NP, Bevan J (1991) Torsade de pointes and terodiline. *Lancet* **338**: 633.

Anon (1988) Prenylamine withdrawn in UK. *Scrip* (England), No. 1300, p. 26.

Anon (1991a) Terodiline (Micturin): Adverse cardiac reactions. *Dear Doctor/Pharmacist* letter dated 25 July 1991. London: Committee on Safety of Medicines.

Anon (1991b) Withdrawal of terodiline. *Current Problems*, Issue 32, pp. 1–2. London: Committee on Safety of Medicines.

Anon (1993) Effects of terodiline on urinary incontinence among older non-institutionalised women. Terodiline in the Elderly American Multicenter Study Group. *J Am Geriat Soc* **41** 915–22.

Anon (1997a) Points to consider: the assessment of the potential for QT interval prolongation by non-cardiovascular medicinal products. *Committee for Proprietary Medicinal Products (CPMP/986/96)*. London: EMEA, 17 December 1997.

Anon (1997b) Note for guidance on the investigation of drug interactions. *Committee for Proprietary Medicinal Products (CPMP/EWP/560/95)* London: EMEA, 17 December 1997.

Anon (1998a) Clinical investigation of chiral active substances. CPMP Guideline (CPMP/3501/91) In: *The Rules Governing Medicinal Products in the*

European Union EUDRALEX, Vol. 3C: Efficacy Guidelines. Brussels: European Commission, pp. 381–91.

Anon (1998b) The extent of population exposure to assess clinical safety for drugs intended for long-term treatment of non-life-threatening conditions. CPMP Guideline (CPMP/ICH/375/95). In: *The Rules Governing Medicinal Products in the European Union EUDRALEX, Vol. 3C: Efficacy Guidelines* Brussels: European Commission, pp. 121–5.

Bayer R, Schwarzmaier J, Pernice R (1988) Basic mechanism underlying prenylamine-induced torsade de pointes: differences between prenylamine and fendiline due to basic actions of the isomers. *Curr Med Res Opin* **11**: 254–72.

Boyd G (1990) A correction to "An apparent fatal overdose of terodiline". *J Anal Toxicol* **14**: 194.

Brynne N, Dalén P, Alván G, Bertilsson L, Gabrielsson J (1998) Influence of CYP2D6 polymorphism on the pharmacokinetics and pharmacodynamics of tolterodine. *Clin Pharmacol Ther* **63**: 529–39.

Brynne N, Forslund C, Hallén B, Gustafsson LL, Bertilsson L (1999) Ketoconazole inhibits the metabolism of tolterodine in subjects with deficient CYP2D6 activity. *Br J Clin Pharmacol* **48**: 564–72.

Castenfors H, Hedenstiarna G, Glenne P-O (1975) Pilot study of the effects of terodiline chloride (Bicor) in obstructive pulmonary disease. *Eur J Clin Pharmacol* **8**: 197–200.

Cattini RA, Makin HL, Trafford DJ, Vanezis P (1989) An apparent fatal overdose of terodiline. *J Anal Toxicol* **13**: 110–12.

Connolly MJ, Astridge PS, White EG, Morley CA, Campbell-Cowan J (1991) Torsade de pointes, ventricular tachycardia and terodiline. *Lancet* **338**: 344–5.

Davis SW, Brecker SJ, Stevenson RN (1991) Terodiline for treating detrusor instability in elderly patients. *Br Med J* **302**: 1276.

Dessertenne F (1966) La tachycardie ventriculaire á deux foyers oppoœes variable. *Arch Mal Coeur Vaiss* **59**: 263–72.

Fischer-Rasmussen W (1984) Evaluation of long-term safety and clinical benefit of terodiline in women with urgency/urge incontinence. A multicentre study. *Scand J Urol Nephrol Suppl* **87**: 35–47.

Ford GA, Wood SM, Daly AK (2000) CYP2D6 and CYP2C19 genotypes of patients with terodiline cardiotoxicity identified through the yellow card system. *Br J Clin Pharmacol* **50**: 77–80.

Geelen P, Drolet B, Rail J, Berube J, Daleau P, Rousseau G, Cardinal R, O'Hara GE, Turgeon J (2000) Sildenafil (Viagra) prolongs cardiac repolarization by blocking the rapid component of the delayed rectifier potassium current. *Circulation* **102**: 275–77.

Geitl Y, Spahn H, Knauf H, Mutschler E (1990) Single

and multiple dose pharmacokinetics of R-(−)- and S-(+)-prenylamine in man. *Eur J Clin Pharmacol* **38**: 587–93.

Hall GC, Chukwujindu J, Richardson J, Lis Y, Wild RN (1993) Micturin (terodiline) hydrochloride, torsade de pointe and other arrhythmias—a study using the VAMP database. *Pharmacoepidemiology and Drug Safety* **2**: 127–132.

Hallén B, Bogentoft S, Sandquist S, Strömberg S, Setterberg G, Ryd-Kjellén E (1989) Tolerability and steady-state pharmacokinetics of terodiline and its main metabolites in elderly patients with urinary incontinence. *Eur J Clin Pharmacol* **36**: 487–93.

Hallén B, Gralls M, Brotell H, Strömberg S (1990) Pharmacokinetics of terodiline and a major metabolite in dogs with a correlation to a pharmacodynamic effect. *Pharmacol Toxicol* **66**: 373–81.

Hallén B, Gabrielsson J, Palmér L, Ekström B (1993) Pharmacokinetics of R(+)-terodiline given intravenously and orally to healthy volunteers. *Pharmacol Toxicol* **73**: 153–8.

Hallén B, Karlsson MO, Strömberg S, Norén B (1994) Bioavailability and disposition of terodiline in man. *J Pharmaceut Sci* **83**: 1241–46.

Hallén B, Gabrielsson J, Nyambati S, Johansson A, Larsson E, Guilbaud O (1995) Concomitant single-dose and multiple-dose pharmacokinetics of terodiline in man, with a note on its enantiomers and major metabolites. *Pharmacol Toxicol* **76**: 171–7.

Hartigan-Go K, Bateman ND, Daly AK, Thomas SHL (1996) Stereoselective cardiotoxic effects of terodiline. *Clin Pharmacol Ther* **60**: 89–98.

Hashimoto K, Nakagawa Y, Nabata H, Imai S (1978) *In vitro* analysis of Ca-antagonistic effects of prenylamine as mechanisms for its cardiac actions. *Arch Int Pharmacodyn Ther* **273**: 212–21.

Haverkamp W, Breithardt G, Camm AJ, Janse MJ, Rosen MR, Antzelevitch C, Escande D, Franz M, Malik M, Moss A, Shah R *et al.* (2000) The potential for QT prolongation and proarrhythmia by non-antiarrhythmic drugs: clinical and regulatory implications. Report on a Policy Conference of the European Society of Cardiology. *Eur Heart J* **21**: 1216–31.

Hoglund P, Paulsen O, Bogentoft S (1989) No effect of terodiline on anticoagulation effect of warfarin and steady-state plasma levels of warfarin enantiomers in healthy volunteers. *Ther Drug Monit* **11**: 667–73.

Inman W, Clarke J, Wilton L, Pearce G, Vendhuis GJ (1993) PEM Report No 2: Terodiline. *Pharmacoepidemiology and Drug Safety* **2**: 287–319.

Iravani VJ, Melville GN (1975) Effect of terodiline on bronchial muscles and on tracheobronchial clearance in the rat. *Arzneimittelforschung* **25**: 415–7 [Article in German].

Jones SE, Ogura T, Shuba LM, McDonald TF (1998) Inhibition of the rapid component of the delayed-rectifier K+ current by therapeutic concentrations of the antispasmodic agent terodiline. *Br J Pharmacol* **125**: 1138–43.

Karlén B, Andersson K-E, Ekman G, Strömberg S, Ulmsten U (1982) Pharmacokinetics of terodiline in human volunteers. *Eur J Clin Pharmacol* **23**: 267–70.

Larsson-Backström C, Arrhenius E, Sagge K (1985) Comparison of the calcium antagonistic effects of terodiline, nifedipine and verapamil. *Acta Pharmacol Toxicol* **57**: 8–17.

Lindeke B, Ericsson O, Jonsson A, Noren B, Strömberg S, Vangbo B (1987) Biotransformation of terodiline. III. Opposed stereoselectivity in the benzylic and aromatic hydroxylations in rat liver microsomes. *Xenobiotica* **17**: 1269–78.

McLeod AA, Thorogood S, Barnett S (1991) Torsade de pointes complicating treatment with terodiline. *Br Med J* **302**: 1469.

Natsukawa T, Matsuzaki T, Hayashi S, Ukai Y, Yoshikuni Y, Kimura K (1998) Comparison of the effects of NS-21 and terodiline on the QTc interval in dogs. *Gen Pharmacol* **30**: 137–42.

Norén B, Strömberg S, Ericsson O, Lindeke B (1989) Biotransformation of terodiline V. Stereoselectivity in hydroxylation by human liver microsomes. *Chem Biol Interactions* **71**: 325–37.

Noronha-Blob L, Prosser JC, Sturm BL, Lowe VC, Enna SJ (1991) (+/−)-Terodiline: an M1-selective muscarinic receptor antagonist. In vivo effects at muscarinic receptors mediating urinary bladder contraction, mydriasis and salivary secretion. *Eur J Pharmacol* **201**: 135–42.

Norton P, Karram M, Wall LL, Rosenzweig B, Benson JT, Fantl JA (1994) Randomized double-blind trial of terodiline in the treatment of urge incontinence in women. *Obstet Gynecol* **84**: 385–91.

Paar WD, Brockmeier D, Hirzebruch M, Schmidt EK, von Unruh GE, Dengler HJ (1990) Pharmacokinetics of prenylamine racemate and enantiomers in man. *Arzneim Forsch* **40**: 657–61.

Peters D (1984) Terodiline in the treatment of urinary frequency and motor urge incontinence. A controlled multicentre trial. *Scand J Urol Nephrol Suppl* **87**: 21–33.

Picard R, Auzepy P, Chauvin JP (1971) Syncopes a repetition au cours d'un traitement prolonge par la prenylamine (Segontine 60). *Presse Med* **79**: 145.

Postlind H, Danielson A, Lindgrén A, Andersson SHG (1998) Tolterodine, a new muscarinic receptor antagonist, is metabolized by cytochromes P450 2D6 and 3A in human liver microsomes. *Drug Metab Dispos* **26**: 289–93.

Pressler ML, Warner MR, Rubart M, Rardon DP, Zipes DP (1995) In vivo and in vitro electrophysio-logic effects of terodiline on dog myocardium. *J Cardiovasc Electrophysiol* **6**: 443–54.

Priori SG (1998) Exploring the hidden danger of noncardiac drugs. *J Cardiovasc Electrophysiol* **9**: 1114–6.

Rodenkirchen R, Bayer R, Mannhold R (1980) On the stereospecific negative inotropic action of prenylamine. *Naunyn-Schmiedeberg's Arch Pharmacol* **313** (Suppl): R41.

Salle P, Rey JL, Bernasconi P, Quiret JC, Lombaert M (1985) Torsades de pointe. Apropos of 60 cases. *Ann Cardiol Angeiol* (Paris) **34**: 381–8.

Shah RR (1999) Drug-induced hepatotoxicity: pharmacokinetic perspectives and strategies for risk reduction. *Adverse Drug React Toxicol Rev* **18**: 181–233.

Shah RR (2000) The influence of chirality on drug development. *Future Prescriber* **1**: 14–17.

Shah RR, Midgley JM, Branch SK (1998) Stereochemical origin of some clinically significant drug safety concerns: lessons for future drug development. *Adverse Drug React Toxicol Rev* **17**: 145–90.

Shuba LM, Kasamaki Y, Jones SE, Ogura T, McCullough JR, McDonald TF (1999) Action potentials, contraction, and membrane currents in guinea pig ventricular preparations treated with the antispasmodic agent terodiline. *J Pharmacol Exp Ther* **290**: 1417–26.

Sofowora G, Dishy V, Roden D, Wood AJJ, Stein CM (2001) The effect of sildenafil on QT interval in healthy men. *Clin Pharmacol Ther* **69**: 67 (abstract PIII-11).

Stewart DA, Taylor J, Ghosh S, Macphee GJ, Abdullah I, McLenachan JM, Stott DJ (1992) Terodiline causes polymorphic ventricular tachycardia due to reduced heart rate and prolongation of QT interval. *Eur J Clin Pharmacol* **42**: 577–80.

Thomas SHL, Hartigan-Go K (1996) Disposition of R(+)- and S(−)-terodiline in healthy man. *Clin Pharmacol Ther* **59**: 160 (PII-6).

Thomas SH, Higham PD, Hartigan-Go K, Kamali F, Wood P, Campbell RW, Ford GA (1995) Concentration dependent cardiotoxicity of terodiline in patients treated for urinary incontinence. *Br Heart J* **74**: 53–6.

Veldhuis GJ, Inman WHE (1991) Terodiline and torsades de pointes. *Br Med J* **303**: 519.

Waldo AL, Camm AJ, deRuyter H, Friedman PL, MacNeil DJ, Pauls KF, Pitt B, Pratt CM, Schwartz PJ, Veltri EP for the SWORD Investigators (1996) Effect of d-sotalol on mortality in patients with left ventricular dysfunction after recent and remote myocardial infarction. *Lancet* **348**: 7–12.

Wibell L (1968) Terodiline in angina pectoris—a controlled study of a new drug. *Acta Soc Med Ups* **73**: 75–80.

Wild RN (1992) Micturin and torsade de pointes—experience of a post-marketing alert. *Pharmacoepidemiology and Drug Safety* **1**: 147–50.

Yoshihara H, Yasumoto R, Kishimoto T, Maekawa M, Horii A, Nishijima T, Sugimoto T, Kashiwara N, Tsujita M, Senjyu M, *et al.* (1992) Clinical study of terodiline hydrochloride for the treatment of urinary frequency and urinary incontinence, and its cardio-vascular adverse effect. Hinyokika Kiyo **38**: 967–72 [Article in Japanese].

12

Nomifensine and Haemolytic Anaemia

PETER D. STONIER

HPRU Medical Research Centre, University of Surrey, Guildford, UK

J. GUY EDWARDS

Khon Kaen University, Khon Kaen and Prince of Songkla University, Hat Yai, Thailand

INTRODUCTION

Nomifensine was introduced by Hoechst AG into clinical practice in West Germany in 1976 and into the United Kingdom the following year. It was thought to have the advantages over older tricyclic antidepressants of causing less sedative, anticholinergic, cardiac and epileptogenic effects. The drug was withdrawn almost a decade later in January 1986 because of the occurrence during treatment of acute immune haemolytic anaemia associated with serious clinical sequelae. In the United Kingdom these included three fatalities, occurring in 1985.

This chapter discusses the response of the company to a drug alert in the post-marketing phase. With the benefit of hindsight several years later, this might seem a relatively straightforward task; it was a clear-cut case of increased recognition of a potentially life-threatening Type B adverse reaction, acute immune haemolytic anaemia. Although reported in small numbers, the unpredictability and speed of onset of the reaction precluded advice to doctors on early diagnosis and treatment. It was this, as much as the distressing condition and the consequences of medical and surgical interven-

tion (including exploratory laparotomies), that prompted the manufacturer to withdraw the product in the interests of patient safety.

Until the company made its announcement on 22 January 1986 in full consultation with the regulatory authorities, there had been no suggestion in the medical literature, the general or medical press or any other media that the drug should be withdrawn from use. Whilst the product withdrawal was coordinated worldwide, this account of the events leading up to the withdrawal relates only to the situation in the United Kingdom (Stonier, 1992).

Over the years since the withdrawal those with legal, political and consumer interests were able to come to their own conclusions about the product and the activities of prescribers, regulators and the manufacturer, which turned nomifensine into something of an international "affair" (Schönhöfer, 1991).

BACKGROUND

Nomifensine was first introduced in Germany in 1976 and in the United Kingdom in 1977 and was

Pharmacovigilance. Edited by R.D. Mann and E.B. Andrews
© 2002 John Wiley & Sons, Ltd

finally registered in 98 countries. It was a novel chemical entity, a tetrahydroisoquinoline, unrelated chemically to any other antidepressant. Like tricyclic antidepressants, however, its supposed mode of action was the inhibition of the presynaptic reuptake of biogenic amines in the brain, enhancing their concentration with the aim of combating depression (thought to be mediated by a relative deficiency of these amines). Nomifensine was also a powerful inhibitor of the reuptake of dopamine, with lesser effects on noradrenaline and, through its metabolites, on serotonin (Nicholson and Turner, 1977).

Its preclinical properties, which were confirmed in clinical use, showed the drug to have few anticholinergic and sedative effects. It was therefore a possible safer alternative to tricyclic antidepressants, which could be especially troublesome when taken in overdose. Nomifensine proved to be well tolerated in overdose and was not associated with significant cardiotoxicity or epileptogenic activity. These properties meant that the drug was potentially useful in certain depressive disorders, notably retarded depression, and in certain subgroups, such as those associated with cardiovascular disease and epilepsy, It was also considered to be of value in the treatment of elderly depressed patients and, through its dopaminergic properties, patients with early Parkinson's disease.

Depression is a very common condition with approximately one in seven general practitioner (GP) encounters being a follow-up appointment of a patient with depressive symptoms, and one in 25 encounters a new case. Only 10% of cases seen by GPs are referred to psychiatrists (Beaumont, 1984). The mainstays of pharmacological treatment during the 1980s, the tricyclic antidepressants and monoamine oxidase inhibitors, were associated with a considerable number of adverse reactions in most physiological systems (Edwards, 1981).

Nomifensine joined mianserin as a representative of a new generation of antidepressants that caused fewer side effects. Other drugs of this category introduced into practice at or near this time were maprotiline, viloxazine, tryptophan, zimeldine, trazodone and lofepramine, each with its own subsequent history of benefit and risk.

In the decade up to 1980 the total number of deaths from drug poisoning in England and Wales remained steady at about 3000 per year, two-thirds of which occurred outside hospital. During this time the proportions due to different groups of drugs changed considerably, with deaths due to barbiturates falling by half, and those due to analgesics and tricyclic antidepressants doubling. In 1980 tricyclic antidepressants were second only to barbiturates in causing death by poisoning (Crome, and Chand, 1980). An antidepressant with low toxicity in overdose would thus have life-saving potential if a patient, despite all efforts at prevention, decided to attempt suicide with the medication. Nomifensine proved to be exceptionally well tolerated in overdose in a number of published reports (Crome, and Chand, 1980; Garnier et al., 1982; Ali and Crome 1984).

HAEMOLYTIC ANAEMIA

Drug-induced haemolytic anaemia results from a type II immune reaction in which antibodies to the drug or its metabolite(s) attack blood cells. Antigens on the cell's surface combine with antibody and complement to stress the cell to the point of destruction. The cell damage causes anaemia. There is an increased production of bilirubin, although a healthy liver can excrete six times the normal load before unconjugated bilirubin accumulates in the plasma; jaundice is therefore mild. Severe haemolysis can result in prerenal uraemia and renal failure. Other related immunological reactions are referred to below.

POST-MARKETING EXPERIENCE 1977–82

Figure 12.1 shows the market data for nomifensine in the United Kingdom. Unit sales are shown in terms of defined daily doses of 100 mg. This terminology was not routinely used in 1979/1980 and was only adopted by the World Health Organisation (WHO) in January 1992 as an international standard denominator for calculating incidence. The numbers of prescription were provided by the Committee on Safety of Medicines (CSM) from the Prescription Pricing Authority,

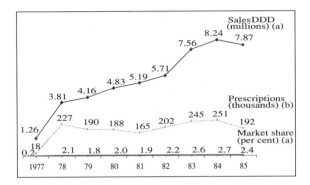

Figure 12.1. Market data for nomifensine in the United Kingdom. DDD = defined daily dose of 100 mg of nomifensine. (a) Source: UK manufacturer; (b) Source: CSM.

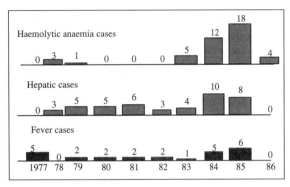

Figure 12.2. Incidences of reports of haemolytic anaemia, hepatic events and fever associated with nomifensine submitted to the UK manufacturer 1977–1986.

and the percentage UK market share achieved by nomifensine is shown; the total represents all antidepressant prescribing including generic compounds.

Figure 12.2 shows the incidence of reports of haemolytic anaemia, hepatic events and fever over time.

Nomifensine was first marketed as a 25 mg capsule formulation on 10 October 1977, whilst the 50 mg capsule was made available on 1 January 1979. Between 1978 and 1979 four reports of acute or chronic haemolytic anaemia occurring during treatment with nomifensine were received by the manufacturer (Table 12.1). The patients were females with an age range of 25–64 years. Three of them were taking 150 mg nomifensine

daily. Each had a different history of exposure and onset of haemolytic anaemia.

The type of haemolytic anaemia was characterised as chronic or acute, depending on the pattern of symptoms, their severity and the presence or absence of intravascular haemolysis. The symptoms of chronic-onset haemolytic anaemia included lethargy, fatigue and breathlessness, whilst the acute presentation of the condition involved backache, loin pain, jaundice and haematuria and, in certain cases, fever, renal failure and cardiorespiratory collapse. The Coombs' (anti-globulin) test was positive in all four cases. All of the patients had received concomitant medication, although it was considered to be non-contributory. When nomifensine

Table 12.1. First reports of haemolytic anaemia received by the UK manufacturer 1978–1979.

Date notified	Demographic data	Dose	Exposure	Type	Exposure time to provoking dose	Coombs' test	Outcome
29.08.78	Female aged 43 years	50 mg tds	1	Chronic	4 months	IgG+++	Full recovery
20.11.78	Female aged 25 years	2 g	2	Overdose		IgG	Full recovery
28.11.78	Female aged 54 years	50 mg tds	2	Chronic	5 months	IgG+	Full recovery
25.06.79	Female aged 64 years	50 mg tds	1	Acute	21 days	C₃d	Full recovery

was stopped the patients made a full and uneventful recovery.

The first documented report of haemolytic anaemia, published in the *Lancet*, came from France. This was a case of immune haemolytic anaemia and acute renal failure in a 50-year-old woman, who was diagnosed in May 1978 (Bournerias and Habibi, 1979). She had had seven episodes of malaise, chills, pain and fever of 2–4 h duration that were accompanied by dark urine and transient jaundice.

During one of the episodes in July 1978, she had had oliguria. At this time, she had a positive Coombs' test and a haemoglobin level of 10 g/dl. Before the episode, she had been treated for an unrelated illness with levomepromazine, diazepam and nomifensine. She made an uneventful recovery on stopping the medication. The serum of the patient demonstrated an antibody that agglutinated red blood cells only in the presence of nomifensine. The authors called for immunological studies for anti-nomifensine antibodies in patients on long-term treatment.

Another case of acute haemolysis and renal failure (following an overdose of nomifensine) was published the following year (Prescott *et al.*, 1980) (see Table 12.1) and three others from outside the United Kingdom were published in 1981–1982 (Eckstein *et al.*, 1981; Habibi *et al.*, 1981). One of these cases had intravascular haemolysis during treatment with nomifensine (Lyllof *et al.*, 1982).

Although these reports were of concern it was not considered at the time that nomifensine was more liable to cause haemolytic anaemia than other marketed drugs. However, heightened vigilance was recommended and the manufacturer initiated a number of retrospective and prospective immunological studies. These investigations failed to provide support for a cause-and-effect relationship between nomifensine and haemolytic anaemia. Some patients with haemolytic anaemia had a negative Coombs' test, while other patients with a positive Coombs' test did not have haemolysis. Nevertheless, in view of the suspected link between the antidepressant and the blood dyscrasias, haemolytic anaemia was included among the side effects listed in the January 1981 data sheet.

Between 1981 and 1982 there were three more UK cases of haemolytic anaemia reported to the Department of Health and Social Security (DHSS). They had not been referred to the manufacturer. They occurred among patients who had received a total of 990 000 prescriptions for nomifensine. This suggested an incidence of only about 1 per 150 000 patients, and thus no regulatory action was considered necessary (CSM Update, 1986; Mann, 1988).

These reports did not provide a consistent basis for any general announcement concerning the safety of nomifensine from the company or from a regulatory authority. They placed nomifensine at worst with a group of marketed drugs associated with haemolytic anaemia. This included stibophen, quinidine, paracetamol, penicillin, sulphonamides, tolbutamide, chlorpromazine, tetracycline, cephalosporins, insulin, rifampicin, hydralazine, streptomycin, triamterene and probenecid for immune haemolytic anaemia, and amongst methyldopa, mefenamic acid, flufenamic acid and levodopa given for autoimmune haemolytic anaemia.

Nevertheless, the company acted on the reports to institute both retrospective and prospective studies in Germany, France, the United Kingdom and Austria, in order to determine potential groups at risk. Between January 1979 and June 1980, 312 patients in these studies who had been treated for more than three months with nomifensine were given a Coombs' test, and sera from 220 patients were subjected to intensive immunological investigations. Even with these studies, the results did not prove a causative link with nomifensine. The Coombs' test proved to be inappropriate as a prediction of possible groups at risk amongst nomifensine users. Some patients without haemolysis had a positive Coombs' test and later several patients with haemolytic anaemia were found to have a negative Coombs' test.

In the course of time, supportable evidence for attributing haemolytic anaemia to nomifensine was produced, and in January 1981 this addition to the UK data sheet was agreed: "Haemolytic anaemia has also been reported in rare cases as has a rise in body temperature". This also appeared in the *ABPI Data Sheet Compendium* in October 1981.

Concern over the occurrence of haemolytic anaemia and the other serious reactions led to a number of additional immunological investigations, and this work in due course provided further evidence for the immunological basis of the haemolytic anaemia reaction (Walti *et al.*, 1983; Miescher, 1985; Salama and Mueller-Eckhardt, 1985).

Salama *et al.* (1984) demonstrated a nomifensine-dependent antibody that reacted exclusively to its *ex vivo* antigen (fresh serum of a volunteer who had taken a therapeutic dose of the drug), but not to nomifensine itself. The investigators later showed an "extraordinary heterogeneity" of antibody response following the ingestion of the antidepressant. Of 19 samples only five were primarily reactive to nomifensine. The majority reacted in the presence of one or more metabolite and *ex vivo* antigens, indicating specificity for an unidentified early or late metabolite.

All samples belonged to the IgG or IgM class or both and were capable of activating complement. At least one sample had two nomifensine-dependent red blood cell antibodies, while one had platelet antibodies. The latter explained the occurrence of purpura alongside the haemolysis. It is of interest also that seven of the 19 patients had signs of transient renal insufficiency, while six had increased levels of serum transaminase (type not specified; Salama and Mueller-Eckhardt, 1985).

Previously (in September 1978, published April 1979) the data sheet had been amended to draw attention to the association of nomifensine with fever. There had been several reports of this in Germany and five reports were submitted to the UK manufacturer in 1977. The data sheet stated that there had been "rare cases of rise in body temperature which returned to normal when the drug was withdrawn".

The data sheet of 1981 also drew attention to the association of nomifensine with changes in liver enzymes by stating that:

> In rare cases, increases in liver enzymes (serum transaminases and alkaline phosphatase) have been observed.

As a result of receiving four reports of haemolytic anaemia in 1978–1979, the manufacturer undertook the following actions:

- Full investigation of each case report. The normal company operating procedure involved acquiring full information on each case from the prescribing doctor, if necessary visiting the doctor to discuss the case and being accompanied on such visits by medical personnel from the central drug safety department of the company headquarters.
- All cases to be reported to the parent company and the UK DHSS.
- Re-appraisal of all preclinical work and clinical trials to see whether there was any evidence of blood dyscrasias. None was found.
- Retrospective and prospective immunological studies. These produced no consistent results related to the clinical use of the drug.
- Sales representatives to be informed of publications and investigative activities in order to respond appropriately to enquiries.
- Data sheet changes with international agreement relating to fever, haemolytic anaemia and the liver

POST-MARKETING EXPERIENCE 1983–1986

The increasing incidence of haemolytic anaemia from 1983 might appear to have been related to the launch of the 100 mg single daily dose formulation on 31 January 1983 (see Figure 12.1). However, no evidence emerged to support this. It appears that new additional sales were generated by this launch and that the associated promotion may have made doctors more aware of nomifensine. Prescriptions, sales and market share increased in 1983 by 21%, 32% and 18%, respectively. This, together with the data sheet changes and literature reports, may have served to alert doctors to the association of unusual symptoms with the use of nomifensine.

Reports of other severe untoward events that could have had an immunological basis also appeared in the literature in 1984–1985: thrombocytopenia (Green *et al.*, 1984), hepatitis (Vaz *et al.*, 1984), alveolitis (Hamm *et al.*, 1985) and a systemic lupus erythematosus (SLE)-like reaction (Garcia-Morteo and Maldonado-Cocco, 1983; Schönhöfer and Groticke, 1985). Those appearing in the British medical literature could possibly have contributed to an increased awareness amongst prescribers of adverse events associated with the drug. The first fatal case of immune haemolysis was published in 1985 (Sokol *et al.*, 1985) and two other cases were reported later the same year (Hamm *et al.*, 1985; Schönhöfer and Groticke, 1985).

In the early- to mid-1980s following the withdrawal of benoxaprofen and the recognition of problems with other non-steroidal anti-inflammatory drugs, together with promotion of the government's Yellow Card scheme, there was an increasing acceptance amongst doctors of the need to report adverse experiences with commonly prescribed drugs. In September 1983, the antidepressant zimeldine was withdrawn from the market following the identification of a serious neurological disorder, the Guillain–Barré syndrome. The publicity given to this may have affected the reporting of adverse events to drug therapy, including nomifensine.

The purpose of showing the comparative incidences of fever, hepatic reactions and haemolytic anaemia in Figure 12.2 is not to suggest any common underlying pathology to these three conditions; none has ever been substantiated. It is to indicate that, whilst reporting rates of haemolytic anaemia and hepatic problems (enzyme changes, jaundice or hepatitis) significantly increased with time, this was not the case with reports of febrile reactions. The incidence of these never reached the same levels as in some other countries, for example Germany. Cases in the United Kingdom in which fever was associated with haemolysis were catalogued in the haemolytic anaemia group.

Table 12.2 shows the UK manufacturer's total database of 296 events; this is to be compared with the CSM's Yellow Card database of 543 suspected adverse reactions. The company had 45 reports of haemolytic anaemia of which 43 were thought to be associated with the drug. This is to be compared with the CSM's 59 reports of which 49 contained sufficient information to attribute nomifensine as the probable, or a possible, cause. Forty-five of the 49 (92%) patients were women, although females received only 71% of the prescriptions for the drug. Some of the subjects, who had had a previous course of nomifensine without experiencing unwanted effects, developed acute haemolytic

Table 12.2. Nomifensine adverse events reported to the UK manufacturer 1977–1986.

Adverse event	Total number of reports
Haematological	
Aplastic anaemia	1
Increased bleeding time	1
Leucopenia	1
Thrombocytopenia	4
Positive Coombs' test	16
Haemolytic anaemia	45
Hepatic disorders	
Jaundice	27
Abnormal liver function tests	12
Hepatitis	6
Hepatic necrosis	1
General	
Pyrexia	13
Influenza-like symptoms	12
Allergic reactions	3
Other	12
Renal	
Interstitial nephritis	1
Other	5
Autonomic	3
Skin	21
Central nervous system	72
Cardiovascular	18
Endocrine	1
Gastrointestinal	17
Musculo-skeletal	1
Respiratory	1
Overdoses	2
Total	296

anaemia on recommencing treatment, while others developed haemolytic anaemia after months or years of continuous use. In 18 patients the haemolysis was severe: 11 of them developed renal failure and four died. Although haemolytic anaemia was the most frequently reported serious adverse reaction, concern was also expressed over other untoward effects (CSM Update, 1986).

From 1983 onwards, there was a steady rise in the number of reports of haemolytic anaemia to the UK manufacturer, with five reports in 1983, 12 in 1984 and 18, including three fatalities, in 1985. The first nomifensine-associated fatality in the United Kingdom was reported on 10 February, the second was reported on 31 March and the third on 10 April 1985. The three cases were discussed with the DHSS on 1 May 1985.

The first of these fatal cases was published in the *British Medical Journal* in August 1985 (Sokol *et al.*, 1985). The patient was a 36-year-old female who collapsed one hour after taking one 100 mg tablet. She had been treated with nomifensine for one week but stopped taking it because of dizziness. There was no jaundice or haematuria. On examination, she was conscious, but pale, cyanosed and shocked. Her blood pressure was 90/50 mmHg and her pulse was 90/min. Haematological tests showed spontaneous red cell agglutination, with free haemoglobin in the plasma, and the following results: haemoglobin 5 g/dl, bilirubin 4 μmol/l, and lactate dehydrogenase 1071 IU/I. The patient

had severe acidosis. Acute intravascular haemolysis was diagnosed. Attempts at resuscitation failed and the patient died. Immunological investigations showed a positive Coombs' test with antisera to IgG, IgM and C1. The serum contained cold-reacting auto-antibodies and pan-antibodies. In the presence of nomifensine, the antibodies led to the agglutination of red cells.

The proposed mechanism was that drug and antibody combined to form loose immune complexes that attached themselves to the red cells and activated complement. Complement activation led to haemolysis, disseminated intravascular coagulation and the shock–lung syndrome.

Between January 1983 and mid-June 1985, the DHSS was aware of 29 reports of haemolysis in 592 000 prescriptions—approximately one in 1 : 20 000 prescriptions (CSM Update, 1986).

In July 1985, the CSM's bulletin, *Current Problems* highlighted the dangers of newer

Table 12.3. Nomifensine: events and assessments leading to withdrawal (Edwards, 1997b).

Year	Events/assessments	References
1976	Nomifensine launched on to market in Germany	
1977	Nomifensine launched on to market in the United Kingdom	
1978–1979	Four cases of haemolytic anaemia reported to UK manufacturer	Stonier (1992)
1979–1981	Published reports of haemolytic anaemia ± renal failure	Bournerias and Habibi (1979) Prescott *et al.* (1980) Eckstein *et al.* (1981) Habibi *et al.* (1981)
	Demonstration of nomifensine-dependent antibody	Salama *et al.* (1984)
1984–1985	Published reports of Thrombocytopenia Hepatitis alveolitis (fatal) SLE[a]-like reaction (fatal)	Green *et al.* (1984) Vaz *et al.* (1984) Hamm *et al.* (1985) Schönhöfer and Groticke (1985)
1985	Published reports of fatal case of immune haemolysis Promotion of nomifensine discontinued "Dear Doctor" letter, United Kingdom "Red Hand" letter, Germany Estimated incidence of haemolytic anaemia June: 1 in 20 000 November: 1 in 4000	Sokol *et al.* (1985) Stonier (1992) CSM Update (1986)
1986	Nomifensine withdrawn from market	

[a]SLE = systemic lupus erythematosus.

antidepressants, and presented a summary of adverse drug reactions to nomifensine. A new data sheet was published with information submitted in October 1984. This stated:

> In rare cases, haemolytic anaemia and abnormal liver function tests with or without clinical jaundice have been observed. These reactions subside within a short time of discontinuing Merital (nomifensine) but may recur if it is taken again.

In September 1985, there were joint discussions between the company and the DHSS on a complete revision of the data sheet. On 24 September, the current data sheet was put in abeyance pending the outcome of these discussions and all promotion of nomifensine ceased.

On 30 September 1985, the company issued a "Dear Doctor" letter warning of the serious adverse reactions reported internationally; this letter was a version of a similar "Red Hand" letter issued at the same time by the parent company in Germany.

On 7 December 1985, the "CSM Update" on antidepressants, published in the *British Medical Journal*, summarised the comparative adverse reaction reports on all antidepressants (CSM Update, 1985).

On 16 December 1985, the *Drug and Therapeutics Bulletin* published an article "Trouble with nomifensine" after several revisions since the first draft in May. This was followed by a number of newspaper reports on the drug.

Between mid-June and the end of November 1985, the DHSS was aware of 25 reports of haemolysis in 96 000 prescriptions (1:4000; CSM Update, 1986). This was the first time that the incidence had increased to a level above 1:10 000 (the accepted WHO definition of a rare incidence), giving rise to a situation in which the benefits of the drug could not longer be said to outweigh the risks of haemolytic anaemia.

Four further cases of haemolytic anaemia were reported to the company in January 1986. One of these patients subsequently died. The UK data contributed to the on-going appraisal of nomifensine being undertaken by the parent company, and this led to the product's withdrawal from world-wide markets on 22 January 1986.

Table 12.3 summarises the events and assessments leading to the withdrawal of nomifensine 10 years after its first market launch.

DISCUSSION

Compared with the pharmacoepidemiological methodologies available today, the measures and methods employed in monitoring the adverse effects of noimifensine were those used in the normal clinical and laboratory assessments of haemolytic anaemia; more specialised immunological investigations into the relationship between nomifensine and the dyscrasia; and epidemiological observations. The last of these was not straightforward in the case of nomifensine because, as discussed, there was a very low rate of reported cases up until the increase in the mid-1980s. This undoubtedly led to the delay in establishing a cause-and-effect relationship between nomifensine and haemolytic anaemia.

It was considered that the rapid escalation of spontaneous reporting could have been due to increased awareness among doctors resulting from reports of haemolytic anaemia in the literature, changes in the data sheets, and encouragement to make use of the CSM's Yellow Card system. It could also have been partly due to the increased promotion, sale and market share of nomifensine that occurred at the time. Furthermore, an impetus may have come from the withdrawal from the market of benoxaprofen (and increasing recognition of problems associated with other non-steroidal anti-inflammatory agents) during the early to mid-1980s. The neurological problems caused by zimeldine also occurred during the early 1980s and may have contributed to heightened concern over, and increased reporting of, adverse reactions in general (Edwards, 1997a).

Altogether, nomifensine was associated with eight deaths before its withdrawal in the United Kingdom. Three of these were associated with haemolytic anaemia (a fourth haemolytic anaemia-associated fatality occurred after the product was withdrawn), and one each with a cardiac arrythmia, an overdose of nomifensine in conjunction with lithium, the Stevens-Johnson syndrome, hepatic necrosis and a cerebrovascular accident.

The "CSM Update" in 1986 outlined the basis for the risk–benefit discussion, which took place late in 1985 when for the first time the incidence of haemolytic anaemia in the United Kingdom was greater than 1 in 10 000 prescriptions. However, reports of other adverse events remained modest.

Hoechst UK's total database was only 55% of the CSM's, but it contained 76% of all haemolytic anaemia reports and 88% of evaluable reports. For hepatic events, the company had 46 reports of which 44 (96%) were thought to be associated with the drug. This compared with the CSM's 51 (86%) reports, but for fever the company had only 25 reports compared with the CSM's 48 (52%). Thus, for perceived serious events, it appeared that prescribers felt more compelled to contact the company directly. For haemolytic anaemia and hepatic events the manufacturer received over 75% of the reports that formed the CSM's database, compared with approximately 50% for all other adverse reactions, including fever. This supports the view that the company was aware of a greater proportion of serious events than the average reporting rate to the company.

Despite some obvious associations such as increased prescribing, increased awareness of nomifensine after the launch of the 100 mg single daily dose tablet, and literature and media reports, the exact reason for an increase in reports of haemolytic anaemia during 1984 and 1985 was never established, nor were the reasons for the timespan of around nine years from the first introduction of nomifensine to the emergence of a drug safety warning signal that could reasonably be acted upon.

It is possible to compare side effect evaluation between 1976–1986 and subsequent years. The current system of evaluation with its heightened awareness amongst healthcare professionals (and indeed society at large) of drug safety risks of marketed products has, at least in part, been the result of the lessons learnt first-hand from problems with former products. These include nomifensine.

The evaluation of nomifensine relied wholly on spontaneous reporting systems with their known inadequacies of incompletely reported data, lack of population data to allow for the calculation of incidence rates and estimates of sub-groups at risk; poor international coordination of drug safety databases; and the need for confidentiality hampering collaboration between the manufacturer and the regulatory authorities at least in the early stages.

Nevertheless, the risk–benefit appraisal of nomifensine was made through a continuing dialogue between the company and the regulatory authority, taking into account time-honoured but rudimentary indicators of risk and benefit. For the company, these included the general properties of nomifensine in relation to older and newer antidepressants; overdose data; market uptake of the single daily dose; crude adverse drug reaction incidence calculations from prescriptions and sales volume; publications in the medical literature and media reports; and comparisons with other drug classes. Specific aspects of nomifensine that were of special concern included the rising incidence of reports of acute immune haemolytic anaemia and the incidence of fatalities.

Of some interest today is what might have been the true effect of a consideration of overdose data on the risk–benefit appraisal of nomifensine, had the successful appeal against the threatened suspension of mianserin using such data been heard earlier (Brahams, 1990). Concern was expressed with mianserin over the number of reports to the CSM of granulocytopenia and agranulocytosis occurring during treatment with this antidepressant and it was at risk of being suspended. However it was given a reprieve as a result of a comparative Prescription Event Monitoring study that was unable to detect any drug-attributable blood dyscrasias and concluded that, if mianserin did cause them, the incidence would probably be in the range of one per 10 000 to one per 100 000 patients. It was also shown that the risks of overdose of mianserin were considerably less than that of amitryptiline (Inman, 1988, 1991).

Between 1977 and 1984 74 patients taking an overdose of nomifensine, 28 of them nomifensine alone, were reported to the London Centre of the National Poisons Information Service, Guys Hospital (Ali and Crome, 1984). The most common symptom, either with nomifensine alone or in combinations with other drugs (benzodiazepines, alcohol and/or tricyclic antidepressants) was drowsiness. There were no reports of convulsions or cardiac arrhythmias in those who took nomifensine alone and all cases made satisfactory recoveries. It was concluded that nomifensine overdose had few clinical sequelae and that there was a notable absence of the complications seen with tricyclic antidepressants.

The nomifensine appraisal might have benefited in a small way, too, from today's pharmacoepidemiological databases and case–control studies. These would have added strength at an earlier stage to incidence calculations, and allowed the incidence to be compared with the background incidence in the community. However, even today there is no rare disease registry that provides the background incidence of haemolytic anaemia in the general population.

Since the mid-1980s, the computerisation of data in the international pharmaceutical industry and the regulatory agencies has greatly facilitated the establishment of drug safety databases and the speed and extent of international reporting, accrual and comparison of pharmacovigilance data. Pharmacoepidemiological databases, such as the Prescription Event Monitoring of the Drug Safety Research Unit (DSRU), the General Practice Research Database (GPRD), the Medicines Evaluation and Monitoring Organisation (MEMO) and Record Linkage are now available to study, contemporaneously and retrospectively, the cause-and-effect relationship of apparently drug-linked events (Mann, 2001).

There has been a concomitant increase in regulation and legislation concerning the formal recording and reporting of suspected adverse events. The application of Good Clinical Practices (GCP), through the International Conference on Harmonisation (ICH), today formalises all aspects of clinical trials of medicines both before and after licensing. It remains hypothetical, however, whether these would have aided the assessment of nomifensine between 1977 and 1986.

A further area of development has been the increased awareness within companies of the need to develop issues management strategies and teams to coordinate the response to matters such as specific drug safety alerts. These bring together all the relevant company resources from medical, regulatory, manufacturing, quality assurance, legal and commercial departments at a local and international level to address matters raised by, for example, the increased reporting of a rare side effect. This enables a much more cooperative and proactive relationship to develop between the company, the regulatory authorities and the media in order to resolve the issues in a timely and diligent manner. Whilst such an approach was taken in the case of nomifensine, it was perhaps more reactive than might be the case today. It remains speculative whether a more formal and rehearsed international issue and relationship management strategy would have helped to shorten the timescale from first alert to the final withdrawal of the drug.

Nomifensine was associated with a rising incidence of a serious life-threatening Type B reaction, namely acute immune haemolytic anaemia. The reasons for the rising incidence are not known, although greater doctor recognition and willingness to report, possibly stimulated by literature reports and the media, were undoubtedly factors involved. The immunology was uncertain throughout because of the variety of case presentations, severity and outcomes, and conflicting laboratory findings.

Because of difficulties in predicting the haemolytic reaction, distinguishing its initial symptoms from those of other disorders, and the variable serological findings, it was impossible to offer firm advice on early diagnosis and treatment.

The drug was withdrawn from sale in the interests of patient safety, even though nomifensine was a well-established antidepressant in many countries, in some of which the problems were thought to be an "acceptable" risk when seen in relation to the drug's benefits. The decision to withdraw nomifensine was made by physicians employed by the company when, despite the uncertainty, the severity and clinical sequelae of the haemolytic reaction were fully appreciated. It is arguable whether the science of pharmacoepidemiology or the procedures of pharmacovigilance as practised today would have impacted on that decision in either January 1986 or indeed in 2001.

Whilst the professionals who make judgements about risk and benefit of a medicine must be aware of both population statistics and individual patient concerns, the decisions on action to ensure the continued safety for some patients without denying the benefits of an established medicine for others will always be demanding. In this context, the decisions of a company to withdraw its product from the market or of a regulatory authority to revoke the marketing authorisation will remain the most difficult of all.

REFERENCES

Ali C, Crome P (1984) The clinical toxicology of nomifensine: an update. In: Rees WL, Priest RG, eds, *RSM International Congress and Symposium Series No. 70.* Oxford: Oxford University Press, pp. 121–3.

Beaumont G (1984) An overview of depression and its treatment with nomifensine in a general practice. In: Rees LW, Priest RG, eds, *RSM International Congress and Symposium Series No. 70.* Oxford University Press, pp. 63–9.

Bournerias F, Habibi B (1979) Nomifensine-induced immune haemolytic anaemia and impaired renal function. *Lancet* **2**: 95–6.

Brahams D (1990) Safety in overdose and drug licensing. *Lancet* **1**: 343–4.

Committee on Safety of Medicines (1985) *Current Problems* **15**: July.

Crome P, Chand S (1980) The clinical toxicology of nomifensine: comparison with tricyclic antidepressants. In: Stonier PD, Jenner FA, eds, *RSM International Congress and Symposium Series No. 25.* London: Academic Press, pp. 55–8.

CSM Update (1985) Adverse reactions to antidepressants. *Br Med J* **291**: 1638.

CSM Update (1986) Withdrawal of nomifensine. *Br Med J* **293**: 41.

Drug and Therapeutics Bulletin (1985) Trouble with nomifensine. *Drug and Therapeutics Bulletin* **23**: 98–100.

Eckstein R, Riess H, Sauer H, *et al.* (1981) Immunhämolytische Anämien mit Nierenversagen nach Nomifensineinnahme. *Klinsche Wochenschrift* **59**: 567–9.

Edwards, JG (1981) Unwanted effects of psychotropic drugs and their mechanisms. In: Van Praag HM, Lader MH, Raphaelson OJ, Sacher EJ, eds, *Handbook of Biological Psychiatry. Part VI. Practical*

Applications of Psychotropic Drugs and Other Biological Treatments. New York: Marcel Dekker, pp. 1–38.

Edwards JG (1997a) Withdrawal of psychotropic drugs from the market: I. From thalidomide to zimeldine. In: Hindmarch I, Stonier PD, eds, *Human Psychopharmacology: Measures and Methods.* Chichester: Wiley, Volume 6, Chapter 12, pp. 199–214.

Edwards JG (1997b) Withdrawal of psychotropic drugs from the market: II. From nomifensine to remoxipride. In: Hindmarch I, Stonier PD, eds, *Human Psychopharmacology: Measures and Methods.* Chichester: Wiley, Volume 6, Chapter 13, pp. 215–33.

Garcia-Morteo O, Maldonado-Cocco JA (1983) Lupus-like syndrome during treatment with nomifensine. *Arthritis Rheumatism* **26**: 936.

Garnier R, Delaby F, Benzaken C, *et al.* (1982) Acute poisoning by nomifensine. *Journal de Toxicologie Médicale* **2**: 141–4.

Green PJ, Naorose-Abidi SMH, *et al.* (1984) Nomifensine and thrombocytopenia. *Br Med J* **288**: 830.

Habibi B, Cartron JP, Bretagne M, *et al.* (1981) Anti-nomifensine antibody causing immune haemolytic anaemia and renal failure. *Vox Sang Jaarg* **40**: 79–84.

Hamm H, Aumiller J, Bohmer R, *et al.* (1985) Alveolitis associated with nomifensine. *Lancet* **1**: 1328–29.

Inman WHW (1988) Blood disorders and suicide in patients taking mianserin or amitriptyline. *Lancet* **323**: 90–2.

Inman WHW (1991) *PEM News*, No. 7. Southampton: Drug Safety Research Unit.

Lyllof K, Jersild C, Bacher T, Slot O (1982) Massive intravascular haemolysis during treatment with nomifensine. *Lancet* **2**, 41.

Mann RD (1988) Lessons from nomifensine. *Lancet* **2**: 1490–1.

Mann RD (2001) Monitoring the safety of medicines. In: Luscombe D, Stonier PD, eds, *Clinical Research Manual.* Chapter 8, pp. 8.1–8.58. Euromed Communications, Haslemere, England (First published 1994; Chapter update 2001).

Miescher PA (1985) Nomifensine-induced allergic reactions. *Lancet* **2**: 551–2.

Nicholson PA, Turner P (1977) Proceedings of a Symposium on Nomifensine—January 1977. *Br J Clin Pharmacol* **4** (Suppl.2).

Prescott LF, Illingworth RN, Critchley JAJH, *et al.* (1980) Acute haemolysis and renal failure after nomifensine overdose. *Br Med J*, **281**: 1392–93.

Salama A, Mueller-Eckhardt C, Kissel K, *et al.* (1984) *Ex vivo* antigen preparation for the serological detection of drug-dependent antibodies in immune haemolytic anaemias. *Br J Haematol* **58**: 525–31.

Salama A, Mueller-Eckhardt C (1985) The role of metabolic-specific antibodies in nomifensine-dependent immune haemolytic anaemia. *New Eng J Med* **313**: 469–74.

Schönhöfer PS, Groticke J (1985) Fatal necrotising vasculitis associated with nomifensine. *Lancet* **2**: 221.

Schönhöfer PS (1991) The nomifensine affair. *Lancet* **2**: 1448.

Sokol RJ, Hewitt S, Brooker DJ, *et al.* (1985) Fatal immune haemolysis associated with nomifensine. *Br Med J* **291**: 311–12.

Stonier PD (1992) Nomifensine and haemolytic anae-mia—experience of a post-marketing alert. *Pharmacoepidemiology and Drug Safety* **1**: 177–85.

Vaz FG, Singh R, Nurazzaman M (1984) Hepatitis induced by nomifensine. *Br Med J* **289**: 1268.

Walti M-L, Neftel K, Cohen M, *et al.* (1983) Demonstration of drug-specific IgE and IgG antibodies using RIA: clinical importance as shown with nomifensine (Alival). *Schweizerische Medizinische Wochenschrift* **113**: 1865–7.

Part II
SIGNAL GENERATION

13

WHO Programme—Global Monitoring

I. RALPH EDWARDS AND STEN OLSSON
Uppsala Monitoring Centre, Stora Torget 3, Uppsala, Sweden

HISTORY

The Programme was established in 1968 as a pilot project with the participation of 10 countries that had organised national pharmacovigilance systems at that time. The intent was to develop international collaboration to make it easier to detect rare adverse drug reactions (ADRs) not revealed during clinical trials. The international drug monitoring centre was moved from the World Health Organisation (WHO) headquarters in Geneva, Switzerland, to a WHO Collaborating Centre for International Drug Monitoring in Uppsala, Sweden, in 1978. This was the result of an agreement between WHO and the government of Sweden by which Sweden assumed the operational responsibility for the Programme. WHO headquarters, Geneva, retained the responsibility for policy matters. The Collaborating Centre is often referred to as the Uppsala Monitoring Centre (UMC).

It is easiest to record the history of pharmacovigilance as a series of milestones that led to the introduction of new concepts or the re-thinking of old concepts within the discipline. A chronological list of these milestones is listed in Table 13.1. It is interesting to note that up to and including the benoxaprofen ("Opren") incident in 1989, changes

in drug safety procedures were implemented as a result of drug disasters that had a high media profile. The responses to these disasters constituted a major re-thinking of drug safety issues. Since the benoxaprofen incident, there have been a number of drug withdrawals related to safety issues, but these have been managed much more effectively and expeditiously. It may seem that we now have safety systems in place that enable effective action to be taken globally before disturbing numbers of patients are affected. However, it is ironic that the recent pill scare in the United Kingdom may have caused more distress because of a rapid regulatory response to a safety issue. Since the benoxaprofen incident, the main changes made in pharmacovigilance have been proactive improvements involving fine-tuning of regulatory systems and the adoption of better epidemiological techniques often associated with improvements in information technology (IT).

PRESENT PROGRAMME STRUCTURE

The number of national centres which are active members of the WHO Programme has increased, in 10 years, from 28 to the present 67 countries,

---

Pharmacovigilance. Edited by R.D. Mann and E.B. Andrews

Table 13.1. Some important milestones in pharmacovigilance.

Milestone	Issue	Linked development	Other development
Elixir of sulphanilimide (1937)	Formulation defect results in poisoning	Improvements in pharmaceutical regulation	
Thalidomide (1961)	Phocomelia in children of mothers who took this apparently safe drug	National and international collections of ADR reports	Yellow card system, UK, 1964 WHO Programme on International Drug Monitoring, 1968—attempt to create automatic signal generation ("Black box")
Clioquinol (1969)	New clinical syndrome reported from Japan (SMONS)	Ethnic susceptibility and drug use issues raised	More realisation of complexity in drug safety Early work on pharmacogenetics
Oral contraceptives (1970s)	Venous thromboembolism	Controversy over epidemiological findings, and acceptance, finally, of their importance	
Practolol (1975)	New clinical syndrome, recognised by UK expert (oculo- muco-cutaneous)	Realisation that spontaneous reporting will not pick up "events", not easily recognised as caused by drugs	Prescription event monitoring introduced—Intensive Medicines Monitoring Programme in New Zealand and Prescription Event Monitoring in the UK Causality algorithms developed
WHO Collaborating Centre for Drug Monitoring, Uppsala (1978) founded	No "black box" signal detection solution found	Enhanced "clinically useful outputs"—critical terms, WHO- ART, WHO-DD, quarterly summaries	National collaboration enhanced under WHO Programme
Non-steroidal anti-inflammatory drugs (NSAIDs) (~1980–)	Blood dyscrasias, GI bleeding a serious public health problem: high background incidence a problem	Development of pharmacoepidemiology	Bayesian methods introduced
Benoxaprofen (1982)	Unusual photosensitivity Liver necrosis in the elderly UK takes action to remove drug from the market without US knowing	US saw the need to have international industry ADR information—CIOMS[a] I Need to have rapid alert system between agencies necessity for regular reporting	CIOMS II at risk groups WHO Programme invites more expert help WHO Programme begins to work towards greater openness France introduces regionalisation and a causality algorithm Start of thinking towards ICH

Table 13.1. *Continued.*

Milestone	Issue	Linked development	Other development
Fenoterol-beta agonists (1989) (previous sympathomimetic deaths in 1970s)	Linked to death in asthma in case–control studies	Signals from case– control studies debated strongly	Use of databases/nested studies becomes more accepted
EU and ICH (~1990–)	Common European policies on pharmacovigilance promoted US, EU and Japan work on harmonised drug regulation	Rapid alert and common international decisions on signals. Development of harmonised methods (ICH) and projects, e.g. EPRG (European Pharmacovigilance Research Group)	
ADR Signal Analysis Project (ASAP) (1994)	International spontaneous report rates available from IMS and used in international signal analysis in WHO Programme	Drug use data more widely used in drug safety	Increasing use of clinical databases
Bayesian Neural Network (1997)	An automated signal detection method with statistical information to aid expert opinion, in WHO Programme		Proportional reporting ratios (UK and Netherlands) Other statistical methods (USA and Australia)
Third generation oral contraceptives (1997)	A small absolute increase in risk of death causes "pill scare", followed by abortions and unwanted pregnancies	Focus on the need for good communications practice and consequence evaluation	Re-opens debate on issues of evidence in pharmacovigilance

[a]Council for International Organisation of Medical Sciences.

and the database has grown from over 600 000 reports to over 2.8 million.

At the time of writing, an additional six countries have formally applied for membership and they are considered associate members while the issue of technical compatibility of their reports with the WHO requirements is established. Member countries and associate member countries are listed in the Table 13.2.

In each country, a national centre, designated by the competent health authority, is responsible for the collection, processing and evaluation of adverse reaction case reports submitted by health professionals. Information obtained from these reports is passed back to the professionals on a national basis, but is also submitted to the WHO centre for inclusion in the international database. Collectively the centres annually provide 200 000–250 000 individual reports to the WHO of reactions suspected of being drug-induced.

Case reports submitted to the WHO centre according to an agreed format are checked for technical correctness and then incorporated in the international database in a weekly routine. The material is screened at least four times a year for new and serious reactions as well as the reporting frequencies of associations of particular interest. Many additional examinations of the data are made on an *ad hoc* basis.

Table 13.2. WHO member and associate member countries.

Country	Year of entry	Country	Year of entry
Member countries			
Argentina	1994	Korea, Rep of	1992
Australia	1968	Malaysia	1990
Austria	1991	Mexico	1998
Belgium	1977	Morocco	1992
Bulgaria	1975	Netherlands	1968
Canada	1968	New Zealand	1968
Chile	1996	Norway	1971
China, PR	1998	Oman	1995
Costa Rica	1991	Philippines	1995
Croatia	1992	Poland	1972
Cuba	1994	Portugal	1993
Cyprus	2000	Romania	1976
Czech Republic	1992	Russia	1998
Denmark	1968	Singapore	1993
Estonia	1998	Slovak Republic	1993
Fiji Islands	1999	South Africa	1992
Finland	1974	Spain	1984
France	1986	Sweden	1968
Germany	1968	Switzerland	1991
Greece	1990	Tanzania	1993
Hungary	1990	Thailand	1984
Iceland	1990	Tunisia	1993
India	1998	Turkey	1987
Indonesia	1990	United Kingdom	1968
Iran	1998	United States	1968
Ireland	1968	Venezuela	1995
Israel	1973	Vietnam	1999
Italy	1975	Yugoslavia Fed Rep	2000
Japan	1972	Zimbabwe	1998
Additional member countries			
Armenia	2001	Macedonia	2001
Brazil	2001	Peru	2002
Egypt	2001	Sri Lanka	2000
Ghana	2001	Uruguay	2001
Latvia	2001		
Associate member countries			
Bahrain		Netherlands Antilles	
Jordan		Pakistan	
Moldovia		Ukraine	

CURRENT WORK

- The database of the WHO Programme is a unique reference source used in many different situations. When a national centre receives the first report of an unfamiliar drug–reaction association the WHO database is often consulted to find out whether a similar observation has been made elsewhere in the world. If so, the initial signal may be strengthened. National centres are provided with an annual reference document providing summary figures of suspected drug–reaction associations reported to WHO. On-line search facilities are also at the disposal of national centres for up-to-date checking of the reporting situation.

From the database, cohorts of patients affected by similar kinds of drug-associated reactions may be retrieved. By looking for common features in these reports, risk factors and hypotheses for underlying mechanisms may be revealed.

- In 1998 a new methodology developed at the Uppsala Monitoring Centre (UMC) using a Bayesian Confidence Propagation Neural Network (BCPNN) in analysing the database, was put into routine use. The concept of data mining (not random data dredging!) is now operating to support all countries in their work. It is based on artificial intelligence using a Bayesian logic system. It has been fully validated and is under continuous development (Bate, 2000; Bate et al., 1998a, 1998b, 2000; Lindquist, 2000; Lindquist et al., 1999; Orre et al., 2000).

A combination of automatic signalling devices and scanning by experienced medical personnel is considered most advantageous to fulfil successfully the original aim of the programme, i.e. the early identification of new ADRs. This method provides a quantitative measure of the strength of association of a drug–reaction combination in the database. Combinations that occur more frequently than expected as compared with the generality of the database are highlighted.

When the new data has been processed and entered into the ADR database, a BCPNN scan is run to generate statistical measurements for each drug–ADR combination. The resulting Combinations database (Combination: *ADR data elements occurring together in ADR reports*) is made available to national centres, and to pharmaceutical companies, in the latter case including only information on the company's own patented products. The database is presented in a computerised form which facilitates searching and sorting of the information.

An associations database (Association: *Combinations selected from a database on a quantitative basis*) is generated by selecting those combinations that pass a pre-set threshold. Based on the results of the test runs of the BCPNN, the threshold level for associations is that of the lower 95% confidence limit of the Information Component (IC) value crossing zero when a new batch of reports is added.

All associations are followed automatically for two years, the data being checked at six-monthly intervals. After the final listing, an association may be reintroduced for another two-year follow-up. The associations are also copied to a cumulative log file (history file), which will serve as a filter to exclude combinations that have in previous quarters passed the threshold level. This will prevent drug–ADR combinations with a confidence limit fluctuating around zero from being fed into the review process repetitiously.

A panel of experts has been established to analyse reactions pertaining to particular body systems. The associations database is sent to the expert review panel for evaluation. Before distributing the database, associations are checked against standard reference sources (e.g. Physician's Desk Reference (PDR), Martindale), and the published literature (using, for example, *Medline* and *Reactions Weekly*). This facilitates the review and identifies those associations that are, if not generally known, at least identified previously.

Searching and sorting of the associations data can be done, not only on drug, ADR and the various statistical measurements, but also on System Organ Class (SOC) and on therapeutic drug groups using the Anatomical–Therapeutic–Chemical (ATC) classification. To ensure that there are at least two reviewers per SOC, we intend to extend the panel of reviewers from today's 30 experts to around double over the next few years.

To the Associations stage, the process is purely quantitative, but clinical knowledge and judgement is necessary for the evaluation of associations, and is provided by the national centres and expert reviewers. Short summaries of their findings are circulated to participating national centres in a memorandum called "Signal". An investigation has demonstrated that the WHO Programme is successful in finding new drug–adverse reaction associations at an early stage and in providing useful information about them to national centres.

Individualised sections of the Signal document will be provided to companies on a subscription basis (only on their patented products). To aid the expert reviewers, and also to facilitate interpretation of the information presented in the Signal document, a set of guidelines is being established. As with the associations, all signals will be automatically reassessed on a six-monthly basis, for two years, with a possibility of re-introduction for follow-up, and also copied to a history file for easy tracking. With the new follow-up procedures we have introduced a mechanism by which signals can be re-evaluated following new information. This enables, for example, renewed consideration of associations for which there initially was not enough information to merit signalling. Signals that are later supported by new evidence can also be highlighted. The nature of the signal will determine what measures need be taken in terms of follow-up.

A larger numbers of variables than the routine drug–ADR combinations can also be considered using the Bayesian approach, as described above. One of the advantages of a neural network, as used in the BCPNN, is that it can search for patterns of associations between fields that are not determined a priori: it can find novel complex relationships. One of the outcomes of these analyses may be to identify patient subgroups that may be at particularly high risk of getting a specific adverse reaction when they have taken a specific drug. Another possibility is to establish that a drug safety problem is related to a particular country, or region, or a certain time period. By further developing the BCPNN methodology for the analysis of the large amount of data in the WHO database, it is expected that hitherto unrevealed risk factors for the development of drug related ailments may be detected.

- The UMC has an important role to play as a communication centre—a clearing house for information on drug safety at the service of drug regulatory agencies, pharmaceutical industry, researchers and other groups in need of drug safety information. Requests for special database searches and investigations are received from these parties at a rate of around 275 per year. In addition, flexible on-line retrieval programmes are made available by which the database users may perform a variety of standardised searches by themselves. Access for non-member parties is subjected to confidentiality restrictions agreed by Programme members. Some countries maintain the right to refuse the release of their own information if they so wish. Use of the information released is subject to a caveat document as to its proper use. Detailed manuals for the on-line service and the customised retrievals on request are available from the Uppsala centre.

National centres were provided with an *Adverse Reactions Newsletter* on a three-monthly basis from 1982 to 1999. The *Newsletter* contained reviews of national adverse reaction bulletins and news of drug problems being investigated in various countries, supplemented by figures from the WHO register. It was recently decided to incorporate this information into the *WHO Pharmaceuticals Newsletter*, distributed by the Health Technology and Pharmaceuticals department of WHO headquarters, leading to a wider distribution of the information to all member countries of WHO.

Uppsala Reports is the name of a bulletin which is made freely available to all interested parties by the UMC. It provides an easy-to-read account of news about pharmacovigilance, the WHO Programme, its members and services.

Communications within the WHO Programme has improved with the increasing use of electronic communications media. The UMC is maintaining an e-mail discussion group called "Vigimed", which allows for rapid exchange of information around the world on drug safety matters. Membership is restricted to persons connected to national pharmacovigilance centres.

The internet home page of the WHO Programme (http://www.who-umc.org) was introduced in 1996. It is intended to be developed into a dynamic tool for communications with all clients of the UMC. Recently, internet-based seminars and training courses were introduced on the UMC web site.

- International comparisons of drug safety reporting have been made (Lindquist, 1990; Lindquist and Edwards, 1993). These comparisons have shown important differences in country profiles of reporting. The differences between countries may be due to a variety of factors. Some of the differences may be purely technical but others may relate to differences in medical practice, the use of medical terms, societal influences such as media interest (Mills and Edwards, 1999). Sometimes the indications, doses of medicines and/or the routes of administration may be significant ((Lindquist *et al.*, 1996). It is sometimes alleged that these findings are not signals, but this is to take a narrow view of a "signal" as simply a previously unreported medicine/ADR association, rather than to consider that any significant new evidence on a medicine-related risk is a signal (see WHO definition–Edwards, 1997).
- Definitions for a variety of pharmacovigilance terms have been proposed and accepted widely (Edwards, 1997). Within the WHO Programme a number of definitions of commonly used terms, such as adverse reaction, side effect, adverse event, signal, have been worked out. These definitions contribute to a harmonised way of communicating both inside and outside the Programme (Edwards and Biriell, 1994).
- Guidelines for signal finding have been proposed and widely accepted (Edwards *et al.*, 1990). It is an important concept that a medicine related signal from spontaneous reports should be considered starting with the seriousness of the apparent signal and then appraising both the quantity of reports as well as the strength/quality of the information in those reports. Because the quality of information on a report is limited does not necessarily mean that the observation underlying it is less

valid: but it does mean that objective assessment may be difficult or impossible. Assessing the weight of reported evidence is a complex clinical decision, which has further been aided by definitions of "certain", "probable", "possible", etc. (Edwards, 1997).

- The idea of the possibility of an exhaustive data set being stored was initiated, and has become the ICH E2B project. A new WHO database containing all the fields is completed (see below) (CIOMS, 1995; Lindquist, 1998). First with CIOMS and then with ICH, we have developed a comprehensive set of data fields, which have been included in our new database, which is now undergoing acceptance tests. In this data model much more detailed information on each case may be stored and case reports may also, in principle, be received directly from drug companies. Other software to support the functions of national centres is also being developed. Our new database has great complexity, and it seems unlikely that many of the available fields will be completed until a "paperless" system comes into operation in several countries. The new database is fully compatible with the old one, so that we can use them in a parallel fashion during an introductory period. To provide flexibility for users with varying requirements and sophistication is a great challenge, but we are hopeful that the new database will pave the way for the international availability of much more useful case data, without recourse to the original provider for more details. Along with the provision of the new database (which is offered as a single-stop repository for industry reports, rather than their sending them to each national centre), we are planning to give more active support to national centres over their IT development. Many delays in the transmission of reports to the WHO are secondary to a variety of technical issues, which must be minimised.
- Biennial Uppsala, and regional, training courses have been introduced.

To foster education and communication in pharmacovigilance, the WHO Centre offers every second year, a two-week training course in Adverse Reactions and Adverse Reaction Monitoring in Uppsala to which 25 healthcare professionals are accepted. The course is in two consecutive modules. The first is focused on spontaneous monitoring and the practicalities of managing a drug monitoring centre. This section also offers hands-on experience in using the database of the WHO Programme. The final module is an introduction to wider issues in pharmacoepidemiology.

There is an increasing trend towards local and regional meetings and courses in pharmacovigilance. The WHO Programme often takes part in such meetings, particularly those organised in developing countries, to provide support and technical advise. UMC staff are commonly invited all over the world to speak at professional meetings.

- Every year representatives of national centres are invited to a meeting arranged jointly by WHO and one of the participating countries. At these meetings technical issues are being discussed, both in relation to how to improve global drug monitoring in general and concerning individual drug safety problems. Since the meetings have very high attendance rates they are important for the establishment and maintenance of personal relationships subsequently contributing to good communications.
- The requirements for a new ADR terminology were set out including the need for definitions (Edwards et al., 1993a, 1993b). The WHO Programme has developed a standardised adverse reaction terminology (WHO-ART) and a comprehensive index of reported drugs (WHO-DD), both of which have a utility beyond their importance to the monitoring system. These tools are used in the pre-marketing safety area, as well as for post-marketing studies by many pharmaceutical companies. WHO-ART has also been adopted by the International Programme on Chemical Safety as the medical terminology to describe poisoning incidents.

The *WHO Drug Dictionary* is unique in its coverage of drugs marketed throughout the world. It is available in paper print, as computer files or on CD. The UMC is developing it further to incorporate more detailed information and make it compatible with the pre-standard proposed by the European Committee for Standardisation (CEN).

The Centre is also working with XML standards for its terminologies and dictionaries, as well as supporting such work with ICD10. The use of XML versions of terminologies will greatly enhance their combined utility and availability, for example, by internet.

- The use of IMS drug-use denominator data was made possible for international pharmacovigilance (Lindquist and Edwards, 1997; Lindquist *et al.*, 1994, 1996, 1997). There is a general need to quantify adverse reaction information. The WHO centre is working jointly with IMS International to analyse adverse reaction reports together with drug use data from different countries. This allows national differences in reporting rates to be further analysed for reasons that may be due to differences in indications for use, medical practice and demographics, etc. It is hoped that this type of analysis of international data will serve as a guide to the need for more precise pharmacoepidemiological investigations.

- The concept of benefit–risk analysis was refined for drug safety (Edwards *et al.*, 1996). Benefit–risk analysis is more than the subjective opinion of a group of experts and is in its infancy for drug therapy. The needs of managed care and the adoption of guidelines for therapy in all therapeutic areas mean that there needs to be satisfactory methods for measuring benefits and risks in clinical practice for all major therapeutic interventions, so that they may be compared. They must be updated regularly.

Safety must be seen as relative: there is no absolute safety. The relativity is in the risk or harm that one medicine causes compared with another and in the risk or harm caused by a drug in relation to its benefits. Andrew Herxheimer (personal communication) has pointed out that there is a lack of symmetry in the expression "benefit–risk", since benefit is actuality, whereas risk is potentiality, harm being the corresponding symmetrical term

for actual damage. The recognition of the balance between terms is important. Benefits of medicines are generally based on hard scientific evidence from clinical trials, and are taken as fact or a high probability of effectiveness (although the medicine may perform differently, usually less well than expected, in the uncontrolled patient population that makes up ordinary clinical practice. Even if the patient being treated is well represented by the trial population, it may be difficult to predict the outcome in that individual.) Harm, above a certain incidence, is measurable in clinical trials, but we have much less information on safety than we need, because clinical trials are not well designed to elicit information about adverse effects. Additional information comes from individual case reports of varying quality and quantity and from observational studies, which are not consistently performed with all drugs and all ADRs. Information on harm is therefore often based on uncontrolled material. The observational material, reports or studies, is susceptible to various biases to different degrees. It may therefore be more useful to use the potential term, because from the patient's point of view the usually single benefit can be explained in close-to-precise terms, but the negative side of the equation is at best made of probabilities and more often made up of unquantified evidence and opinion.

In the future, the Human Genome Project, and other investigations into genetic variance, must be linked to our knowledge of ADRs and, in particular, idiosyncratic ADRs so that we are able to be more predictive about issues of drug safety.

- The concept and needs for benefit–risk communication have been explored and developed. One of the widely quoted outcomes was the "Erice Declaration" which proposes principles for such communication (Bowdler, 1997; Edwards and Hugman, 1997; Edwards, 1999; Edwards *et al.*, 2000). With the aim of improving communications in pharmacovigilance, initiatives have been taken to call together representatives of all major groups involved in the provision of drug safety information. The Erice report on communicating drug safety information sets out the basis for further development in this area. The UMC is collaborating with the CIOMS to work out detailed recommendations on good communication practices in pharmacovigilance.

- *National Pharmacovigilance Systems—Country Profiles and Overview* (Olsson, 1999) is an important publication useful to many people who wish to know who's who and what's where in pharmacovigilance. We are also considering a web version of this as well as much more information and analysis of activity.

- The idea of monitoring herbal medicines and classifying them has been introduced and is operating (Farah, 1998; Farah *et al.*, 2000a, 2000b; Lindquist *et al.*, 2000). In response to the challenge to safety monitoring offered by traditional herbal remedies, the UMC has taken initiatives to improve the classification systems for such medicines. In a joint project with institutions in the United Kingdom and the Netherlands, a system compatible with the ATC system used for modern, synthetic medicines is being developed. Input from experts from all parts of the world, representing different therapeutic traditions, is indispensable for this project. The database is far enough advanced to be finding some herbal signals and allow us to respond to queries using an extensive literature resource as well as ADR reports. Collaboration is commencing with South Africa, the United States and Germany.

- The need for new pharmacovigilance approaches to deal with the aggressive global marketing of drugs has been identified: see below (Edwards, 2000).

- There have been 86 publications in 10 years actively involving UMC staff

- An Anniversary Symposium was held in 1998 to commemorate 20 years of the UMC in Sweden. It was attended by about two hundred delegates.

- Developments within WHO have led to a meeting of an expert group to produce an advocacy document for pharmacovigilance which has the tentative title of: "The value of pharmacovigilance" and subsidiary title of: "In public health and patient care". The results of this meeting will be made available and will set the scene for much to be done in the future.

WHAT IS STILL MISSING—WHAT WE MUST DO IN THE FUTURE

The pharmaceutical industry is poised on the edge of new opportunities and challenges in the new millennium (Edwards, 2000). Better and faster ways to develop new medicines clearly afford one opportunity, but the real excitement is in the area of genetic knowledge and manipulation, which allows unprecedented interference with disease processes. The industry is faced with challenges to become ever more profitable and this has resulted in what might be called management experiments of re-structuring, merging, out-sourcing, virtual companies, and so on. There is an aim to market medicinal products globally and fast. Even recreational drugs are a possible legitimate consideration for the pharmaceutical industry in the future. All of this has implications for the safety of medicines, and the most obvious issue is that the rapid exposure of large numbers of people to novel products, which might have profound effects for ill as well as good.

Many publications attest to the high proportion of hospital admissions that are related to drug injury. Most other diseases do not come close to drug injury as a cause for morbidity. Moreover, it seems likely that about half of these events are avoidable. A chronological examination of the literature on drug-related morbidity makes it clear that this public health problem is not decreasing. Why is this?

More drugs become available on the market all the time, and this may itself be a factor in keeping the incidence of drug-related morbidity high. In addition, there can be a higher reporting rate for adverse effects associated with new drugs (the Weber effect). This comes about because of clinical interest in the new drug, the possibility of a novel ADR profile, as well as effects which may have come about because of lack of clinical inexperience with the agent (e.g. first dose hypotension with calcium antagonists, dependence and withdrawal with selective serotonin reuptake inhibitors.

Multiple drug use may result in adverse interactions, causing ADRs or lack of efficacy (Meyboom *et al.*, 2000a, 2000b). Not only does polypharmacy occur when a single physician is treating compound disease processes, but with increasing specialisation more than one doctor may be prescribing without another's knowledge. In addition, the patient may be taking over-the-counter medications and herbal preparations. Treating compound disease also requires consideration of the interaction of concomitant disease on drugs used for the target illness. More patients are treated for multiple serious illnesses: elderly patients need specific consideration in this respect, and a larger part of the population of most countries is in the geriatric age group.

Fraudulent drugs may cause problems of lack of efficacy (Meyboom et al., 2000a, 2000b) and issues relating to adverse effects resulting from excipients. This growing problem, which affects developed and developing countries, needs a different approach to pharmacovigilance. Certainly there are many countries which still need to develop effective drug regulation.

Misdiagnosis, bad prescribing, bad dispensing and other poor practice leads to drug injury, but there may be correctable reasons for this poor performance. It is clear that the pressure is mounting on doctors and other health professionals. The technical and professional complexity of their work is increasing and to this we must add an increasing administrative and bureaucratic load. Undergraduate medical training does not devote sufficient time to drug safety and post-graduate education is too frequently concerned with the latest therapy and the importance of being up to date in the scholarly rather than practical sense. There is unending pressure on doctors, including the threat of litigation for even the most genuine of errors by the most careful of doctors. Patients are increasingly informed on medical matters and are encouraged, quite rightly, to understand and be active partners in their therapy instead of passive subjects. Unfortunately, the reliability of information sources is very variable, including a huge amount of information accessible to patients on the internet. Increasingly, therefore, doctors are required to justify their advice on therapy and even to undo confusion because of conflicting information.

There may be more reasons why drug-induced injury continues to be a public health problem, but it seems clear that much of it relates to fundamental issues of health professional education and working circumstances. The rest has to do with more drugs, more technical innovation and increasing information overload.

There are five broad activities that are essential to pharmacovigilance. These are:

- suspected ADR signal generation and formation of hypotheses,
- analysis of all issues around the signal, particularly confirmation (or refutation) of hypotheses, estimation of the size of the risk and whether susceptible patients exist,
- consideration of possible changed benefit-to-risk issues in therapy,
- communication of information to health professionals and patients in a useful way and possible regulatory action,
- consequence evaluation.

Each of the above steps will be considered below in relationship to some change, critical to make more progress. A basic assumption is that, since drug therapy very rarely constitutes epidemic risks, public health is very much concerned with securing the best benefit–risk for minority groups as well.

DRUG SAFETY SIGNALS

Suspected ADR signals may be related to a new drug or to the way in which any drug is used in the community. Since many hospital admissions are caused by avoidable ADRs, we should take much more notice of reports of known ADRs to older drugs, and generally regard any ADR report as something that has concerned a reporter enough to send it! This means not just concentrating on adverse reactions to new drugs (serious, unexpected), but to encourage health professionals and consumers to report any significant adverse effect relating to drug therapy. We need to provide the right climate for health professionals to be observant and critical in their diagnoses and therapy, so that they do not miss any piece of new information that may make therapy safer. IT and data mining can improve the transfer and analysis of the additional reports, respectively. In addition, it will be necessary to widen the scope of reporting to include adverse reactions to herbal and other traditional remedies, drug misuse, abuse, poisoning and overdose, and unexpected lack of effect, if we really wish to tackle the public health issues surrounding drug therapy comprehensively.

Multipurpose health databases should be used to monitor for drug safety signals much more than they are at present. Such databases should be planned so that appropriate data can be captured. Reports from consumers should be acted upon, both with a response to the individual and to the general public where appropriate.

SIGNAL ANALYSIS AND IMPACT-HYPOTHESIS TESTING

Very many signals are produced, and our ability to analyse them is limited. Currently, there seems to be little consistency over what signals will be considered further. Serious signals that appear to be new, and relate to new drugs, usually elicit regulatory action. Less serious signals that may none the less have an important impact on morbidity and compliance may not be investigated so rigorously even when the numbers build up. Epidemiological studies may take months to years to perform during which time thousands of patients may be exposed to the signalled risk.

This period of new signal analysis is rarely made transparent, and controversies tend to linger. Almost the whole effort of this vast collection machinery for clinical case report information is directed towards finding new ADR signals. Little use is made of the data for other signal work, such as:

- finding at-risk groups (e.g. do some ADRs occur disproportionately with age?)
- interactions (do known reactions occur more frequently with certain medicine combinations?)
- ADRs related to usage (e.g. do certain reactions occur more frequently in certain countries? at higher doses?)

This is not surprising, since the quantity of data is so large and most national centers have few resources. Several needs are apparent if we are to meet the challenges of the future. Amongst the most important are:

- to encourage clinicians to report clinically relevant experience
- to give advice about the diagnosis and management of ADRs
- to improve the rapid transmission of quality information to national centres and industry, and thence to the WHO database
- to find ways of supporting the examination of large amounts of disparate information
- to be able to bridge the gap between a tentative signal from raw ADR data and observational studies that use specific protocols.

BENEFIT TO RISK ANALYSIS

Much of the debate about comparative benefit and risk is bedevilled by failures of logic and definition (for example clearly differentiating between "harm" and "risk") and the use of different criteria in different situations. It is very important that these issues are identified in any critical review of information. The UMC developments in this area involve:

- promotion of the principle that responsible safety information must involve an element of benefit–risk analysis
- the further development of definitions that are acceptable to the WHO collaborating national centres
- to develop much further on the CIOMS IV guidelines on the principles of benefit–risk comparison (Lindquist and Edwards, 1993)
- the development or promotion of methods that will enhance more rigorous benefit–risk analysis, for example
  — comparing like with like (Edwards and Biriell, 1994)
  — the use of best-case and worst-case analysis for uncertain safety information
  — international analysis to highlight and to determine reasons for differences in reporting of ADRs (Mills and Edwards, 1999)

— analysis of ADR reports for comparator medical products when important safety signals are raised (Lindquist *et al.*, 1996)

COMMUNICATION OF BENEFIT–RISK INFORMATION

Currently, the emphasis of communication is on deciding whether a drug should be available or not and communicating that information, and the provision of official information in summaries of product characteristics (SPCs) and their equivalents, or in formularies. Decisions are made by regulators and the industry and their professional advisers as a result of a debate that is not transparent to consumers in most countries. Medicines are somewhat different from most other consumer products, in so far as patients generally do not have the ability, either because of lack of knowledge or insight, to make good choices about their own treatment. The question then arises as to whether health professionals, as learned intermediaries, have the correct or sufficient information on the benefits and risks of drugs from information that is readily available during clinical practice, e.g. reference books and SPCs.

Patient information leaflets are now promoted by some authorities, such as the EU and industry. These moves seem reasonable, but there must be a review of their effectiveness.

Communication to health professionals on adverse reactions needs to give some idea of their likelihood, severity and possible outcome to be useful to a clinician, and, of course, their patients. Little of this information is made available, nor is the level of certainty made clear on the evidence for most reactions.

CONSEQUENCE ANALYSIS

As far as possible, the likely consequences of a response to a safety concern should be considered before the action is undertaken. Input should be sought from experts in communication science, patient groups, practising health professionals and others when trying to predict consequences. This knowledge should guide choices between the options for action available. For example, a consequence analysis should be planned before a warning about a drug is given out or the drug is taken off the market. This analysis should be in two parts: an early investigation designed to ensure that the expected effect was achieved, so that a correction or reinforcement can be applied as necessary, and a later evaluation to ensure that a positive response is maintained. The UMC has previously looked at the way in which the signals it produces have been used in national centres (Edwards and Fucik, 1996).

COLLABORATION WITH OTHER ORGANISATIONS

Co-operation with organisations interested in developing early signals of significance is of importance to achieve a safer drug therapy. The International Society for Pharmacoepidemiology (ISPE) is specifically interested in the science of pharmacovigilance and the CIOMS is pivotal in bringing interested parties together to mount various collaborative projects. Much support has been given to the International Society of Pharmacovigilance (ISOP) which is gaining increasing international status. The Centre also supports the European Pharmacovigilance Research Group which has allowed regulators and drug safety specialists from a variety of European countries to come together to plan co-ordinated drug safety exercises. Initiatives like these may pave the way for a much more logical development and investigation of drug safety signals world-wide.

JOINING THE WHO PROGRAMME

Considering the sensitive nature of the data being collected within the Programme, countries contributing such data to the scheme have agreed on certain requirements that should be complied with by countries wishing to join. Collaborating with WHO, being an organisation for co-operation between member states, also requires a certain administrative structure of the drug monitoring activity. The basic requirements are:

● General acquaintance with the methodology of spontaneous monitoring. A country joining the

WHO Programme must have a programme for collection of spontaneous adverse reaction reports in place.
- A national centre for pharmacovigilance must be designated and recognised by the Ministry of Health (or equivalent).
- Technical competence to fulfill reporting requirements to WHO. Case reports collected in the national drug monitoring programme must be submitted to the WHO Programme in a defined format.

The UMC has published *Safety Monitoring of Medicinal Products: Guidelines for Setting-up and Running a Pharmacovigilance Centre* (WHO and Uppsala Monitoring Centre, 2000) and argues the case for good pharmacovigilance practice (Meyboom, 2000).

For further information please contact:
World Health Organisation
Health Technology and Pharmaceuticals
CH-1211 Geneva 27
Switzerland
telephone   +41-22 7912111
telefax   +41-22 7910746
e-mail   couperm@who.ch

WHO Collaborating Centre for International Drug Monitoring (the Uppsala Monitoring Centre)
Stora Torget 3
S-753 20 Uppsala
Sweden
telephone   +46-18 656060
telefax   +46-18 656080
e-mail   info@who-umc.org

CONCLUSIONS

The discipline of pharmacovigilance has developed and improved over the years. Much information on drug safety is now collected and subject to expert analysis and review. However, drug-induced morbidity remains a leading cause of hospital admission in several countries. A number of improvements have been mentioned, but the primary immediate need is for effective and efficient communication to health professionals.

This will need a paradigm shift from a gaze focused only on finding novel ADRs to new drugs, to a concentration on finding the problems associated with drug use in the community and how to improve it.

Health professions are criticised for many deficiencies, one of which is drug-related injury, but in our view society does not equip the health professions with the right resources to improve their performance. On the contrary, health professionals work under increasingly difficult circumstances in many countries. As far as drug safety is concerned, the provision of much better information for health professionals and the time for them to analyse and use the information is the main challenge for the near future. Only then can patients feel that they have the best chance of rational, individually tailored treatment, the best chance of not experiencing ADRs, the best chance of having unavoidable ADRs diagnosed and the best chance of important clinical experiences of ADRs being reported and used for future improvements.

ACKNOWLEDGEMENTS

The UMC serves the national centres in the WHO Collaborating Programme for International Drug Monitoring, and we are indebted to them for information and collaboration over the years.

REFERENCES

Bate A (2000) "Validating" automated signal detection methods used in spontaneous reporting systems. In: *16th International Conference on Pharmacoepidemiology*. Barcelona.
Bate A, *et al.* (1998a) A Bayesian neural network method for adverse drug reaction signal generation. *Eur J Clin Pharmacol* **54**: 315–21.
Bate A, *et al.* (1998b) Identifying and quantifying signals automatically. *Pharmacoepidemiology and Drug Safety* 7 (Suppl 2).
Bate A, Lindquist M, Orre R, Meyboom R, Edwards R (2000) Automated classification of signals as group effects or drug specific on the WHO database. In: *8th Annual Meeting European Society of Pharmacovigilance*. Verona: Elsevier.

Bowdler J (1997) *Effective Communications in Pharmacovigilance*, Vol. 1, 1st edn. Birmingham, England: W. Lake Ltd.

CIOMS (1995) *Harmonization of Data Fields for Electronic Transmission of Case–Report Information Internationally*. Geneva: CIOMS.

Edwards IR (1997) Pharmacological basis for adverse drug reactions. In: Speight T, Holford N, eds., *Avery's Drug Treatment*. Auckland: Adis International Ltd, pp. 261–99.

Edwards IR (1999) Spontaneous reporting—of what? Clinical concerns about drugs. *Br J Clin Pharmacol* **48**: 138–41.

Edwards IR (2000) The accelerating need for pharmacovigilance. *J R Coll Phys Lond* **34**(1): 48–51.

Edwards IR, Biriell C (1994) Harmonisation in pharmacovigilance. *Drug Safety* **10**: 93–102.

Edwards IR, Fucik H (1996) Impact and credibility of the WHO adverse reaction signals. *Drug Inf J* **30**(2): 461–4.

Edwards IR, Hugman B (1997) The challenge of effectively communicating risk–benefit information. *Drug Safety* **17**(4): 216–27.

Edwards IR, Wiholm B-E, Martinez C (1996) Concepts in risk–benefit assessment. *Drug Safety* **15**(1): 1–7.

Edwards IR, *et al.* (1990) Quality criteria for early signals of possible adverse drug reactions. *Lancet* **336**: 156–8.

Edwards IR, *et al.* (1993a) Proposed improvement to the WHO Adverse Reaction Terminology (WHO-ART). *Pharmacoepidemiology and Drug Safety* **2**: 177–84.

Edwards IR, *et al.* (1993b) Towards a new adverse event dictionary. *Pharmacoepidemiology and Drug Safety* **2**: 175–6.

Edwards IR *et al.* (2000) Understanding and communication of key concepts in therapeutics. In: *Moments of Truth—Communicating Drug Safety*. Verona: Elsevier.

Farah MH (1998) Consumer protection and herbal remedies. *WHO Drug Information* **12**(3): 141.

Farah MH. (2000a) Key issues in herbal pharmacovigilance. *Adverse Drug Reactions J* **2**(2): 105–9.

Farah MH, *et al.* (2000b) International monitoring of adverse health effects associated with herbal medicines. *Pharmacoepidemiology and Drug Safety* **9**: 105–12.

Lindquist M, Edwards IR (1993) Adverse drug reaction reporting in Europe: some problems of comparison. *Int J Risk Safety Med* **4**: 35–46.

Lindquist M, Edwards IR (1997) Risks of non-sedating antihistamines. *Lancet* **349**: 1322.

Lindquist M (1990) Uses and limitations of a global reporting pool. In: *Meeting on Methods for the Detection and Study of Unwanted Drug Effect*. Kiel, Germany, 26–29 Nov.

Lindquist M (1998) The WHO Programme for International Drug Monitoring: the present and future. In: Mitchard M, ed., *Electronic Communication Technologies*. pp. 527–49.

Lindquist M (2000) Signal detection using the WHO international database. In: *8th Annual Meeting European Society of Pharmacovigilance*. Verona: Elsevier.

Lindquist M, *et al.* (1994) Pharmacovigilance information on an old drug—an international study of spontaneous reports on Digoxin. *Drug Investigation* **8**: 73–80.

Lindquist M, *et al.* (1996) Omeprazole and visual disorders: seeing alternatives. *Pharmacoepidemiology and Drug Safety* **5**: 27–32.

Lindquist M, *et al.* (1997) How does cystitis affect a comparative risk profile of tiaprofenic acid with other non-steroidal antiinflammatory drugs? An international study based on spontaneous reports and drug usage data. *Pharmacol Toxicol* **80**: 211–17.

Lindquist M, *et al.* (1999) From association to alert—a revised approach to international signal analysis. *Pharmacoepidemiology and Drug Safety* **8**: S15–S25.

Lindquist M, Farah MH, Edwards R (2000) Monitoring of herbal medicines. In: *Clinical Pharmacology and Therapeutics*. Florence: Blackwell.

Meyboom RHB (2000) The case for good pharmacovigilance practice. *Pharmacoepidemiology and Drug Safety* **9**: 335–6.

Meyboom RHB, Lindquist M, Flygare AK, Biriell C, Edwards IR (2000a) Should therapeutic ineffectiveness be reported as an adverse drug reaction? In: *8th Annual Meeting European Society of Pharmacovigilance*. Verona: Elsevier.

Meyboom RHB, Lindquist M, Flygare A-K, Biriell C, Edwards RI (2000b) The value of reporting therapeutic ineffectiveness as an adverse drug reaction. *Drug Safety* **23**(2): 95–99.

Mills A, Edwards IR (1999) Venous thromboembolism and the pill. *Human Reproduction* **14**(1): 7–10.

Olsson S, ed. (1997) *National Pharmacovigilance Systems*. Uppsala: Uppsala Monitoring Centre.

Orre R, *et al.* (2000) Bayesian neural networks with confidence estimations applied to data mining. *Computational Statistics and Data Analysis* **34**(8): 473–93.

WHO and Uppsala Monitoring Centre (2000) *Safety Monitoring of Medicinal Products*. Uppsala: WHO and Uppsala Monitoring Centre.

14

Regulatory Pharmacovigilance in the EU

PATRICK C. WALLER

Post-Licensing Division, Medicines Control Agency, London, UK

PRIYA BAHRI

European Agency for the Evaluation of Medicinal Products (EMEA), London, UK

INTRODUCTION AND HISTORICAL PERSPECTIVE

Modern drug regulation in Europe began in the 1960s in the wake of the occurrence of several thousand cases (most of them in Europe) of phocomelia, a congenital limb abnormality which was caused by exposure to thalidomide during pregnancy (Burley, 1988). In response to this tragedy spontaneous adverse drug reaction (ADR) reporting schemes were developed with the aim of providing signals of unexpected hazards. Also legislation was passed to provide regulatory controls on safety, quality and efficacy of medicines through systems of standards for development and manufacturing, authorisation, pharmacovigilance and inspection. In Europe, the first Community Directive on medicines was enacted in 1965 (Council Directive 65/65/EEC) and laid down basic principles relating to these systems, which are still operational at the turn of the millennium. In particular, safety, quality and efficacy are the criteria through which medicines are regulated and other factors, such as cost, are not taken into account in decisions relating to the granting of a marketing authorisation.

Despite the extensive requirements for evidence on quality, efficacy and safety which are necessary to gain a marketing authorisation, pharmacovigilance remains a high priority for regulatory authorities in the European Union (EU). Although the quality and efficacy of a medicine are generally well described at the time of authorisation, conclusions on the adverse effect profiles of medicines from clinical trials are limited by the numbers and selectivity of patients included in such trials, their duration, and the relatively controlled conditions under which they are conducted. Safety in practice can only be assessed after marketing and it is well recognised that hazards may emerge at any time during the life of a product. Hence there is a need to monitor continuously the safety of all marketed medicines indefinitely. The overall objectives of regulatory pharmacovigilance (Waller et al., 1996) are summarised in Table 14.1.

Spontaneous reporting schemes continue to underpin such monitoring throughout the EU and have proved successful in identifying many

---

Pharmacovigilance. Edited by R.D. Mann and E.B. Andrews
© 2002 John Wiley & Sons, Ltd

Table 14.1. Objectives of regulatory pharmacovigilance.

---

1. Long-term monitoring of drug safety in clinical practice to identify previously unrecognised drug safety hazards or changes in the adverse effect profiles.
2. Assessment of the risks and benefits of licensed medicines, in order to take action to improve drug safety.
3. Provision of information to users to optimise safe and effective use of their medicines.
4. Monitoring the impact of any action taken.

---

important safety issues. However, both false positives and false negatives have occurred, one of the most striking examples of the latter being the failure to identify the oculomucocutaneous syndrome induced by practolol at an early stage (Felix et al., 1974). Specific limitations of spontaneous reporting schemes include underreporting, and uncertainty about causality and frequency. Thus many other sources of information are also used. There is increasing emphasis on epidemiological studies and the use of databases such as the UK General Practice Research Database (Wood and Waller, 1996; Walley and Mantgani, 1997) and the Dutch PHARMO system (Herings, 1993) in order to evaluate the safety of marketed medicines.

During the early 1990s closer co-operation between Member States developed as proposals for a more closely integrated regulatory system were formulated. Ultimately this led in 1995 to the establishment of the European Agency for the Evaluation of Medicinal Products (EMEA) and to a new regulatory system that includes procedures for a centralised authorisation and multiple identical authorisations through mutual recognition. These systems have had a considerable impact on the operation of pharmacovigilance in the EU. Although pharmacovigilance continues to be based on national systems, particularly in terms of data collection and expertise, there is central co-ordination through the EMEA and the Pharmacovigilance Working Party (PhVWP) of the Committee for Proprietary Medicinal Products (CPMP). This involves agreed standards and procedures, and systems for exchanging information and decision-making, which are described further below.

LEGAL BASIS, PRINCIPLES AND ORGANISATION OF THE EU PHARMACOVIGILANCE SYSTEM

The concept of pharmacovigilance was introduced into the legislation of the EU in 1993 through a Council Directive (Council Directive 93/39/EEC amending Council Directive 75/319/EEC). EU medicines legislation has since been codified into a single Directive (2001/83/EC) in which pharmacovigilance is covered in Title IX (Articles 101–108). Council Directives have the objective of harmonising the national legislation of the Member States of the EU, and Member States are bound to implement these legal provisions into their national legislation. However, pharmacovigilance systems already existed in most Member States. These vary according to differences in historical development and the organisation of the national healthcare systems. Table 14.2 summarises the organisational features of these national systems. All are an integral part of the respective national drug regulatory agency except in Luxembourg (for which spontaneous reports are submitted to one of the French regional centres). Through the EU legislation their activities are specified with regard to medicinal products authorised for use on their territory, as follows:

- to collect information about ADRs that occur under normal conditions of use;
- to obtain information on consumption data;
- to collate information on misuse and abuse;
- to evaluate this information scientifically; and
- to ensure the adoption of appropriate regulatory decisions.

Practice has shown that pharmacovigilance needs to be conducted with a view to how the product is used in ordinary clinical practice. This includes use outside the terms of the marketing authorisation. Experience gained during the post-authorisation phase may also provide valuable input into the evaluation of medicinal products at the stage of application for marketing authorisation, if there are chemical or pharmacological similarities with authorised products.

Table 14.2. National pharmacovigilance systems in the European Union (Olsson, 1999).

Member State and year of joining the European Union	Year of establishing the national pharmacovigilance centre	Status of spontaneous reporting of ADR cases by health professionals	Procedure for compilation of ADR cases occurring in this Member State	Procedure for assessment of ADR cases and other data and decision-making for nationally authorised medicinal products	Main tool of communication of safety information to healthcare professionals/general public
Austria 1995	1987	Mandatory	Nationwide reporting to national centre	Case assessment by single expert of national centre and advisory committee, recommendations on regulatory action by advisory committee (meets 4×/year)	Press releases routinely published in professional journals
Belgium 1951	1976	Voluntary	Nationwide reporting to national centre	Case assessment and recommendations by advisory committee (meets 2–4×/month) to medicines commission which proposes regulatory action	Monthly bulletin for health professionals, press releases
Denmark 1973	1968	Voluntary	Nationwide reporting to national centre	Case assessment by single expert of national centre, sometimes by ADR advisory committee, recommendations on regulatory action by ADR advisory committee (meets 1×/month) and medicines licensing committee	Press releases and publications in scientific journals
Finland 1995	1966	Voluntary	Nationwide reporting to national centre, major hospitals operate additional ADR monitoring systems and submit them to the national centre	Case assessment by single expert and minor regulatory action by national centre, recommendations on major regulatory action by committee on safety and efficacy	Bi-monthly drug bulletin for health professionals, press releases
France 1951	1975	Mandatory	Reporting by health professionals to regional centre (31 regional hospital-based centres), compiled at national centre, reporting by marketing authorisation holders to national centre	Case assessment by single expert at regional centre, signal generation and further assessment by national centre, signal evaluation on causal relationship by advisory committee (meets every second month), validation of their opinion by technical committee, recommendations on regulatory action by national commission, sometimes validated by the marketing authorisation commission	Press releases

(continued)

Table 14.2. *Continued.*

Member State and year of joining the European Union	Year of establishing the national pharmacovigilance centre	Status of spontaneous reporting of ADR cases by health professionals	Procedure for compilation of ADR cases occurring in this Member State	Procedure for assessment of ADR cases and other data and decision-making for nationally authorised medicinal products	Main tool of communication of safety information to healthcare professionals/ general public
Germany 1951	1978	Voluntary	Reporting by health professionals to the drug commission of health professionals for transmission to the national centre, reporting by marketing authorisation holders to national centre	Case assessment by single expert at national centre, sometimes by advisory committee, recommendations on regulatory action by advisory committee (meets at least every second month)	Press releases routinely published in professional journals
Greece 1981	1986	Mandatory	Nationwide reporting to national centre	Case assessment by single expert at national centre and an advisory committee, recommendations on regulatory action by pharmacovigilance committee (meets 1–2×/month)	Press releases and publications in scientific journals
Ireland 1973	1969	Voluntary	Nationwide reporting to national centre	Case assessment and signal generation at national centre, further assessment and recommendations on regulatory action by committee on drug usage and adverse reactions (meets 2×/month)	Drug bulletin for health professionals
Italy 1951	1980	Mandatory	Nationwide reporting to national centre; major hospitals and universities operate additional ADR monitoring systems and submit them to the national centre	Case assessment by single experts at national centre, further assessment and recommendation on regulatory action by national drug committee (meets 1×/week) and higher health council (meets 1×/month)	Drug bulletin for health professionals

Luxembourg 1951	See text				
The Netherlands 1951	1963	Voluntary	Reporting to five hospital-based regional centres under control of national centre for transmission to national centre	Case assessment in co-operation between national and regional centres, further assessment in consultation with advisory committee for transmission of recommendations to medicines evaluation board	Press releases and publications for health professionals
Portugal 1986	1992	Mandatory	Nationwide reporting to national centre, establishment of regional centres planned	Case assessment and signal evaluation by advisory committee (meets on demand), recommendation on regulatory action by pharmacovigilance committee	Quarterly drug bulletin for health professionals, press releases
Spain 1986	1983	Mandatory	Reporting to 18 regional centres under control of national centre for transmission to national centre	Case assessment by an advisory committee, recommendation on regulatory action by pharmacovigilance committee (meets 4×/year)	Half-yearly to quarterly drug bulletin for health professionals, press releases
Sweden 1995	1965	Mandatory	Reporting to national centre and regional centres under control of national centre	Case assessment by single expert or advisory committee, recommendation on regulatory action by advisory board (meets 4×/year) and implementation by national centre, recommendation on withdrawal of marketing authorisation by drugs advisory board	Press releases
United Kingdom 1973	1964	Voluntary	Reporting to four regional centres or national centre as applicable	Case and further assessment at national centre, advice from pharmacovigilance advisory subcommittee (meets 5×/year), recommendation on regulatory action by safety advisory committee (meets 2×/month)	Quarterly drug bulletin to health professionals

The national pharmacovigilance systems of the Member States together form the pharmacovigilance system in the EU, co-operating in a network structure under the co-ordination of the EMEA and in liaison with the European Commission. Also included are Norway, Iceland and Liechtenstein, which are not members of the EU but are part of the European Economic Area (EEA) (EEA Joint Committee, 1999). Within this network structure all parties have their roles and responsibilities for the surveillance of medicinal products. These roles and responsibilities vary depending on the route of marketing authorisation of the product in the EU and are defined in Directive 2001/83/EC and Council Regulation (EEC) No. 2309/93. These are described in guidance documents which were developed during the 1990s for competent authorities and marketing authorisation holders in consultation with Member States and interested parties (Table 14.3). These guidelines are in accordance with recommendations

Table 14.3. Guidance documents developed by the regulatory pharmacovigilance system of the European Union at Community level (European Commission, 2001).

- Procedure for Competent Authorities on the Undertaking of Pharmacovigilance Activities
- Rapid Alert System (RAS) and Non-Urgent Information System (NUIS) in Human Pharmacovigilance
- Conduct of Pharmacovigilance for Centrally Authorised Products
- Crisis Management Plan regarding Centrally Authorised Products for Human Use
- Conduct of Pharmacovigilance for Medicinal Products Authorised Through the Mutual Recognition Procedure
- Standard Operating Procedure (SOP) on Referrals in accordance with the Provisions of Council Directive 75/319/EEC in the case of Safety Concerns related to Medicinal Products Marketed in the European Union
- Principles of Providing the World Health Organisation with Pharmacovigilance Information
- Notice to Marketing Authorisation Holders
- Note for Guidance on Electronic Exchange of Pharmacovigilance Information for Human and Veterinary Medicinal Products in the European Union

Explanatory note: This constitutes an updated list as of time of going to press. These guidance documents are subject to continuous review and revised documents are announced for publication by the European Commission.

agreed at the International Conference on Harmonisation of Technical Requirements for Registration of Pharmaceuticals for Human Use (ICH). They have been revised in the light of experience and are available in a compiled format (European Commission, 2001).

The EMEA is a Community Agency, i.e. a public authority of the EU set up by a Community act of secondary legislation (Council Regulation (EEC) No. 2309/93) with its own legal personality (Bodies of the European Union, 2000). The objective of the EMEA is the protection and promotion of human and animal health in the EU by fulfilling, *inter alia*, the following tasks with respect to human medicines:

- the co-ordination of the scientific evaluation of the safety, quality and efficacy of medicinal products that have been applied for a central marketing authorisation with the aim of facilitating the access to effective and safe innovative medicinal products throughout the EU; and
- the co-ordination of post-authorisation safety of medicinal products through the pharmacovigilance network.

The EMEA pools scientific expertise from the Member States for the evaluation of medicinal products, and to provide advice on drug research and development programmes (European Agency for the Evaluation of Medicinal Products, 2001). More specific to pharmacovigilance, the tasks of the EMEA include the following:

- co-ordination of the supervision (including pharmacovigilance activities) of medicinal products authorised in the EU;
- provision of access to information on ADRs reported for medicinal products marketed in the EU by means of a data-processing network which can be accessed by all Member States, the EMEA and the Commission (a project known as EudraVigilance);
- maintenance of and variations to the terms of the marketing authorisation for centrally authorised products;
- management of referral procedures for nationally authorised products leading to Commission

Decisions binding in all Member States when there is a safety concern which impacts on public health in the Community; and
- provision of recommendations on measures necessary to ensure safe and effective use of these products.

Much of the work of the EMEA is done within its scientific committees. For medicines used in humans this is the CPMP. This committee is supported by several expert working parties, one of which is the PhVWP. The PhVWP currently meets eight times per year at the EMEA and provides a forum for scientific discussion of product and product-class-related safety issues leading to recommendations on harmonised and synchronised action. These are ultimately implemented either by the European Commission following a CPMP Opinion for centrally authorised products, or by national competent authorities. The PhVWP also takes the lead in the development of pharmacovigilance guidelines.

In order to facilitate, in addition, a continuous exchange of information between regulators in the EEA, in particular with regard to changes in the benefit–risk balance possibly requiring major regulatory action, but also for signal evaluation, the so-called Rapid Alert–Non-Urgent Information System has been established. Records of this information flow are maintained centrally by the EMEA and followed up by the PhVWP at each of their meetings. The principles and procedures of this system are presented in a Note for Guidance (European Commission, 2001, Part I, Chapter 2.1). Guidance for the electronic submission of case reports on ADRs in relation to medicinal products authorised in the EU is provided (European Commission, 2001, Part III).

Pharmaceutical companies holding marketing authorisations in the EU have various obligations in the area of pharmacovigilance which are laid down in Title IX of Directive 2001/83/EC and Council Regulation (EEC) No. 2309/93 and elaborated further in guidelines (European Commission, 2001). In particular, marketing authorisation holders must employ a qualified person who is

responsible for:

- establishing and maintaining a system that collects and collates all suspected adverse reactions;
- the preparation of periodic safety update reports; and
- responding to requests for additional information from competent authorities.

In addition, marketing authorisation holders are obliged to report serious suspected adverse reactions in accordance with the legislation and guidance cited above to competent authorities within 15 days ("expedited reports").

THE PROCESS OF REGULATORY PHARMACOVIGILANCE IN THE EU

Regulatory pharmacovigilance is dependent on the availability of information on the clinical effects of medicines in representative populations as used in normal practice. In addition to systems for collecting and handling suspected ADRs, processes for generating and investigating signals are necessary. All potentially important hazards are investigated with a view to taking appropriate action based on the available scientific evidence. The most important outputs of the process are actions to promote safer use of medicines. These include, for example, introducing warnings, contraindications, information on adverse effects or changes to dosing recommendations. Indications or methods of supply may be also restricted, although withdrawal of a medicinal product from the market on safety grounds is relatively unusual (Jefferys et al., 1998). Informing users and explaining the reasons for the action taken is a critical determinant of the effectiveness of these measures. The process of regulatory pharmacovigilance is summarised in Figure 14.1.

DETECTION OF ADRS

Potentially important drug safety issues can be identified at any stage of drug development. In the post-authorisation phase they are particularly

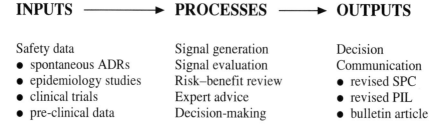

INPUTS ⟶ **PROCESSES** ⟶ **OUTPUTS**

Safety data	Signal generation	Decision
• spontaneous ADRs	Signal evaluation	Communication
• epidemiology studies	Risk–benefit review	• revised SPC
• clinical trials	Expert advice	• revised PIL
• pre-clinical data	Decision-making	• bulletin article

Figure 14.1. Regulatory pharmacovigilance.

likely to be identified in the first few years after marketing, although new issues also arise with long-established drugs. In order to ensure that safety problems which have not been recognised or fully understood pre-marketing are handled promptly, proactive processes are used for screening emerging data for potential issues and bringing together all the available information from multiple sources. In regulatory practice, a signal is an alert from any available source that a medicine may be associated with a previously unrecognised hazard, or that a known hazard may be quantitatively (e.g. more frequent) or qualitatively (e.g. more serious) different from existing expectations.

The commonest source for identification of significant drug safety concerns arising with marketed medicines is spontaneous suspected adverse reaction reporting. These are individual case reports from health professionals of adverse events which the reporter considers *may* be related to the medicine(s) being taken. Reporters are not asked to provide all adverse events that follow administration of the medicine but to selectively report those which they suspect were adverse reactions. There is frequently confusion between the terms "adverse event" and "adverse reaction" which can be avoided by using the term "*suspected adverse reaction*" when referring to a case or series of cases reported through a spontaneous reporting scheme. The term "adverse event" should be used in the context of studies where all events are being collected regardless of where or not they are suspected to be related to a drug. This approach is underpinned by standard definitions given in European legislation (Title I of Directive, 2001/83/EC) and is also consistent with defini-

tions proposed by the ICH in guideline E2A (D'Arcy and Harron, 1995).

Although formal studies of drug safety are particularly used in the investigation of signals generated by methods such as spontaneous ADR reporting (i.e. hypothesis-testing), they may also provide the initial evidence producing a safety concern. Signals may also be detected from other sources such as literature reports and from screening of the international spontaneous reporting database operated by the Uppsala Monitoring Centre in Sweden, a Collaborating Centre of the World Health Organization (Uppsala Monitoring Centre, 1998), to which all EU Member States contribute data. Whatever the source of the signal, the aim is to identify it as rapidly as possible. The next steps are to inform other Member States, gather further information and conduct an evaluation.

EVALUATION OF PHARMACOVIGILANCE ISSUES

When there is sufficient evidence of a hazard to warrant further investigation, detailed consideration is given to causality, possible mechanisms, frequency and preventability. Assessment of these issues may require new epidemiological studies, but the hypothesis may be strengthened or weakened using immediately available sources of retrospective information such as worldwide spontaneous reporting, published literature and epidemiological databases.

The broad principles relating to post-authorisation studies have been set out in guidelines for pharmaceutical companies (European Commission, 2001, Part I, Chapter 1). When new data become available from purpose-designed studies it is important that they are reviewed in the context of the existing data. An assessment is made of whether and how the new evidence changes the previous evaluation, focusing particularly on the strength of the evidence for a drug-related association and possible approaches to prevention. In the latter respect, detailed analysis of the data to identify possible risk factors for the hazard is important.

The output of an evaluation is an assessment report that brings together the key information on the hazards and facilitates discussion of the risks and benefits of the medicine and possible measures which may facilitate safe use. Experts in pharmaco-epidemiology and relevant therapeutic areas are consulted and involved in such discussions both at national and EU level.

DECISION-MAKING AND RISK MANAGEMENT

The objective of the EU competent authorities is to take regulatory actions which are justified by scientific evidence, and allow users to make informed decisions and to use medicines safely. Sometimes the balance of risks and benefits will be sufficiently clear to allow firm recommendations (such as contraindications), whilst in other situations less directive advice will be warranted.

The types of action which may be taken vary according to potential means of preventing the adverse reaction. In particular, hazards may be minimised by targeting the drug at patients least likely to be at risk of the ADR and by specifically contraindicating it in patients with identifiable risk factors. Dose and duration of treatment are often important issues since the risk of many hazards is related to one or both of these parameters. It is quite common for dosage regimens to change during the post-marketing period in response to safety concerns and many drugs have been initially recommended at doses higher than necessary. In re-evaluating dose in response to a safety concern, consideration is also given to the evidence of efficacy at lower doses.

The identification of a new ADR or the accumulation of important new evidence about a recognised reaction leads to a need to make changes to the product information, and hence to vary the marketing authorisation(s). Variations to marketing authorisations on safety grounds may be proposed by the competent authority or pharmaceutical company. Regardless of who proposes the changes, there is exchange of information and discussion between the parties before a variation is submitted in order to facilitate rapid implementation. When the competent authorities and companies are in agreement about the nature and impact of a drug safety issue, changes can be made on a voluntary basis by the marketing authorisation holder. However, if the companies do not agree about the actions required, then the competent authorities may exercise compulsory powers. Exceptionally, when the issue has urgent public health implications the authorities may act rapidly, without a right of appeal by the company, to immediately withdraw the product(s) from the market by suspension of the authorisation(s) or to change the product information.

COMMUNICATION

Communicating information to users of medicinal products is a vital step in the process of handling a safety issue with a marketed medicine. The distribution of safety information may be targeted at specialists or generalists or both, other relevant health professionals and at patients. A particularly important aim in communications about drug safety is to ensure that essential information is clearly conveyed and not obscured by other less important information. Every effort is therefore made to word the key facts and recommendations unambiguously.

The key principles with patient information are that it should, in substance, be the same as the information provided to health professionals and it should be presented in language that the patient can understand. Good patient information adds to and reinforces the main issues that should be discussed between health professionals and patients, and does not make statements which could interfere with that relationship.

An important consideration is how quickly information needs to be made available to users.

A new life-threatening adverse reaction requires immediate communication, whereas the addition of information relating to a non-serious ADR could be added at the next routine revision of the product information. In the EU there is a mechanism for an immediate (i.e. within 24 hours) measure to restrict use or provide essential additional information on urgent safety grounds (Commission Regulation (EC) No. 541/95; Commission Regulation (EC) No. 542/95). Subsequently such changes are followed by a variation using standard procedures.

Any change to the marketing authorisation and product information which has significant safety implications is actively drawn to the attention of the relevant health professionals, usually by circulating the new product information under cover of a "Dear Doctor/Pharmacist" letter. When the changes being made are vital for ensuring patient safety they are implemented very quickly, and it is normal practice to make information available to the media and general public through press releases and/or the internet.

The EU competent authorities recognise that successful communication about drug safety is a vital component of the pharmacovigilance process. This is a particular challenge because of the need to translate messages into all the official languages used in the EU (currently 11) and considerable attention is being paid to improving this aspect of the process.

FUTURE CHALLENGES

Changes to pharmacovigilance aspects of EU legislation were recently put forward in Commission Directive 2000/38/EEC and these have been codified into Directive 2001/83/EC. In the longer term, medicines legislation is currently under review by the Commission with the resultant changes likely to be implemented in 2005. However, it does not seem likely that there will be fundamental changes to the basic system described above. The most important challenges will probably result from EU enlargement involving Central and Eastern European countries. Steps have already been taken to involve them in medicines regulation and pharma-

covigilance activities through an initiative known as the Pan-European Regulatory Forum (PERF). In this context it will be particularly important to have in place agreed standards for the conduct of pharmacovigilance for all the parties involved. The PhVWP is currently developing such standards through an initiative known as Good Pharmacovigilance Practice (GVP). Particular efforts are also being put into the completion of the electronic information network through the EudraVigilance project, allowing for the exchange of pharmacovigilance information between all stakeholders (EMEA, national competent authorities and marketing authorisation holders).

One important limitation of all current pharmacovigilance systems is the difficulty in measuring the effects of the actions taken. It will be particularly important for EU competent authorities to address this using the available electronic epidemiological databases. Expectations of consumers in respect of drug safety have increased considerably in recent years (Asscher *et al.*, 1995) and are likely to continue to do so. In order to meet these expectations, processes will need to become even more transparent and to be demonstrably effective. Communication tools also need to be improved and it will be important that both competent authorities and pharmaceutical companies ensure full compliance with their pharmacovigilance obligations.

CONCLUSIONS

The system of pharmacovigilance established in the EU aims to promote the safe use of medicines in clinical use thereby protecting public health. During the 1990s existing pharmacovigilance systems in Member States have been brought together to form a Community-wide system that currently covers a population of about 350 million people. The main challenges of the next decade include preparing for expected EU enlargement and the increasing expectations of consumers. In order to meet these challenges, and to efficiently add further value in the protection of public health, the system is continuing to evolve, particularly in response to scientific progress and technological developments.

ACKNOWLEDGEMENTS

We would like to thank Stella Blackburn and Noël Wathion for helpful comments on an earlier draft. The views expressed in this chapter are those of the authors and not necessarily those of their respective employers.

REFERENCES

Asscher AW, Parr GD, Whitmarsh VB (1995) Towards safer use of medicines. *Br Med J* **311**: 1003–5.

Bodies of the European Union (2000) Internet-publication of information accessible at `http://europa.eu.int/agencies`.

Burley DM (1988) The rise and fall of thalidomide. *Pharmaceut Med* **3**: 231–7.

Commission Directive 2000/38/EC of 5 June 2000 amending Chapter Va (Pharmacovigilance) of Council Directive 75/319/EEC on the approximation of provisions laid down by law, legislation or administrative action relating to medicinal products. In *Official Journal of the European Communities*, Office for Official Publications of the European Communities, Luxembourg, L139, pp. 28–30.

Commission Regulation (EC) No. 541/95 of 10 March 1995 concerning the examination of variations to the terms of a marketing authorisation granted by a competent authority of a Member State. In *Official Journal of the European Communities*, Office for Official Publications of the European Communities, Luxembourg, L55, pp. 7–14.

Commission Regulation (EC) No. 542/95 of 10 March 1995 concerning the examination of variations to the terms of a marketing authorisation falling within the scope of Council Regulation (EEC) No. 2309/93 (1995). In *Official Journal of the European Communities*, Office for Official Publications of the European Communities, Luxembourg, L55, p. 15.

Council Directive 65/65/EEC of 26 January 1965 on the approximation of provisions laid down by law, regulation or administrative action relating to medicinal products (1965). In *Official Journal of the European Communities*, Office for Official Publications of the European Communities, Luxembourg, 022, pp. 3–12.

Council Directive 75/319/EEC of 20 May 1975 on the approximation of provisions laid down by law, regulation or administrative action relating to medicinal products as amended (1993). In *Pharmaceutical Legislation: Medicinal Products for Human Use*, Office for Official Publications of the European Communities, Luxembourg (1998), pp. 41–63.

Council Directive 93/39/EEC of 14 June 1993 amending Directives 65/65, 75/318/EEC and 75/319/EEC in respect of medicinal products (1993). In *Official Journal of the European Communities*, Office for Official Publications of the European Communities, Luxembourg, L 214, pp. 22–30.

Council Regulation (EEC) No. 2309/93 of 22 July 1993 laying down Community procedures for the authorisation and supervision of medicinal products for human and veterinary use and establishing a European Agency for the Evaluation of Medicinal Products (1993). In *Official Journal of the European Communities*, Office for Official Publications of the European Communities, Luxembourg, L 214, pp. 0001–21.

Directive 2001/83/EC of the European Parliament and of the Council of 6 November 2001 on the Community Code relating to medicinal products for human use. In *Official Journal of the European Communities*, Office for Official Publications of the European Communities, Luxembourg, L 311, pp. 67–128.

D'Arcy PF, Harron DWG (1995) Background to the Conference. In: *Proceedings of the Third International Conference on Harmonisation, Yokohama*. Belfast: Queen's University, pp. 1–14.

EEA Joint Committee (1999) Decision No. 74/1999. In: *Official Journal of the European Communities*, Office for Official Publications of the European Communities, Luxembourg, 9 November 2000, pp. 65–6.

European Agency for the Evaluation of Medicinal Products (2001) About us. Internet-publication accessible at `http://www.emea.eu.int`.

European Commission (2001) Volume 9 of the Rules Governing Medicinal Products in the European Union—Pharmacovigilance. Internet-publication accessible at `http://pharmacos.eudra.org`.

Felix RH, Ive FA, Dahl MCG (1974) Cutaneous and ocular reactions to practolol. *Br Med J* **iv**: 321.

Herings RMC (1993) PHARMO: a record linkage system for postmarketing surveillance of prescription drugs in The Netherlands. Dissertation, Universiteit Utrecht.

International Conference on Harmonisation of Technical Requirements for Registration of Pharmaceuticals for Human Use (ICH) (1994) Clinical safety data management: Definitions and standards for expedited reporting (ICH E2A).

Jefferys DB, Leakey D, Lewis J, Payne S, Rawlins MD (1998) New active substances authorized in the United Kingdom between 1972 and 1994. *Br J Clin Pharmacol* **45**: 151–6.

Olsson S, ed (1999) *National Pharmacovigilance Systems*. Uppsala: WHO Collaborating Centre for International Drug Monitoring.

Uppsala Monitoring Centre (1998) *A Network for Safety*. Uppsala: WHO Collaborating Centre for International Drug Monitoring.

Waller PC, Coulson RA, Wood SM (1996) Regulatory

pharmacovigilance in the United Kingdom: Current principles and practice. *Pharmacoepidemiology and Drug Safety* **5**: 363–75.

Walley T, Mantgani A (1997) The UK General Practice Research Database. *Lancet* **350**: 1097–9.

Wood SM, Waller PC (1996) Record linkage databases for pharmacovigilance: a UK perspective. In: *Databases for Pharmacovigilance*. Walker SR, ed., Carshalton: Centre for Medicines Research, pp. 47–54.

15

Spontaneous Reporting—UK

SARAH DAVIS AND JUNE M. RAINE

Post-Licensing Division, Medicines Control Agency, London, UK

INTRODUCTION

In the United Kingdom, the Licensing Authority responsible for medicines for human use consists of ministers, including the Secretary of State for Health. The Authority's executive function in the control of medicines is performed on a day-to-day basis by the UK Medicines Control Agency (MCA). The Agency's primary objective is to safeguard public health by ensuring that medicines on the UK market meet appropriate standards of safety, quality and efficacy.

While the quality and efficacy of a medicine are fairly well defined at the time of licensing, the clinical trials conducted in support of a licence application can only provide limited data on a medicine's safety profile; the safety profile of a medicine in normal clinical use can only be fully assessed after it has been marketed. The Post Licensing Division of the MCA is responsible for monitoring the safety of all licensed medicines in the United Kingdom, in order to identify and investigate possible hazards and take appropriate action to minimise the risks and maximise the benefits to users, thus protecting public health. Although data from a wide range of sources are used (Waller *et al.*, 1996), it is the UK's spontaneous reporting scheme (commonly known as the "Yellow Card Scheme") that is the cornerstone of the monitoring process.

The aim of this chapter is to inform the reader about the past, present and future of the Yellow Card Scheme. First, the background to the Yellow Card Scheme since its introduction in the 1960s is outlined, including examples of the safety hazards identified from spontaneous reporting, and some of the problems faced by the Scheme in past years. Secondly, we describe some of the recent initiatives implemented in order to tackle these problems, focusing on areas such as widening the reporting base and facilitation of reporting. Finally, we outline some of the possible future directions for the Yellow Card Scheme that are intended to allow it to continue to fulfil its key role in pharmacovigilance in the years to come.

BACKGROUND

INTRODUCTION OF THE YELLOW CARD SCHEME

The public health importance of controls on the safety of medicines was dramatically brought to the attention of the public in the early 1960s, by the thalidomide tragedy. In the wake of this tragedy,

Pharmacovigilance. Edited by R.D. Mann and E.B. Andrews
© 2002 John Wiley & Sons, Ltd

many countries introduced systems for the systematic collection of reports of adverse drug reactions. In the United Kingdom, the Committee on Safety of Drugs (now the Committee on Safety of Medicines; CSM) was set up. One of the responsibilities of this new committee was to collect and disseminate information relating to adverse effects of drugs (Griffin, 1992). To address this objective, the UK's spontaneous reporting scheme was introduced in 1964, when Sir Derrick Dunlop (the chairman of the Committee on Safety of Drugs) wrote to all doctors and dentists in the United Kingdom to announce the launch of the new Scheme (Griffin and Weber, 1992).

In his milestone letter, Sir Derrick asked "every member of the medical/dental profession in the United Kingdom" to report "promptly details of any untoward condition in a patient which might be the result of drug treatment" and stated that "All the reports or replies that the Committee receive from doctors/dentists will be treated with complete professional confidence by the Committee and their staff."

This established four key principles of the scheme, namely:

1. *Suspected* adverse reactions should be reported; reporters do not need to be certain or to prove that the drug caused the reaction.
2. It is the responsibility of all doctors and dentists to report.
3. Reporters should report without delay.
4. Reports could be made and would be treated in confidence.

Reports were to be made on specially provided yellow reporting forms, a supply of which was provided with Sir Derrick's letter. The significance of the yellow colour of the card is no more than that there was by coincidence a large supply of yellow paper unutilised at that time; however, as a result, the scheme has come to be known as the Yellow Card Scheme. In the almost 40 years since the introduction of this scheme, the design of the reporting form has changed progressively, to include guidelines on reporting and ask for additional specific pieces of information (e.g. Lawson, 1990; Griffin and Weber, 1992; Anon,

2000a). Reports are also received via the pharmaceutical industry, which has a statutory obligation to report suspected adverse reactions (Waller *et al.*, 1996). The CSM continue to be responsible for the Yellow Card Scheme, which is now run on the Committee's behalf by the MCA, using the specialised Adverse Drug Reactions On-line Information Tracking (ADROIT) database to facilitate rapid processing and analysis of reports and detection of signals of drug safety hazards. The CSM's Regional Monitoring Centres (RMCs), introduced in the 1980s, provide valuable support for the running of the Scheme in Merseyside, the Northern region, Wales and the West Midlands (e.g. Houghton *et al.*, 1996).

PURPOSE AND ACHIEVEMENTS OF THE YELLOW CARD SCHEME

It is generally accepted (e.g. Amery, 1999) that it is not possible to detect all the adverse effects of a medicine during the pre-marketing clinical trials, because of a number of factors. First, trials are generally small (on average 1500 patients for a new drug substance); although they will detect common side effects, particularly those that are predictable from the pharmacology of the drug, they are too small to detect side effects that occur rarely (incidence of 1 in 10 000 or less). Additionally, medicines are used in clinical trials in a very controlled manner—they are given for a limited duration, to carefully selected patients who are closely monitored. This is in complete contrast to the manner in which the medicine may be used once marketed, when it may be used in patient populations for which it was not intended, may be given for long periods of time, and in combination with other medicines.

It is therefore vital to monitor the safety of medicines as used in routine clinical practice throughout their marketed life, in order to detect those side effects that are not identified through clinical trials. The best established way to do this is to collect reports of suspected adverse drug reactions (ADRs) via a spontaneous reporting scheme such as the Yellow Card Scheme.

All spontaneous reporting schemes, including the Yellow Card Scheme, have a number of limitations, perhaps the most significant of which is under-reporting (e.g. Griffin and Weber, 1992; see the section on weaknesses below). Despite this, such schemes have a proven track record as an "early warning" system for the identification of new drug safety hazards. Examples of drug safety hazards identified through spontaneous reporting have been described previously (e.g. Rawlins, 1988b; Griffin and Weber, 1992); recent examples of ADRs identified through the Scheme are shown in Table 15.1.

WEAKNESSES

As mentioned previously, all spontaneous reporting schemes have a number of limitations; these

have been documented previously (e.g. Rawlins et al., 1992; Meyboom et al., 1997a, 1997b). The limitation of most concern is the issue of under-reporting: it is clear from a number of studies that only a small proportion of ADRs are ever reported to the regulatory authorities, both in the United Kingdom (e.g. Smith et al., 1996; Sweis and Wong, 2000), and in other countries (e.g. Chan and Critchley, 1994; Moride et al., 1997; Alvarez-Requejo et al., 1998).

Under-reporting of ADRs is clearly of concern, since it may lead to under-estimation of the significance of a particular reaction. This is compounded by the fact that the magnitude of under-reporting is variable; studies have suggested that levels of reporting are influenced by factors

Table 15.1. Important early warnings of new adverse reactions identified since 1995 and the resultant UK actions in respect of marketing authorisations/product information.

Year	Drug (product)	Adverse reaction	Resultant action
1995	Tramadol (Zydol▼)[a]	Psychiatric reactions	Warnings
1995	Cyproterone acetate (Cyprostat, Androcur)	Dose-related hepatotoxicity	Restricted indications and requirement for hepatic function monitoring
1995	Quinolone antibiotics	Tendonitis, tendon rupture	Improved warnings
1995	Tacrolimus (Prograf▼)	Hypertrophic cardiomyopathy	Warnings, dose reduction and monitoring requirements
1996	Alendronate (Fosamax▼)	Severe oesophageal reactions	Warnings and revised dosing instructions
1997	Clozapine (Clozaril)	GI obstruction	Improved warnings
1997	HIV protease inhibitors	Hyperlipidaemia and fat re-distribution	Improved warnings and monitoring recommendations
1998	Isotretinoin (Roaccutane)	Psychiatric reactions	Improved warnings
1998	Sertindole (Serdolect▼)	Sudden cardiac death	Drug withdrawn
1999	Aristolochia in Chinese herbal remedies	Renal failure	Aristolochia banned
1999	Human clottable protein concentrate (Quixil▼)	Fatal neurotoxic reactions following unlicensed use in neurosurgery	Increased warnings
2000	Cisapride (Prepulsid, Alimix)	Serious cardiovascular reactions, including QT prolongation	Use suspended
2001	Bupropion (Zyban▼)	Seizures	Strengthened warnings and revised dosing instructions

[a] ▼ Black Triangle drug at the time the major safety issue was identified.

such as the seriousness of the reaction, whether the reaction is labelled, the length of time a drug has been on the market, and promotion or publicity about the medicine or the reaction (Rawlins, 1988a; Griffin and Weber, 1992; Smith et al., 1996; Haramburu et al., 1997; Moride et al., 1997; Alvarez-Requejo et al., 1998). There is also evidence to suggest that levels of reporting may vary between different groups of doctors, with hospital doctors reporting less frequently than general practitioners (GPs) (Bateman et al., 1992; Eland et al., 1999).

Various studies have attempted to establish the reasons for under-reporting; recent surveys of attitudes to reporting of ADRs suggest that lack of time, and uncertainty as to whether the reaction was caused by a drug are among the most common factors in deterring reporting (Belton et al., 1995; Eland et al., 1999; Sweis and Wong, 2000). Another factor identified by some groups was concern about breaching patient confidentiality (Bateman et al., 1992; Sweis and Wong, 2000).

Average ADR reporting rates for the Yellow Card Scheme (e.g. reports per million inhabitants per year) are among the highest in the world (e.g. Edwards, 1997), especially when compared with other countries with a large population (Griffin, 1986). However, a survey in 1984 (Speirs et al., 1984) found that only 16% of doctors who were eligible to report suspected ADRs to the Scheme had actually submitted a Yellow Card between 1972 and 1980. More recent figures are more encouraging; an analysis of the reporters of Yellow Cards submitted between 1992 and 1995 showed that around one-third of practising doctors submitted a report during this four-year period. However, it is clear that many doctors do not contribute to the Yellow Card Scheme; this is unlikely to be simply because these doctors do not see patients who have experienced an adverse reaction.

REPORTING VOLUMES

The number of reports received via the Yellow Card Scheme between 1964 and 2001 is shown in Figure 15.1. It can be seen that the annual number of reports received has risen significantly since the introduction of the Scheme, with notable increases

in reporting being seen in the mid 1970s and again in 1986. The first of these increases coincided with the withdrawal of practolol following its association with oculomucocutaneous syndrome, the introduction of the CSM drug safety bulletin *Current Problems in Pharmacovigilance*, and the inclusion of a yellow page in prescription pads used by GPs, reminding them to report ADRs. The second increase is thought to have resulted from the increased availability of Yellow Cards to doctors, following their inclusion in the British National Formulary (BNF) which is supplied to all doctors, and in prescription pads (Rawlins, 1988a).

There was a significant change in the early 1990s when the annual number of Yellow Cards received declined from a peak of just over 20 000 to an annual average of around 17 000 in the mid to late 1990s. A number of factors may be responsible for contributing to this decline; for instance, the number of Yellow Cards submitted on forms included in GPs' prescription pads has fallen dramatically in the past 10 years (these "FP10" forms comprised 10% of all UK reports received in 1991, compared with 0.1% in 2001), suggesting a move from hand-written prescriptions to increasing use of computerised practice systems. Additional factors may include the increasing demands on doctors' time and concerns over confidentiality, as evidenced by surveys of factors affecting reporting as described above.

GP focus groups have been used by the MCA to examine understanding of, and attitudes to, ADRs and reporting via the Yellow Card Scheme. The key findings were broadly in line with published surveys of attitudes to adverse reaction reporting, namely that GPs were too busy to report, and that they were uncertain about how to distinguish adverse reactions from adverse events. Additionally, there was some concern about confidentiality issues associated with supplying patient details, and uncertainly about where ADR reports were sent and how the information would be used.

In 2000, there was a dramatic rise in the number of Yellow Cards received, with over 33 000 reports received during this 12-month period. This can largely be accounted for by the reporting of a large number of suspected adverse reactions to meningitis C vaccines, administered to children under the age

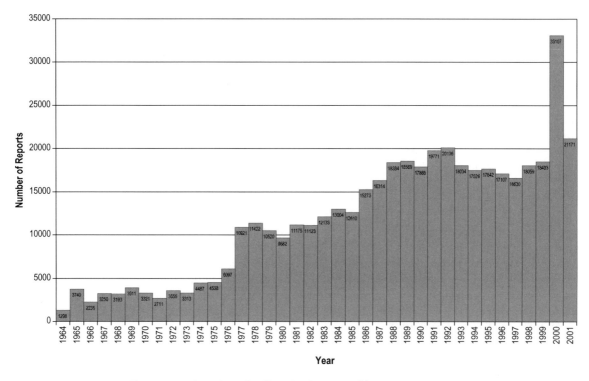

Figure 15.1. Number of Yellow Cards received by year since 1964.

RECENT INITIATIVES TO ENHANCE THE SCHEME

of 18 in a nation-wide immunisation campaign. An estimated 18.5 million doses of vaccine were distributed in just over a year. Even when reports for this vaccine are excluded, there was a 16% rise in the number of Yellow Cards received in 2000 compared with 1999.

In 2001, following completion of the meningitis C immunisation campaign, the number of Yellow Cards received returned to previous levels, with approximately 21 000 received during this 12-month period. Although this represents a small fall (1.3%) in the number of reports received when compared with reports received in 2000 excluding meningitis C vaccine reports, it is encouraging that reporting is still at higher levels compared with the late 1990s, when typically 17 000–18 000 reports were received each year. One possible explanation is that the high levels of reporting of suspected ADRs for meningitis C vaccines seen in 2000 may have led to an increased general awareness of ADRs and the need to report them via the Yellow Card Scheme. It remains to be seen if this upturn in reporting will be maintained in future years.

Although the importance of the Yellow Card Scheme in protecting public health, by monitoring the safety of medicines in routine practice, is not in dispute, there is a need to tackle continually the issue of under-reporting by addressing some of the factors highlighted in the section on weaknesses above. The environment in which the Scheme operates is very different now, compared with the 1960s. There is ever-increasing public and media interest in the availability of medicines and their safety, new medicines are delivered more rapidly to the market place than ever before, and more medicines are available without a doctor's prescription. Additionally, it is clear that the roles of pharmacists and nurses have evolved over recent years. For pharmacists, an increasing role in patient care is due at least in part to the increasing range of medicines being made available without prescription. Nurses are now able to prescribe some medicines, and have increasing involvement in the routine care of patients in the community, particularly in the management of chronic conditions. These changing roles now place pharmacists and nurses in a position in which they are increasingly likely to encounter suspected adverse reactions.

A number of initiatives have been undertaken recently in order to try to address a number of the issues raised in the section on weaknesses above. These initiatives fall into three main groups; initiatives aimed at increasing the general reporting base, those aimed at increasing reporting in particular areas where under-reporting is of particular concern, and those aimed at facilitation of reporting. Finally, recent developments in data protection legislation have resulted in the introduction of anonymised Yellow Card reporting. Initiatives in each of these areas are described below.

The potential impact of any change to the Scheme has been assessed in relation to its effectiveness in detecting previously unrecognised drug safety hazards. Simply increasing the number of reports is not alone of particular value; the objective is to receive Yellow Card information of suitable quality to enable detailed assessments of individual cases to be made as part of the investigation of potential safety hazards. Furthermore, although absolute numbers of reports are important for the identification of new hazards, it is paramount that reports of serious ADRs are collected, since these are more likely to impact on the balance of risks and benefits of the medicine than reports of more minor side effects. An increase in the number of reports received also has resource implications. Yellow Cards are processed rapidly, according to published targets, in order to ensure that data from the reports are available as quickly as possible for inclusion in the signal generation process. Any large increase in the volume of reports will slow down the time taken to process the reports and may increase the signal-to-noise ratio.

WIDENING THE YELLOW CARD REPORTING BASE

Pharmacist Reporting

For many years, pharmacists have been recognised as reporters to national spontaneous reporting schemes in a number of countries (Griffin, 1986), and there is published evidence suggesting a role for both hospital and community pharmacists in the monitoring and reporting of ADRs (e.g. Roberts et al., 1994; Smith et al., 1996).

The CSM's RMCs have played a key role in conducting pilot studies into the potential contribution of hospital and community pharmacists to the Yellow Card Scheme. A pilot scheme for hospital pharmacist reporting, conducted by the Northern RMC, showed that, in comparison with hospital doctors, hospital pharmacists submitted a higher proportion of reports of serious ADRs, and reports from the two groups of reporters were of similar quality. Additionally, a survey of consultants whose patients had been the subject of a pharmacist report during the pilot study showed a high level of support for the continuation of the scheme (Lee et al., 1997). This study led in April 1997 to the extension of the Yellow Card Scheme nation-wide to include reporting by hospital pharmacists (Anon, 1997a). A subsequent evaluation of hospital pharmacist reports made in the first year following this extension generally confirmed the findings of the pilot study, and indicated that reports received from hospital pharmacists were additional to those received from hospital doctors, rather than simply replacing them (Davis et al., 1999). Following the nation-wide extension, by the end of 2001, in excess of 4800 reports had been received directly from hospital pharmacists; in 2001, approximately 6.2% of Yellow Cards were submitted by this group.

A pilot study of community pharmacist reporting was conducted by all four RMCs; an evaluation of reports received during the first 12 months of the pilot showed that community pharmacists submitted reports which were comparable to those received from GPs, with regard to both the quality of the reports and the seriousness of reactions reported. Furthermore, community pharmacists submitted a higher proportion of reports for herbal products compared with GPs (Davis and Coulson, 1999). An attitudinal survey carried out in Wales, one of the areas in which the pilot study was conducted, demonstrated a high degree of support among both GPs and community pharmacists for a role of the latter group in reporting suspected ADRs to the Yellow Card Scheme

(Houghton *et al.*, 1999). In light of these findings, and the assumption that community pharmacists are well placed to inform patients about, and be made aware of, any ADRs experienced in association with "over the counter" products, nation-wide reporting by community pharmacists was introduced in November 1999 (Anon, 1999). Following this extension, by the end of 2001 the MCA had received almost 900 reports directly from community pharmacists; in 2001, around 2% of Yellow Cards were received from this group.

SPECIALIST THERAPEUTIC AREAS

As mentioned above, there is some evidence to suggest that hospital doctors report less frequently than GPs (Bateman *et al.*, 1992; Eland *et al.*, 1999). This may result in under-reporting being a particular problem for medicines where treatment is initiated and monitored by hospital specialists. In addition, in certain situations or patient groups, data to support the safe and effective use of medicines is particularly limited. For such areas of particular concern, an increase in the number of relevant reports may not be achieved simply by increasing the overall reporting base. Rather, in such areas, an approach has been taken to target existing reporting groups to improve the reporting of reactions relevant to these areas. Described here are recent initiatives aimed at improving reporting of ADRs in three areas of particular interest: drugs used in the treatment of HIV/AIDS, ADRs in children, and those associated with herbal products, including unlicensed remedies.

The HIV Reporting Scheme

Since the mid 1990s a number of important new drugs have become available for the treatment of individuals infected with HIV. Some of these drugs have been licensed on the basis of clinical trials that involved small numbers of patients and were designed to show changes in surrogate markers of HIV disease. This meant that at the time of licensing there was very limited safety data available for these drugs.

Following their introduction onto the UK market, it was noted that relatively few suspected ADRs were being reported in the United Kingdom for these anti-retroviral treatments, despite the fact that new safety issues were being identified from world-wide safety data.

In order to address this, the HIV reporting scheme, an extension of the Yellow Card Scheme, was launched in November 1997 by the MCA and CSM in collaboration with the Medical Research Council HIV Clinical Trials Centre (Anon, 1998a). The scheme targeted specialist health professionals (doctors, nurses and pharmacists) working with people infected with HIV; these health professionals were asked to report suspected ADRs on specific reporting forms which did not request the name of the patient, in order to allay concerns over patient confidentiality which might be a serious deterrent to reporting for this particular patient group.

The introduction of this scheme resulted in a significant increase in the number of UK reports of suspected ADRs associated with anti-retroviral drugs: for instance, during the seven months prior to the launch of the scheme, 112 reports were received, compared with 207 during the seven months following the launch (Anon, 1998b). Ongoing promotion of the scheme, including the production of a regular newsletter, is aimed at maintaining the effectiveness of this initiative.

Suspected ADRs in Children

There has been significant public interest expressed in the safety of medicines used in children; particular concern surrounds the safety of medicines which are not specifically licensed for use, or are used "off label" (i.e. for unlicensed indications) in this patient group (Wells, 1996). Despite the lack of firm evidence of safety and efficacy in children of medicines licensed for use in adults, such medicines may well be used when treating children, especially where no licensed alternatives exist. Safety and efficacy in children cannot be assumed simply based on data from studies in adults; for instance, children differ from adults in terms of their pharmacokinetics (Reed, 1996; Leeder, 1996). It is possible that the adverse reaction profile of a medicine in children may differ from that in adults, and it is therefore particularly important to collect suspected ADR reports in this area. However, it is notable that under-18-year-olds make up around 20% of the population, but that the proportion of Yellow Card reports received for this age group is somewhat lower (approximately 8% in 1997 and 1998).

To investigate whether unlicensed or "off label" use of medicines in children was leading to adverse reactions, and whether such reactions were being reported, a pilot scheme to stimulate reporting of suspected ADRs in children was set up in the Trent NHS region in September 1998; this scheme targeted paediatricians and hospital pharmacists.

An analysis by the MCA of this pilot scheme, two years following its introduction, showed that there was an increase in the absolute numbers of hospital reports of suspected ADRs in children received from the Trent region. Since the time covered by this analysis overlapped significantly with the nation-wide meningitis C vaccination campaign, it was perhaps not surprising that the majority of reports received were of suspected ADRs associated with this vaccine. However, when reports for meningitis C vaccine were excluded, it was notable that the underlying rate of paediatric reporting in the Trent region had remained relatively static between 1994 and 2000, and was comparable with national reporting rates for suspected ADRs in children; additionally a relatively low proportion (less than 30%) of reports related to serious reactions. Broader initiatives are being planned, building on the experience gained in the pilot scheme.

Unlicensed Herbal Remedies

A survey of the use of complementary and alternative medicine in the United Kingdom found that 20% of adults interviewed had used such treatments in the past year, and it was estimated that the annual expenditure on these treatments in the United Kingdom may exceed £1.5 billion (Ernst and White, 2000). Although some herbal products are licensed for use, there is a large variety of unlicensed herbal preparations, including traditional Chinese and Ayurvedic remedies, which are increasingly available. Herbal products may be perceived as "natural" and therefore safe

by the general public; many products are available on general sale in pharmacies and health food shops and are likely to be used by patients to self medicate without prior consultation with their health professional.

Until 1996, the Yellow Card Scheme collected reports of suspected ADRs to licensed herbal products only; in 1995, less than 0.2% of Yellow Cards received related to such products. In October 1996, the Yellow Card Scheme was extended to include reporting for unlicensed herbal remedies, following a report from Guy's Hospital Toxicology Unit on potentially serious adverse reactions associated with herbal remedies (Anon, 1996). Although levels of reporting remain low, there has been an almost two-fold increase in the reporting of suspected ADRs to herbal remedies (around 40 reports per year until 1998; more than 70 reports in 2001), with such reports accounting for 0.4% of reports received in 2001. This information is important in monitoring the safety of herbal products, many of which are unlicensed and therefore unregulated, and in evaluating how such products might interact with licensed medicinal products, e.g. the recently reported interactions between the herbal remedy St John's Wort and a number of medicines including the oral contraceptive pill (Anon, 2000d). It is important that efforts continue to be made to stimulate reporting in this area, in light of the large usage of unlicensed herbal remedies; it is likely that community pharmacists may play an important role in reporting in this area (Davis and Coulson, 1999).

FACILITATION OF REPORTING—NEW TECHNOLOGY AND MEDIA

It seems self-evident that making reporting easier may increase levels of reporting; this is demonstrated by the rise in reporting in the mid 1980s following the move to make Yellow Cards readily available by including them in the BNF and in GP's prescription pads. This is supported by the fact that lack of time has been found to be one of the main factors in deterring ADR reporting in various studies (Bateman et al., 1992; Belton et al., 1995; Sweis and Wong, 2000), including the MCA's work with GP focus groups.

In addition to increasing time pressures on health professionals, the recent expansion in the use of information technology means that the majority of GP practices, hospitals and pharmacies are now using computers as a routine tool in their daily work. In light of this, it is recognised that the paper Yellow Card may no longer be the most convenient method of reporting. Electronic reporting of suspected ADRs to the MCA is now routine for a small number of pharmaceutical companies who have been submitting reports via the MCA's ADROIT Electronically Generated Information Service (AEGIS) since 1995. Following on from this initiative, the MCA is currently piloting the use of electronic reporting for health professionals. Working with the GP practice software companies EMIS and Meditel, electronic reporting has now been made available to all users of these systems, either by the electronic submission of reports via a modem, or semi-automated completion of an electronic Yellow Card which is printed out and posted to the MCA. This pilot scheme was introduced in mid-1998 (Anon, 1997b); to date almost 1800 GP electronic reports have been received, and these reports comprised approximately 2.5% of UK reports received in 2001.

THE ANONYMISED YELLOW CARD

One of the key principles of the Yellow Card Scheme is that reports are submitted and handled in complete confidence. Concerns about confidentiality might deter both doctors (Bateman et al., 1992) and pharmacists (Sweis and Wong, 2000) from submitting Yellow Cards; this issue was also highlighted by the GP focus group work.

Until 2000, patient names/dates of birth, as requested on the Yellow Card and recorded on the ADROIT database, were used in correspondence only with the original reporter to enable them to identify the patient—for instance, letters acknowledging receipt of, or requesting additional information on a suspected ADR reported to the Yellow Card Scheme. Additionally, this information was also useful in the identification of duplicate reports. Names and dates of birth were not used for any other purposes.

An anonymised reporting form was first used in the HIV reporting initiative, as described above, because of particular concerns regarding confidentiality in this patient group. However, patients rights to privacy are now guarded by data protection legislation based in European legislation; this issue was recently highlighted by the General Medical Council's Guidelines on confidentiality (General Medical Council, 2000). This has led to the introduction of an "anonymised" Yellow Card in September 2000 (Anon, 2000b, 2000c), which asks for the initials and age (rather than name and date of birth) of the patient. In addition, the "anonymised" Card asks reporters to include an identification number or code for the patient; this should enable the reporter, but not the MCA to identify the patient, and is used in correspondence between the MCA and the reporter. The use of such an identifier was introduced in order to address concerns that "anonymised" reporting might lead to a reduction in our ability to detect duplicate reports and to obtain follow-up information from the original reporter. After six months, over 6000 suspected adverse reactions had been reported to the MCA on the "anonymised" reporting form; of these, around 77% of forms included an entry in the patient "identification number" field.

FUTURE DIRECTIONS FOR THE YELLOW CARD SCHEME

The Yellow Card Scheme is operating in a changing environment, particularly with regard to the roles of health professionals: this has led to the recent introduction of pharmacist reporting, as described above. The roles and responsibilities of nurses in relation to the provision of medicines to, and the care of, patients are also rapidly developing: this is illustrated by the introduction of nurse prescribing and the provision of medicines under Patient Group Directions.

If health professionals other than doctors and dentists are given the responsibility for providing medicines, it is arguable that they should be able to report any suspected ADRs experienced by patients in their care. There is some published evidence to suggest that nurses may have a role to play in the spontaneous reporting of suspected ADRs (Hall *et al.*, 1995; Smith *et al.*, 1996; Van den Bemt *et al.*, 1999), although a lack of knowledge about adverse effects of medicines was identified by nurses in one study as a major constraint to their participation (Hall *et al.*, 1995).

During the UK campaign to vaccinate against meningitis C, school nurses were the main body of health professionals administering the vaccine. When the campaign began, nurses began to submit spontaneously significant numbers of Yellow Card reports; the CSM subsequently recommended that nurses should be allowed to report suspected ADRs for meningitis C vaccine for the duration of this important public health campaign. Nurse reports received during the vaccination campaign have been used by the MCA to evaluate the potential contribution which this group might make to the Yellow Card Scheme. This evaluation also considered the findings of a pilot study of nurse reporting which has recently been conducted by the CSM's RMC in Merseyside (Morrison-Griffiths, 2000).

The evaluation of nurse reporting suggested that nurses report similar levels of serious reactions to other health professionals and that, with appropriate formal training, their reports are of similar quality to those received from doctors. Based on these findings, the MCA are currently in discussion with the Chief Nursing Officer and other relevant groups from the wider Department of Health in order to develop a strategy for the introduction of nurse reporting, focusing on the implementation of educational programmes which will help to ensure the success of any future nurse reporting initiatives. Any such initiatives will be publicised widely at an appropriate time.

In addition to generally extending the reporting base for the Yellow Card Scheme, it will be necessary to continue to target reporting in areas of special interest, such as those discussed in the section on initiatives above. Since they were set up, the CSM's RMCs have been important in conducting pilot studies of reporting, and have gained valuable experience in the implementation of local initiatives designed to stimulate awareness of, and reporting to, the Yellow Card Scheme (e.g.

Houghton *et al.*, 1996). These initiatives include the production of newsletters, training materials for use in presentations to health professionals on the Yellow Card Scheme, and, in Wales, the introduction of a distance learning pack on ADR reporting for pharmacists and doctors. It is likely therefore that the RMCs will continue to play a role in the development of the Yellow Card Scheme, including initiatives to target areas of special interest. In the future it may be beneficial to consider increasing the RMCs coverage of the United Kingdom, either by extending existing RMCs to cover a larger target area, or by the establishment of RMCs in new target areas.

It is worth mentioning two approaches which have been suggested as ways to enhance reporting, but which are not at present under consideration as future directions for the Yellow Card Scheme. The first of these is payment for the completion of Yellow Cards. This issue has been raised with the MCA by doctors, both directly and through the GP focus groups mentioned above; however, it is not known whether the introduction of remuneration for the completion of a Yellow Card would result in an increase in high quality reports of serious reactions. Above all, reporting of suspected ADRs may be considered to be part of the professional responsibilities of the health professionals involved and for this reason, payment for the completion of Yellow Cards would be inappropriate.

The second approach concerns the voluntary nature of the Yellow Card Scheme. France, Norway and Sweden have all introduced compulsory reporting of suspected serious ADRs to the regulatory authority (Moore *et al.*, 1985; Wilholm *et al.*, 1994) whereas in the majority of countries, including the United Kingdom, reports are submitted on a voluntary basis by health professionals. Although it would be expected that legislation to make reporting compulsory should increase the number of reports received, reporting rates are not clearly or consistently higher in countries where compulsory reporting has been introduced, compared with the United Kingdom (Griffin, 1986; Wilholm *et al.*, 1994). Furthermore, the introduction of statutory obligations for health professionals to report would be almost impossible to enforce: there is no easy and systematic mechanism for identifying the suspected ADRs that should have been reported, especially since the decision to report depends on the health professional's suspicion of causation. To date, the MCA has not identified a case for the introduction of compulsory reporting in the United Kingdom.

The long-term future will be based on developing electronic reporting and information exchange. Although the MCA has received electronic reports of suspected ADRs from a small group of pharmaceutical companies since 1995, this continues to be a focus for development. Within the European Union, there is a pilot plan for the implementation of electronic submission of individual case reports, following the standards set out in the International Conference of Harmonisation (ICH) E2B guideline "Data elements for the electronic transmission of individual case safety reports" (EMEA, 2000). Of equal importance will be the development of electronic communication between regulatory authorities and health professionals, which should include a mechanism for electronic reporting of suspected ADRs. With increasing use of computerised software systems by GP practices, hospitals and pharmacies, the inclusion of Yellow Cards on such systems might be one approach, as in the current pilots described above. There are a number of such GP systems; it may be more useful to provide a single method by which all health professionals involved with the Yellow Card Scheme can submit suspected ADR reports, potentially via internet-based reporting. It will be necessary to be able to ensure the secure transmission of reports, through a widely available system; it is possible that future development of the NHSnet may provide a suitable medium for electronic reporting of suspected ADR reports.

Finally, no attempt to improve the effectiveness of the Yellow Card Scheme can be effective unless it is communicated clearly to the health professionals involved with the Scheme. Ongoing communication with reporters will be critical to the success of any future developments of the Scheme. In particular, improved feedback—rapid, relevant and targeted to the reporter—will be essential.

CONCLUSIONS

The Yellow Card Scheme has been in existence for almost four decades. Despite its limitations, which are common to all spontaneous reporting schemes, it has a proven track record in the identification of previously unrecognised safety hazards. The Scheme has undergone continual evaluation and development over the years, and this will continue in the foreseeable future. This will ensure that the Scheme will continue to fulfil its central role in UK pharmacovigilance in the changing climate in which it operates, whilst continuing to adhere to the key principles defined by Sir Derrick Dunlop at the inception of the Scheme—spontaneity and speediness, confidentiality, and, above all, the commitment of health professionals to report their suspicions in the interest of protecting public health.

ACKNOWLEDGEMENTS

The authors would like to thank all the doctors, dentists, coroners and pharmacists who have supported the Yellow Card Scheme over the past 38 years.

REFERENCES

Alvarez-Requejo A, Carvajal A, Bégaud B, Moride Y, Vega T, Martin Arias LH (1998) Under-reporting of adverse drug reactions. Estimate based on a spontaneous reporting scheme and a sentinel system. *Eur J Clin Pharmacol* **54**: 483–8.

Amery WK (1999) Why there is a need for pharmacovigilance. *Pharmacoepidemiology and Drug Safety* **8**: 61–4.

Anon (1996) Extension of Yellow Card scheme to unlicensed herbal remedies. *Current Problems in Pharmacovigilance* **22**: 10.

Anon (1997a) Pharmacists' adverse drug reaction reporting to start on April 1. *Pharmacol J* **258**: 330–1.

Anon (1997b) Electronic yellow card in GP computer prescribing systems. *Current Problems in Pharmacovigilance* **23**: 10

Anon (1998a) HIV adverse drug reactions reporting scheme. *Current Problems in Pharmacovigilance* **24**: 3.

Anon (1998b) HIV ADR reporting scheme. The first seven months. *HIV ADR Reporting Scheme News* **August 1998**: 1.

Anon (1999) "Yellow card" reporting now allowed for all community pharmacists. *Pharmacol J* **263**: 776.

Anon (2000a) An updated Yellow Card for the new millennium. *Current Problems in Pharmacovigilance* **26**: 12.

Anon (2000b) Updated "yellow card" launched. *Pharmacol J* **265**: 387.

Anon (2000c) Yellow card updated to protect privacy. *Scrip* **2575**: 6.

Anon (2000d) Reminder: St John's wort (Hypericum perforatum) interactions. *Current Problems in Pharmacovigilance* **26**: 6–7.

Bateman DN, Sanders GLS, Rawlins MD (1992) Attitudes to adverse drug reaction reporting in the Northern Region. *Br J Clin Pharmac* **34**: 421–6.

Belton KJ, Lewis SC, Payne S, Rawlins MD, Wood SM (1995) Attitudinal survey of adverse drug reaction reporting by medical practitioners in the United Kingdom. *Br J Clin Pharmacol* **39**: 223–6.

Chan TYK, Critchley JAJH (1994) Reporting of adverse drug reactions in relation to general medical admissions to a teaching hospital in Hong Kong. *Pharmacoepidemiology and Drug Safety* **3**: 85–89.

Davis S, Coulson RA, Wood SM (1999) Adverse drug reaction reporting by hospital pharmacists: the first year. *Pharmacol J* **262**: 366–7.

Davis S, Coulson R (1999) Community pharmacist reporting of suspected ADRs: (1) The first year of the yellow card demonstration scheme. *Pharmacol J* **263**: 786–8.

Edwards IR (1997) Adverse drug reactions: finding the needle in the haystack. *Br Med J* **519**: 500.

Eland IA, Belton KJ, van Grootheest AC, Meiners AP, Rawlins MD, Stricker BHCh (1999) Attitudinal survey of voluntary reporting of adverse reactions. *Br J Clin Pharmacol* **48**: 623–7.

EMEA (2000) Joint pilot plan for the implementation of the electronic transmission of individual case safety reports between the EMEA, national competent authorities, and the pharmaceutical industry (Doc. Ref. EMEA/CPMP/PHVWP/2058/99). EMEA Joint pilot implementation plan. Document Reference: *EMEA/CPMP/PhPWP/1383/00 FINAL*.

Ernst E, White A (2000) The BBC survey of complementary medicine in the UK. *Complementary Therapies in Medicine* **8**: 32–6.

General Medical Council (2000) Confidentiality: protecting and providing information. www.gmc-uk.org/standards/standards-framework.htm

Griffin JP (1986) Survey of the spontaneous adverse drug reaction reporting schemes in fifteen countries. *Br J Clin Pharmacol* **22**: 83S–100S

Griffin JP (1992) Medicines control within the United Kingdom. In: Griffin JP, ed., *Medicines: Regulation, Research and Risk*, 2nd edn. Belfast: The Queen's University.

Griffin JP, Weber JCP (1992) Voluntary systems of adverse reaction reporting. In: Griffin JP, ed., *Medicines: Regulation, Research and Risk*, 2nd edn. Belfast: The Queen's University.

Hall M, McCormack P, Arthurs N, Feely J (1995) The spontaneous reporting of adverse drug reactions by nurses. *Br J Clin Pharmacol* **40**: 173–5.

Houghton JE, Pinto Pereira LM, Woods FJ, Richens A, Routledge PA (1996) The Welsh adverse drug reactions scheme: experience of a UK regional monitoring centre. *Adverse Drug React Toxicol Rev* **15**: 93–107.

Houghton J, Woods F, Davis S, Coulson R, Routledge PA (1999) Community pharmacist reporting of suspected ADRs: (2) Attitudes of community pharmacists and general practitioners in Wales. *Pharmacol J* **263**: 788–91.

Haramburu F, Bégaud B, Moride Y (1997) Temporal trends in spontaneous reporting of unlabelled adverse drug reactions. *Br J Clin Pharmacol* **44**: 299–301.

Lawson DH (1990) The yellow card: mark II. *Br Med J* **301**: 1234.

Lee A, Bateman DN, Edwards C, Smith JM, Rawlins MD (1997) Reporting of adverse drug reactions by hospital pharmacists: pilot scheme. *Br Med J* **315**: 519.

Leeder JS (1996) Developmental aspects of drug metabolism in children. *Drug Inf J* **30**: 1135–43.

Meyboom RHB, Egberts ACG, Edwards IR, Hekster YA, de Koning FHP, Gribnau FWJ (1997a). Principles of signal detection in pharmacovigilance. *Drug Safety* **16**: 355–65.

Meyboom RHB, Hekster YA, Egberts ACG, Gribnau FWJ, Edwards IR (1997b). Causal or casual? The role of causality assessment in pharmacovigilance. *Drug Safety* **17**: 374–89.

Moore N, Paux G, Bégaud B, Biour M, Loupi E, Boismare F, Royer RJ (1985) Adverse drug reaction monitoring: doing it the French way. *Lancet* **9** (November): 1056–58.

Moride Y, Haramburu F, Requejo AA, Bégaud B. (1997) Under-reporting of adverse drug reactions in general practice. *Br J Clin Pharmacol* **43**: 177–81.

Morrison-Griffiths S. (2000) Adverse drug reaction reporting by nurses. *M Phil Thesis*. University of Liverpool.

Rawlins MD (1988a) Spontaneous reporting of adverse drug reactions I: the data. *Br J Clin Pharmacol* **26**: 1–5.

Rawlins MD (1988b) Spontaneous reporting of adverse drug reactions II: uses. *Br J Clin Pharmacol* **26**: 7–11.

Rawlins MD, Fracchia GN, Rodriguez-Farré E. (1992) EURO-ADR: pharmacovigilance and research. A European perspective. *Pharmacoepidemiology and Drug Safety* **1**: 261–8.

Reed MD (1996) The ontogeny of drug disposition: focus on drug absorption, distribution and excretion. *Drug Information J* **30**: 1129–34.

Roberts PI, Wolfson DJ, Booth T.G (1994) The role of

pharmacists in adverse drug reaction reporting. *Drug Safety* **11**: 7–11.

Smith CC, Bennett PM, Pearce HM, Harrison PI, Reynolds DJM, Aronson JK, Grahame-Smith DG (1996) Adverse drug reactions in a hospital general medical unit meriting notification to the Committee on Safety of Medicines. *Br J Clin Pharmacol* **42**: 423–9

Speirs CJ, Griffin JP, Weber JCP, Glen-Bott M. (1984) Demography of the UK adverse reactions register of spontaneous reports. *Health Trends* **16**: 49–52.

Sweis D, Wong ICK (2000) A survey on factors that could affect adverse drug reaction reporting according to hospital pharmacists in Great Britain. *Drug Safety* **23**: 165–72.

Van den Bemt PML, Egberts ACG, Lenderink AW, Verzijl JM, Simons KA, van der Pol WSCJM, Leufkens HGM (1999) Adverse drug events in hospitalized patients. A comparison of doctors, nurses and patients as sources of reports. *Eur J Clin Pharmacol* **55**: 155–8.

Waller PC, Coulson RA, Wood SM (1996) Regulatory pharmacovigilance in the United Kingdom: current principles and practice. *Pharmacoepidemiology and Drug Safety* **5**: 363–75.

Wells TG (1996) Underserved therapeutic classes: examples which should not be ignored in infants and children. *Drug Information J* **30**: 1179–86.

Wiholm B-E, Olsson S, Moore N, Wood S. (1994) Spontaneous reporting systems outside the United States. In Strom BL, ed., *Pharmacoepidemiology,* 2nd edn. Chichester: Wiley.

16

Spontaneous Reporting—France

NICHOLAS MOORE

Department of Pharmacology, Université Victor Segalen, Bordeaux, France

CARMEN KREFT-JAIS AND ALBAN DAHNANI

Agence Française de Sécurité Sanitaire des Produits de Santé (AFSSAPS), St Denis, France

THE FRENCH PHARMACOVIGILANCE SYSTEM

The French Pharmacovigilance System has a number of features that make it stand out: it is based upon a network of 31 Regional Pharmacovigilance Centres, co-ordinated by the Pharmacovigilance Unit of the French Agency (AFSSAPS). Regional Pharmacovigilance Centres and AFSSAPS are connected via a national database, which contains adverse drug reactions (ADRs) reported by healthcare professionals. All reports are assessed before entry into the national database, with a common imputability method. The French organisation is based on a decentralised collection and validation of safety data through the Regional Pharmacovigilance Centres and a centralised evaluation and decision-making process at the AFSSAPS.

HISTORY

To understand the way it functions, and some of the differences with other countries' pharmacovigilance systems, a little history is necessary. After the problem with thalidomide, and the other early drug safety scandals or scares, a number of clinical toxicologists and pharmacologists, usually associated with Poison Control Centres (Paris, Lyon, Marseilles) decided to set up units to inform their physicians of the risks of drugs, and provide for a local place to report ADRs. In 1973, a national centre was set up by the national order of physicians in collaboration with the French pharmaceutical manufacturers association. The same year, six experimental pharmacovigilance centres were created in France. Over the years, more pharmacologists joined the first ones, and the network of centres appeared. The heads of these centres, at the time without any official remit, met regularly during meetings of the French Association of Pharmacologists. As this network evolved, they had to work out common methodologies. From the mid-1970s the centres were officially recognised, the regular meetings started taking place at the Ministry of Health, and a unit was set up there to co-ordinate activities. In 1979 a decentralised system was put in place with a network of 15 centres, which was thereafter extended to 29 in 1984 and 31 in 1994. Since

Pharmacovigilance. Edited by R.D. Mann and E.B. Andrews

1984 prescribers and marketing authorisation holders (MAHs) have been required to report ADRs. The national database was rejuvenated in 1985 so that online input became possible, and it could be accessed from all centres. In 1994 the Pharmacovigilance Unit was transferred to the French Medicines Agency (now Agence Française de Sécurité Sanitaire des Produits de Santé, AFSSAPS). Good Pharmacovigilance Practices were evolved and sent to every prescriber in the country. To implement the new European legislation, two decrees came into force which defined the general organisation of the French pharmacovigilance system: the decree of March 1995 on general principles and the decree of May 1995 that especially related to human blood products.

The important point in this short history is that the system actually grew from the ground up, rather from the top down as in most other countries. At the present time, the 31 Regional Centres have a duty to collect and record ADR reports, and input them into the common database, after rapid causality assessment. The Heads of the Regional Pharmacovigilance Centres meet monthly at the AFSSAPS in the Technical Committee, a working group set up to prepare the work of the National Pharmacovigilance Commission (Advisory Board). The Technical Committee is responsible for co-ordinating the collection and evaluation of information on ADRs, conducting surveys and providing recommendations that are forwarded to the National Pharmacovigilance Commission, which recommends action to the Director of the Agency, to prevent or eliminate drug-related accidents (Table 16.1). This structure is in fact pretty close to that of the European system.

The Pharmacovigilance Unit of AFSSAPS is in charge of the co-ordination of the Regional Centres' activities, the organisation of meetings held by the Technical Committee and the National Pharmacovigilance Commission, the receipt and the evaluation of pharmacovigilance data sent by MAH and the exchange of information with other competent authorities (the European Agency for the Evaluation of Medicinal Products (EMEA), other Member States, the World Health Organisation (WHO), the Food

Table 16.1. A comparison of French and European systems.

France	vs.	Europe
Prescribers, MAH		Prescribers, MAH
Signal		Rapid Alert System
31 Regional Centres		15 National Centres
Technical Committee		CPMP Pharmacovigilance Working Party
National Commission		CPMP
Head of Agency		European Commission

and Drug Administration (FDA), etc.). It also monitors the fulfilment of the legal obligations of each partner involved in this system, especially to ensure that the reporting requirements are fulfilled.

REGIONAL CENTRES

Regional Centres are located in departments of clinical pharmacology or clinical toxicology in the University Hospitals. They each have a defined geographical region of intervention which is included along with their address and phone numbers in the *Vidal Drug Dictionary*.

They have several missions (Moore *et al.*, 1985):

● Collecting and recording reports of ADRs
● Providing information on ADRs to healthcare professionals, but also to the local hospital director(s) (e.g. in formulary boards), and to the Agency, as required
● Conducting research on drug-related risks.

Regional Pharmacovigilance Centres are established through a convention between the Agency and the University Hospital. They are financed by the Agency on the basis of performance, which includes not only the number of reports received and questions answered, but also collective activities and scientific publications.

The University Hospitals also contribute to their financing by seconding personnel, and by providing material support, the latter varying according to the Hospital. Personnel in the Centres can be financed through the university and hospital (professors, practitioners, assistants, interns and medical or pharmacy students), and through the Agency grants.

Regional Centres have a scientific association, included within the French Pharmacological Society, which organises yearly scientific meetings within the yearly French Pharmacological Society Meeting in the spring, and other workshops or thematic meetings in the fall, and co-sponsors with the Agency and the French Pharmaceutical companies yearly methodology workshops.

SOURCE AND MANAGEMENT OF REPORTS

Reports to regional centres come from several sources:

- Spontaneous reports sent by healthcare professionals. There is no official form for reporting ADRs to Regional Centres. Centres usually have their own forms (commonly devised) on to which the information is transferred, and in which raw data (e.g. photocopies of lab tests or hospital discharge letters) can be stored.
- Reports gathered during clinical rounds: since the Regional Centres are in reference hospitals, the appropriate departments (internal medicine, haematology, dermatology, hepatology, for instance) can be regularly visited or contacted for hospitalised drug-related cases. These departments sometimes have "drug staffs" where drug-related problems can be discussed with the team from the Department of Pharmacology. In addition, pharmacy students in the clinical wards are often used as pharmacovigilance relays.
- A large number of reports come from the requests for information by health professionals, i.e. the drug information centre activity. Though a fair number of these questions concern pre-emptive information (what can I prescribe this pregnant women with this condition?), about half concern new medications and suspected drug reactions, usually under the form "has this ever been reported before?" These actually usually correspond to a specific patient, the prescriber asking the Centre for

help in solving a diagnostic problem, where a drug may possibly be involved. The dialogue that ensues between the pharmacologist and the clinician will usually help solve the problem. Since the interaction occurs early, the pharmacologist can suggest further action, such as diagnostic tests, or drug dechallenge, which will improve the case's information content. In this interaction, the clinician receives help for a specific problem, and the Regional Centre receives a case with better information (Moore, 2001).

This activity is viewed as a service rendered to local healthcare professionals, making them more willing to call and report. This will also have an influence on the type of reports retrieved, since physicians are more likely to call in for unusual, severe or unexpected events than for well-known ones, which after all is the main objective of spontaneous reporting systems.

After assessment for causality using the French imputation method (see below) (Bégaud et al., 1985), reports are input to the national pharmacovigilance database at the Regional Centre. Mean time from receiving the case to input is a few days, with priority given to serious reports, which are identified as such in the database. Centres are required to report all serious reactions to the Agency within 15 days. At any time, every Centre can access the complete database, which is located in the Pharmacovigilance Unit of the Agency.

Though there are no automated alerting processes functioning routinely on the database at this time, it is customary when a new report comes in, especially if it concerns a recently marketed drug, or if the event is serious and unexpected, to query the base for similar cases, possibly using the case–non-case approach (Montastruc et al., 2000; Moore et al., 1993, 1997), to generate some measure of reporting disproportionality that could be indicative of an impending problem. Serious reports are automatically retrieved from the database at the Agency on a daily basis and forwarded from the Agency to the relevant MAH, and in the case of centrally authorised products to the European Medicines Evaluation Agency (EMEA) as required by European regulations.

Pharmaceutical Companies

Pharmaceutical companies also have to comply with the European regulations, including 15-day transmission of serious ADRs occurring on French territory to the Agency, and the submission of Periodic Safety Update Reports (PSURs) according to defined periodicity. Reports from industry are received at the Agency, and input manually to a separate database, which can for the moment be accessed only at the Agency. The whole database system is presently being overhauled to provide electronic data transfer to and from industry, in order to avoid manually re-entering data or sending reports.

ALERT MANAGEMENT

Alerts can arise from individual case reports at the regional level, because of the number or nature of the reports or because of reporting disproportionality. Alerts may also originate from other competent European authorities through the Rapid Alert System or from FDA alerts, from literature data or any other source. Possible domestic alerts are reviewed within the Technical Committee for attribution.

The Technical Committee is presided over by the Chairman of the National Pharmacovigilance Commission, and includes a representative of each Regional Centre (usually its director). The Pharmacovigilance Unit of the Agency ensures the secretariat of both the National Commission and the Technical Committee. There is no industry representative on the Technical Committee.

During each committee meeting, current problems are reviewed, results of ongoing investigations are presented, methodological matters broached, and new investigations decided upon and attributed. Whenever it is decided that a problem should be investigated, a Centre is designated to take responsibility for the investigation (rapporteur). This can be an "unofficial investigation" or an "official investigation". In the former case, the Rapporteur Centre looks at all cases reported to the Centres, and at other sources of information, to recommend whether the alert is or is not worthy of official investigation. If not, it is usually shelved, or kept under distant surveillance in case it reactivates. The MAH is not formally involved in unofficial investigations.

An official investigation can be initiated because of an alert (at the national or European level), or can be systematic in the case of a new drug class, for instance, or if specific problems are anticipated when a drug is put on the market.

When an official investigation is decided upon, the marketing authorisation holders concerned are informed and instructed to make contact with the designated Rapporteur Centre. The rules for these official investigations are outlined in the Good Pharmacovigilance Practices (AFSSAPS, 1994). In brief, the cases reported to the Regional Centres and to the MAH are pooled. Duplicates are identified and resolved. All cases are reviewed together by the MAH and the Centre, with the help of external experts as necessary, and causality is reassessed, using more specific criteria, such as those devised in consensus conferences, national or Council for International Organizations of Medical Sciences (CIOMS)-supported. The population exposure to medication is estimated from sales data, or from more precise data if available, resulting in reporting rates, usually given in number of cases reported per treatment-months of product sold. This estimation is done for the various levels of causality and seriousness. Additionally, indications of risk factors such as age, concomitant diseases or medication are looked for.

The assessment report written by the Rapporteur Centre on the investigation is sent to the MAH for comments, and presented to the Technical Committee. The Technical Committee ensures that the investigation has been carried out properly, validates it or not and submits it for examination to the National Commission, usually after a consultation meeting with the MAH, where the MAH's proposals or comments are discussed.

The National Pharmacovigilance Commission is composed of representatives of health authorities and research bodies, clinicians, toxicologists, pharmacologists, pharmacists, a representative of the ministry for consumers and a representative of the pharmaceutical industry. It can be supplemented and guided as needed by invited experts. The

Rapporteur Centre presents the assessment report, in the presence of the MAH representatives, who are invited to comment and make their proposals. These are then discussed, first in the presence, then in the absence of the MAH. The final recommendation of the Commission is presented to the Director of the Agency. In the case of centrally authorised products, the Commission's recommendation is forwarded to the Committee for Proprietary Medicinal Products (CPMP) of the EMEA and other member states for possible further action.

The French pharmacovigilance system provides an active participation at the European level which relies on a close co-operation between Member States ensuring a common evaluation and management of safety concerns.

These processes are relatively similar to the European processes, except that there seems to be greater interaction and co-operation with the MAHs. This is built into the system, and may be related to the fact that many of the industry pharmacovigilance personnel have been trained in the Regional Centres. In addition there are many programs to enhance industry-centred communications, such as commonly organised training courses, and yearly workshops. In fact, the industry is a recognised part of the system, which has been officially designed as including the Agency, its Pharmacovigilance Unit and the Commissions it harbours, the Regional Centres, and the Industry Pharmacovigilance Departments.

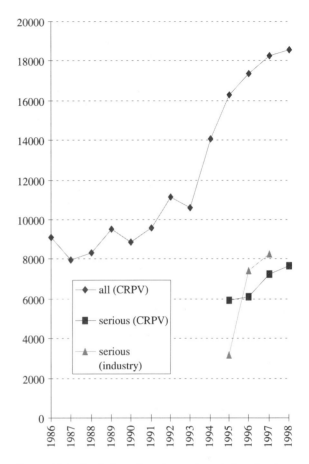

Figure 16.1. Evolution of yearly number of all and serious reports to Regional Centres for Pharmacovigilance (CRPV) and serious reports to industry.

RESULTS

In 1998 (Figure 16.1):

- The Regional Centres received 18 590 reports that were entered in the national database: 7635 (41%) were serious. Industry transmitted about the same number of serious reports to the Agency (8261 reports in 1997).
- There were 32 099 requests for information, 6552 of which became reports.
- 195 investigations were ongoing or initiated (systematic or alert-based), resulting in 84 reports to the Technical Committee, and 46 European Alerts. In addition, there were 78 investigations related to marketing authorisation re-evaluations for over-the-counter (OTC) switches or product information changes at the request of the MAH.
- Centre personnel taught 954 hours of initial training (medical, pharmacy or other), 957 hours of complementary training (e.g. in master-level courses), and 533 hours continuing medical education.
- There were 193 peer-reviewed publications, 193 didactic or review publications (such as this one), and 285 presentations in scientific meetings.

In 2000:

- 17 063 ADR reports (7853 serious) have been collected by the Regional Pharmacovigilance

Centres which also conducted 116 national pharmacovigilance investigations.

- 53 237 serious ADR reports have been sent by the pharmaceutical companies to the Pharmacovigilance Unit of the Agency, of which 13 845 came from France, including follow-up reports and duplicates. In addition, the Pharmacovigilance Unit received 2180 PSURs from the companies.

THE FRENCH IMPUTABILITY METHOD

This method was first devised in 1978 (Dangoumau *et al.*, 1978), revised in 1985 (when it was published simultaneously in French and in English) (Bégaud *et al.*, 1985). It is the only imputability (causality assessment) method to have legal status. It is probably one of the most widely used, if not *the* most widely used, imputability method, having been applied to more than 100 000 reports, and yet it remains widely misunderstood.

The method was derived when the regional network was developing, to ensure that all the Centres worked and assessed reports in reasonably the same way. It has a few basic principles, designed to ensure the highest possible sensitivity when used routinely on incoming reports. It is because of this that the term "causality assessment" may not really be applicable in that it is not causation *per se* that is assessed, but the possibility of involvement, a subtle distinction.

BASIC PRINCIPLES

The basic principles are

- That the causality be judged only on the data present in the case, in abstraction of all published data concerning the drug–reaction association. Each case is judged on its own merits (intrinsic imputability) to ensure maximal identification of possible new reactions. This also ensures time-independent classification. Previous publications and labelling, which vary over time, are only indicated, and are not an integral part of the imputability.

- That the causality be assessed on each drug–reaction pair presented by the patient at the time of the event, or that could be involved (such as previously stopped medication that could result in unidentified withdrawal symptoms).

This method is thus very dependent on the Regional Centre/drug information centre system, where there is early interaction with the reporter, so that information can be accrued in real-time, rather than having to judge a case *a posteriori* on incomplete information as is usually the case in most paper-based spontaneous reporting systems where the reporter has already made up his mind on causality when reporting, and information is only present on the drug suspected by the reporter who often has no formal pharmacological or ADR-assessment training.

The method relies on a set of criteria that are, in fact, common to all causality assessment methods, so that it is easy to reapply other causality methods if the proper information has been obtained. It is perforce very general in its definition of criteria, and much attention has been devoted to refining definitions of these criteria for specific reactions, and even for specific drug–reaction associations (Habibi *et al.*, 1988; Fournier *et al.*, 1989; Roujeau *et al.*, 1989; Vigeral *et al.*, 1989; Benichou, 1990; Benichou and Solal Celigny, 1991).

There are six main criteria, three for chronology (time sequence), and three for semiology (signs and symptoms). These are:

TIME SEQUENCE ANALYSIS

The criteria include challenge, dechallenge and rechallenge.

- *Challenge* can be classified into "very suggestive" (when there is an obvious temporal association between drug administration and the onset of the reaction, such as anaphylaxis during intravenous drug injection), impossible (when the drug is given after event onset), and compatible (other cases). The "impossible" category is especially pertinent, since it justifies knowing the reason for which the drug was given to eliminate protopathic bias, the pre-scribing of a drug for early symptoms of the event later reported as a reaction (e.g. agranu-locytosis attributed to an antibiotic that was prescribed for the sore throat and fever that are the first signs of agranulocytosis, or stomach cancer and H2 antagonists prescribed for undiagnosed dyspepsia).

- *Dechallenge* can be suggestive when the reaction abates when the drug is stopped. It can be non-conclusive when there is no assessable dechal-lenge (e.g. drug not stopped, or patient dies), or there is no information on dechallenge, or the reaction is irreversible (renal failure, death), or specific treatment was applied to the reac-tion, etc. It is against the role of the drug if the reaction persists (if reversible) when the drug is stopped, within pharmacokinetic constraints.
- *Rechallenge* is positive when the reaction recurs when the patient takes the drug again (for whatever reason, bearing in mind recur-rent protopathic bias), negative when the reaction does not recur when the drug is taken again at the same dose, for the same duration, with the same concomitant diseases and medication (a rare event), and not assessable in all other cases.

Information on challenge, dechallenge and rechal-lenge is input into the appropriate three-way table, which results in a grade from C0 (drug excluded) to C3 (very suggestive time association or positive rechallenge) (Table 16.2).

SIGNS AND SYMPTOMS

Signs and symptoms are graded in much the same way. Three criteria are assessed;

- Pharmacological plausibility: are the signs and symptoms suggestive of a pharmacological effect of the drug (i.e. a type A reaction), that could be reproduced experimentally?
- Other causes: have other reasonable causes for the event been looked for and eliminated? By reasonable, one means most (90%?) of the usual causes for the disease. There has been much discussion on what reasonable means, and this is probably where the consensus conference criteria are most useful.
- Is there a laboratory test that is specific to the drug–reaction pair, and is it positive or negative? The criteria for specificity may vary. For example, if there were signs of toxicity, elevated or null plasma concentrations of a drug would qualify (within pharmacokinetic timeframes, of course). This would not apply for an allergic reaction, though null plasma concentration with sufficient sensitivity could perhaps qualify as a negative laboratory test if it effectively eliminates drug exposure within the appropriate timeframe.

Again, the results are fed into a three-way table (Table 16.3), resulting in a semiology grading from S1 (doubtful) to S3 (very suggestive). Most cases are S2 (non-specific reaction, no other reasonable cause, no specific laboratory test), or S1 (same but

Table 16.2. Chronological imputability.

	Challenge						
	Very suggestive			Compatible			Impossible
Rechallenge	R+	R0	R−	R+	R0	R−	
Dechallenge:							
• Suggestive	C3	C3	C1	C3	C2	C1	C0
• Inconclusive	C3	C2	C1	C3	C1	C1	C0
• Unsuggestive	C3	C1	C1	C1	C1	C1	C0

Table 16.3. Semiological imputability.

	Signs and symptoms					
	Very suggestive of drug involvement or interaction			Compatible		
Lab test	L+	L0	L−	L+	L0	L−
Alternate non-drug explanation:						
• Absent	S3	S3	S1	S3	S2	S1
• Possible or present	S3	S2	S1	S3	S1	S1

other causes not looked for usually because reaction to the drug is known, and all signs abated when the drug was stopped, before further investigations were made).

This method is not very precise, and is probably much less specific than other methods, and especially the Bayesian approaches. It has a number of merits, however:

- It is more of a triage method, and can be applied extremely rapidly in the vast majority of cases if there is the appropriate information.
- It is, in fact, extremely useful to ensure that the proper information on a case report is retrieved on an ongoing basis. Using the causality method on a routine basis helps tremendously in making sure all relevant information is retrieved when discussing a case with a reporter. In this it improves the quality of the data, and the later application of any causality method, be it the same with refined criteria, as would be used in an official investigation, or any other, since all methods rely on mostly the same information.
- Its use by all persons involved in the system facilitates communication, by the use of a common language. This was and remains indispensable in a network-based system, where harmonisation of practice is essential.

In conclusion, the French System is based on a number of specific items, which made its success, and should be included or at least understood in other systems that want to use a Regional Centre approach:

- The existence of a real network, where alert investigation is done in the Regional Centres, which are not only a glorified mailbox sending data into a distant administrative black box, never to see them again.
- The use of common procedures, to ensure quality of data, including the use of the causality method.
- The integration of the Centres in clinical pharmacology and in the local life of the regional hospitals, with emphasis on the information centre function, as a continuing

resource for healthcare professionals: retrieving good cases is just a by-product of good information.

REFERENCES

Agence Française de Sécurité Sanitaire des Produits de Santé (AFSSAPS) (1994) Bonnes pratiques de Pharmacovigilance. In: http://agmed.sante.gouv.fr/htm/5/5000.htm; Accessed 4 May 2001.

Bégaud B, Evreux JC, Jouglard J, Lagier G (1985) Imputation of the unexpected or toxic effects of drugs. Actualization of the method used in France. *Therapie* **40**(2): 111–18.

Benichou C (1990) Criteria of drug-induced liver disorders. Report of an international consensus meeting. *J Hepatol* **11**(2): 272–6.

Benichou C, Solal Celigny P (1991) Standardization of definitions and criteria for causality assessment of adverse drug reactions. Drug-induced blood cytopenias: report of an international consensus meeting. *Nouv Rev Fr Hematol* **33**(3): 257–62.

Dangoumau J, Evreux JC, Jouglard J (1978) Method for determination of undesirable effects of drugs. *Therapie* **33**(3): 373–81.

Fournier M, Camus P, Benichou C, Danan G, Bégaud B, Castot A, *et al.* (1989) Interstitial pneumopathies: criteria of drug side-effects. Results of consensus meetings. *Presse Med* **18**(27): 1333–6.

Habibi B, Solal-Celigny P, Benichou C, Castot A, Danan G, Lagier G, *et al.* (1988) Drug-induced hemolytic anemia. Results of consensus conferences. *Therapie* **43**(2): 117–20.

Montastruc JL, Chaumerliac C, Desboeuf K, Manika M, Bagheri H, Rascol O, *et al.* (2000) Adverse drug reactions to selegiline: a review of the French pharmacovigilance database. *Clin Neuropharmacol* **23**(5): 271–5.

Moore N (2001) The role of the clinical pharmacologist in the management of adverse drug reactions. *Drug Safety* **24**(1): 1–7.

Moore N, Biour M, Paux G, Loupi E, Bégaud B, Boismare F, *et al.* (1985) Adverse drug reaction monitoring: doing it the French way. *Lancet* **2**(8463): 1056–8.

Moore N, Kreft-Jais C, Haramburu F, Noblet C, Andrejak M, Ollagnier M, *et al.* (1997) Reports of hypoglycaemia associated with the use of ACE inhibitors and other drugs: a case/non-case study in the French pharmacovigilance system database. *Br J Clin Pharmacol* **44**(5): 513–8.

Moore N, Noblet C, Joannides R, Ollagnier M, Imbs JL, Lagier G (1993) Cough and ACE inhibitors. *Lancet* **341**(8836): 61.

Roujeau JC, Beani JC, Dubertret L, Guillaume JC, Jeanmougin M, Danan G, et al. (1989) Drug-induced cutaneous photosensitivity. Results of a consensus meeting. *Therapie* **44**(3): 223–7.

Vigeral P, Baumelou A, Benichou C, Castot A, Danan G, Kreft-Jais C, et al. (1989) Drug-induced renal insufficiency. Results of consensus meetings. *Nephrologie* **10**(3): 157–61.

17

Spontaneous Reporting—USA

DAVID J. GRAHAM, SYED R. AHMAD AND TONI PIAZZA-HEPP
Office of Drug Safety, Center for Drug Evaluation and Research, US Food and Drug Administration, Rockville, USA

INTRODUCTION

The US Food and Drug Administration (FDA) is responsible not only for approving drugs for marketing, but also for monitoring their safety after marketing (Kennedy *et al.*, 2001). Drug approvals are based on data obtained from clinical trials that are oftentimes limited in size and duration, and that have excluded patients with other therapies or comorbidities from study (Rogers, 1987). After marketing, new information relating to drug safety usually becomes available as product use becomes more widespread, and on occasion this may alter the benefit–risk profile of a drug (Friedman *et al.*, 1999).

In the United States, pharmacovigilance is regarded as those aspects of drug safety monitoring and assessment that are related to or dependent upon voluntarily reported cases of adverse drug reactions (ADRs), or that relate to other activities, the primary purpose of which is the generation of a signal or hypothesis of a potential drug–adverse effect association. This perspective considers pharmacoepidemiology as being more closely related to population-based, systematic investigations that may range in complexity from purely descriptive to rigorous hypothesis-testing studies. There is admittedly a gray zone whereby the two approaches blend together.

There are many ways by which drug safety signals arise. The most common is through voluntary or spontaneous case reporting to regional or national pharmacovigilance centers, such as the FDA. Case reports and small case series from the medical literature also contribute. Other potential sources of safety concerns include pre-clinical animal testing, pre-marketing clinical trials, experience with other drugs in the same class and experience from other national centers around the world. The clinical pharmacology of the drug itself, its pharmacokinetics (absorption, distribution, metabolism and excretion) and pharmacodynamics, may raise other concerns related to organ-specific toxicity or drug–drug interactions.

ADR REPORTING IN THE UNITED STATES

The FDA continues to assess the benefit–risk profile of approved drugs throughout the life of the drug, primarily on the basis of ADR case reports (GAO/HEHS, 2001). In the United States,

---

Pharmacovigilance. Edited by R.D. Mann and E.B. Andrews

ADR case reports are voluntarily sent to the FDA or the drug's manufacturer by healthcare professionals and consumers (Johnson and Barash, 1991). Drug manufacturers are legally required to submit all ADR reports they receive to the FDA. Under current US regulations (21 CFR 314.80), reports of "serious" ADRs not presently listed in the drug product's labeling must be submitted to the FDA within 15 calendar days of the company's receipt of them. For regulatory purposes, a "serious" report is defined as one describing an ADR that is life-threatening or that leads to death, hospitalization, disability, congenital anomaly, or is an "important medical event". Reports meeting the regulatory definition of "serious" but describing events already listed in product labeling, as well as all reports with non-serious outcomes are submitted to the FDA on a periodic basis that varies depending on the market age of the product.

The FDA has maintained a computerized repository of these voluntarily reported ADRs since 1969 (Kennedy et al., 2000). This repository and the system to manage it have grown and changed since then. In recent years, the FDA has received over 250 000 reports annually and the total number in the database exceeds 2.5 million, covering all marketed prescription drug products in the United States. For most over-the-counter (non-prescription) products, manufacturers are not required to submit ADR case reports to the FDA.

The ADR database has evolved over the years as computer and information technologies have improved. The most recent modification occurred in 1997 when the FDA redesigned the database, now referred to as the Adverse Event Reporting System (AERS) and shifted from using Coding Symbols for Thesaurus of Adverse Reaction Terms (COST-ART) to Medical Dictionary for Regulatory Activities (MedDRA) coding terminology (Brown et al., 1999). These changes were implemented for several reasons. Agreements reached through the International Conference on Harmonization (ICH) necessitated a restructuring of the database in order to meet international standards for electronic submission of ADR reports. This "ICH compatibility" should facilitate information exchange with industry and with other national pharmacovigilance centers (Green, 1998). Furthermore, electronic submission of ADR reports will greatly enhance the efficiency and accuracy of the data entry process. From a pharmacovigilance perspective, the AERS should result in higher quality data and greater immediate access to this data by those who review or work with the case reports.

ADR REPORTS REVIEW PRACTICES AT THE FDA

Each serious unlabeled ADR report, every serious ADR report (labeled or unlabeled) submitted directly to the FDA by health professionals or consumers, and reports describing specific pre-determined "important" medical events are electronically transferred to the computer "in-box" of one of approximately 20 safety evaluators, who review them on a daily basis. The safety evaluators are primarily trained clinical pharmacists who are assigned to cover specific groups or classes of drugs. Over time, they acquire in-depth familiarity with the products they monitor.

In reviewing these case reports the primary focus is placed on identifying previously unrecognized serious ADRs. When such a report is identified, a computer search is made of the entire AERS database for reports of similar cases with the drug in question. These cases are reviewed for clinical content and completeness. If important information is missing or supporting medical records are needed for some cases, the safety evaluator contacts the reporter, usually a health professional, to obtain the needed data. This is a time-consuming but essential process, especially when faced with a serious ADR associated with a widely used medicine. In parallel with these activities, a literature review is performed, national drug usage data is obtained and, frequently, an epidemiologist within the office conducts an investigation of background incidence rates and risk factors for the clinical event of interest. For example, a case series of pancreatitis in association with use of a particular drug product might be supplemented by incidence data from a population-based, randomized survey conducted by the US National Center for Health Statistics.

After a case series is assembled and follow-up completed, it is analyzed for drug-relatedness. Several factors are important to this assessment. Temporal association describes the relationship between drug exposure and event. If the adverse effect preceded the drug exposure, the drug cannot have caused the effect. If the reaction resolves with the withdrawal of the drug, the "dechallenge" is positive; if the reaction reoccurs with the re-initiation of the drug, the "rechallenge" is positive. Dechallenge is often cited as evidence of drug-relatedness. However, the lack of resolution (negative dechallenge) should not be viewed as evidence against an association. Many adverse effects, once initiated, follow a course of their own. This is especially apparent with certain blood dyscrasias, serious skin reactions and acute liver failure. Positive rechallenge has traditionally been cited as strong evidence of drug association. Our experience suggests that the absence of reoccurrence should not be taken as evidence against the association. For most recognized and serious ADRs, rechallenge is not intentionally performed.

The timing of onset of the ADR after the beginning of drug use may provide clues as to possible mechanisms (short latency: anaphylaxis; long latency: cirrhosis). It is also important to note if other explanations for the adverse effect are present such as underlying disease states or other medications. A profound hypotensive episode shortly prior to development of acute liver failure may be the causative factor rather than the drug the patient was taking. Alternatively, the natural course of the patient's medical condition(s) may be associated with the event of interest. Additionally, other medications taken by the patient may be linked to the ADR. Disease states and/or other drugs may therefore cloud or confound the relationship between a particular drug and event, complicating the assessment of case reports. Finally, clinical and laboratory features of the ADR and its progressive unfolding may also provide information that distinguishes it from underlying or other disease processes (Meyboom et al., 1997). For example, myopathy is a recognized consequence of HIV infection, but can also result from zidovudine, used in the treatment of HIV/AIDS. Zidovudine-induced myopathy was found to be due to damaged muscle mitochondria, distinguishable from HIV myopathy based on the presence of "ragged-red" fibers in biopsy specimens from affected patients (Dalakas et al., 1990).

The safety evaluator usually stratifies the cases into those with more complete information in which other potential explanations are absent or extremely remote, cases with incomplete information, and cases with other risk factors or potential explanations for the adverse event. The case material is evaluated in combination with drug usage data, epidemiologic information and the published literature. In general, a signal results if there are higher-quality, unconfounded cases plus supporting cases with less complete information or confounding factors present. There is no "threshold" number of cases required to indicate the significance of a potential signal; medical judgement is used in each situation. An analysis of the safety issue is presented to the medical reviewing division responsible for ongoing regulation of the drug. A decision is then made about whether the signal is strong enough to warrant a regulatory action such as changes in product labeling, further study, issuance of a public health advisory, restriction of use or market withdrawal.

METHODS OF SIGNAL DETECTION AND REFINEMENT

CASE SERIES

The most common approach to signal development is based on the evaluation of a series of case reports. Although several criteria (described above) are used in this review, no formal causality assessment algorithm is followed. A number of such algorithms have been reported in the literature, but these suffer from important liabilities including inflexibility, lack of sensitivity and lack of validation (Pere et al., 1986; Frick et al., 1997). They are also oftentimes difficult and time consuming to use, may tend to discount even remotely confounded cases and may place excess weight on the presence of positive rechallenge.

Because the AERS database draws on the cumulative experience of over 270 million people, it is a rich source of clinical material. A physician in practice may see one case of a rare or unusual drug reaction, and may perhaps even publish the case. The advantage of a centralized ADR repository is that it offers the potential of much greater case numbers, and with that comes the capacity to describe the spectrum and natural history of the reaction and to identify risk factors for its occurrence.

Several examples help to illustrate this. Based on a review of 121 cases of seizure reported with alprazolam, the importance of the duration of drug use and the sudden cessation of therapy were identified as risk factors for seizure occurrence (Graham, 1989). The "epidemic curve" derived from these case reports strongly suggested benzodiazepine withdrawal as the underlying mechanism (Figure 17.1). Evaluation of 95 reported cases of hemolysis with use of the antibiotic temafloxacin resulted in the discovery of hemolytic-uremic syndrome with this drug and identified prior fluoroquinolone use as a strong risk factor for development of this life-threatening complication (Blum et al., 1994). More recently, a review of 43 cases of acute liver failure reported with the use of troglitazone described the clinical spectrum and natural history of this disorder (Graham and Green, 1999). Of note, this analysis provided evidence of the inability to predict who was at risk or how to prevent this often fatal reaction. In another instance, a review of 58 case reports

suggested a possible association between use of the antifungal, itraconazole, and the development of congestive heart failure (Ahmad et al., 2001). No evidence of a similar signal was observed with the other azole fungicides.

PROPORTIONAL DISTRIBUTIONS

This approach to signal identification and refinement is similar in concept to proportional morbidity ratios (Rothman and Greenland, 1998). Basically, the number of reports of a given ADR or of a group of ADR terms is viewed as a proportion of all ADRs reported for that drug. The resulting measure can serve to highlight specific drug reactions or show a clustering of different reactions, all of which affect a particular organ or body system. Of perhaps greater utility, a drug's proportional distribution can be compared with that of other drugs in the same pharmacologic class or with drugs from other classes used to treat the same indication. From this type of analysis, one might observe that a particular antibiotic has a relatively high proportion of skin-related ADRs compared with other class members. As with proportional morbidity ratios, proportional distributions are useful in a qualitative sense, revealing potential "problem areas" for a drug. However, they do not contribute to our understanding of ADR incidence.

REPORTING RATES

In its simplest form, a reporting rate is the number of reported cases of a particular ADR divided by some measure of the suspect drug's utilization, usually the number of dispensed prescriptions. As such, they are not true rates but convention refers to them thus. An epidemiologic modification of the reporting rate "denominator" employs an estimate of the total person-time of exposure to the drug in the general population, rather than the total number of dispensed prescriptions.

The reporting rate of an ADR can be compared between different drugs. A review of case reports identified a signal of pulmonary fibrosis with the anti-androgen, nilutamide, used in the treatment

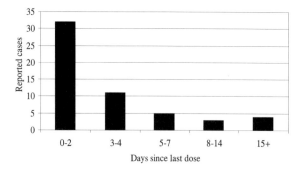

Figure 17.1 Reported cases of seizure by time since stopping alprazolam use.

of prostate cancer. Reporting rates, adjusted for market age and calendar time, were calculated for this drug and two other anti-androgens marketed in the United States for the same indication (Ahmad *et al.*, 2000). This analysis found a much higher reporting rate with nilutamide and led to changes in product labeling.

Reporting rates must be interpreted carefully because they are not incidence rates. True rates incorporate the element of time and depend upon the complete ascertainment of the event being measured within a defined population (Clayton and Hills, 1993). These requirements do not hold for reporting rates. Using person-time rather than prescription number as the denominator of the reporting rate still does not give rise to an incidence rate because most ADRs are not reported, and hence the reporting rate will seriously underestimate the true incidence. The failure of most ADRs to be reported to the FDA or other pharmacovigilance centers is referred to as underreporting. This is the single greatest limitation of using spontaneous case reports to monitor drug safety. After an ADR occurs, a series of barriers must be overcome if this event is to reach the "in-box" of a safety evaluator. These are (a) recognition and correct diagnosis of the clinical event; (b) attribution of that event to a drug exposure; and (c) registration of the event (filing a report) with the drug company or the FDA (Graham *et al.*, 2000). These barriers generally reduce the level of reporting of serious ADRs to the range of 1%–10% (Inman and Adelstein, 1969; Inman and Weber, 1986; Scott *et al.*, 1987; Rogers *et al.*, 1988; Belton *et al.*, 1995; Eland *et al.*, 1999).

OBSERVED-TO-EXPECTED ANALYSIS

A natural extension of the concept of reporting rates is the technique of observed-to-expected analysis. This approach to signal refinement is more epidemiologic in nature than the above described methods. To employ this approach, it is necessary to have an estimate of the background rate for the clinical event of interest in the general population. Such rate information may be found in published literature or possibly through other

sources such as the US National Center for Health Statistics (La Grenade *et al.*, 2000).

The other piece of information that must be obtained is an estimate of the total exposure-time to the drug of interest within the population. This estimate is usually derived from data estimating the total number of prescriptions dispensed for a specific drug, along with an estimate of the average prescription length in days. At the FDA, such data are usually available through a contract with a commercial drug-utilization data vendor. This information is sometimes supplemented by drug-utilization data obtained through the FDA's Cooperative Agreement Program. This program provides access to large, automated claims data from population-based healthcare plans (Graham *et al.*, 2000).

Two examples illustrate this method. Returning to nilutamide and pulmonary fibrosis, the person-time of drug exposure in the US population was estimated using commercially available data (Ahmad *et al.*, 2000). The background rate for "idiopathic" pulmonary fibrosis was obtained from a population-based epidemiologic study (Coultas *et al.*, 1994), and was applied to the accumulated person-time of exposure to nilutamide. This analysis found that the number of spontaneous case reports of pulmonary fibrosis with this drug was 15-fold greater than expected.

An evaluation of ADR reports for clozapine found 47 reports of myocarditis and cardiomyopathy, with a sizable proportion occurring within the first few months of starting therapy. A literature review produced a population-based estimate for fatal myocarditis of 4 per million person-years (Murray and Lopez, 1992). To determine the total US exposure-time to clozapine, FDA epidemiologists turned to the US National Clozaril Registry and obtained the number of patients ever treated with the drug (Honigfeld *et al.*, 1998). The cumulative patient-time for the first month of drug use was calculated and an estimate of the expected number of fatal cases of myocarditis derived. This analysis showed a 321-fold excess in fatal reports of myocarditis in the first month of clozaril use (La Grenade *et al.*, 2001).

This method works best when the background rate for the clinical event of interest is very low. In the above examples, the background rates were in the range of a few per 100 000 to a few per million per year. With more common events, such as myocardial infarction or asthma, the expected number of cases becomes large, thereby greatly reducing the signal-to-noise ratio. Because of the presence of large-scale underreporting of ADR cases, the lack of an excess number of reports over the number expected cannot be interpreted by itself as invalidating the signal. However, the strength of the method is demonstrated in those situations where the reported number ("observed") is close to or exceeds the expected number. Because of underreporting, the actual level of risk is much greater than that obtained. In such instances, one has moved beyond signal towards establishing an association.

"CASE–CONTROL" ANALYSES

Another approach for signal development borrows heavily from the case–control method of standard clinical epidemiology (Breslow and Day, 1980; Kahn and Sempos, 1989). The simplest variant of this approach identifies all ADR cases describing a particular event of interest within a national center's pharmacovigilance database. These will serve as "cases" in the analysis. All other reports in the database serve as non-cases or "controls". Reports listing the drug under investigation are classified as "exposed", regardless of their status as a case or non-case. Similarly, reports not listing the drug of interest are "unexposed". A two-by-two table is created and an odds ratio is calculated as the cross-products ratio $((a*d)/(b*c))$ (Table 17.1). Moore et al. (1997) used this approach to chart the emergence of a signal and its progression over a period of months.

A modified version of this approach has been developed at the Medicines Control Agency in the United Kingdom (Wilholm et al., 2000). The proportional reporting ratio is calculated from the same two-by-two table as with the case–non-case method above. However, instead of deriving a cross-product ratio, a ratio of proportions among

Table 17.1

	Case (ADR of interest)	Non-case (all other ADR reports)	
Exposed	a	b	$a+b$
Unexposed	c	d	$c+d$

the exposed and unexposed is computed, analogous to the epidemiologic concept of relative risk $((a/(a+b))/(c/(c+d)))$.

The above two approaches rely solely upon data contained within the national pharmacovigilance database. A third variant supplements case reports data with population-based data obtained from large automated healthcare databases (Graham et al., 2000). This method was helpful in assessing the effect of daily dose and cumulative duration of use on the risk of experiencing withdrawal seizures following abrupt cessation of the benzodiazepine, alprazolam (Graham, 1989). A nested case–control design was used for this study, with all cases and non-cases exposed to alprazolam. From the AERS database, all cases of seizure reported with alprazolam were reviewed and data on daily dose and duration of use abstracted. Reports were coded into binary categories for each of these two potential risk factors (dose: >4 mg/d vs. ⩽4 mg/d; duration: >4 months vs. ⩽4 months), and the proportion of cases in each category was calculated. From a population-based healthcare database, the proportional distribution of alprazolam users in each of the dose and duration categories was obtained. A two-by-two table was created in which each of the four cells contained the relevant proportion from the 121 AERS seizure reports ("cases") and from the general population of alprazolam users ("controls"). The resulting cross-products ratio yielded an odds ratio of 39 for seizure risk with higher dose alprazolam use (Table 17.2).

An advantage of this approach is that an unbiased measure of exposure is obtained from a general population of drug users that can usually be assumed to be representative of all users nationally. It thereby serves as an unbiased

Table 17.2.

	Seizure reports "cases"	General population "controls"
>4 mg/d	0.67	0.012
≤4 mg/d	0.33	0.988

Table 17.3. Life-table estimation of reporting rates of acute liver failure with trovafloxacin.

Interval (days)	No. cases	Days of follow-up	Interval hazard rate (per 10^6 person-years)
1–60	14	60	45
9–60	11	52	73
11–60	7	50	168
15–60	5	46	326
31–60	2	30	1912

estimate of the source population from which the reported cases emerge. If the probability of the ADR being reported is unlikely to be influenced by the exposure of interest (e.g. dose), a reasonable estimate of the relative risk may be obtained. In this circumstance, underreporting does not affect the observed result.

SURVIVAL ANALYSIS

One final technique, recently developed to enhance the information content of spontaneous case reports data, employs principles of time-to-event and survival analysis to the evaluation of ADR reports (Kahn and Sempos, 1989; Graham and Green, 1999). The technique requires access to nationally representative population-based drug use data in order to model the pattern of duration of use in the general population. In a clinical trial or longitudinal observational cohort study, patients who drop out before study completion are censored at that point in time and only the time during which they were in the study is considered in the analysis (Meinert, 1986). Life-table techniques are a common means of accurately accounting for changes in the size of the population at risk resulting from withdrawals (Clayton and Hills, 1993; Kelsey et al., 1996). By use of this method, one can calculate interval-specific reporting/hazard rates (e.g. for the first month, fifth month or twelfth month of product use) as well as the cumulative risk of an ADR being reported through a given point in time such as after one or three years of continuing drug use.

The method is complex but useful. It was used to demonstrate the association between risk of developing acute liver failure and the duration of use of trovafloxacin, a fluoroquinolone antibiotic. Over about a two-year period, the FDA received 14 reports of acute liver failure associated with

trovafloxacin use (Public Health Advisory, 1999). In an effort better to characterize the contour and magnitude of risk over time, the survival technique was used. For comparison purposes, the background incidence rate for acute liver failure due to "idiopathic" causes was previously estimated at one case per million per year (Graham and Green, 1999). Based only on *reported* cases, the relative risk of acute liver failure was increased from the start of therapy and increased rapidly with increasing duration of exposure (Table 17.3).

THE VALUE AND FUTURE OF PHARMACOVIGILANCE IN THE UNITED STATES

It is not an exaggeration to state that pharmacovigilance is the cornerstone of postmarketing drug safety activities in the United States, and will likely remain so for the foreseeable future. Nearly all postmarketing labeling changes related to drug toxicity are based on spontaneous case reports. The same holds true for drug withdrawals. Since 1980, there have been 18 major prescription drug withdrawals in the United States. Of these, spontaneous case reports and their analysis were a critical informational component contributing to the withdrawal decision in 16. The two exceptions were encainide and flosequinan, where randomized clinical trials identified the increased mortality risk conferred by these approved drugs (Echt et al., 1991; Massie et al., 1993). This should not be a surprise because patients with cardiac arrhythmias under treatment for those arrhythmias will sometimes experience sudden death due to arrhythmias, and death is not infrequent among patients with congestive heart failure. In situations where the underlying disease being treated and the ADR resulting from treatment are the same, only a well-conducted randomized trial will convincingly establish the drug–ADR association.

While the utility of case reports is undeniable, there is much that might be done to improve and expand their value. Strategies to improve the level of reporting of serious ADRs need to be developed. The proverb about "strength in numbers" also applies to pharmacovigilance. A few reports may provide a sufficient basis upon which to modify a product's label. However, important information regarding the magnitude and duration of risk as well as risk factors for ADR occurrence is more easily and reliably discovered through careful analysis of a larger series of cases. Hand in hand with the value of a larger numbers of serious case reports is improved quality and completeness of those reports. The more clinically detailed a series of reports is, the greater the range of analytic possibilities. The value of this for regulatory decision-making and risk management efforts cannot be overstated. How to achieve these goals in an environment of immense time constraints and litigation fear is an important challenge for the future.

Another area of potentially great public health value is the expansion of current pharmacovigilance practice to include other venues and types of ADRs. In the United States, the focus of pharmacovigilance has been on the rapid identification of serious *unlabeled* events. Many, if not most of these fall into the category of "unexpected" or "idiosyncratic" and have been referred to as type B reactions (Meyboom *et al.*, 1997). This is an important endeavor but from a population perspective, the bulk of drug-related morbidity and mortality is due to type A reactions, that is, those that represent an extension of the drug's pharmacology. The problem is great enough to represent one of the leading causes of mortality in the United States (Lazarou *et al.*, 1998).

Pharmacovigilance strategies in this arena might lead to the identification of "problem areas" and provide the basis for more effective intervention and prevention.

Finally, advances in technology over the past decade and the advent of the ICH process have created an environment where global pharmacovigilance is now conceivable. A remaining challenge is to make this a reality.

REFERENCES

Ahmad SR, Graham DJ, Toyer DP, Wassel R, Mann M (2000) Comparison of pulmonary toxicity risks with anti-androgens (abstract). *Pharmacoepidemiology and Drug Safety* 9: S121.

Ahmad SR, Singer SJ, Leissa BG (2001) Congestive heart failure associated with itraconazole. *Lancet* 357: 1766–7.

Belton KJ, Lewis SC, Payne S, Rawlins MD, Wood SM (1995) Attitudinal survey of adverse drug reaction reporting in the United Kingdom. *Br J Clin Pharmacol* 39: 223–6.

Blum MD, Graham DJ, McCloskey CA (1994) Temafloxacin syndrome: review of 95 cases. *Clin Infect Dis* 18: 946–50.

Breslow NE, Day NE (1980) *Statistical Methods in Cancer Research: The Analysis of Case–Control Studies*. Lyon: IARC Scientific Publications.

Brown EG, Wood L, Wood S (1999) The medical dictionary for regulatory activities (MedDRA). *Drug Safety* 20: 109–17.

Clayton D, Hills M (1993) *Statistical Models in Epidemiology*. New York: Oxford University Press.

Coultas DB, Zumwalt RE, Black WC, Sobonya RE (1994) The epidemiology of interstitial lung diseases. *Am J Respir Crit Care Med* 150: 967–72.

Dalakas MC, Illa I, Pezeshkpour GH, Laukaitis JP, Cohen B, Griffin JL (1990) Mitichondrial myopathy caused by long-term zidovudine therapy. *New Engl J Med* 322: 1098–1105.

Echt DS, Liebson PR, Mitchell LB, Peters RW, Obias-Manno D, Barker A, *et al.* (1991) Mortality and morbidity in patients receiving encainide, flecainide and placebo. *New Engl J Med* 324: 781–8.

Eland IA, Belton KJ, van Grootheest AC, Meiners AP, Rawlins MD, Stricker BHCh (1999) Attitudinal survey of voluntary reporting of adverse drug reactions. *Br J Clin Pharmacol* 48: 623–7.

Frick PA, Cohen LG, Rovers JP (1997) Algorithms used in adverse drug reaction reports: a comparative study. *Ann Pharmacother* 31: 164–7.

Friedman MA, Woodcock J, Lumpkin MM, Shuren JE, Hass AE, Thompson LJ (1999) The safety of newly approved medicines: do recent market removals mean there is a problem? *J Am Med Assoc* 281: 1728–34.

GAO/HEHS (2000) *Adverse Drug Events: The Magni-*

tude of Health Risk is Uncertain Because of Limited Incidence Data. GAO/HEHS-00-21, January.

Graham DJ (1989) Epidemiologic Review of Spontaneous Case Reports of Withdrawal Seizures, Physiologic Dependence and Death Reported with Alprazolam, with Special Attention to Effects of High Dose and Longer Duration Use. Rockville, MD: Psychopharmacologic Drugs Advisory Committee Meeting, Food and Drug Administration, September 20.

Graham DJ, Green L (1999) Epidemiology of Hepatotoxicity with Troglitazone. Bethesda, MD: Metabolic-Endocrine Drugs Advisory Committee Meeting, Food and Drug Administration, March 26.

Graham DJ, Waller PC, Kurz X (2000) View from regulatory agencies. In: Strom BL, ed., Pharmacoepidemiology, 3rd edn. Wiley: New York, pp. 109–24.

Green G (1998) Regional initiatives, past, present and future in the US. In: D'Arcy PF, Harron DWG, eds, Proceedings of the Fourth International Conference on Harmonisation, Brussels 1997 Belfast: Queen's University, pp. 425–9.

Honigfeld G, Arellano F, Sethi J, Bianchini A, Schein J (1998) Reducing clozapine-related morbidity and mortality: 5 years experience with the Clozaril National Registry. J Clin Psychiatry 59 (Suppl 3): 3–7.

Inman WHW, Adelstein AM (1969) Rise and fall of asthma mortality in England and Wales in relation to use of pressurized aerosols. Lancet 2: 279–85.

Inman WHW, Weber JCP (1986) The United Kingdom. In: Inman WHW, ed., Monitoring for Drug Safety, 2nd edn. Lancaster: MTP Press Ltd, pp. 13–47.

Johnson JM, Barash D (1991) A review of postmarketing adverse drug experience reporting requirements. FDC Law J 46: 665–72.

Kahn HA, Sempos CT (1989) Statistical Methods in Epidemiology. New York: Oxford University Press.

Kelsey JL, Whittemore AS, Evans AS, Thompson WD (1996) Methods in Observational Epidemiology, 2nd edn. New York: Oxford University Press.

Kennedy DL, Goldman SA, Lillie RB (2000) Spontaneous reporting in the United States. In: Strom BL, ed., Pharmacoepidemiology, 3rd edn. New York: Wiley, pp. 151–74.

La Grenade L, Graham DJ, Trontell A (2000) Fatal myocarditis with clozapine. New Engl Med, in press.

La Grenade L, Kornegay C, Graham DJ (2000) Using publicly available data to derive background rates when evaluating adverse drug reaction reports (abstract). Pharmacoepidemiology and Drug Safety 9: S70–1.

Lazarou J, Pomeranz BH, Corey PN (1998) Incidence of adverse drug reactions in hospitalized patients: a meta-analysis of prospective studies. J Am Med Assoc 279: 1200–5.

Massie BM, Berk MR, Brozena SC, Elkayam U, Plehn JF, Kukin ML, et al. (1993) Can further benefit be achieved by adding flosequinan to patients with congestive heart failure who remain symptomatic on diuretic, digoxin, and an angiotensin converting enzyme inhibitor? Circulation 88: 492–501.

Meinert CL (1986) Clinical Trials: Design, Conduct and Analysis. New York: Oxford University Press.

Meyboom RHB, Egberts ACG, Edwards RI, Hekster YA, de Koning FHP, Gribnau WJ (1997) Principles of signal detection in pharmacovigilance. Drug Safety 16: 355–65.

Moore N, Kreft-Jais C, Haramburu F, Noblet C, Andrejak M, Ollagnier M, et al. (1997) Reports of hypoglycemia associated with the use of ACE inhibitors and other drugs: a case–not case study in the French Pharmacovigilance System database. Br J Clin Pharmacol 44: 513–18.

Murray CJ, Lopez AD (1992) Global health statistics: a compendium of incidence, prevalence, and mortality estimates for over 200 conditions. In: Global Burden of Disease and Injury Series, Vol. 11. Boston: Harvard University Press, pp. 1–33.

Pere JC, Bégaud B, Haramburu F, Albin H (1986) Computerized comparison of six adverse drug reaction assessment procedures. Clin Pharmacol Ther 40: 451–61.

Public Health Advisory (1999) Trovan (trovafloxacin/alatrofloxacin mesylate) and risk of liver failure. Food and Drug Administration, June 9. Available from: http://www.fda.gov/cder/news/trovan/trovan-advisory.htm.

Rogers AS (1987) Adverse drug events: identification and attribution. Drug Intell Clin Pharm 21: 915–20.

Rogers AS, Israel E, Smith CR (1988) Physician knowledge, attitudes and behavior related to reporting adverse drug events. Arch Intern Med 148: 1596–1600.

Rothman KJ, Greenland S (1998) Modern Epidemiology, 2nd edn. Philadelphia, PA: Lippincott-Raven, pp. 76–7.

Scott HD, Rosenbaum SE, Waters WJ, Colt AM, Andrews LG, Juergens JP, et al. (1987) Rhode Island physicians' recognition and reporting of adverse drug reactions. RI Med J 70: 311–6.

Wiholm BE, Olsson S, Moore N, Waller P (2000) Spontaneous reporting outside the US. In: Strom BL, ed., Pharmacoepidemiology, 3rd edn. New York: Wiley, pp. 175–92.

18

Algorithms

JOHN A. CLARK

Galt Associates, Inc., Sterling, VA, USA

INTRODUCTION

Assessments of the clinical circumstances of individual patient adverse events (AEs) have been important components of health care product monitoring programs every since systematic AE surveillance was first proposed in the early 1960s (Finney, 1963). Reliance on such methods is based on the view, shared by many safety professionals, that careful analysis of the diagnostic data found in AE reports can help to find causal product–AE relationships. In the 1970s and 1980s, signalling procedures based on the medical interpretation of individual patient experiences came to be described by the word "imputation", meaning an evaluation that summarizes the causally-related features pertaining to a single patient's AE (Venulet, 1984). It has been suggested that imputology can be an effective surveillance strategy for individual patient reports arising from studies (Emanueli and Sacchetti, 1980; Jones, 1987), medical literature case reports (Venning, 1983; Rossi and Knapp, 1984), and spontaneous sources (Jones, 1994; Stephens, 1999) (see Table 18.1), all three of which contribute to both premarketing and postmarketing pharmacovigilance. Individual patient reports from clinical studies are useful in postmarketing

surveillance when large phase IV trials are conducted for a product, and, conversely, individual patient reports from spontaneous sources are useful in premarketing surveillance when marketing is initiated outside of a product development territory. This chapter considers the use of imputation methods to evaluate patient AE experiences that come from any of these sources, focusing on their use both as report database screening devices for "interesting" product–AE pairs during the signal detection (report-based) phase of AE surveillance, as well as their value in analyzing series of cases of the same product–AE during the signal evaluation (case-based) phase of AE surveillance (see Chapter 19, Overview—Spontaneous Signalling).

Table 18.1. Data sources for single patient imputation methods.

Human studies (published or unpublished) • From clinical studies • From epidemiologic studies
Literature case reports • Single case reports • Case series
Spontaneous reports

Pharmacovigilance. Edited by R.D. Mann and E.B. Andrews

THE USE OF IMPUTATION-BASED METHODS IN ADVERSE EVENT SIGNALLING PROGRAMS

GENERAL CONSIDERATIONS

Imputation Methods

The term "imputation method" can be defined as any monitoring procedure based on individual patient test results, the aim of which is to differentiate a monitored product cause from other causes for an AE. Throughout health care product surveillance, imputation-derived procedures (e.g. causality assessments) are either mandated by regulation (Code of Federal Regulations), or are encouraged by international agreements, such as those pertaining to expedited individual patient AE reporting (ICH E2A) or periodic safety update reports (ICH E2C) (European Agency for the Evaluation of Medicinal Products, 1995, 1997). However, while well accepted in the regulatory sense, imputation-based methodology has never been well rationalized epidemiologically, and a definitive theory through which imputation-based methodology can be implemented has not yet evolved. A useful alternative, as is followed in this chapter, is to view imputation methodology functionally, i.e. relative to its purpose within a comprehensive AE surveillance scheme. The parameters of imputation-based methodology can then be discussed in terms of their intended effect, such as their appropriateness for implementing a particular step in the signalling process.

From the surveillance perspective, two general uses for imputation can be identified (see Table 18.2 and Figure 18.1). The first, imputation screening, involves the automated examination of product-specific report databases with imputation-based instruments in order to find "interesting" product–AE pairs (Venulet, 1992). Like all identification signalling methods, screening imputation examines collections of AE reports, selecting only certain product–AEs for subsequent scrutiny (see the section Imputation Screening (Causality) Assessments in Chapter 19). The second, case series imputation, applies imputation methods to a product–AE case series to see if evidence favoring

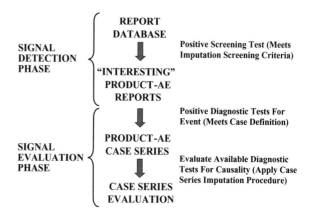

Figure 18.1 Use of imputation methods to carry out two-phase signalling.

further action exists. Like other case series formation methods, case series imputation is intended to summarize the aggregate evidence in favor of a product–AE relationship that is exhibited by a group of cases, i.e. a group of reports that meet a case definition (see the section Spontaneous Signalling Methods Used at the Case Series Formation Step in Chapter 19). While the use of imputation methods for these two purposes was not clearly delineated in the past, it has recently been pointed out and discussed by Meyboom (Meyboom *et al.*, 1997b; Meyboom, 1998).

Regardless of functional intent, imputation methods are dependent on report quality (accuracy and completeness (Edwards *et al.*, 1990)), which differs from one data source to the next. Individual patient reports from clinical trials are usually well documented on standardized data forms and offer access to medical records. On the other hand, patient reports from studies can also be limited by investigators' perceptions of reportable content, the lack of data following closure of a trial, and the forwarding of a large number of reports for which a medical rationale may be lacking. Literature case reports are characterized by rigorous editorial expectations. However, the publication process does not impose any clearly definable minimum standard, is not applied uniformly, and, in general, not does not provide for peer review of actual medical records (Venulet, 1985). While spontaneous individual patient reports frequently lack sufficient detail to provide

Table 18.2. Two uses for imputation in adverse event surveillance schemes.

	Imputation screening	Case series imputation
Applied to	Single reports in a report database	Multiple cases in an assembled case series
Signalling step	Identification (screening)	Case series formation
Purpose	Screen for "interesting" product–AE pairs	Summarize evidence in favor of product–AE relationships
Resource expenditure	Semi- or fully-automated	Time and resource intensive
Depends on	Systematically entered data fields pertaining to tests for causality	Applicable case definition
Report case requirements	Must meet minimum requirements to be a screenable report	Must meet a case definition to be included in an analysis

value and are often documented with practitioner opinions only, prescriber-selected patient reports have repeatedly proven effective in finding important safety outcomes. Additionally, follow-up activities can compensate for initial deficiencies in spontaneous reports by seeking out and acquiring supporting medical documentation (Clark et al., 1990). Thus, each of the three major reporting environments that give rise to individual patient reports are associated with strengths and limitations, and each has come to occupy a complementary niche in health care monitoring systems.

The Role of Imputation Methods in AE Surveillance Programs

Defining a logical role for the use of imputation methodology in AE surveillance programs has been complicated by its historical development. Single report imputation methodology was first published in the medical literature in the 1970s, a time that coincided with the adoption of early computerized expert systems into medical practice. Most of this work pertained to single AE occurrences (as distinct from a series of the same AE in different patients), originated in academic settings, and was not designed to address the needs of surveillance systems (Irey, 1976a; Karch and Lasagna, 1977; Kramer et al., 1979; Naranjo et al., 1981). Influenced by these trends, AE-

oriented imputation instruments were developed primarily as single occurrence, medical diagnostic aids, and were only subsequently adapted for use in surveillance databases.

Since the main focus of AE surveillance is to find product–AE pairs for possible public health interventions, and not to establish medical diagnoses in individual patients, the published imputation literature is only indirectly applicable to AE surveillance systems. At present, in-depth, single report imputation procedures in AE monitoring are essentially limited to satisfying regulatory requirements (Bégaud and Royer, 1986) or addressing special project needs. For imputation methods to become widely applicable as screening imputation tools, they would have to be simplified for automated or semi-automated use, and would have to be adapted to a report database environment (Venulet, 1992).

Likewise, the bulk of imputation-based methodology involves the assessment of product–AEs on a case-by-case basis, and is also minimally applicable to case series imputation procedures. While single cases of exceptional value can rarely become pertinent signalling evidence (Meyboom et al., 1997a), case series imputation is almost always based on multiple patient occurrences of the same AE (Meyboom et al., 1997b). Except in highly unusual circumstances, product–AE associations have generally not been proposed on the basis of one known patient experience. For imputation methods to become widely applicable as case series imputation procedures, they would have to be extended from one to multiple cases, and would have to produce results that are interpretable from a population viewpoint.

Imputation, Causality, and Causality Assessments

Since imputation addresses causally oriented data by way of defined procedures, it has become closely identified with the phrase "causality assessment". Unfortunately, the word "causality" is confusing because it describes at least six different, but loosely related, concepts: (1) etiologic (causal) certainty, (2) epidemiologic causality, (3) retrodictive causality, (4) operational causality (causality assessment procedures), (5) regulatory causality, and (6) legal causality. Without clarification, the meaning of the word "causality" is too general to be of value when describing AE surveillance procedures or results.

Imputation screening procedures are specialized methods for rating operational causality. Their purpose is to screen surveillance databases for suspected product–AE pairs. In contrast, case series imputation methods are best grouped together with epidemiologic methods, since they are intended to clarify, however imperfectly, epidemiologic propositions. (As a result of constraints related to data quality and completeness, the term "pre-epidemiology" has sometimes been used in place of the word "epidemiology" to describe their use (Wartenberg and Greenberg, 1993).) Case series imputation is one of several case series formation signalling methods, all of which assess potential product-AE relationships through the analysis of incompletely reported case series (see Chapter 19).

Etiologic (Causal) Certainty

Etiologic certainty accepts without qualification the retrodictive causal proposition that an AE occurring in a particular patient would not have happened as and when it did unless a specified product exposure had occurred (Hutchinson and Lane, 1989; Kramer and Lane, 1992). This is equivalent to the statement that a particular product caused a particular AE to occur in a specific patient. A causal versus a non-causal AE in this sense amounts to acceptance or rejection of an absolute etiologic proposition, and is reducible to either "yes" or "no". It is widely accepted, however, that causation for a given AE type is multifactorial and variable, so that, in a given individual, the extent and nature of the causal constellation is unknown (Rothman and Greenland, 1998). Although the word "causal" continues to be used in the sense of etiologic certainty, this concept is no longer scientifically viable as a causal model.

Epidemiologic Causality

Over the course of the twentieth century, epidemiologic causality gradually displaced etiologic certainty as the prevailing causal model for medical applications. Epidemiologic causal models possess time–space context and counterfactuality (Greenland and Rothman, 1998). Time–space context implies that rates or proportions pertaining to safety outcomes can be ascertained and compared across product exposures because the temporal and geographical limits of the model are explicitly defined. This, in turn, means that epidemiologic causality refers to aggregate comparisons, and need not be ascribed to any particular case. Epidemiologic causality also depends on the notion of counterfactuality, i.e. determining what would have happened to a particular group of cases under the scenarios of both an index and alternative exposure. Since both scenarios cannot occur simultaneously, the observer must have confidence that another aggregate case experience (such as a control group) can be substituted for one of the two counterfactual scenarios as a comparative standard. Taken together, time–space context and counterfactual reasoning allow causal propositions to be formally evaluated by comparing model-based test statistics vis-à-vis their expected values. Epidemiologic models allow safety professionals to quantify the strength of probabilistic evidence in favor of a product–AE relationship, rather than relying on personal judgment to formulate absolute responses on a case-by-case basis.

Retrodictive Causality

Individual cases of product–AEs can also be considered in a counterfactual paradigm that has been assessed in its most detailed way with a Bayesian causal/non-causal odds model (Lane *et al*., 1987; Kramer and Lane, 1992) (see Figure 18.1). The Bayesian odds model uses individual case information and epidemiologic data to assess individual cases. The resulting quantity, which is applicable to a particular case only, can theoretically demonstrate the strength of probabilistic evidence in favor of a product–AE causal argument for a single patient (i.e. it addresses a retrodictive causal proposition). Unfortunately, systematic formal statistical testing of retrodictive causal propositions is unrealistic in surveillance environments for two major reasons. First, the Bayesian odds model requires existing epidemiologic data pertaining to product–AE causality. But in AE surveillance, such data usually do not exist, or, if they do, often represent only a "best guess" estimate. Second, the sensitivities and specificities for available diagnostic testing for causality for a particular case can be difficult to quantify. Problems with data availability may account for why authors analyzing specific retrodictive causal hypotheses have not recommended formal statistical testing procedures for individual product–AE cases *vis-à-vis* an expected value, and have, instead, treated the results as if the underlying variability of the estimate was not calculable (Lane *et al*., 1987; Ghajar *et al*., 1989). Given these difficulties, from the surveillance viewpoint the Bayesian odds model and its derivatives are best considered to be forms of operational causality (see below), and not as models that offer precise solutions to retrodictive causal propositions (Hutchinson and Lane, 1989).

Operational Causality

Causality assessment procedures are a group of methods by which single cases can be considered in a counterfactual model for the purpose of generating operational causal ratings (Venulet, 1992). All operational causality instruments are based on the Bayesian principle that individual patient data can modify an assessor's pre-existing view of a causal association between a particular etiologic alternative and an AE to obtain a more accurate final impression of a particular patient's adverse experience. The operational rating that results from this process can then be used to categorize individual patient product–AEs along an arbitrary continuous or ordinal scale. Although such ratings provide causal information within the scale defined by the observer, they are not referable to a time–space context, and cannot mathematically relate individual patient causality to a larger causal concept by way of formal hypothesis testing. From the surveillance perspective, operational causality ratings are useful as triaging methodologies (i.e. imputation screening tools) that help to focus subsequent analytic activity on high priority patient experiences.

Regulatory Causality

Regulatory causality means the use of an operational causality instrument to explicitly define one or more categories as "causal" for reporting purposes. Since regulatory causality depends on how the results of an operational instrument are further defined as a basis for reporting actions, it is not necessarily equivalent to the results of any specific operational causality assessment. Regulatory causality implies that a reporting entity has defined a procedure in order to comply with territorial requirements.

Legal Causality

In the context of product–AEs, legal causality means the designation of an AE as causal during proceedings conducted by a court possessing appropriate jurisdiction (Freilich, 1984). This legal view of causality may or may not coincide with any other view of causality that is formulated on either an aggregate or individual case basis. The usual purpose of a jurisprudential causal debate pertaining to a health care product is to adjudicate claims against manufacturers that have been filed by an individual or group under product liability law.

A GENERAL MODEL FOR IMPUTATION-BASED METHODS

Bayesian Odds Model

The odds form of Bayes' equation is useful as a general model upon which imputation-based methodology can be designed (see Figures 18.2 and 18.3). In the Bayesian causal/non-causal odds model, existing epidemiologic data determine a prior odds of product causation versus non-product causation that is available to the safety analyst at the outset of the procedure. It has been suggested that the prior odds can be approximated

Posterior odds = Prior odds × Summary likelihood ratio

$$\frac{\Pr(D \rightarrow AE \mid B,C)}{\Pr(D \not\rightarrow AE \mid B,C)} = \frac{\Pr(D \rightarrow AE \mid B)}{\Pr(D \not\rightarrow AE \mid B)} \times \frac{\Pr(C \mid D \rightarrow AE)}{\Pr(C \mid D \not\rightarrow AE)}$$

The best estimate for a particular case (*C*) of the ratio of posterior probabilities (posterior odds) that the AE (*AE*) was caused by (*D*→*AE*) or was not caused by (*D*⇸*AE*) the evaluated product (*D*) can be calculated by multiplying the same ratio in the absence of case information (prior odds=prior probability of causality divided by the prior probability of non-causality) times a summary likelihood ratio. A summary likelihood ratio is the ratio of the probabilities that a case such as the one examined (*C*) would occur if the product was causal versus if the product was non-causal. The prior odds is conditional on baseline (*B*) information, while the posterior odds is conditional both on baseline and case (*B,C*) information. Reproduced from Clark *et al.* (2001), *Epidemiologic Reviews* 23(2), 191–210, Fig. 2, with permission from Oxford University Press.

Figure 18.2. The Bayesian odds model for evaluating the probability of causality versus non-causality in single product–AE cases.

The prior odds (lower limit) [*] can be estimated as
$$\frac{I_c}{I_{nc}} \approx \frac{(I_e - I_u)}{I_u} = \frac{RD}{I_u}$$

Likelihood ratios (*LR*) can be estimated as:

Dichotomous test for causality, positive result:
$$\frac{\text{sensitivity}}{1 - \text{specificity}}$$

Dichotomous test for causality, negative result:
$$\frac{1 - \text{sensitivity}}{\text{specificity}}$$

Multiple (≥2) independent dichotomous tests: $LR_1 \times LR_2 \times \ldots$

[*]This prior odds estimation assumes that $I_{nc} = I_u$ (see text for details). RD = incidence rate difference; I_c = product causal incidence rate; I_{nc} = product non-causal incidence rate; I_e = product exposed incidence rate; I_u = product unexposed incidence rate; LR = likelihood ratio.

Figure 18.3. Estimating the parameters of the Bayesian odds model.

by dividing the incidence rate difference for the AE between product-exposed and product-unexposed groups by the product-unexposed incidence rate (Kramer, 1988a) (see Figure 18.3). If this quantity, also referred to as the relative excess rate, is used to estimate the prior odds, then the analyst must make a counterfactual assumption that the product-unexposed incidence rate is an acceptable approximation for the product-exposed, non-causal incidence rate, which may be incorrect (Greenland and Rothman, 1998). Since product exposure could accelerate the onset of AE occurrences that result from multifactorial (including product) causation, the product-unexposed incidence rate could be greater than the product-exposed, non-causal incidence rate. For the purposes of this discussion, we note that the prior odds is a useful theoretical construct that expresses an initial expectation of relative causal/non-causal occurrence in product-exposed patients, and whose true value can be estimated as greater than or equal to the relative excess rate.

In the Bayesian odds paradigm, the prior odds is then multiplied by one or more likelihood ratios derived from case diagnostic data (see Figure 18.2). This result, called the posterior odds, represents a theoretical final view of relative product causality versus other causality after all relevant case information has been incorporated. Each likelihood ratio is the mathematical expression of a specific test result for product causality that was available for that case (a positive rechallenge test, for example). The likelihood ratio for a positive test result for a dichotomous test is equal to the test's sensitivity divided by 1 − specificity (Kramer, 1988b) (see Figure 18.3). The sensitivity (true positive rate) for a test is the probability of obtaining a positive test result in a population of causal cases, while the quantity 1 − specificity (false positive rate) of a test is the probability of obtaining a positive test result in a population of non-causal cases. The product of all likelihood ratios for all available tests for causality forms a single summary likelihood ratio for that AE occurrence. If no diagnostically applicable information is available for a particular AE occurrence, then the Bayesian odds model assumes a summary likelihood ratio of one.

Implications of the Bayesian Odds Model for Imputation Methods Design

In the event of a positive test result, the likelihood ratio for a dichotomous test must be greater than 1 as long as both test sensitivity and specificity are >0.5. Hence, appropriately selected, positive tests increase the posterior odds favoring product–AE causality regardless of the prior odds value. This implies that imputation screening would logically be directed toward finding cases in which the summary likelihood ratio for that case is greater than one. Screening for AEs likely to have a high prior odds due to, for example, a low non-causal incidence rate, is also an appealing strategy, but does not involve individual case diagnostic information, and is therefore not a form of imputation screening. Thus, an examination of the Bayesian odds model suggests that imputation screening methods are essentially procedures that look for "interesting" product–AEs by finding individual AE reports that possess one or more diagnostically relevant tests for causality.

In contrast, case series imputation methodology represents a pre-epidemiologic approach to the summarization of causal evidence in a product–AE case series. Such methods depend on both the prior odds (epidemiologic data) and the summary likelihood ratios (individual case testing) for all cases in the case series. In designing and using case series imputation methods, safety evaluators will need to focus both on the refinement of estimates affecting the prior odds (e.g. background incidence rates), as well as estimates for the sensitivity and specificity of tests for causality that were performed for all cases in the case series. Since empirical data pertaining to these quantities are often not available, case series imputation frequently becomes an exercise in which analogous and simulated data are used to support a product-AE causal argument (Lane *et al.*, 1987; Ghajar *et al.*, 1989).

Tests for Event Versus Tests for Causality

The Bayesian odds model underscores the fundamentally conditional nature of diagnostic testing in case series imputation procedures (Naranjo and Lanctôt, 1991). Such testing is a two-step process in which diagnostic tests for an AE are first applied to establish a product–AE case, following which diagnostic tests for causality are interpreted (see Figure 18.1). Tests for the event (AE) establish reports as cases, while interpretation of tests for causality alter the conditional probabilities that pertain to at least two potential causes for such cases. In AE surveillance, two alternative causes, the monitored product versus all other (background) causes, are usually considered.

Both the identification of a product-event (acceptance of a report as a case), and the summarization of evidence concerning product versus non-product causality are quantitatively dependent on the sensitivity and specificity of the aggregate testing that was used by the evaluator for those purposes. Since summary tests for event are generally quite accurate, physician diagnoses that are provided in AE reports are often taken at face value, as long as reasonable supporting descriptions are available. In contrast, tests for causality can be more difficult to interpret, and frequently lack empirical validation data concerning their sensitivity and specificity. As a consequence, the results of tests for causality are usually carefully scrutinized by product monitors prior to their acceptance.

Tests for causality can be further divided into chronological tests (time to onset, dechallenge, rechallenge tests), tests based on clinical manifestations (features of the case that suggest product rather than background causation), and tests based on physical–chemical linkage of the AE with the monitored product (Kramer *et al.*, 1979). Physical–chemical linkage can be directly accomplished, in particular, by high suspect product serum levels or the presence of a product moiety in pathologic specimens, but would also encompass immunologic testing such as *in vitro* challenge tests, skin tests, and antibody-related testing that have an appropriate positive predictive value for product causality. Risk factors could also be used as tests for causality, provided that their ability to differentiate product causality from other causes for the AE was adequate. Although the assumed sensitivities and specificities of tests for causality are difficult to formulate explicitly, the safety analyst should carefully weigh any evidence that might influence the derivation of a best estimate, since the summary likelihood ratio for each AE occurrence is a function of these quantities.

IMPUTATION SCREENING (CAUSALITY) ASSESSMENTS

RATIONALE AND APPROACH TO IMPUTATION SCREENING

Imputation screening involves the use of imputation-based procedures to find "interesting" product–AEs in an AE report database. Imputation screening procedures have four basic attributes: (1) application on a report-by-report basis, (2) amenability to automation or semi-automation, (3) sensitivity and specificity for finding "interesting" product–AEs, and (4) focus on finding reports possessing summary causality testing that favors the monitored product (i.e. a summary likelihood ratio greater than one) (see Table 18.3, Part A). Those imputation screening procedures that are selected for actual use should exhibit the features of a good screening test as they apply to the imputation screening environment, namely: (1) easy to use, (2) generalizable to many product–AE pairs, (3) capable of producing reproducible (uniform, reliable) output, and 4) associated with a low false positive rate (see Table 8.3, Part B). In the presence of a declining or low prevalence of

Table 18.3. Features of database imputation screening instruments.

A. Basic features
- Applied on a report-by-report basis
- Amenable to automation or semi-automation
- Associated with a sensitivity and specificity for finding "interesting" product–AE pairs
- Finds reports for which positive tests for causality have been reported

B. Desirable features
- Ease to use
- Generalizable to many product–AE pairs
- Capable of producing uniform output
- Associated with a low false positive rate

"interesting" product–AE pairs, imputation screening can exhibit a high false positive rate. This circumstance leads to a low efficiency rating, and is inconsistent with the operational realities of AE surveillance programs.

For the past four decades, imputation methods have undergone continuous change, much of which has focused on individualizing them for use in medical diagnosis (Lane et al., 1987; Stephens, 1999). To the degree that this was successful, imputation instruments became more applicable for diagnosis, but less applicable as screening methods. The first imputation procedures devised in the 1960s depended entirely on subjective judgments made by physicians or other health care professionals (MacDonald and Mac-Kay, 1964). In the 1970s, this evolved into formalized procedures based on rules in which assessor subjectivity was applied more uniformly through the use of algorithms or questionnaires (Irey, 1976a, 1976b). In the early 1980s, statistical modelling was first applied to imputation problems when Bayesian methodology was introduced (Lane, 1984; Auriche, 1985), while, in the late 1980s, AE–specific approaches were first proposed (Bénichou and Celigny, 1991). Since that time, more complex statistical procedures, such as decision support algorithms, have also been suggested (Hoskins and Manning, 1992). Of these five groups of published methods by which single report imputation screening could potentially be performed (subjective, generalized rule-based, Bayesian odds model, AE-specific rule-based, and non-Bayesian statistical models), practical limitations have led to the widespread use of subjective and generalized rule-based methodology only. AE-specific rule-based methods and Bayesian and non-Bayesian statistical models have had essentially no systematic use as screening devices in databases comprised of individual patient reports.

Three important functional issues have been raised about the applicability of single report imputation methods to AE data: (1) the effect of missing, unobtainable, or erroneous data elements (Irey, 1976, 1976b; Venulet, 1986; Meyboom and Royer, 1992); (2) the isolation of a single product out of a list of multiple potential causes (Meyboom and Royer, 1992); and (3) the value of imputation in generating signals of previously undescribed product–AE pairs (Meyboom, 1998: Stephens, 1999). The first issue, data integrity, is especially pertinent to report-by-report assessments because individual patient report data are often incomplete or inaccurate (Edwards *et al.*, 1990; Funch *et al.*, 1993; Sicker *et al.*, 1998). Additionally, many reports are not useful sources for contributory data elements because the product–AE pair is not amenable to classical imputation procedures (e.g. dechallenge evaluation in the presence of a non-resolving AE) (Stephens, 1999). The second issue, selection of a single product for monitoring focus in the presence of multiple potential product contributors, is frequently encountered in individual patient reports (Kramer, 1986; Meyboom and Royer, 1992). In general, imputation methods tend to have less value as the complexity of either the disease or treatment background increases. The third issue, initial discovery value, arises because operational causality assessments always depend to some degree on expectations shaped by prior experience. However, it has been well documented that important new spontaneous signals can originate from settings where prior experience is limited or misleading, thereby resulting in a delay in signal recognition (Inman, 1993).

IMPUTATION SCREENING (CAUSALITY) ASSESSMENTS

Subjective Judgment

Subjective imputation (also called "global introspection" (Kramer, 1986), "unstructured clinical judgment" (Jones, 1994), or "striking case method" (Amery, 1999)), involves the assignment of a causal rating to an individual spontaneous AE report based on medical diagnostic experience (MacDonald and MacKay, 1964). Subjective assessments have usually involved classification into multiple categories, such as the designations "documented", "probable", "possible", and "doubtful" that were first proposed in the 1960s and are still used in modified form in AE evaluations today (Cluff *et al.*, 1964; Seidl *et al.*, 1965). Subjective judgment probably remains the

most widely used method by which imputation screening is performed in AE surveillance programs (Meyboom and Royer, 1992; Jones, 1994; Hartmann *et al.*, 1997; Amery, 1999).

Subjectively generated imputation assessments have been shown to be associated with high levels of intra- and inter-rater variability (Karch *et al.*, 1976; Koch-Weser and Greenblatt, 1976; Koch-Weser *et al.*, 1977; Blanc *et al.*, 1979; Naranjo *et al.*, 1981), and can produce results that differ substantially from results derived using rules (Miremont *et al.*, 1994). This imprecision appears to be largely related to the many factors that affect any particular AE occurrence, making reproducibility (i.e. uniformity of the result with repetition) difficult to achieve in the absence of an algorithm (Kramer, 1986; Jones, 1994). It is interesting to note, however, that subjective assessments performed by assessors with longstanding professional relationships are not necessarily less uniform than those based on formalized procedures (Grohmann *et al.*, 1985). Such examples probably reflect the tacit adoption and systematic use of non-written rules by a group of evaluators.

Generalized Rule-Based Methods

Generalized rule-based methods (also called standardized assessment methods (Hutchinson *et al.*, 1983; Hutchinson, 1986) or standardized decision aids (Naranjo, 1986)), involve rating a product–AE occurrence using a questionnaire or algorithm (Lane *et al.*, 1987; Hutchinson and Lane, 1989; Jones, 1994; Meyboom *et al.*, 1997b). Over the past three decades, a large number of such instruments have been published (Irey, 1976a, 1976b; Karch and Lasagna, 1977; Kramer *et al.*, 1979; Naranjo *et al.*, 1981; Stephens, 1999). All rule-based methods contain three basic components that have been designed by an expert (see Figure 18.4): (1) a set of structured responses to questions, (2) a weighting algorithm that translates question-specific values into a summary value, and (3) a scaling algorithm that equates summary value ranges to imputation ratings (probable, possible, etc.) (Hutchinson, 1986). Evidence has been published that rule-based methods can reduce intra- and inter-rater variability as compared with subjective judgment, thereby

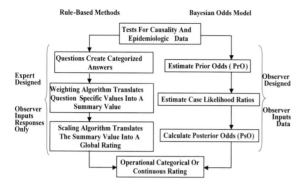

Figure 18.4. Steps used in two kinds of single report formal imputation procedures.

addressing one of the objections to the use of subjective judgment (Hutchinson *et al.*, 1979; Naranjo *et al.*, 1981; Busto *et al.*, 1982).

Several limitations of rule-based methods in identifying product–AE relationships have been described that are based on both applied and theoretical considerations (Hutchinson, 1986). First, unlike results obtained in optimal settings, the use of rule-based methods in actual surveillance environments may not significantly improve inter-rater variability beyond that obtainable subjectively (Leventhal *et al.*, 1979; Grohmann *et al.*, 1985; Louik *et al.*, 1985; Schmidt *et al.*, 1986). Additionally, rule-based methods do not reliably discriminate between proximate imputation categories (e.g. "probable" vs. "possible") when measured against a gold standard (Meyboom, 1998). These observations suggest that, even when complex and diagnostically oriented, generalized rule-based methods possess a limit of resolution that is quickly reached following implementation in actual surveillance environments.

Second, the scoring of product–AE test sets by several raters can differ widely, even when the same rule-based procedure is being used (Case and Oszko, 1991). Such residual inter-rater variability appears to be associated with questions that require more subjective input on the part of the user (Hutchinson *et al.*, 1983). The phenomenon of residual variability reflects the fact that subjectivity is homogenized, not eliminated, through the use of assessment rules (Hutchinson, 1986; Hutchinson and Lane, 1989).

Third, when applied to the same product–AE test set, the use of different rule-based methods can create widely divergent scores (Michel and Knodel, 1986; Péré *et al.*, 1986). Of the design components involved, this divergence appears to relate mostly to the use of different weighting assumptions for causality criteria (Venulet, 1984; Frick *et al.*, 1997). Theoreticians have also pointed out the impossibility of validation or inter-method translation of assessment scores derived from different rule-based instruments since a "gold standard" cannot be defined for these purposes (Hutchinson and Lane, 1989). Both of these observations underline the inappropriateness of the word "standardized" when referring to rule-based methodology, since such instruments are, themselves, not standard, nor do they result in standard output. Rule-based methods are better thought of as a group of independently designed expert systems that evaluate individual patient AE data in a similar manner (Hutchinson and Lane, 1989).

Fourth, little attention has been given to designing and validating generalized rule-based methods that are appropriate as imputation screening devices. Most published methods, for example, have not adequately addressed the need for simplicity, and essentially no data have ever been described that formally evaluate screening efficiency in a database population of heterogeneous product–AE pairs. Thus, the most important problem facing the use of imputation at the identification (screening) step of AE signalling remains the design of a reasonably simple, automated or semi-automated, broadly applicable procedure that can be calibrated to achieve acceptable sensitivity and specificity values. In the absence of this developmental step, manufacturers and agencies will likely continue to use a variety of published and unpublished instruments to meet their database screening needs.

AE-Specific Rule-Based Methods

In part in reaction to the residual subjectivity of generalized rule-based methods, some researchers have developed algorithms that are specific to particular AEs (Benichou, 1990; Danan and

Benichou, 1993). Such AE-specific rule-based methods are designed by a consensus of expert clinicians, thereby producing an increased response specificity (Meyboom *et al.*, 1997b). While this may be useful from a diagnostic perspective, it markedly restricts applicability by forcing the user to maintain a library of AE-specific instruments for predefined safety outcomes. No examples have been published in which AE-specific rule-based methods have been systematically compared with generalized rule-based methods, or have been used for imputation screening in AE surveillance programs.

Bayesian Odds Model

The most individualized formal imputation method devised thus far for evaluating single report content, Bayesian AE analysis, was introduced into the medical literature by Lane and Auriche (Lane, 1984; Auriche, 1985) (see Figures 18.2, 18.3, and 18.4, and text above). In the odds form of the Bayesian expression, the prior odds (the best initial estimate among exposed patients of the ratio of probabilities favoring causality vs. noncausality) is multiplied by one or more likelihood ratios. Likelihood ratios are formed by dividing the probability for a risk factor or test result (usually a temporal test) under a causal scenario by the probability for the same risk factor/test result under a non-causal scenario. The product of the prior odds and all pertinent likelihood ratios results in a posterior odds for product versus non-product causality that incorporates all known relevant epidemiologic and report information. For a spontaneous report, the posterior odds can be interpreted as the best estimate for the odds in favor of product causality, taking into account the limitations of external data sources, report content, and report quality (Lane, 1986a, 1986b; Lane *et al.*, 1987).

The Bayesian odds model has several limitations that reduce its appeal as a database screening instrument. First, Bayesian assessments are time intensive, requiring a large number of assumptions and calculations (Jones, 1994). Although Naranjo and Lanctôt have pointed out that the Bayesian odds model, once populated

with reference data, is straightforward to implement in subsequent drug problems involving the same AE type (Naranjo and Lanctôt, 1993), the time resources involved in its systematic implementation will likely always be significant. Second, the results of Bayesian case report evaluations have been compared with laboratory evidence (lymphocyte toxicity assay) in patients who experienced dermatological and/or hypersensitivity reactions. In this cross comparison, which was based on AEs amenable to Bayesian imputation, the Bayesian odds model had a high sensitivity (i.e. high true positive rate) for detecting allergic individuals (Naranjo *et al.*, 1994). (Because few patients with negative lymphocyte toxicity assays were available for study, the specificity was essentially not calculable.) Third, and perhaps most importantly, the Bayesian odds model is individualized according to each situation in which it is applied, and therefore has essentially no generalizability as a screening device. The finding that Bayesian assessments exhibit relatively low correlations to rule-based methods (Lanctôt and Naranjo, 1995) is a reflection of this attribute, since Bayesian methodology does not use a weighting algorithm, but instead relies upon report-specific epidemiologic estimates and case data modelling that are strongly influenced by empirical observation. These factors (time intensive, high sensitivity, and high level of individualization) all suggest that the Bayesian odds model is a diagnostic, not a screening, methodology and is unlikely to be successful as an imputation screening method.

Non-Bayesian Statistical Models

Decision analysis modelling has also been suggested as a single AE report assessment methodology (Hoskins and Manning, 1992). Like the Bayesian odds model, decision analysis requires the safety professional to specify a large number of (conditional) probabilities, as well as to define their corresponding utilities (quantified relevance to the model) (Kramer, 1988c). Thus, as currently recommended for single AE report data, decision analysis also appears to be best suited for diagnostic, rather than for screening purposes.

CASE SERIES IMPUTATION

RATIONALE AND APPROACH TO CASE SERIES IMPUTATION

Case series imputation evaluates the aggregate case diagnostic evidence in a case series to create an argument supporting a potential relationship between a product and an AE. The concept of case series imputation, coming after and based on report-based signalling, is inherent in AE surveillance schemes, and has occasionally been noted by experts in AE surveillance methods (Venulet, 1984; Bégaud, 1994). In recent years this distinction has been emphasized by Meyboom, who has pointed out the difference between using imputation to identify "interesting" adverse events, versus using it to review case series of suspected product–AE pairs (Meyboom et al., 1997b; Meyboom, 1998). Case series imputation methods are characterized by four main attributes: (1) use of a case definition that specifies which reports are to be included in the case series, (2) analytic orientation and time intensiveness, (3) focus on summarization of evidence derived from (usually) multiple cases, and (4) use of pre-epidemiologic methodology to generate or strengthen hypotheses pertaining to specific product–AE relationships (see Tables 18.2 and 18.4).

Like all case series formation methods, case series imputation requires that the evaluator devise a case definition that is defensible from a medico-epidemiologic perspective (Clark et al., 1990; Blum et al., 1994; Meyboom et al., 1997b). Although accepting reports at face value may sometimes be reasonable, the importance of careful definition of cases is underlined by the relatively low rate of case validation frequently observed at the time of follow-up (Funch et al., 1993; Sicker et al.,

Table 18.4. Basic features of case series imputation instruments.

- Based on cases (i.e. reports that meet a case definition)
- Time intensive
- Represents a summarization of diagnostic causal evidence of all cases in a case series
- Uses pre-epidemiologic methodology to address product–AE relationships

1998). Following the application of a case definition to candidate reports, the resulting case series is examined for the presence of tests for causality, and the aggregate testing evidence is summarized as formally as the data permit. Case series imputation procedures often serve as the focal point around which a variety of relevant observations can become incorporated into a comprehensive safety evaluation, in particular the number of cases, data consistency, relationships pertaining to time and dose, biologic plausability, analogous observations involving other products, and the nature and quality of the data (Bégaud et al., 1994; Meyboom, 1998).

From the time AE surveillance systems were first established, the most important safety-related actions that have resulted from health care product surveillance, including product withdrawals, have come from an examination of reported case series. Many of these analyses incorporated some type of description of case causal diagnostic features (Inman, 1993; McEwen, 1999). Reliance by safety monitors on the aggregate testing for causality contained in a case series has undoubtedly been influenced by the substantial under-reporting that is typical of passive (spontaneous and literature) AE reporting systems. In the presence of a non- or marginally quantitative signalling argument, aggregate diagnostic evidence from multiple cases offers a complementary rationale by which AE surveillance can be systematically performed. For example, the halothane–hepatitis experience demonstrated early on how case series containing instances of positive tests for causality (the time-to-onset patterns of repeat positive rechallenge) can justify important public health warnings, even in the absence of a clear-cut quantitative argument (Inman and Mushin, 1974). Despite such contributions, relatively few product–AE case series imputation methods (as opposed to single case imputation methods) have ever been published, and literature reviews devoted to this subject are virtually non-existent. One of the challenges facing researchers within the AE surveillance community is to develop a better understanding of how case series imputation has contributed to public health actions, and to incorporate these lessons into an improved and more expansive case series imputation methodology.

Case series imputation methods can be classified as: subjective, generalized rule-based, retrospective Bayesian, and AE-specific rule-based. Subjectively imputed case series (no written imputation assessment rules) have been used as long as case series of safety outcomes have been utilized for decision-making by the medical community (McEwen, 1999). In the 1980s, rule-based methods were first proposed as a basis for defining product–AE case series criteria (Food and Drug Administration, 1987), while, in the 1990s, the first Bayesian method for analyzing a product–AE case series was published (Naranjo et al., 1990, 1990b). The slow rate of developmental evolution for imputation-oriented procedures probably derives to a great extent from the difficulties that are confronted when sensitivity and specificity data for tests for causality must be combined across multiple cases (Clark et al., 2000). At present, case series imputation continues to consist mostly of descriptions of the prevalence of causality testing in a case series using either descriptive statistical or non-statistical (narrative) means. Widely accepted methods for mathematically combining imputation-based evidence in favor of product–AE causality in a multiple product–AE case series have not yet been published.

CASE SERIES IMPUTATION METHODS

Subjective Case Series

With subjective case series an evaluator diagnostically interprets case causal information without formally specifying rules. As a result, the development of subjectively imputed case series is strongly influenced by an evaluator's individual medical and epidemiologic judgment. As with individual report imputation, subjective assessments of case series are probably the most common way in which associative evidence for product–AE relationships is summarized.

Generalized Rule-Based Case Series

Rule-based case series are created when either minimum, uniform, or a range of causal diagnostic criteria are applied to candidate reports to create and analyze a case series. A traditional approach to this problem is to include cases using an explicit case definition, following which the cases are examined in aggregate for evidence for causality (Clark et al., 1990). A minimum, uniform approach can also be accomplished by applying a generalized rule-based procedure to reports and only accepting high level ratings that are defined by tests for causality as cases ("definite" and "probable", for example) so that imputational value is included in the case series at the time it is generated (George et al., 1998). These strategies establish per-case minimum standards upon which a subsequent summarization of product–AE causal data is based, regardless of the number of cases that are eventually included.

Two published generalized rule-based case series imputation methods that use both imputation and case number features to define case series are the monitored adverse reaction and the quality criteria grading method of Edwards (Food and Drug Administration, 1987; Edwards et al., 1990). The monitored adverse reaction procedure uses a combination of operational causality ratings (as determined by the FDA's rule-based imputation method) and case number to construct a case series with minimum imputation plus numerical features. The FDA's published rule-based method defines a probable case as the presence of positive dechallenge information, a possible case as the presence of "reasonable" temporal sequence, and a remote case as a temporal relationship of any nature (Jones, 1982; Turner, 1984). A monitored adverse reaction is then said to exist if a high-quality case series with any of the following attributes is noted: (1) at least one probable case, (2) at least two possible cases, (3) at least one possible and five remote cases, or (4) at least 10 remote cases (Food and Drug Administration, 1987). The quality criteria grading system of Edwards creates a rule-based case series by specifying imputation, numerical, and/or quality criteria (Edwards et al., 1990). An index case means that either positive rechallenge information is available or the case exhibits no confounding variables, a substantial case means that 11 key variables (which include the six key variables that define feasible cases below) are available for that case, and a feasible case means that six key variables are available for that case. A publishable signal is then said to exist if any combination of at least three index case equivalents are present, where one index case, two substantial cases, or four feasible cases constitute an equivalent. Both the monitored adverse reaction and the Edwards procedure allow the safety evaluator to compensate for decreasing numbers of cases by overweighting key cases with significant diagnostic value, and both are intended as starting points for a case series imputation analysis.

Retrospective Bayesian Analysis

A case series approach based on Bayesian methodology has also been described that is referred to as retrospective Bayesian analysis (Naranjo *et al.*, 1990a, 1990b). In the retrospective Bayesian method, a single estimate for the prior odds for the case series as a whole is estimated from the reported series. Following examination of the included cases, each case is then reassessed in the light of data from all cases, and a calculation of the posterior odds for the entire case series is obtained. A Bayesian-like solution has also been proposed that creates a modified standardized reporting ratio by weighting each possible causal test result sequence for the case series by the number of cases assigned to that stratum (Clark *et al.*, 2000).

AE-Specific Rule-Based Case Series

Rule-based, AE-specific (also called etiologic-diagnostic (Meyboom *et al.*, 1997b)) case series are generated when AE-specific, rule-based methods, which may contain imputation criteria, are applied to candidate reports to generate a case series. Rule-based, AE-specific case series therefore include the concepts of both consensus-developed case definition and causal diagnostic value, and are thought to be well suited for defining and imputing case series data (Meyboom *et al.*, 1997b; Meyboom, 1998). AE-specific case definitions have typically concentrated on the surveillance of AEs known to be frequent complications of health care product use, such as drug-

induced liver injury or hematologic cytopenias (Bénichou, 1990; Benichou and Celigny, 1991; Danan and Benichou, 1993).

SELECTING IMPUTATION-ORIENTED METHODS FOR A PRODUCT-SPECIFIC ADVERSE EVENT SURVEILLANCE PROGRAM

Screening imputation can be carried out on complete sets of AE reports, or can be made more efficient by the antecedent use of sorting measures that produce important AE report subsets for imputation screening review (e.g. the alert (15-day) or designated medical events sorting methods). In selecting imputation screening instruments for use in an AE surveillance database, the characteristics of a good screening test should be kept in mind (ease of use, generalizability, uniformity of result, and low false positive rate). The selected methods should be adaptable to systematic use with AE surveillance data models, and should allow the rapid insertion of an imputation rating into the records of key reports during typically defined workflows. In modifying existing instruments for this purpose, the safety professional will want to define a screening strategy that increases the operational ratings of reports that contain positive tests for causality. False positive rates can be kept low: by increasing the stringency of criteria needed to obtain a high rating, by periodically assessing the results of imputation screening, and adjusting the "set point" of the screening imputation instrument as needed. While maintenance of a low false positive rate could increase the number of false negatives that remain undetected in the AE report database, it should be emphasized that imputation screening is only one of several strategies by which periodic AE database screening is performed, and that AE report database screening will be carried out on a repeat basis (Venulet, 1988). In the presence of a product–AE relationship, false negatives that remain undetected using imputation criteria will likely become detectable either through other non-imputation-based means of product–AE identification, or at the time of subsequent screening evaluations.

Likewise, case series imputation is only one of several possible case series formation strategies that can be used by the safety evaluator to summarize evidence in favor of a product–AE relationship. For example, the standardized reporting ratio, which compares the number of reported cases with the number of expected incident cases, is an important complementary numerical approach (Tubert *et al.*, 1991) (see Chapter 19). In creating case definitions, the safety evaluator can use purely AE-associated criteria, or can require as well imputation-related criteria through the use of either generalized or AE-specific rule-based methods. The final construction of a case series may also involve numerical and report quality criteria. When summarizing aggregate tests for causality, it is useful to identify which tests were used, the number of patients to whom each was applied, and the evaluator's impression of test sensitivity and specificity. The results of positive rechallenge tests, tests that provide physical–chemical linkage with the monitored product, and clinical manifestations indicating spatially localized exposures followed by a localized effect will probably have the greatest discriminative ability, and would therefore warrant the greatest emphasis in final interpretation.

REFERENCES

Amery WK (1999) Signal generation from spontaneous adverse event reports. *Pharmacoepidemiology and Drug Safety* 8: 147–50.

Auriche M (1985) Approache bayésienne de l'imputabilité des phénomènes indésirables aux médicaments. *Therapie* 40: 301.

Bégaud B (1984) Standardized assessment of adverse drug reactions: the method used in France. *Drug Inf J* 18: 275–81.

Bégaud B, Moride Y, Haramburu F (1994) Quality improvement and statistical calculations made on spontaneous reports. *Drug Inf J* 28: 1187–95.

Bégaud B, Royer RJ (1986) The regulatory perspective. *Drug Inf J* 20: 409–12.

Benichou C (1990) Criteria of drug-induced liver disorders. Report of an international consensus meeting. *J Hepat* 11: 272–6.

Benichou C, Celigny PhS (1991) Standardization of definitions and criteria of causality assessment of adverse drug reactions. *Int J Clin Pharmacol Ther Tox* 29: 75–81.

Blanc S, Leuenberger P, Berger JP, Brooke EM, Schelling JL (1979) Judgements of trained observers on adverse drug reactions. *Clin Pharmacol Ther* 25: 493–8.

Blum MD, Graham DJ, McCloskey CA (1994) Temafloxacin syndrome: review of 95 cases. *Clin Inf Dis* 18: 946–50.

Busto U, Naranjo CA, Sellers EM (1982) Comparison of two recently published algorithms for assessing the probability of adverse drug reactions. *Br J Clin Pharmacol* 13: 223–7.

Case B, Oszko MA (1991) Use of an algorithm to evaluate published reports of adverse drug reactions. *Am J Hosp Pharm* 48: 121–2.

Clark JA, Klincewicz SL, LaFrance NL (2000) A Bayesian method for the evaluation of case series of adverse reactions (Abstr). *Pharmacoepidemiology and Drug Safety* 9 (Suppl): S33.

Clark JA, Klincewicz SL, Stang PE (2001) Spontaneous adverse event signaling methods: classification and use with health care treatment products. *Epidemiol Rev* 23: 191–210.

Clark JA, Zimmerman HJ, Tanner LA (1990) Labetalol hepatotoxicity. *Ann Int Med* 113: 210–3.

Cluff LE, Thornton GF, Seidl LG (1964) Studies on the epidemiology of adverse drug reactions. I. Methods of surveillance. *J Am Med Assoc* 188: 976–83.

Code of Federal Regulations (US), Section 312.32.

Danan G, Benichou C (1993) Causality assessment of adverse reactions to drugs—I. A novel method based on the conclusions of international consensus meetings: application to drug-induced liver injuries. *J Clin Epidemiol* 46: 1323–30.

Edwards IR, Lindquist M, Wiholm BE, Napke E (1990) Quality criteria for early signals of possible drug reactions. *Lancet* 336: 156–8.

Emanueli A, Sacchetti G (1980) An algorithm for the classification of untoward events in large scale clinical trials. *Agents Actions* 7: 318–22.

European Agency for the Evaluation of Medicinal Products (EMEA), Committee for Proprietary Medicinal Products (1995) *ICH Topic E2A: Clinical Safety Data Management: Definitions and Standards for Expedited Reporting (CPMP/ICH/377/95)*. London: EMEA, p. 2/10.

European Agency for the Evaluation of Medicinal Products (EMEA), Committee for Proprietary Medicinal Products (1997) *ICH Topic E2C: Clinical Safety Data Management: Periodic Safety Update Reports for Marketed Drugs* (CPMP/ICH/288/95) London: EMEA, pp. 6/22, 15/22–17/22.

Food and Drug Administration (FDA), Center for Drugs and Biologics (1987) *Reports Evaluation Branch Manual*. Rockville: FDA, pp. 23–23a.

Finney DJ (1963) An international drug safety program. *J New Drugs* **3**: 262–5.

Freilich WB (1984) Legal perspectives in causality assessment. *Drug Inf J* **18**: 211–7.

Frick PA, Cohen LG, Rovers JP (1997) Algorithms used in adverse drug event reports: a comparative study. *Ann Pharmacother* **31**: 164–7.

Funch D, Dreyer NA, Bassin LG, Crawley JA, Brickley MG, Walker AM (1993) The validity of case reports in a pharmacoepidemiologic study. *Post Marketing Surveillance* **7**: 283–9.

George JN, Raskob GE, Shah SR, Rizvima MA, Hamilton SA, Osborne S, Vondracek T (1998) Drug-induced thrombocytopenia: a systematic review of published case reports. *Ann Int Med* **129**: 886–90.

Ghajar BM, Lanctôt KL, Shear NH, Naranjo CA (1989) Bayesian differential diagnosis of a cutaneous reaction associated with the administration of sulfonamides. *Semin Dermatol* **8**: 213–8.

Greenland S, Rothman KJ (1998) Measures of effect and association. In: Rothman KJ, Greenland S, eds., *Modern Epidemiology*. Philadelphia: Lippincott-Raven, pp. 51–6.

Grohmann R, Dirschedl P, Scherer J, Schmidt LG, Wunderlich O (1985) Reliability of adverse drug reaction assessment in psychiatric inpatients. *Eur Arch Psychiatr Neurol Sci* **235**: 158–63.

Hartmann K, Ciorciaro C, Kuhn M (1997) Signal generation in a non-EU country. *Pharmacoepidemiology and Drug Safety* **6** (Suppl 3): S13–S19.

Hoskins RE, Manning S (1992) Causality assessment of adverse drug reactions using decision support and informatics tools. *Pharmacoepidemiology and Drug Safety* **1**: 235–49.

Hutchinson TA (1986) Standardized assessment methods for adverse drug reactions: a review of previous approaches and their problems. *Drug Inf J* **20**: 439–44.

Hutchinson TA, Flegel KM, HoPingKong H, Bloom WS, Kramer MS, Trummer EG (1983) Reasons for disagreement in the standardized assessment of suspected adverse drug reactions. *Clin Pharmacol Ther* **34**: 421–6.

Hutchinson TA, Lane DA (1989) Assessing methods for causality assessment of suspected adverse drug reactions. *J Clin Epidemiol* **42**: 5–16.

Hutchinson TA, Leventhal JM, Kramer MS, Karch FE, Lipman AG, Feinstein AR (1979) An algorithm for the operational assessment of adverse drug reactions. II. Demonstration of reproducibility and validity. *J Am Med Assoc* **242**: 633–8.

Inman B (1993) 30 years in postmarketing surveillance. A personal perspective. *Pharmacoepidemiology and Drug Safety* **2**: 239–58.

Inman WHS, Mushin WW (1974) Jaundice after repeated exposure to halothane: an analysis of reports to the Committee on Safety Of Medicines. *Br Med J* **1**: 5–10.

Irey NS (1976a) Tissue reactions to drugs. *Am J Path* **82**: 616–47.

Irey NS (1976b) Adverse drug reactions and death: A review of 827 cases. *J Am Med Assoc* **236**: 575–8.

Jones JK (1982) Adverse drug reactions in the community health setting: approaches to recognizing, counseling, and reporting. *Fam Comm Health* **5**: 58–67.

Jones JK (1987) A Bayesian approach to causality assessment. *Psychopharm Bull* **23**: 395–9.

Jones JK (1994) Determining causation from case reports. In: Strom BL, ed., *Pharmacoepidemiology*, 2nd edn. New York: Wiley, pp. 365–78.

Karch FE, Lasagna L (1977) Toward the operational identification of adverse drug reactions. *Clin Pharmacol Ther* **21**: 247–54.

Karch FE, Smith CL, Kerzner B, Mazzullo JM, Weintraub M, Lasagna L (1976) Adverse drug reactions: a matter of opinion. *Clin Pharmacol Ther* **19**: 489–92.

Koch-Weser J, Greenblatt DJ (1976) The ambiguity of adverse drug reactions (Abstr). *Clin Pharmacol Ther* **19**: 110.

Koch-Weser J, Sellers EM, Zacest R (1977) The ambiguity of adverse drug reactions. *Eur J Clin Pharmacol* **11**: 75–8.

Kramer MS (1986) Assessing causality of adverse drug reactions: global introspection and its limitations. *Drug Inf J* **20**: 433–7.

Kramer MS (1988a) *Clinical Epidemiology and Biostatistics*. New York: Springer-Verlag, pp. 266–7.

Kramer MS (1988b) *Clinical Epidemiology and Biostatistics*. New York: Springer-Verlag, pp. 201–19.

Kramer MS (1988c) *Clinical Epidemiology and Biostatistics*. New York: Springer-Verlag, pp. 220–35.

Kramer MS, Lane DA (1992) Causal propositions in clinical research and practice. *J Clin Epidemiol* **45**: 639–49.

Kramer MS, Leventhal JM, Hutchinson TA, Feinstein AR (1979) An algorithm for the operational assessment of adverse drug reactions: I. Background, description, and instructions for use. *J Am Med Assoc* **242**: 623–32.

Lanctôt KL, Naranjo CA (1995) Comparison of the Bayesian approach and a simple algorithm for assessment of adverse drug events. *Clin Pharmacol Ther* **58**: 692–8.

Lane DA (1984) A probabilist's view of causality assessment. *Drug Inf J* **18**: 323–30.

Lane DA (1986a) The logic of uncertainty: measuring degree of belief. *Drug Inf J* **20**: 445–53.

Lane DA (1986b) The Bayesian approach to causality assessment: an introduction. *Drug Inf J* **20**: 455–61.

Lane DA, Kramer MS, Hutchinson TA, Jones JK, Naranjo C (1987) The causality assessment of adverse drug reactions using a Bayesian approach. *Pharmaceut Med* **2**: 265–83.

Leventhal JM, Hutchinson TA, Kramer MS, Feinstein AR (1979) An algorithm for the operational assessment of adverse drug reactions. III. Results of tests among clinicians. *J Am Med Assoc* **242**: 1991–4.

Louik C, Lacouture PG, Mitchell AA, Kauffman R, Lovejoy FH, Yaffe SJ, Shapiro S (1985) A study of adverse reaction algorithms in a drug surveillance program. *Clin Pharmacol Ther* **38**: 183–7.

MacDonald MG, MacKay BR (1964) Adverse drug reactions: experience of Mary Fletcher Hospital during 1962. *J Am Med Assoc* **190**: 1071–4.

McEwen J (1999) Adverse reactions—a pesonal view of their history. *Int J Pharm Med* **13**: 269–77.

Meyboom RHB (1998) Causality assessment revisited. *Pharmacoepidemiology and Drug Safety* **7**: S63–S65.

Meyboom RH, Egberts AC, Edwards IR, Hekster YA, de Koning FHP, Gribnau FWJ (1997a) Principles of signal detection in pharmacovigilance. *Drug Safety* **16**: 355–65.

Meyboom RH, Hekster YA, Egberts AC, Gribnau FW, Edwards IR (1997b) Causal or casual? The role of causality assessment in pharmacovigilance. *Drug Safety* **17**: 374–89.

Meyboom RHB, Royer RJ (1992) Causality classification at pharmacovigilance centres in the European Community. *Pharmacoepidemiology and Drug Safety* **1**: 87–97.

Michel DJ, Knodel LC (1986) Comparison of three algorithms used to evaluate adverse drug reactions. *Am J Hosp Pharm* **43**: 1709–14.

Miremont G, Haramburu F, Bégaud B, Péré JC, Dangoumau J (1994) Adverse drug reactions: physicians' opinions versus a causality assessment method. *Eur J Clin Pharmacol* **46**: 285–9.

Naranjo CA (1986) A clinical pharmacologic perspective on the detection and assessment of adverse drug reactions. *Drug Inf J* **20**: 387–93.

Naranjo CA, Busto U, Sellers EM, Sandor P, Ruiz I, Roberts EA, Janecek E, Domecq C, Greenblatt DJ (1981) A method for estimating the probability of adverse drug reactions. *Clin Pharmacol Ther* **30**: 239–45.

Naranjo CA, Kwok MCO, Lanctôt, KL, Zhao HP, Spielberg SP, Shear NH (1994) Enhanced differential diagnosis of anticonvulsant hypersensitivity reactions by an integrated Bayesian and biochemical approach. *Clin Pharm Ther* **56**: 564–75.

Naranjo CA, Lanctôt KL (1991) Recent developments in computer-assisted diagnosis of putative adverse drug reactions. *Drug Safety* **6**: 315–22.

Naranjo CA, Lanctôt KL (1993) Bayesian evaluation of sequential cases of neutropenia. *Pharmacoepidemiology and Drug Safety* **2**: S1–S6.

Naranjo CA, Lanctôt KL, Lane DA (1990a) The Bayesian differential diagnosis of neutropenia associated with antiarrhythmic agents. *J Clin Pharmacol* **30**: 1120–7.

Naranjo CA, Lane D, Ho-Asjoe M, Lanctôt KL (1990b) A Bayesian assessment of idiosyncratic adverse reactions to new drugs: Guillain-Barré Syndrome and zimeldine. *J Clin Pharmacol* **30**: 174–80.

Péré JC, Bégaud B, Haramburu F, Albin H (1986) Computerized comparison of six adverse drug reaction assessment procedures. *Clin Pharmacol Ther* **40**: 451–61.

Rossi AC, Knapp DE (1984) Discovery of new adverse drug reactions. A review of the Food and Drug Administration's Spontaneous Reporting System. *J Am Med Assoc* **252**: 1030–3.

Rothman KJ, Greenland S (1998) Causation and causal inference. In: Rothman KJ, Greenland S, eds., *Modern Epidemiology*. Philadelphia, PA: Lippincott-Raven, pp. 7–28.

Schmidt LG, Dirshedl P, Grohmann R, Scherer J, Wunderlich O, Muller-Oerlinghausen B (1986) Consistency of assessment of adverse drug reactions in psychiatric hospitals: a comparison of an algorithmic and an empirical approach. *Eur J Clin Pharm* **30**: 199–204.

Seidl LG, Thornton GF, Cluff LE (1965) Epidemiological studies of adverse drug reactions. *Am J Pub Health* **55**: 1170–5.

Sicker Th, Hoffmann A, Hoffmann H (1998) Individual case assessment of venous thromboembolic events suspected to be associated with combined oral contraceptives. Experience of reevaluating individual case histories on Valette®. *Pharmacoepidemiology and Drug Safety* **7** (Suppl): S109–S10.

Stephens MDB (1999) Causality assessment and signal recognition. In: Stephens MDB, Talbot JCC, Routledge PA, eds., *Detection of New Adverse Drug Reactions*. London: Macmillan Reference Ltd (UK), pp. 297–318.

Tubert P, Bégaud B, Haramburu F, Péré JC (1991) Spontaneous reporting: how many cases are required to trigger a warning? *Br J Clin Pharmacol* **32**: 407–8.

Turner WM (1984) The Food and Drug Administration algorithm. Special workshop–regulatory. *Drug Inf J* **118**: 259–66.

Venning GR (1983) Identification of adverse reactions to new drugs. I: What have been the important adverse reactions since thalidomide? *Br Med J* **286**: 199–202.

Venulet J (1984) Aspects of standardization as applied to the assessment of drug-event associations. *Drug Inf J* **18**: 199–210.

Venulet J (1985) Informativity of adverse drug reactions data in medical publications. *Drug Inf J* **19**: 357–65.

Venulet J (1986) Incomplete information as a limiting factor in causality assessment of adverse drug reactions and its practical consequences. *Drug Inf J* **20**: 423–31.

Venulet J (1988) Possible strategies for early recognition of potential drug safety problems. *Adv Drug React Ac Pois Rev* **1**: 39–47.

Venulet J (1992) Role and place of causality assessment. *Pharmacoepidemiology and Drug Safety* **1**: 225–34.

Wartenberg D, Greenberg M (1993) Solving the cluster puzzle: clues to follow and pitfalls to avoid. *Stat Med* **12**: 1763–70.

19

Overview—Spontaneous Signalling

JOHN A. CLARK

Galt Associates, Inc., Sterling, VA, USA

STEPHEN L. KLINCEWICZ

Johnson and Johnson Pharmaceutical Research and Development LLC, Titusville, NJ, USA

PAUL E. STANG

Galt Associates Inc., Blue Bell, PA, USA, and University of North Carolina School of Public Health, Chapel Hill, NC, USA

INTRODUCTION

Since the systematic recording of pharmaceutical product-related adverse events (AEs) was first proposed by Finney after the thalidomide tragedy, regulators, public health organizations, and manufacturers have been faced with the difficult task of interpreting postmarketing AE signals that arise from health care product surveillance programs (Finney, 1963, 1964, 1965). Health care product monitoring is based on data from four major data sources: spontaneous reports, medical literature case reports or case series, human studies, and pharmacologic or toxicologic experiments (European Agency for the Evaluation of Medicinal Products, 1995, 1997) (see Table 19.1). Of these, spontaneous reporting is typically the largest contributor (Faich et al., 1987; Faich, 1996). The term "spontaneous" refers to unsolicited AE reports that are forwarded to manufacturers or regulators, pertain to individual patients, and are not derived from either the medical literature or studies. Spontaneous reporting systems have become the foundation of postmarketing surveillance programs because of the high volume of information they supply, their low maintenance costs, and their demonstrated usefulness when supervised by experienced evaluators (Bégaud et al., 1994a). This chapter summarizes and integrates the published literature pertaining to spontaneous signalling methods and AE surveillance program design.

While the emphasis in this chapter is on how spontaneous reports can be used to generate signals, safety professionals should note that the terms "spontaneous" and "signalling" are not equivalent. Spontaneous reports are only one data source from which postmarketing AE signals can be generated. With the exception of the circumstance in which a safety outcome is hypothesized a priori and then tested using a study design, any source of relevant data with a bearing on a marketed product's risk profile can give rise to postmarketing AE signals (Meyboom et al., 1997a; Waller and Lee, 1999).

Pharmacovigilance. Edited by R.D. Mann and E.B. Andrews
© 2002 John Wiley & Sons, Ltd

Table 19.1. Data sources for AE surveillance programs.

Spontaneous reports
● To manufacturers
● To regulatory agencies

Literature case reports
● Single case reports
● Case report series

Studies (published or unpublished)
● Clinical studies
● Epidemiologic studies

Pre-clinical and toxicological data
● *In vitro* experiments
● Animal models
● Toxicologic studies

This point also extends to signalling logic itself, since similar signalling methods can often be applied to AE information arising from different data sources. This is particularly true for individual patient reports from spontaneous, literature, and study environments, all three of which are subject to report forwarding under the same general regulatory scheme, and are usually organized by manufacturers and regulators in the same "spontaneous" database. Thus, safety evaluators should recognize that, while this discussion focuses on signalling from spontaneous reports, overlap is considerable among the various postmarketing data sources and the signalling methods that are applied to them.

SPONTANEOUS AE SIGNALS, SIGNALLING METHODS, AND SIGNALLING PROGRAMS

THE RATIONALE FOR SPONTANEOUS AE SIGNALLING

It is now well accepted that spontaneous reporting programs contribute to the comprehensive risk assessment of health care products as they are actually used in medical practice (Faich, 1986; Carson *et al.*, 1994; Council of International Organization of Medical Sciences, 1998; Abenheim *et al.*, 1999; Institute of Medicine, 1999; Food and Drug Administration, 1999). However, it has also been established that spontaneous evaluations are

speculative at their outset. Consequently, prior to wide acceptance, spontaneous assessments require demonstration of consistency using multiple methods, and may require confirmation from non-spontaneous data sources. Spontaneous methodology should therefore not be regarded as generating precise estimates (the calculation of incidence rates, for example), but, rather, as providing the constituents of signalling arguments (Goldman, 1998) (see Figure 19.1). In the public health literature, such activities are sometimes referred to as "pre-epidemiology" to distinguish them from the more formalized logic of observational studies (Wartenberg and Greenberg, 1993).

SPONTANEOUS AE SIGNALS

The primary focus of spontaneous safety data review is the detection of AE signals, which can be defined as any potential product–AE relationship that deserves further attention (including clarification of a product–AE relationship that has already been described) (Lindquist *et al.*, 1999). While newly discovered product–AE causal pairs are generally the most important findings of AE surveillance programs, a causal argument is not the only kind of relationship that has been investigated using spontaneous reports. Other potentially important observations include the identification of non-causal associations, the clinical spectrum of a product–AE pair, the patient subtypes and medical circumstances associated with a product-induced adverse reaction, clues to the mechanism of action by which product

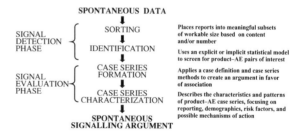

Figure 19.1. Steps in the spontaneous AE signalling process. Reproduced from Clark *et al.* (2001), *Epidemiologic Reviews* 23(2), 191–210, Fig. 1, with permission from Oxford University Press.

exposure leads to an adverse reaction, factors associated with the initiation of reporting behavior, and unintended benefits that can be developed as secondary indications (Bateman *et al.*, 1986; Hart *et al.*, 1987; Rawlins, 1988; Moride *et al.*, 1997; Tubert-Bitter *et al.*, 1998).

SPONTANEOUS AE SIGNALLING METHODS

Spontaneous AE signals are generated when statistical or non-statistical methods are applied to spontaneous AE data (Venulet, 1973). Although the manner in which a particular drug–AE pair comes to attention (spontaneous AE signalling method) has sometimes been used synonymously with the subject matter that was identified (spontaneous AE signal), signalling methods are better defined as procedures that are independent of content. This convention is consistent with the observation that particular spontaneous AE signals are often generated simultaneously by more than one signalling method (Inman, 1970; Meyboom *et al.*, 1997a). AE signalling methods can be applied to report/case sets numbering from one to thousands, range in applicability from extremely limited to nearly universal, and encompass a variety of functions from simple sorting procedures for creating workable subsets of reports (Finney, 1971a; Amery, 1999) to complex analyses of case series that eventually come to be regarded as definitive (Blum *et al.*, 1994).

SPONTANEOUS AE SIGNALLING PROGRAMS

The spontaneous component of an AE signalling program is created when one or more spontaneous signalling methods are applied systematically to the AE reports for a particular product (Royall, 1971; Venulet, 1988). Spontaneous signalling programs are administered by international agencies (e.g. the World Health Organization (WHO), by national bodies (e.g. individual country regulators), by regional surveillance programs (e.g. regional pharmacovigilance units in France and Spain), and by manufacturers (e.g. manufacturer-based drug safety departments). In the past, for convenience, such signalling programs have usually been carried out as standardized regimens that were applied uncritically to multiple drugs. However, since AE signals are ultimately interpreted in the context of a particular product (Finney, 1965), spontaneous AE signalling programs are essentially product-specific (the term "product" means one or more dosage forms that are monitored together as a distinct entity). In general, the inclusion of a signalling method in a spontaneous AE signalling program should address an applicable epidemiologic, medical, or regulatory design principle and should be consistent with the International Conference on Harmonization E2A and E2C guidances (European Agency for the Evaluation of Medicinal Products, 1995, 1997; International Society for Pharmacoepidemiology, 1996).

SPONTANEOUS SIGNALLING STEPS, DATA STRATEGIES, AND PROGRAM DESIGN

SPONTANEOUS SIGNALLING ARGUMENTS

Report Phase Signalling (Signal Detection)
Versus Case Phase Signalling (Signal Evaluation)

It is useful to classify spontaneous signalling methods around several broad functional steps that comprise signalling arguments, namely sorting, identification, case series formation and case series characterization (see Figure 19.1 and Table 19.2). The first two steps (sorting and identification) are based on reports, while the second two (case series formation and characterization) are based on only those reports that meet a case definition. The report-based steps and case-based steps are sometimes referred to as the signal detection and signal evaluation phases, respectively. Report phase followed by case phase signalling programs probably evolved from the basic attributes of spontaneous surveillance: (1) the large number of different product–AE pairs that are reported for any given product; (2) the relatively small number of product–AE pairs that are found to be important from a surveillance perspective; and (3) the need to carefully examine spontaneous report data prior to the initiation of

Table 19.2. Classification of spontaneous report signalling methods by functional step and data strategy.

Functional steps	Data strategies		
	Qualitative intra-product	Quantitative	
		Intra-product	Inter-product
Sorting	*Qualitative sorting methods* ● Key content methods	*Quantitative sorting methods* ● Subjective judgment ● Cutoff criteria	
Identification	*Imputation screening assessments* ● Subjective judgment ● Rule-based methods ● Statistical models	*Intra-product quantitative identification methods* ● Serial (increased frequency) identification methods ● Temporospatial cluster identification methods	*Inter-product identification methods* ● 2 × 2 table count methods ● Bayesian data mining methods
Case series formation	*Intra-product qualitative case series formation methods* ● Subjective case series ● Rule-based case series ● Retrospective Bayesian analysis	*Intra-product quantitative case series formation methods* ● Standardized reporting ratio ● Associative case–control study	*Inter-product case series formation methods* ● Spontaneous cohort design ● Spontaneous case–control design
Case series characterization	*Intra-product qualitative case series characterization methods* ● Descriptive case distribution	*Intra-product quantitative case series characterization methods* ● Numerator-only case distribution ● Rate/proportion-based case distribution ● Characterization case–control study	*Inter-product case series characterization methods* ● Comparative case distribution

Reproduced from Clark *et al.* (2001), *Epidemiologic Reviews*, 23(2), 191–210, Table 1, with permission from Oxford University Press.

safety labelling changes or other responses. These considerations suggest that spontaneous AE surveillance programs must be able efficiently to narrow a large number of reported product–AE pairs to a short list of high priority candidates, from which resource intensive case series are then compiled (Institute of Medicine, 1999).

Signalling Steps

In the sorting step (a report-based step), reports are assigned to subsets using data management tools (see Figure 19.1). The aim of sorting is to break down an undifferentiated collection of reports into meaningful subsets of manageable size. In the identification step (a report-based step) an explicit or implicit statistical model is used to select product–AE pairs for further scrutiny. Identification is therefore a form of screening in which a database of product–AE reports, each containing at least one product–AE pair, is screened for relationships that are "interesting". In the case series formation step (a case-based step), a report series of a single product–AE pair is compiled and is evaluated according to a case definition. Case series formation involves: (1) creation of a reasonably homogenous product–AE report series; (2) exclusion of reports that do not meet minimum criteria; (3) creation of a multiple case series that has medico-epidemiologic meaning; and (4) summarization of the resulting evidence in favor of a product–AE relationship. In the case series characterization step (a case-based step) the case series is further examined for patterns and disproportions. The purpose of case series characterization is, to the extent possible, to identify biologic mechanisms, risk factors, and features that are related to reporting behaviour.

SPONTANEOUS SIGNALLING DATA STRATEGIES

The development of signalling arguments can be accomplished using at least three different data strategies: intra-product qualitative methods, intra-product quantitative methods, and inter-product quantitative methods (see Table 19.2). Qualitative methods assess one or more content elements of a particular report or case series, while quantitative methods apply procedures involving numbers, proportions, or rates to groups of reports or cases. Both qualitative and quantitative methods are ultimately concerned with identifying and describing potentially associative (but not necessarily causal) relationships, but do so using different logical frameworks (Kramer and Lane, 1992).

Quantitative data strategies can be further subdivided into intra-product and inter-product procedures. Intra-product methods generate signals by examining spontaneous reports in the context of the index (monitored) product and its user population, while inter-product methods work by comparing spontaneous reporting for the index product to spontaneous reporting for another product(s) (Bégaud et al., 1994a). Unlike intra-product methods, which can be either qualitative or quantitative, the inter-product methods that have been described to date are all quantitative. Intra- versus inter-product logic is a fundamental feature of spontaneous signalling method design and has been a factor throughout the history of its development (Rawlins, 1988).

DESIGNING SPONTANEOUS SIGNALLING PROGRAMS

In order to generate fully formed signalling arguments on a timely, ongoing basis, one or more AE signalling methods must be deployed in a logical design that facilitates the refinement of collections of raw reports into finished spontaneous signals. To accomplish this, report-based procedures, which are amenable to automation, are first used to create a list of "interesting" product–AE pairs (Finney, 1965, 1974; DuMouchel, 1999). Then, case-based procedures, which are time intensive and epidemiologic in orientation, are used to refine these suggestions into full-fledged arguments. This sequence corresponds roughly to the concepts of "hypothesis generating" and "hypothesis strengthening" that have been invoked to explain signalling methodology (Meyboom et al., 1997a). In establishing spontaneous signalling programs, it makes sense for the evaluator to select signalling methods that can meet monitoring program requirements, including: (1) type of spontaneous reporting system providing the report data; (2) appropriateness of particular data strategies; (3) applicability of the proposed methods to the monitored product and its use; and (4) complementarity and non-duplication of function among methods selected for the program.

SPONTANEOUS SIGNALLING METHODS

SPONTANEOUS SIGNALLING METHODS USED AT THE SORTING STEP

Sorting procedures are data management screens that create report sets of regulatory and/or epidemiologic interest. Historically, they have been considered a form of signalling (Bégaud et al., 1994a), although their results are almost always re-examined through the application of additional techniques. Sorting methods are the basic data management tools of spontaneous signalling, and are probably the most common signalling procedures used in health care product surveillance. The careful inclusion of report sorting in a product-specific surveillance program is generally believed to be important in enhancing its effectiveness (European Agency for the Evaluation of Medicinal Products, 1997).

Qualitative Sorting (Key Content) Methods

Qualitative sorting by key content selects subsets of reports for further examination that contain content elements of interest from a regulatory, medical, or report quality perspective (Hartmann et al., 1997). Qualitative sorting allows an evaluator to break down a large reporting universe into smaller, more meaningful parcels, which can then be considered separately by safety professionals. Perhaps the most important qualitative sorting methodology is the well-known alert (or 15-day) report, which depends on the AE seriousness and local labelling data fields that are added to spontaneous reports by manufacturers (Venulet, 1988). Key content methods often focus as well on data fields believed to possess diagnostic value (e.g. positive dechallenge or rechallenge), important outcomes (Finney, 1971a; Venulet, 1988) (e.g. fatal, life-threatening), previously unreported AE types (Royall, 1971; Royall and Venulet, 1972), or AE types of high interest (Hartmann et al., 1997), such as those included in the Food and Drug Administration's (FDA) partial listing of designated medical events (Food and Drug Administration, 2000).

Quantitative Sorting Methods

Subjective Judgment

The first published quantitative sorting method was based on a subjective impression of excessive report numbers (the "pigeon hole" signal of Napke) (Napke, 1968). Although a formal evaluation of subjective quantitative signalling has not been published, the same limitations that are seen with subjective methods in general (i.e. increased intra- and inter-observer variability) would be expected to apply (see the section Imputation Screening (Causality) Assessments below).

Cutoff Criteria

Cutoff signalling methods refer to procedures that detect an arbitrary number of reports of a product–AE pair. While unrefined, cutoff criteria have long been regarded as useful mechanisms for directing resources (Finney, 1971a; Royall, 1971; Venulet, 1973; Hartmann et al., 1997; Lindquist et al., 1999). Simple approaches such as cutoff methods may be the only reasonable quantitative approach for drug-specific AE surveillance programs that accumulate few reports, since, in this setting, more elaborate procedures are often not feasible.

SPONTANEOUS SIGNALLING METHODS USED AT THE IDENTIFICATION STEP

Identification procedures apply explicit or implicit statistical models to one or more spontaneous reports in order to screen for product–AE pairs of interest. Much of the published statistical research concerning AE signalling methodology has been directed toward developing methods that are used at this step. Like sorting, the identification step is carried out using reports, not cases, so that the output of such activity is intended to undergo further refinement using case-based methods. It has long been well understood that the use of statistical models at this step is intended to automate the process of finding product–AE pairs that are "suspicious" or "interesting", and does not represent a form of hypothesis testing (Finney, 1971a, 1971b, 1982; DuMouchel, 1999). It is helpful to think of identification procedures as "screening tests" that are applied to report databases in order to find potentially important material.

As noted in Table 19.3, procedures employed at the identification (screening) step of signalling should be: (1) easy to use, (2) generalizable to many product–AE pairs, (3) associated with a low false positive rate, (4) amenable to automation, and (5) capable of producing uniform output. Although achieving all of these objectives simultaneously is

Table 19.3. Characteristics of a good method used at the identification (screening) step of spontaneous signalling.

- Easy to use
- Generalizable to many product–AE pairs
- Associated with a low false positive rate
- Amenable to automation
- Capable of producing uniform output

difficult, program designers can improve the effectiveness of AE database screening programs by increasing the specificity (and, concomitantly, decreasing the sensitivity) of instruments used at the identification step, as illustrated in Figure 19.2.

Panel A of Figure 19.2 emphasizes that the function of the identification step is to look within product–AE databases for the presence of "interesting" safety outcomes. This process is screening-oriented (not patient- or diagnostic-oriented), and is associated with a sensitivity, specificity, positive predictive value, and likelihood ratio for "interesting" safety issues. Panel B of Figure 19.2 demonstrates that, in the presence of a low prevalence of "interesting" product–AE pairs (a typical situation in postmarketing surveillance), the likelihood ratio for those safety outcomes that are identified must be extremely high if a reasonable positive predictive value for the program is to be achieved. This latter attribute is critical because the positive predictive value of the report-based identification step is equivalent to the proportion of safety outcomes selected for intensive, case-based work-up that are subsequently found to be programmatically significant. Failure to maintain this proportion at an acceptable level quickly leads to saturation of evaluative resources, and, in the long run, to an ineffective AE surveillance effort (Institute of Medicine, 1999).

In recent years, much emphasis has been placed on the use of complex statistical models to carry out the identification step of signalling. There is no evidence, however, that departing from the basic idea of report-based screening, as originally articulated by Finney (Finney, 1965, 1974) has improved the efficiency of AE surveillance programs. On the contrary, the design principles discussed above, as well as actual US experience with "increased frequency" methods (see the section Serial Identification Methods below), suggest that statistical modelling will have to be used carefully and employed selectively if excessive false positive rates are to be avoided.

A. Screening For "Interesting" Product AEs

Screening Result		Interesting	
		Yes	No
	Yes	TP = True Positive	FP = False Positive
	No	FN = False Negative	TN = True Negative

Sensitivity = TP / (TP + FN)

Specificity = TN / (TN + FP)

Positive Predictive Value = TP / (TP + FP)

Likelihood Ratio = Sensitivity / (1 − Specificity)

B. Report Phase Positive Predictive Value (PPV)

$$PPV = \frac{(Sensitivity)\,(X)}{(Sensitivity)\,(X) + (1 - Specificity)\,(Y)} \approx \frac{1}{1 + 1/(P\,LR)}$$

PPV = positive predictive value for screening

X = number of "interesting" AEs in product database *

Y = number of "not interesting" AEs in product database *

P = underlying probability of interesting product AE–pairs

LR = likelihood ratio for a positive screen

* X is assumed to be small in comparison to Y

Figure 19.2. The identification step of signalling.

Imputation Screening (Causality) Assessments

Imputation screening assessments use single-report evaluations to identify a signal (i.e. they implement the signalling process by screening for reports that contain diagnostically suggestive information). When used at the identification step to search spontaneous report databases, imputation is not intended to establish or refute product–AE causality, but, rather, like all identification methods, attempts to find promising product–AE pairs (Venulet, 1992; Meyboom et al., 1997a; Stephens, 1999). Thus, the reader should recognize that the use of the term "causality assessment" to describe report-based imputation is misleading. In this chapter we will use instead the term "imputation screening".

Imputation methodology has undergone extensive refinement over the past four decades (Lane et al., 1987; Kramer and Lane, 1992; Naranjo and Lanctôt, 1993). Starting from pure subjectivity, it evolved into formalized procedures based on rules, and then into more specific probabilistic calculations derived from Bayes' Theorem. More complex approaches, such as decision support algorithms, have also been suggested (Hoskins and Manning, 1992). However, essentially no experience exists in which Bayesian or other statistical models have been used systematically to screen spontaneous databases for product–AE signals. Although formal studies are lacking, it is likely that elaborate, diagnostically oriented models will have limited applicability at the identification step of spontaneous signalling due to their complexity and emphasis on individualization.

Subjective Judgment

In the simplest form of imputation screening, subjective assessment (also called global introspection (Kramer, 1986) or unstructured clinical judgment (Jones, 1994)), an evaluator assigns a causal rating to an individual spontaneous AE report based on medical diagnostic experience (MacDonald and MacKay, 1964). Subjective assessments usually have involved classification into imputation categories, such as the designations "documented", "probable", "possible", and "doubtful" proposed in the 1960s and still used in modified form in AE evaluations today (Cluff et al., 1964; Seidl et al., 1965). It has been shown that subjectively generated causality assessments are associated with high levels of intra- and inter-rater variability (Karch et al., 1976; Koch-Weser and Greenblatt, 1976; Koch-Weser et al., 1977; Blanc et al., 1979; Naranjo et al., 1981) and produce results that can differ substantially from imputation methods based on more explicit methods (Miremont et al., 1994). This imprecision stems in large part from the multifactorial nature of AE causality, which makes reproducible evaluations difficult to carry out in the absence of a formal rating procedure (Kramer, 1986). Nonetheless, global introspection probably remains the method most widely used for screening imputation (Meyboom and Royer, 1992; Jones, 1994; Hartmann et al., 1997).

Rule-Based Methods

With rule-based methods (also called standardized assessment methods (Hutchinson et al., 1983;

Hutchinson, 1986) or standardized decision aids (Naranjo, 1986)), evaluation of an individual AE report is scored using a questionnaire or an algorithm (Lane et al., 1987; Hutchinson and Lane, 1989; Bégaud et al., 1994a; Jones, 1994). Rule-based methods have been shown to decrease intra- and inter-rater variability, and can therefore improve the uniformity of ratings that are assigned to candidate reports in spontaneous databases (Hutchinson et al., 1979; Busto et al., 1982). A large number of such generalized, rule-based instruments have been published, beginning with that of Irey (Irey, 1976a, 1976b; Karch and Lasagna, 1977; Kramer et al., 1979; Naranjo et al., 1981). Rule-based methods intended for use with a particular AE have also been developed (Danan and Benichou, 1993). However, there is essentially no published experience in which such AE-specific rule-based methods have been used systematically to screen spontaneous databases.

Several concerns have been raised about the use of rule-based methods that have implications for their value as database screening methodologies (Naranjo and Lanctôt, 1993). These include residual inter-rater variability (Case and Oszko, 1991), poor performance in actual surveillance environments (Leventhal et al., 1979; Grohmann et al., 1985; Louik et al., 1985; Schmidt et al., 1986; Meyboom, 1998), and the lack of inter-method comparability or translation methodologies (Michel and Knodel, 1986; Péré et al., 1986; Hutchinson and Lane, 1989; Frick et al., 1997) (see Chapter 18, Algorithms). The latter observation underlines the inappropriateness of the word "standardized" to describe rule-based methods, since such instruments neither conform to an accepted standard nor produce standard output. Rule-based methods are better thought of as a group of independently designed expert systems that possess similar report assessment features. The biggest problem facing the implementation of rule-based methods as identification procedures in AE report databases is the lack of information to evaluate their performance as screening tests. Given the absence of studies to support the use of any particular approach to screening imputation, health care product manufacturers and regulatory agencies will likely continue to use a multiplicity of instruments (and their modifications) for this purpose.

Bayesian and Other Statistical Models

Bayesian analysis is the most individualized formal imputation method that has been applied thus far to the evaluation of single-report content (Lane, 1984; Auriche, 1985). The odds form of Bayes" expression can be thought of as the underlying statistical model from which more simplistic rule-based methods are derived. The model requires the evaluator to stipulate an initial estimate of the ratio of probabilities favoring causality versus non-causality for a given product–AE pair among exposed patients (the prior odds) (see the section Bayesian Odds Model in Chapter 18). This quantity is then multiplied by AE occurrence-specific likelihood ratios. Each likelihood ratio is formed by dividing the probability for a risk factor or test result (usually a temporal test) under the condition of causality by the probability for the same risk factor/test result under the condition of other causality. The resulting quantity (the posterior odds) is the theoretical best estimate for the odds in favor of product versus other causal explanations, and is calculated for each AE occurrence in each affected patient (Lane, 1984, 1986a, 1986b; Auriche, 1985; Lane *et al.*, 1987).

Bayesian assessments are time-intensive, requiring a large number of assumptions and calculations, and are individualized on a patient-by-patient basis (Jones, 1994). The latter attribute is reflected in relatively low correlations between Bayesian and rule-based assessments. Bayesian methodology is not algorithmic, but instead relies upon report-specific epidemiologic estimates and case data modelling that are strongly influenced by empirical observation (Lanctôt and Naranjo, 1995). Although Bayesian calculations can be automated to an extent (Naranjo and Lanctôt, 1993), they will likely always require significant time input on the part of the operator. These considerations suggest that the Bayesian odds model is fundamentally a diagnostic tool whose primary application is to formally evaluate etiologic alternatives in those unusual situations where single-case diagnosis of safety outcomes is

warranted (investigatory purposes, for example). Thus, as a result of complexity and the need for recomputation on a report-by-report basis, the Bayesian odds model, as well as other statistical procedures that have been proposed for use with spontaneous data (Hoskins and Manning, 1992), have limited applicability as screening tools for AE surveillance programs.

Intra-Product Quantitative Identification Methods

Intra-product quantitative identification methods (serial (increased frequency) methods and temporospatial cluster identification methods) enumerate groups of reports of similar content for the same product over time or time–space in order to identify an AE signal. The statistical models that have been used for serial identification methods have often been based on a two-group Poisson model, while temporospatial cluster identification methods use established clustering procedures to identify localized increases in the reporting rate of a product–AE pair. Past experience indicates that, when applied routinely to collections of spontaneous reports, knowledge of the limitations of serial methodology is important. A good example of this occurred in the United States, where a regulatory requirement for serial signalling was eventually withdrawn as a result of a high "false alarm" (false positive) rate (Food and Drug Administration, 1996, 1997). In contrast to serial methods, procedures that focus on temporospatial clustering identification have received little attention from the AE signalling community, although there are both theoretical and practical bases for the application of these techniques in AE surveillance programs (Moussa, 1978; Jacquez *et al.*, 1996a, 1996b; Clark *et al.*, 1999). AE clustering methodology takes essentially the same approach that is commonly used by public health agencies in the investigation of both product- and non-product-induced disease outbreaks (Jacquez *et al.*, 1996a).

Serial Identification Methods

Spontaneous serial methods monitor the number, proportion, or rate of a reported product–AE pair over time (Finney, 1971a, 1974; Royall, 1971; Royall and Venulet, 1972; Moussa, 1978; Lydick et al., 1990; Tsong, 1992; Praus et al., 1993; Amery, 1994; Lao, 1997). The first such method (Patwary signalling) was based on a current versus historical comparison of the proportion of index-product-attributed AE reports to all-product-attributed AE reports for a particular AE type in a multi-product batch. This "AE-specific, proportion of all products" strategy was subsequently changed to the "product-specific, proportion of all AEs" strategy which is commonly used today. The same statistical procedures can be used to carry out either calculation.

All serial signalling procedures are designed to identify either a sudden departure in a reported rate or proportion relative to prior experience or a sustained increased trend in reporting over time (Lao et al., 1998; Lao, 2000) (see Table 19.4). Methods for detecting spike increases were originally derived from a reporting rate comparison between current versus extensive historical time periods (Finney, 1974), whereas later approaches emphasized comparison between two successive equal time periods (Food and Drug Administration, 1985, 1992; Clark, 1988; Norwood and Sampson, 1988). Unequal time period procedures have also been suggested that involve comparing current to all (i.e. current + past, rather than just past) historical experience (Lao et al., 1998). Trend methods have been published in which a comparison is made over several contiguous time intervals (Finney, 1974; Mandel et al., 1976; Levine et al., 1977; Lao et al., 1998; Lao, 2000), or in which cumulative experience is compared with an externally specified standard (Moussa, 1978). The latter two types of procedures are aimed at ascertaining incremental increases over time and cumulative upward divergence beyond a pre-set

Table 19.4. Kinds of serial signalling methods.

Detection of spikes
● Period-to-period methods
● Long history methods

Detection of gradual increases
● Trend methods
● Cumulative sum methods

---

level, respectively. Although valuable experience and data have accumulated regarding serial signalling methods, there is, at present, no empirical evidence to suggest that any single procedure would be superior as a screening tool in spontaneous databases.

Two acknowledged methods for period-to-period serial testing are the conditional binomial method of Norwood and Sampson (Norwood and Sampson, 1988; Tsong, 1992) and the normal approximation for a difference between two proportions described in the US FDA 1991 reporting guidelines (Food and Drug Administration, 1992). Tsong published an evaluation of six period-to-period increased frequency methods based on simulated false positive rates that showed the FDA's 1991 method to be the optimal procedure of those that were investigated (Tsong, 1992), while Hillson suggested a method in which serial comparisons are adjusted for variations in the lag time between the dates of occurrence and reporting (Hillson et al., 1998). Regardless of what report-based serial test is used, the safety professional should carefully evaluate and adjust for false positive rates, since experience indicates that this is the major limitation associated with serial methodology (Food and Drug Administration, 1996, 1997). A listing of published serial methods is provided in Table 19.5.

Spontaneous serial methods that assume a classical statistical distribution are limited by the presence of geographical clustering (Moussa, 1978; Clark et al., 1999). Specifically, when widely distributed products are monitored using a Poisson-based or negative binomial-based test, geographical clustering of reports (which occurs commonly in spontaneous reporting systems) can be shown to violate the distributional assumption. In the presence of geoclustering, an evaluator should therefore consider replacing Poisson-based or similar serial testing with a procedure that identifies high probability clusters. Other methodologic approaches in this setting include region-based serial testing, in which numerator counts are made of reporters and/or institutions instead of reports (Clark et al., 1999), or the use of specialized probability distributions for reports (Moussa, 1978; Lao, 1997, 2000; Lao et al., 1998).

Table 19.5. Spontaneous serial methods.

Type of method	Test method	References[a]	Comments
Period-to-period	Numerical increase	N/A	Sometimes referred to as safety "shift tables"
			Assumes uniform product usage/reporting
	Doubling	FDA (1985)	1985 FDA "arithmetic" method
	Normal approximation	FDA (1985)	1985 FDA "Poisson" method
			High false alarm rate
	Conditional binomial	Norwood and Sampson (1988)	Exact method, rare event assumption
	Normal approximation	Norwood and Sampson (1988)	Derived by Norwood and Sampson
			1991 FDA method
			Best false alarm rate of those tested
	Normal approximation with Yate's correction	Tsong (1992)	Variant of normal approximation method
	Normal approximation (log transformed data)	Tsong (1992)	Variant of normal approximation method
	Normal approximation (square root transformed data)	Tsong (1992)	Variant of normal approximation method
			High false alarm rate
	Chi-squared with continuity correction	Lao et al. (1998)	Also referred to as "pairwise comparisons"
			Proposed for medical device reports
			Assumes uniform product usage/reporting
			Intended for comparisons when periods are short
	Normal approximation with lag time adjustment	Hillson et al. (1998)	Adjusts for lag time between event occurrence and reporting
Long history	T-test	Finney (1974)	Patwary method
			Comparison of current to past report proportions
	Score standardized to past experience compared to an arbitrary threshold (M-statistic)	Mandel et al. (1976)	Mandel method
			Comparison of current to past mean report numbers (or proportions)
			Specified threshold based on severity of AE
	Negative binomial exact test	Lao et al. (1998)	Proposed for medical device reports
			Detects a cluster of reports during a specified period
			Assumes uniform product usage/reporting
	Binomial–Poisson exact test	Lao (2000)	Comparison of current to all report proportions
			Proposed for medical device reports
			Detects a cluster of reports during a specified period
			Assumes uniform product usage/reporting
			Comparison of current to all report proportions
	Zero-truncated Poisson exact test	Lao (2000)	Proposed for medical device reports
			Detects a cluster of reports during a specified period
			Assumes uniform product usage/reporting
			Comparison of current to all report proportions

(continued)

Table 19.5. *Continued.*

Type of method	Test method	References[a]	Comments
Trend	Chi-squared	Finney (1974)	Comparison of current to ⩾2 past proportions
	Exact probability for specified number of increases	Finney (1974)	Nonparametric comparison of current to ⩾2 past proportions
	Linear trend threshold method of Mandel	Mandel et al. (1976)	Assumes uniform product usage/reporting
	Centre-batch matrix for trend	Mandel et al. (1976)	Comparison of geographically stratified, report means or proportions over sequential batches Uses geographical dispersion of data sources to reduce false positives
	Exact (or, if appropriate, asymptotic) test based on distributions derived from a centre-batch matrix	Levine et al. (1977)	Intended for finding "latent" signals (i.e. detectable centrally but not by peripheral contributors) Uses geographically dispersed trend data Assumes uniform product usage/reporting
	Cox–Stuart non-parametric	Lao et al. (1998)	Proposed for medical device reports Detects a gradual trend in reports Proper interpretation is based on knowledge of product usage
	Graphical smoothing techniques	Lao (2000)	Proposed for medical device reports Use graphical smoothing to visually present reporting trends Assumes uniform product usage/reporting
Cumulative sum	Modified one-sided numerical cumulative sum test (NCST)	Moussa (1978)	Devised by WHO Specified threshold based on severity of AE

[a] Indicates primary footnote reference for that method.
Reproduced from Clark et al. (2001), *Epidemiologic Reviews* 23(2), 191–210, Table 2, with permission from Oxford University Press.

The latter two strategies take geoclustering into account either by eliminating it from the calculation or by incorporating its effects into the assumed probability distribution.

Temporospatial Cluster Identification Methods

A number of product–AE outbreak investigations have been published that arose from reports that were clustered over time and space (Centers for Disease Control, 1984, 1989a, 1989b; Martone *et al.*, 1986; Jolson *et al.*, 1992; Bennett *et al.*, 1995). Consequently, the safety professional may find it desirable to design a method that screens product-specific spontaneous AE reports for the presence of temporospatial clusters. Temporospatial clustering has been seen with lot-associated and other

product defects (Centers for Disease Control, 1984, 1989a; Martone *et al.*, 1986; Jolson *et al.*, 1992), with localized patterns of use/misuse (Bennett *et al.*, 1995), and with events later determined to occur commonly under permissive conditions (Centers for Disease Control, 1989b).

Inter-Product Quantitative Identification Methods

Although first described by WHO researchers in the 1970s, only recently have inter-product identification methods become the subject of intense discussion (Bate *et al.*, 1998a, 1998b; Amery, 1999; DuMouchel, 1999). Such procedures evaluate disproportions found in multiple product reporting systems in order to identify suspected product–AE relationships. Like other identification methods, inter-product identification comparisons yield product–AE pairs that are then further evaluated through the use of more precise techniques (Bate *et al.*, 1998b; DuMouchel, 1999; Lindquist *et al.*, 1999). An increase in the number of products in the computational universe for inter-product quantitative identification methods is associated logically with both improvement in estimates for expected reporting behavior and a reduction in sensitivity to underreporting. Thus, inter-product identification techniques appear to be most useful when applied to large AE reporting systems, such as those found at the regional, national, or international levels.

2 × 2 Table Methods

In the early 1970s Patwary and Finney described an inter-product identification method in which the proportion of all index-product reports containing a specific AE type was compared with the same proportion derived from a multiple product database. They referred to this strategy as "reaction proportion signalling" and applied it to WHO's spontaneous reporting system (Finney, 1974). In 1994, Amery published a similar procedure called the relative adverse drug experience profile, which was applied to a manufacturer's multi-product report database (Amery, 1994, 1999). With these methods, signal identification occurs when standard statistical tests indicate that the product–AE to product–all-AE proportion exceeds an expected value calculated from the reference reporting system under the null assumption of product–AE independence.

The Medicines Control Agency (MCA) has described a procedure called the proportionate reporting ratio (PRR) method. Like the two previous procedures, the PRR portion of this calculation is based on a comparison of the proportion of index product reports that contain a specific AE type with the same proportion from a multi-product universe (Evans, 2000). The PRR is then defined as for reaction proportion signalling (see above). However, unlike the above methods, the PRR methodology selects suspect product–AE pairs by applying combination criteria derived from general experience, such as a PRR > 2 + a chi-square score > 4, in the presence of at least two product–AE reports (Evans, 2000).

Bayesian Data Mining Methods

Two Bayesian data mining procedures have been published that extend inter-product quantitative identification to $M \times N$ tables (Bate *et al.*, 1998a; 1998b; Lindquist *et al.*, 1999; Amery, 1999; DuMouchel, 1999), where M refers to a large set of AEs, and N to a large set of monitored products (see Table 19.6). The first of these, the Bayesian confidence propagation neural network method, was proposed by Bate and colleagues from the WHO (Bate *et al.*, 1998a); the second was developed by DuMouchel with reference to the FDA's spontaneous reporting system (DuMouchel, 1999). A stepwise approach to the development of Bayesian data mining techniques has been described (Louis and Shen, 1999) which involves: (1) the construction of a large $M \times N$ table, where cells contain counts of the 1st through Mth AE for the 1st through Nth product; (2) the creation of a null model that calculates expected counts for each cell; (3) derivation of a statistic that measures deviation beyond the expected value in each cell; and (4) quantification of the relationship between observed and expected counts in each cell to assist in selecting or evaluating product–AE pairs.

The procedure of Bate and colleagues has been carried out for specific product–AE pairs at multiple time points, thereby incorporating interval changes into a time scan. This repeated comparison technique has been proposed as an enhancement of signal detection, since an upward change in the measurement statistic over time implies that increasing "awareness" of a product–AE pair has developed within the reporting system as time progresses. In contrast, DuMouchel's method employs time stratification in the overall model to adjust for secular reporting trends. Its aim is to use all accumulated evidence in the reporting system to rank order suspect product–AE pairs. Both the Bate and DuMouchel methods explicitly recognize that Bayesian data mining is an identification process only, and is not meaningful unless subsequent evaluation takes place.

Table 19.6. Comparison of two Bayesian data mining procedures used in spontaneous report signalling.

	Bayesian Confidence Propagation Neural Network (BCPNN) method[a]	DuMouchel method[b]
Product–AE stratifications (tables)	● Non-stratified	● Stratified by (at least) gender and year of report
Null model	● Product–AE independence	● Product–AE independence
Cell level measurement statistic	● IC (information component) = $\log_2(\Pr[x,y]/\Pr[x]\,\Pr[y])$, where $\Pr(x)$ and $\Pr(y)$ are the report probabilities for the product and AE whose association is under study	● $\Pr(x_a > x_e)$, where x_a is the actual cell count, and x_e is the expected cell count ● $\Pr(x_a > x_e)$ is assumed to derive from the Poisson distribution
Prior distribution for product–AE pairs (specified for a time point)	● $\Pr(x)$, $\Pr(y)$, and $\Pr(x,y)$ are assumed to derive from beta distributions ● Single distribution is assumed ● Can be approximated by the exponential distribution	● Distribution derived empirically ● Based mathematically on a two gamma mixture distribution
Final output	● Product–AE IC statistics that are sufficiently "interesting" ● Time scanning—the IC values are plotted over time	● Ranking of product–AE pairs by degree of "interest"

[a] Bate et al. (1998a).
[b] DuMouchel (1999).
Reproduced from Clark et al. (2001), Epidemiologic Reviews 23(2), 191–210, Table 3, with permission from Oxford University Press.

SPONTANEOUS SIGNALLING METHODS USED AT THE CASE SERIES FORMATION STEP

Case series formation methods are procedures used to create case series evidence in favor of a potential relationship between a product and an AE. The concept of case-based signalling (i.e. signal evaluation), coming after and based on report-based signalling (i.e. signal detection), is inherent in much of the spontaneous methods literature, and dates at least to the early writings of Finney (Finney, 1966). In recent years, this distinction has also been emphasized by Meyboom, who has stressed the difference between the use of imputation to screen for "interesting" AEs, versus its use to form case series for the intensive review of suspected product–AE pairs (Meyboom et al., 1997b). Unlike epidemiologic arguments, the purpose of the case series formation step in signalling is to formalize (to the extent possible) a basis for subsequent regulatory and scientific action, not to provide definitive commentary concerning the nature of underlying

causal relationships. From the signalling perspective, any important potential relationship that can be argued, whether causal or not, is a useful surveillance finding.

Case series formation relies heavily on an evaluator's ability to devise a case definition that specifies the minimum quality and diagnostic criteria needed to designate reports as cases, and that is defensible from the medical and epidemiologic perspectives (Clark et al., 1990; Bégaud et al., 1994a). Although acceptance of spontaneous reports at face value may sometimes be reasonable, the importance of more specific case definitions is underscored by the relatively low rate of case validation at the time of follow-up when spontaneous reports are carefully scrutinized (Funch et al., 1993; Sicker et al., 1998). Bégaud has emphasized that the definition of cases is an arbitrary exercise that can be made more sensitive or more specific, depending on the evaluator's purpose (Bégaud et al., 1994a).

The case series formation step of spontaneous signalling evaluates at least four kinds of information that are provided by a product–AE case series: (1) the number of cases, (2) the aggregate diagnostic features of a (usually) multiple case series, (3) the degree of clinical similarity (or dissimilarity) exhibited by two or more cases, and (4) the presence (or absence) of independent repeatability of cases. In spontaneous reporting systems, an increasing number of product–AE cases is generally regarded as useful in establishing a signalling argument (Tubert *et al.*, 1991; Meyboom *et al.*, 1997a). Likewise, the impact of multiple case aggregate diagnostic features (as opposed to the diagnostic features of any particular case) has also been cited as helpful (Meyboom *et al.*, 1997a). The third type of information, an increased level of "content clustering", is often referred to by public health professionals when distinguishing true from false signals (Jacquez *et al.*, 1996a). And, lastly, a case series provides evidence that the suspect product–AE pair is repetitive if the cases were reported by two or more independent observers (Meyboom *et al.*, 1997a; Clark *et al.*, 1999).

Intra-Product Qualitative Case Series Formation Methods

Spontaneous qualitative association methods can be defined as the application of an imputation method to one or more cases in order to demonstrate that sufficient associative evidence exists for signal generation. The formation of a case series implies that a case definition (i.e. minimum AE diagnostic information) has been applied to candidate reports, although in practice the requirements used are often not specified. Qualitative assessments of case series allow an evaluator to condense a range of imputation results into a descriptive impression, much as an experienced clinician would do when considering multiple cases of a disease. Qualitative association methods can be classified as subjective, rule-based, or retrospective Bayesian.

Subjective case series

Subjective case series are formed when an evaluator designates and analyzes cases using unstructured clinical judgment. As with other purely subjective methods, limitations that derive from subjectivity (e.g. lack of uniformity) would be expected to apply (see the section Imputation Screening (Causality) Assessments above). Subjective assessments of case series are probably the most common way by which associative evidence in favor of product–AE relationships is summarized.

Rule-Based Case Series

Rule-based case series are created when explicit rules are used to designate and/or analyze cases in a case series. The safety analyst typically either creates a case definition that is consistent with medico-epidemiologic principles (Clark *et al.*, 1990), or simply accepts the reporter's diagnosis at face value, perhaps requiring some degree of clinical corroboration. A case definition can also be created by using a rule-based imputation algorithm and designating as cases only those reports that carry high ratings (e.g. only reports rated as "definite" or "probable"). Unlike the report-based procedure screening imputation (see above), AE-specific rule-based methods have considerable applicability to case series formation, because they derive from the results of consensus conferences that are conducted by experts in a particular clinical area (Benichou, 1990; Benichou and Celigny, 1991; Meyboom *et al.*, 1997b). The rule-based case definitions described above produce series that possess minimum uniform criteria across all cases.

Rule-based case series can also be generated by accepting an entire set of reports as cases, provided the series as a whole conforms to defined minimum criteria. Examples of this strategy are the monitored adverse reaction and a quality criteria grading methodology proposed by Edwards (Jones, 1982; Turner, 1984; Edwards *et al.*, 1990). The monitored adverse reaction method allows case series to be created from the range of case diagnostic criteria (as determined by the FDA's rule-based imputation method) that is found in a reported product–AE series of specified length, while the quality criteria grading system of Edwards defines the minimum recommended evidence for a report series to be publishable, given quality criteria and key content (Edwards *et al.*, 1990). These kinds of rule-based case series define minimum requirements for case series as a whole, within which individual cases may be highly variable.

Retrospective Bayesian Analysis

A retrospective Bayesian analysis has been described in which Bayesian methodology is used to construct a spontaneous case series (Naranjo *et al.*, 1990) (see also the section Imputation Screening (Causality) Assessments). In the retrospective Bayesian method, a single estimate for the prior odds that applies to the case series as a whole is calculated using information provided by the series. Following examination of the included cases, each individual case is then reassessed in the light of the aggregated case information from all cases, and a posterior odds for the entire case series as a unit is calculated.

Intra-Product Quantitative Case Series Formation Methods

Intra-product quantitative case series formation methods form an associative argument by comparing the number of reported cases with an expected value. With the standardized reporting ratio (SRR), this is accomplished by comparing an observed number of reported cases with the number of cases expected based on background incidence data. With the associative case–control study, this is accomplished using cases and controls that are based on spontaneous reporting.

The SRR

In SRR analyses, the number of spontaneously reported cases of a product–AE pair (or the case reporting rate) is compared with the expected number of background cases for the same product–AE pair (or the background incidence rate) to see if the actual number of reported cases exceeds the number of cases expected on the basis of chance (Tubert *et al.*, 1991, 1992). The SRR is therefore analogous to a standardized incidence ratio, except that the numerator is formed from reported, not incident, cases. The number of

expected cases is calculated by applying an appropriate background rate schedule to the person-time of the patient group using the product. While background rates are logically derived from a source of data in which cases are fully ascertained, it can also be modified to take into account the supposition that background cases, like reported cases, will also be underreported (Bégaud *et al.*, 1994b). With the latter modification, the number of reported cases is compared with the number of background cases that would have been expected to both occur by chance and be reported.

SRRs are usually expressed either as spontaneous rate ratios or as gross numerical comparisons. With spontaneous rate ratios the number of reported cases is compared with the expected number of incident cases using a Poisson model (Tubert *et al.*, 1991; Bégaud *et al.*, 1994b), while with gross numerical comparisons authors prefer to interpret the reported and expected case counts (or rates) non-statistically (Idanpaan Heikkila *et al.*, 1977; Wysowski and Green, 1995; Wysowski and Fourcroy, 1996). Methods have also been described in which one or more unknown components of the Poisson model are parameterized (Tubert and Bégaud, 1991).

SRRs rely on a case definition for the AE that is applicable to both spontaneously reported cases (the numerator) and an externally derived incidence rate (the denominator). If such a case definition is not feasible, or if a usable external data source is not available, then the method cannot be used. Additionally, if expected reports are made subject to an underreporting factor (which increases the utility of the procedure) a sensitivity analysis is recommended to see how much the underreporting assumption affects the results. Despite these shortcomings, the SRR offers an important advantage over inter-product case series comparisons (see the section Inter-product Case Series Formation Methods below), since any underreporting assumptions that are made by an evaluator are presented explicitly in the calculation. If an evaluator chooses to use a fully ascertained background rate, then false positives due to clustering and underreporting are unlikely explanations for any resulting signals because the comparison standard is both "completely reported and completely clustered".

Associative Case–Control Study

Intra-product associative case–control strategies have also been described in general terms, the aim of which is to support or refute product–AE associations (Martinez and Walker, 1995). To date, very little experience has accumulated in which spontaneously based case-control designs are used as spontaneous signalling techniques.

Inter-Product Case Series Formation Methods

Inter-product case series formation methods evaluate the spontaneous rate or proportion of index product–AE cases *vis-à-vis* the analogous spontaneous rate or proportion for a comparator product, usually over a single comparable time frame. Such procedures seek to provide an understanding of the relative association between product and AE by benchmarking against an "other product" standard. Like other case series formation techniques, inter-product associative methods assume that reports have been validated to the extent necessary to carry out the analysis (i.e. they have met a case definition). In general, the methods employed in two-group comparisons of this type can be classified as spontaneous cohort design methods, spontaneous case–control design methods, and gross numerical comparisons.

In the spontaneous cohort design the distribution of reports between two products is compared with a probabilistic expectation based on unit sales, prescription number, market share, defined daily doses, or estimated exposed patients (Inman and Vessey, 1968; Inman, 1970; Inman *et al.*, 1970; Bergman *et al.*, 1978; Tubert-Bitter and Bégaud, 1993; Lindquist *et al.*, 1997). This model is conceptually equivalent to the two-group Poisson model that is well described in standard texts (Greenland and Rothman, 1998). If exact testing is performed, it has usually been carried out using a conditional binomial procedure (Tubert-Bitter *et al.*, 1996). A spontaneous case–control design has also been described in which a 2×2 contingency table is populated by

using AE and all-other-AE case counts for the index and other products (Rawlins, 1988; Amery, 1994; Figueras *et al.*, 1994; Moore *et al.*, 1995, 1997; Egberts *et al.*, 1997). A version of this has been referred to as the "case/non-case design" or "ADR reporting odds ratio" (Moore *et al.*, 1995, 1997; Egberts *et al.*, 1997), with quantitative evaluation carried out using a standard odds ratio statistic. Some authors have preferred to interpret differences between the reporting rates/proportions of specific AEs to different drugs non-statistically, i.e. by using gross numerical comparison (Rossi *et al.*, 1987; Platt *et al.*, 1988; Mason *et al.*, 1990; Figueras *et al.*, 1994; Stahl *et al.*, 1997). While comparative analyses have typically been carried out over comparable equal-length segments of the marketing cycle, Tsong proposed the use of a Mantel–Haenszel statistic that allows a single summary comparison over multiple analogous time periods of two marketing cycles (Tsong, 1995).

In addition to well-described confounders such as age, gender, intended use, duration of use, and concomitant medications (Sachs and Bortnichak, 1986; Rawlins, 1988), a number of other factors have been suggested that could affect the interpretability of spontaneous comparative signals, including the year(s) of the marketing cycle to be analyzed (Sachs and Bortnichak, 1986; Rossi *et al.*, 1987; Mason *et al.*, 1990), secular trends in reporting (Sachs and Bortnichak, 1986; Rossi *et al.*, 1987; Mason *et al.*, 1990), publicity (Sachs and Bortnichak, 1986), and the effects of product promotion (Sachs and Bortnichak, 1986). Bégaud and Tubert-Bitter have emphasized the conservative interpretation of the reporting rates for two compared products in evaluating such signals (Bégaud *et al.*, 1991, 1994a; Tubert-Bitter *et al.*, 1996); Sachs, Bortnichak and Lawson have noted the effect that reporting biases (such as confounding by indication) may have played in misinterpreting spontaneous comparisons of the rate of gastrointestinal bleeding in patients receiving the drug piroxicam versus other similar anti-inflammatory products (Bortnichak and Sachs, 1986; Sachs and Bortnichak, 1986; Lawson, 1988); and Stang has emphasized the importance of taking confounding by indication into account when interpreting spontaneous report-based analyses (Stang and Fox, 1992).

SPONTANEOUS METHODS USED AT THE CASE SERIES CHARACTERIZATION STEP

Once a product–AE pair that exhibits potentially associative features has been identified, the spectrum of the product–AE case series can often be further described. Case series analyses of the distribution of selected content elements within a drug–AE case series have been called "characterizations" or "identification of risk factors", and have been well described as AE signalling methods (Rawlins, 1986, 1988; Amery, 1994). Case series characterizations usually focus on clinical features, age, gender, and dose and duration of therapy. Such procedures are used to refine and expand an existing AE signalling argument by, for example, demonstrating a reported dose relationship, providing clues to potential explanatory mechanisms, identifying sub-populations at risk, or describing reporting patterns that help distinguish biologic from reporting phenomena.

Case series characterization relies on patterns contained in a spontaneous case series that pertain to report content (especially any relationship between dose and outcome), reporting dates, or the geographical origin of reports. Since characterizations are undertaken after the associative logic of case series formation has been applied, they are based on cases that meet medical and epidemiologic definitions, and do not represent analyses of unrefined spontaneous report data. Case series characterization can provide important insights into both the mechanisms underlying product–AE pairs and the circumstances that led to their reporting.

Intra-Product Qualitative Case Series Characterization Methods

Qualitative summaries of product–AE case series based on spontaneous data have long been well accepted as a characterization methodology (Rawlins, 1988). Case-based descriptive statistics provide a general sense of the information contained in the case series as a unit, generally focusing

on age, gender, dose, and clinical presentation. Analyses of report content distribution for a given drug–AE pair can also provide important clues concerning patient subtypes at high risk and the underlying mechanism of the event, and are an important source for postmarketing data that may eventually be included in the package insert (Wechsler et al., 1998). However, authors such as Rawlins have argued that proposing a correlation between product exposure and a characterized factor is inappropriate unless population use proportions for that factor are available (Rawlins, 1988) (see the section Intra-product Quantitative Case Series Characterization Methods below).

Intra-Product Quantitative Case Series Characterization Methods

"Numerator Only" Case Series Distribution

Within the reported case series, different clinical outcomes may be associated with different age groups, gender, dosage, or concomitant medications (Inman et al., 1970; Bateman et al., 1986; Amery, 1994). Halothane-hepatitis is a classic example of the sometimes substantial impact such "numerator-only" (internal correlative) characterizations can have (Inman and Mushin, 1974). In this instance, a product–AE case series demonstrated a decreasing time-to-onset with increasing numbers of exposures, thereby supporting an associative argument and providing a potential explanatory mechanism (allergy) by which the event could occur. "Numerator only" characterizations are also the basis for many spontaneous registries (e.g. disease or pregnancy outcomes) where the primary interest lies in patterns of relevant features among the cases.

A specialized form of "numerator only" case series distribution occurs when clustering methods are used to examine information contained in the reported case distribution of an AE type over time and/or space (Rossi et al., 1988; Clark and Gross, 1992). Temporal clustering of cases has been associated with publicity-induced reporting effects (Rossi et al., 1988), while geographical clustering of cases by region or country within the same time frame (i.e. tests for spatial clustering) can suggest localized reporting or product-related phenomena (Inman *et al.*, 1970). Temporospatial clustering has already been addressed as a report-based identification method, but could also become apparent subsequently as part of a product–AE characterization.

Rate/Proportion-Based Case Series Distribution

If sufficiently detailed product use data are available, signalling based on selected content characteristics can be enhanced by comparisons with analogous population rates or proportions (Asplund *et al.*, 1983; Rawlins, 1988). This results in a more formalized signal statistic that resembles the rate comparisons of inter-product case series, but differs by being confined to subset comparisons for a single product–AE pair (Inman and Vessey, 1968; Amery, 1994). Although this approach can be biased by the same sensitivity to differential reporting rates and differential clustering that affects the serial identification and inter-product case formation methods, the assumption of similar within-product reporting dynamics is likely reasonable in selected instances. This occurs when the factors that have the greatest impact on reporting rates are not altered substantially by those characteristics that are being examined. (For example, under a usual circumstance of use, the reporting dynamic for a death suspected to be due to an AE is not likely to be significantly altered by the therapeutic dose given.) Rate/proportion-based case series distributions will have limited usefulness if an evaluator has reason to believe that the reporting rate for a product–AE pair by characteristic is related to that characteristic itself.

Characterization Case–Control Study

In addition to the associative case–control design described above, spontaneously reported cases and reporter-selected exposed controls can be used to characterize risk factors. This design is spontaneous in origin (an evaluator obtains data for both cases and non-cases from self-selected reporters), and requires that both cases and non-cases receive the product. Between-group comparisons then

focus on potential risk factors for the development of the syndrome. An excellent example of a characterization spontaneous case–control study, aimed at determining risk factors for the suprofen flank pain syndrome, was published by Strom (Strom *et al.*, 1989).

Inter-Product Case Series Characterization Methods

Quantitative case series characterization methods have rarely been extended to comparative characterizations of two or more products (i.e. to create comparative case series distributions). Such analyses have typically focused on the reported seriousness profile of a particular product–AE pair in cases receiving the index versus another product(s) (Carvajal *et al.*, 1996).

DESIGNING A PRODUCT-SPECIFIC ADVERSE EVENT SURVEILLANCE PROGRAM

The design of a health care product surveillance program should take into account product class effects and indications, the patient user and prescriber populations, and the route of administration. It should also be appreciated that use patterns may change over time, thereby necessitating alterations in the structure of the surveillance program itself. Venulet has published an example in which a product-specific surveillance scheme is designed and diagrammed (Venulet, 1988), while Klincewicz has pointed out the importance of linking product monitoring mechanisms with the periodic safety update report (PSUR) requirements found in the ICH E2C document (Klincewicz *et al.*, 1999). An exhaustive review has also been published recently that focuses on AE signalling methods and AE surveillance program design (Clark *et al.*, 2001).

In selecting sorting methodologies, it is noteworthy that the expedited (serious + unlabelled) report sorting procedure and several PSUR line listings are mandated by regulation, and should therefore be included in essentially all such designs. Sorting methods based on designated medical events would also appear to be appropriate for many spontaneous report data sets, given the regular appearance of a selected list of AE types throughout the history of health care product monitoring. For products that give rise to small numbers of reports, one or two sorting methods will usually be sufficient to address report-based monitoring needs.

The use of automated identification procedures would logically be reserved for larger and more complex report databases. In creating report screening strategies, it is helpful to conceptualize the identification step as the use of screening tests to select "interesting" product–AE pairs for further study. In this view, the use of effective identification procedures for product monitoring resembles the use of screening tests for other public health applications, and implies special attention to false positive rates. The false positive rate for an AE surveillance program can be decreased by selecting identification procedures with a higher specificity (and, therefore, a lower sensitivity), while its false negative rate can be decreased by using multiple identification procedures, each of which operates on a different principle, and by repeat screening on a regular basis. The overall effectiveness of the report phase of an AE surveillance program can be evaluated by calculating the report-based positive predictive value, which is equivalent to the proportion of signal evaluations found at the case-based phase to be "interesting". A lower than desired predictive value suggests that the specificity of the identification methods should be increased.

Experience suggests that, despite past difficulties, there remains a place for both rule-based imputation screening and serial signalling methods in spontaneous AE surveillance programs, but that the use of both of these identification methodologies must be scrutinized carefully. Statistical models are unlikely to be helpful on a widespread basis at the identification step, because such tools are too complex and individualized to be effective as screening tests. Although not employed systematically in the past, screening for temporo-geographical clusters may be effective for certain types of safety outcomes, especially those that are related to product preparation and local circumstances of use.

At present, inter-product identification methods appear to be promising developments for public-health-oriented databases, but would usually not be feasible for manufacturer-specific databases which, in comparison with other product–AE monitoring databases, are relatively small and highly selective.

In constructing case series, evaluators should clearly specify case definitions, and adapt them to the limitations of spontaneous data. When comparing such experience with expectation, the standardized reporting ratio and its modifications remains one of the most valuable tools currently available to program designers. This methodologic approach requires extensive knowledge of background incidence rates that is best confirmed empirically through literature reviews and/or database research. Many program administrators will want to have these resources and pertinent expertise available on an ongoing basis. Product monitors will likely want to regard inter-product comparisons of spontaneously based case series with care. Because of the many biases affecting interpretation, these methods are probably best thought of as a group of public-health-motivated analyses of last resort that are undertaken when better data cannot be acquired in an appropriate time frame.

A review of the literature pertaining to case series characterization methods suggests that, when carried out thoughtfully and represented appropriately, such data can be helpful to prescribers. In formulating characterization analyses, the possibility of a relationship between the characterized feature and the adverse event rate or other endpoint should always be formally considered. In presenting such data, the analyst should also bear in mind the possibility that the characteristics of the reported case series may be different from population-based case series, and commentary that addresses this uncertainty should be provided.

REFERENCES

Abenheim L, Moore N, Begaud B (1999) The role of pharmacoepidemiology in pharmacovigilance. A conference at the 6th ESOP meeting, Budapest, 28 September 1998. *Pharmacoepidemiology and Drug Safety* **8** (Suppl): S1–S7.

Amery W (1994) Analysis of the information in a central ADE database. *Int J Risk Safety Med* **5**: 105–23.

Amery WK (1999) Signal generation from spontaneous adverse event reports. *Pharmacoepidemiology and Drug Safety* **8**: 147–50.

Asplund K, Wiholm, B-E, Lithner F (1983) Glibenclamide-associated hyoglycaemia: a report on 57 cases. *Diabetologia* **24**: 412–7.

Auriche M (1985) Approache bayésienne de l'imputabilité des phénomènes indésirables aux médicaments. *Therapie* **40**: 301.

Bate A, Lindquist M, Edwards IR, Olsson S, Orre R, Lansner A, De Freitas RM (1998a) A Bayesian neural network method for adverse drug reaction signal generation. *Eur J Clin Pharmacol* **54**: 315–21.

Bate A, Lindquist M, Ore R, Edwards R (1998b) Identifying and quantifying signals automatically. *Pharmacoepidemiology and Drug Safety* **7** (Suppl 2): 99(Abstract).

Bateman DN, Rawlins MD, Simpson JM (1986) Extrapyramidal reactions to prochlorperazine and haloperidol in the United Kingdom. *Quart J Med* **59**: 549–56.

Bégaud B, Moride Y, Haramburu F (1994a) Quality improvement and statistical calculations made on spontaneous reports. *Drug Inf J* **28**: 1187–95.

Bégaud B, Moride Y, Tubert-Bitter P, Chaslerie A, Haramburu F (1994b) False-positives in spontaneous reporting. Should we worry about them? *Br J Clin Pharmacol* **38**: 401–4.

Bégaud B, Tubert P, Haramburu F, Moride Y, Salame G, Pere JC (1991) Comparing toxicity of drugs. Use and misuse of spontaneous reporting. *Post Marketing Surveillance* **5**: 69–76.

Benichou C (1990) Criteria of drug-induced liver disorders. Report of an international consensus meeting. *J Hepat* **11**: 272–6.

Benichou C, Céligny PhS (1991) Standardization of definitions and criteria of causality assessment of adverse drug reactions. *Int J Clin Pharmacol Ther Tox* **29**: 75–81.

Bennett SN, McNeil MM, Bland LA, Arduino MJ, Villarino ME, Perrotta DM, Burwen DR, Welbel SF, Pegues DA, Stroud L, Zeitz PS, Jarvis WR (1995) Postoperative infections traced to contamination of an intravenous anesthetic, propofol. *New Engl J Med* **333**: 147–54.

Bergman U, Boman G, Wiholm B-E (1978) Epidemiology of adverse drug reactions to phenformin and metformin. *Br Med J* **2**: 464–6.

Blanc S, Levenberger P, Berger JP, Brooke EM, Schelling JL (1979) Judgements of trained observers on adverse drug reactions. *Clin Pharmacol Ther* **25**: 493–8.

Blum MD, Graham DJ, McCloskey CA (1994) Temafloxacin syndrome: review of 95 cases. *Clin Inf Dis* **18**: 946–50.

Bortnichak EA, Sachs RM (1986) Piroxicam in recent epidemiologic studies. *Am J Med* **81** (Suppl 5B): 44–8.

Busto U, Naranjo CA, Sellers EM (1982) Comparison of two recently published algorithms for assessing the probability of adverse drug reactions. *Br J Clin Pharmacol* **13**: 223–7.

Carson JL, Strom BL, Maislin G (1994) Screening for unknown effects of newly marketed drugs. In: Strom BL, ed., *Pharmacoepidemiology*, 2nd edn. New York: Wiley, pp. 432–47.

Carvajal A, Prieto JR, Requejo AA, Arias LHM (1996) Aspirin or acetaminophen? A comparison from data collected by the Spanish Drug Monitoring System. *J Clin Epidemiol* **49**: 255–61.

Case B, Oszko MA (1991) Use of an algorithm to evaluate published reports of adverse drug reactions. *Am J Hosp Pharm* **48**: 121–2.

Centers for Disease Control (CDC) (1984) Unusual syndrome with fatalities among premature infants. Association with a new intravenous vitamin E product. *Morb Mort Wkly Rep* **33**: 198–9.

Centers for Disease Control (CDC) (1989a) Deaths associated with thiamine-deficient total parenteral nutrition. *Morb Mort Wkly Rep* **38**: 43–6.

Centers for Disease Control (CDC) (1989b) Eosinophilia-myalgia syndrome—New Mexico. *Morb Mort Wkly Rep* **38**: 765–7.

Clark J (1988) *Increased Frequency Reporting*. Rockville: Food and Drug Administration (FDA), Center for Drug Evaluation and Research, p. 4C.

Clark JA, Berk RH, Klincewicz SL (1999) Calculation of the probability of multiplicities in two cell-occupancy models. Implications for spontaneous reporting systems. *Drug Inf J* **33**: 1195–203.

Clark JA, Gross TP (1992) Pain and cyanosis associated with α_1-proteinase inhibitor. *Am J Med* **92**: 621–6.

Clark JA, Klincewicz SL, Stang PE (2001) Spontaneous adverse event signaling methods: classification and use with health care treatment products. *Epidemiol Rev* **23**: 191–210.

Clark JA, Zimmerman HJ, Tanner LA (1990) Labetalol hepatotoxicity. *Ann Int Med* **113**: 210–3.

Cluff LE, Thornton GF, Seidl LG (1964) Studies on the epidemiology of adverse drug reactions. I. Methods of surveillance. *J Am Med Assoc* **188**: 976–83.

Council for International Organizations of Medical Sciences (CIOMS) (1998) *Benefit–Risk Balance for Marketed Drugs. Evaluating Safety Signals*. Geneva: CIOMS, pp. 12–16.

Danan G, Benichou C (1993) Causality assessment of adverse reactions to drugs—I. A novel method based on the conclusions of international consensus meetings. Application to drug-induced liver injuries. *J Clin Epidemiol* **46**: 1323–30.

DuMouchel W (1999) Bayesian data mining in large frequency tables, with an application to the FDA Spontaneous Reporting system. *Am Stat* **53**: 177–90.

Edwards IR, Lindquist M, Wiholm BE, Napke E (1990) Quality criteria for early signals of possible drug reactions. *Lancet* **336**: 156–8.

Egberts ACG, Meyboom RHB, De Koning, FHP, Bakker A, Leufkens HGM (1997) Non-puerperal lactation associated with antidepressant drug use. *Br J Clin Pharmacol* **44**: 277–81.

European Agency for the Evaluation of Medicinal Products (EMEA), Committee for Proprietary Medicinal Products (1995) *ICH Topic E2A. Clinical safety data management. Definitions and standards for expedited reporting (CPMP/ICH/377/95)*. London: EMEA, pp. 4/10–5/10.

European Agency for the Evaluation of Medicinal Products (EMEA), Committee for Proprietary Medicinal Products (1997) *ICH Topic E2C. Clinical safety data management. Periodic safety update reports for marketed drugs* (CPMP/ICH/288/95). London: EMEA, pp. 6/22, 15/22–17/22.

Evans SJW (2000) Pharmacovigilance: a science or fielding emergencies. *Stat Med* **19**: 3199–209.

Faich GA (1986) Adverse-drug-reaction monitoring. *New Engl J Med* **314**: 1589–92.

Faich GA (1996) U.S. Adverse drug reaction surveillance 1989–94. *Pharmacoepidemiology and Drug Safety* **5**: 393–8.

Faich GA, Knapp D, Dreis M, Turner W (1987) National adverse drug reaction surveillance: 1985. *J Am Med Assoc* **257**: 2068–70.

Figueras A, Capella D, Castel JM, Laporte JR (1994) Spontaneous reporting of adverse drug reactions to non-steroidal anti-inflammatory drugs. *Eur J Clin Pharmacol* **47**: 297–303.

Finney DJ (1963) An international drug safety program. *J New Drugs* **3**: 262–5.

Finney DJ (1964) An international drug safeguard plan. *J Chron Dis* **17**: 565–81.

Finney DJ (1965) The design and logic of a monitor of drug use. An international drug safety guard plan. *J Chron Dis* **18**: 77–98.

Finney DJ (1966) Monitoring adverse reactions to drugs—Its logic and its weaknesses. *Proc Eur Soc Stud Drug Tox* **7**: 198–207.

Finney DJ (1971a) Statistical aspects of monitoring for danger in drug therapy. *Meth Inform Med* **10**: 1–8.

Finney DJ (1971b) Statistical logic in the monitoring of reactions to therapeutic drugs. *Meth Inform Med* **10**: 237–45.

Finney DJ (1974) Systematic signalling of adverse reactions to drugs. *Meth Inf Med* **13**: 1–10.

Food and Drug Administration (FDA), Center for Drugs and Biologics (1985) *Guideline For Postmarketing Reporting Of Adverse Drug Reactions*. Rockville, MD: FDA, pp. 11–14.

Food and Drug Administration (FDA), Center for Drug Evaluation and Research (CDER) (1992) *Guidance for Postmarketing Reporting of Adverse Experiences: Drugs*. Rockville, MD: FDA, pp. 3, 27–8.

Food and Drug Administration (FDA) (1996) Postmarketing expedited adverse experience reporting for human drug and licensed biological products: increased frequency reports. *Fed Reg* **61**: 55603–6.

Food and Drug Administration (FDA) (1997) Postmarketing expedited adverse experience reporting for human drug and licensed biological products: increased frequency reports. *Fed Reg* **62**: 34166–8.

Food and Drug Administration (FDA) (1999) *Managing the Risks from Medical Product Use. Creating a Risk Management Framework*. Rockville, MD: FDA, pp. 69–70.

Food and Drug Administration (FDA), Center for Drug Evaluation and Research (2000) The four levels of AERS. FDA Web Page, http://www.fda.gov/cder/aers/slides/index.htm.

Frick PA, Cohen LG, Rovers JP (1997) Algorithms used in adverse drug event reports: a comparative study. *Ann Pharmacother* **31**: 164–7.

Funch D, Dreyer NA, Bassin LG, Crawley JA, Brickley MG, Walker AM (1993) The validity of case reports in a pharmacoepidemiologic study. *Post Marketing Surveillance* **7**: 283–9.

Goldman SA (1998) Limitations and strengths of spontaneous reports data. *Clin Ther* **20** (Suppl C), C40–C44.

Greenland S, Rothman KJ (1998) Introduction to categorical statistics. In: Rothman KJ, Greenland S, eds., *Modern Epidemiology*. Philadelphia: Lippincott-Raven, pp. 237–9.

Grohmann R, Dirschedl P, Scherer J, Schmidt LG, Wunderlich O (1985) Reliability of adverse drug reaction assessment in psychiatric inpatients. *Eur Arch Psychiatr Neurol Sci* **235**: 158–63.

Hart D, Ward M, Lifschitz MD (1987) Suprofen-related nephrotoxicity. *Ann Int Med* **106**: 235–8.

Hartmann K, Ciorciaro C, Kuhn M (1997) Signal generation in a non-EU country. *Pharmacoepidemiology and Drug Safety* **6** (Suppl 3): S13–S19.

Hillson EM, Reeves JH, McMillan CA (1998) A statistical signalling model for use in surveillance of adverse drug reaction data. *J Appl Stat* **25**: 23–40.

Hoskins RE, Manning S (1992) Causality assessment of adverse drug reactions using decision support and informatics tools. *Pharmacoepidemiology and Drug Safety* **1**: 235–49.

Hutchinson TA (1986) Standardized assessment methods for adverse drug reactions. A review of previous approaches and their problems. *Drug Inf J* **20**: 439–44.

Hutchinson TA, Flegel KM, HoPingKong H, Bloom WS, Kramer MS, Trummer EG (1983) Reasons for disagreement in the standardized assessment of suspected adverse drug reactions. *Clin Pharmacol Ther* **34**: 421–6.

Hutchinson TA, Lane DA (1989) Assessing methods for causality assessment of suspected adverse drug reactions. *J Clin Epidemiol* **42**: 5–16.

Hutchinson TA, Leventhal JM, Kramer MB, Karch FE, Lipman AG, Feinstein AR (1979) An algorithm for the operational assessment of adverse drug reactions. II. Demonstration of reproducibility and validity, *J Am Med Assoc* **242**: 633–8.

Idanpaan Heikkila J, Alhava E, Olkinuora M, Palva, IP (1977) Agranulocytosis during treatment with clozapine. *Eur J Clin Pharmacol* **11**: 193–8.

Inman WHW (1970) Role of drug-reaction monitoring in the investigation of thrombosis and "the pill". *Br Med Bull* **26**: 248–56.

Inman WHS, Mushin WW (1974) Jaundice after repeated exposure to halothane. An analysis of reports to the Committee on Safety of Medicines. *Br Med J* **1**: 5–10.

Inman WHW, Vessey MP (1968) Investigation of deaths from pulmonary, coronary, and cerebral thrombosis and embolism in women of child-bearing age. *Br Med J* **2**: 193–9.

Inman WHW, Vessey MP, Westerholm B, Engelund A (1970) Thromboembolic disease and the steroidal content of oral contraceptives. A report to the Committee on Safety of Drugs. *Br Med J* **2**: 203–9.

Institute of Medicine (IOM) (1999) *To Err is Human. Building a Safer Health System.* Washington, DC: National Academy Press, pp. 86, 90–1.

International Society for Pharmacoepidemiology (ISPE) (1996) Guidelines for good epidemiology practices for drug, device, and vaccine research in the United States. *Pharmacoepidemiology* **5**: 333–8.

Irey NS (1976a) Tissue reactions to drugs. *Am J Path* **82**: 616–47.

Irey NS (1976b) Adverse drug reactions and death: a review of 827 cases. *J Am Med Assoc* **236**: 575–8.

Jacquez GM, Waller LA, Grimson R, Wartenberg D (1996a) The analysis of disease clusters, Part I: state of the art. *Infect Contr Hosp Epidemiol* **17**: 319–27.

Jacquez GM, Grimson R, Waller LA, Wartenberg D (1996b) The analysis of disease clusters, Part II. Introduction to techniques. *Infect Contr Hosp Epidemiol* **17**: 385–97.

Jolson HM, Bosco L, Bufton MG, Gerstman BB, Rinsler SS, Williams E, Flynn B, Simmons WD, Stadel BV, Faich GA, Peck C (1992) Clustering of adverse drug events. Analysis of risk factors for cerebellar toxicity with high-dose cytarabine. *J Nat Cancer Inst* **84**: 500–5.

Jones JK (1982) Adverse drug reactions in the community health setting. Approaches to recognizing, counseling, and reporting. *Family Commun Health* **5**: 58–67.

Jones JK (1994) Determining causation from case reports. In: Strom BL, ed., *Pharmacoepidemiology*, 2nd edn. Chichester: Wiley, pp. 365–78.

Karch FE, Lasagna L (1977) Toward the operational identification of adverse drug reactions. *Clin Pharmacol Ther* **21**: 247–54.

Karch FE, Smith CL, Kerzner B, Mazzullo JM, Weintraub M, Lasagna L (1976) Adverse drug reactions: a matter of opinion. *Clin Pharmacol Ther* **19**: 489–92.

Klincewicz SL, Clark JA, Arnold BDCA, Muniz EN, Blake MK (1999) Globalization of the safety sections of the periodic safety update report. *Drug Inf J* **33**: 887–98.

Koch-Weser J, Greenblatt DJ (1976) The ambiguity of adverse drug reactions. *Clin Pharmacol Ther* **19**: 110 (Abstract).

Koch-Weser J, Sellers EM, Zacest R (1977) The ambiguity of adverse drug reactions. *Eur J Clin Pharmacol* **11**: 75–8.

Kramer MS (1986) Assessing causality of adverse drug reactions. Global introspection and its limitations. *Drug Inf J* **20**: 433–7.

Kramer MS, Lane DA (1992) Causal propositions in clinical research and practice. *J Clin Epidemiol* **45**: 639–49.

Kramer MS, Leventhal JM, Hutchinson TA, Feinstein AR (1979) An algorithm for the operational assessment of adverse drug reactions: I. Background, description, and instructions for use. *J Am Med Assoc* **242**: 623–32.

Lanctôt KL, Naranjo CA (1995) Comparison of the Bayesian approach and a simple algorithm for assessment of adverse drug events. *Clin Pharmacol Ther* **58**: 692–8.

Lane DA (1984) A probabilist's view of causality assessment. *Drug Inf J* **18**: 323–30.

Lane DA (1986a) The logic of uncertainty. Measuring degree of belief. *Drug Inf J* **20**: 445–53.

Lane DA (1986b) The Bayesian approach to causality assessment: an introduction. *Drug Inf J* **20**: 455–61.

Lane DA, Kramer MS, Hutchinson TA, Jones JK, Naranjo C (1987) The causality assessment of adverse drug reactions using a Bayesian approach. *Pharmaceut Med* **2**: 265–83.

Lao CS (1997) Application of CUSUM technique and beta-binomial model in monitoring adverse drug reactions. *J Biopharm Stat* **7**: 227–39.

Lao CS (2000) Statistical issues involved in medical device postmarketing surveillance. *Drug Inf J* **34**: 483–93.

Lao CS, Kessler LG, Gross TP (1998) Proposed statistical methods for signal detection of adverse medical device events. *Drug Inf J* **32**: 183–91.

Lawson DH (1988) More about spontaneous reports of suspected adverse drug reactions. *Human Toxicol* **7**: 3–5.

Leventhal JM, Hutchinson TA, Kramer MS, Feinstein AR (1979) An algorithm for the operational assessment of adverse drug reactions. III. Results of tests among clinicians. *J Am Med Assoc* **242**: 1991–4.

Levine A, Mandel SPH, Santamaria A (1977) Pattern signalling in health information monitoring systems. *Meth Inform Med* **16**: 138–44.

Lindquist M, Edwards R, Bate A, Fucik H, Nunes AM, Stahl M (1999) From association to alert—a revised approach to international signal analysis. *Pharmacoepidemiology and Drug Safety* **8** (Suppl): S15–S25.

Lindquist M, Pettersson M, Edwards IR, Sanderson JH, Taylor NEA, Fletcher AP, Schou JS, Savage R (1997) How does cystitis affect a comparative risk profile of tiaprofenic acid with other non-steroidal antiinflammatory drugs. An international study based on spontaneous reports and drug usage data. *Pharm Tox* **80**: 211–17.

Louik C, Lacouture PG, Mitchell AA, Kauffman R, Lovejoy FH Jr, Yaffe SJ, Shapiro S (1985) A study of adverse reaction algorithms in a drug surveillance program. *Clin Pharmacol Ther* **38**: 183–7.

Louis T, Shen W (1999) Discussion. *Am Stat* **53**: 196–8.

Lydick E, Blumenthal SJ, Guess HA (1990) Learning to see. Twenty years of renal adverse experience reporting with Indocin®. *J Clin Res Pharmacoepidem* **4**: 183–9.

MacDonald MG, MacKay BR (1964) Adverse drug reactions. Experience of Mary Fletcher Hospital during 1962. *J Am Med Assoc* **190**: 1071–4.

Mandel SPH, Levine A, Beleno GE (1976) Signalling increases in reporting in international monitoring of adverse reactions to therapeutic drugs. *Meth Inform Med* **15**: 1–10.

Martinez C, Walker A (1995) Hypothesis testing using spontaneous reports as a source for case–control studies. *Pharmacoepidemiology and Drug Safety* **4**: S69.

Martone WJ, Williams WW, Mortensen ML, Gaynes RP, White JW, Lorch V, Murphy D, Sinha SN, Frank DJ, Kosmetatos N, Bodenstein CJ, Roberts RJ (1986) Illness with fatalities in premature infants: association with an intravenous vitamin E preparation, E-Ferol. *Pediatrics* **78**: 591–600.

Mason DH, Bernstein J, Bortnichak EA, Ehrlich GE (1990) Spontaneous reporting of adverse drug reactions. Diclofenac sodium and four other leading NSAIDs. *Int Med* **11**: 103–17.

Meyboom RHB (1998) Causality assessment revisited. *Pharmacoepidemiology and Drug Safety* **7**: S63–S65.

Meyboom RH, Egberts ACG, Edwards IR, Hekster YA, de Koning FHP, Gribnau FWJ (1997a) Principles of signal detection in pharmacovigilance. *Drug Safety* **16**: 355–65.

Meyboom RH, Hekster YA, Egberts AC, Gribnau FW, Edwards IR (1997b) Causal or casual? The role of causality assessment in pharmacovigilance. *Drug Safety* **17**: 374–89.

Meyboom RHB, Royer RJ (1992) Causality classification at pharmacovigilance centres in the European Community. *Pharmacoepidemiology and Drug Safety* **1**: 87–97.

Michel DJ, Knodel LC (1986) Comparison of three algorithms used to evaluate adverse drug reactions. *Am J Hosp Pharm* **43**: 1709–14.

Miremont G, Haramburu F, Bégaud B, Péré JC, Dangoumau J (1994) Adverse drug reactions: physicians' opinions versus a causality assessment method. *Eur J Clin Pharmacol* **46**: 285–9.

Moore ND, Bégaud B, Wiholm BE, Stricker BHCh, Kreft-Jais C (1995) The case/non-case design to generate and assess alerts from pharmacovigilance case–report databases. *Pharmacoepidemiology and Drug Safety* **4** (Suppl 1): S66.

Moore N, Kreft-Jais C, Haramburu F, Noblet C, Andrejak M, Ollagnier M, Bégaud B (1997) Reports of hypoglycaemia associated with the use of ACE inhibitors and other drugs. A case/non-case study in the French pharmacovigilance system database. *Br J Clin Pharmacol* **44**: 513–18.

Moride Y, Haramburu F, Requejo AA, Bégaud B (1997) Under-reporting of adverse drug reactions in general practice. *Br J Clin Pharmcol* **43**: 177–81.

Moussa MAA (1978) Statistical problems in monitoring adverse drug reactions. *Meth Inform Med* **17**: 106–12.

Napke E (1968) Drug adverse reaction alerting program. *Canad Pharm J* **20**: 251–4.

Naranjo CA (1986) A clinical pharmacologic perspective on the detection and assessment of adverse drug reactions. *Drug Inf J* **20**: 387–93.

Naranjo CA, Busto U, Sellers EM, Sandor P, Ruiz I, Roberts EA, Janecek E, Domecq C, Greenblatt DJ (1981) A method for estimating the probability of adverse drug reactions. *Clin Pharmacol Ther* **30**: 239–45.

Naranjo CA, Lanctôt KL (1993) Bayesian evaluation of sequential cases of neutropenia. *Pharmacoepidemiology and Drug Safety* **2**: S1–S6.

Naranjo CA, Lane D, Ho-Asjoe M, Lanctôt KL (1990) A Bayesian assessment of idiosyncratic adverse reactions to new drugs. Guillain–Barré Syndrome and zimeldine. *J Clin Pharmacol* **30**: 174–80.

Norwood PK, Sampson AR (1988) A statistical methodology for postmarketing surveillance of adverse drug reaction reports. *Stat Med* **7**: 1023–30.

Péré JC, Bégaud B, Haramburu F, Albin H (1986) Computerized comparison of six adverse drug reaction assessment procedures. *Clin Pharmacol Ther* **40**: 451–61.

Platt R, Dreis MW, Kennedy DL, Kuritsky JN (1988) Serum sickness-like reactions to amoxicillin, cefaclor, cephalexin, and trimethoprim-sulfamethoxazole. *J Inf Dis* **158**: 474–7.

Praus M, Schindel F, Fescharek R, Schwarz S (1993) Alert systems for post-marketing surveillance of adverse drug reactions. *Stat Med* **12**: 2383–93.

Rawlins MD (1986) Spontaneous reporting of adverse drug reactions. *Quart J Med* **59**: 531–4.

Rawlins MD (1988) Spontaneous reporting of adverse drug reactions. II. Uses. *Br J Clin Pharmacol* **26**: 7–11.

Rossi AC, Hsu JP, Faich GA (1987) Ulcerogenicity of piroxicam. An analysis of spontaneously reported data. *Brit Med J* **294**: 147–50.

Rossi AC, Bosco L, Faich GA, Tanner A, Temple R (1988) The importance of adverse reaction reporting by physicians. Suprofen and the flank pain syndrome. *J Am Med Assoc* **259**: 1203–4.

Royall BW (1971) International aspects of the study of adverse reactions to drugs. *Biometrics* **27**: 689–98.

Royall BW, Venulet J (1972) Methodology for international drug monitoring. *Meth Inform Med* **11**: 75–86.

Sachs RM, Bortnichak EA (1986) An evaluation of spontaneous adverse drug reaction monitoring systems. *Am J Med* **81**: 49–55.

Schmidt LG, Dirshedl P, Grohmann R, Scherer J, Wunderlich O, Muller-Oerlinghausen B (1986) Consistency of assessment of adverse drug reactions in psychiatric hospitals: a comparison of an algorithmic and an empirical approach. *Eur J Clin Pharm* **30**: 199–204.

Seidl LG, Thornton GF, Cluff LE (1965) Epidemiological studies of adverse drug reactions. *Am J Pub Health* **55**: 1170–5.

Sicker Th, Hoffmann A, Hoffmann H (1998) Individual case assessment of venous thromboembolic events suspected to be associated with combined oral contraceptives. Experience of reevaluating individual case histories on Valette®. *Pharmacoepidemiology and Drug Safety* **7** (Suppl): S109–S110.

Stahl MMS, Lindquist M, Pettersson M, Edwards IR, Sanderson JH, Taylor NFA, Fletcher AP, Schou JS (1997) Withdrawal reactions with selective serotonin re-uptake inhibitors as reported to the WHO system. *Eur J Clin Pharmacol* **53**: 163–9.

Stang PE, Fox JL (1992) Adverse drug events and the Freedom of Information Act: an apple in Eden. *Ann Pharmacother* **26**: 238–43.

Stephens MDB (1999) Causality assessment and signal recognition. In: Stephens MDB, Talbot JCC, Routledge PA, eds., *Detection of New Adverse Drug Reactions*. London: Macmillan Reference Ltd (UK), p. 298.

Strom BL, West SL, Sim E, Carson JL (1989) The epidemiology of the acute flank pain syndrome from suprofen. *Clin Pharmacol Ther* **46**: 693–9.

Tsong Y (1992) False alarm rates of statistical methods used in determining increased frequency of reports on adverse drug reaction. *J Biopharm Stat* **2**: 9–30.

Tsong Y (1995) Comparing reporting rates of adverse events between drugs with adjustment for year of marketing and secular trends in total reporting. *J Biopharm Stat* **5**: 95–114.

Tubert P, Bégaud B (1991) Random models for margins of a 2×2 contingency table and application to pharmacovigilance. *Stat Med* **10**: 991–9.

Tubert P, Bégaud B, Haramburu F, Péré JC (1991) Spontaneous reporting. How many cases are required to trigger a warning? *Br J Clin Pharmacol* **32**: 407–8.

Tubert P, Bégaud B, Péré JC, Haramburu F, Lellouch J (1992) Power and weakness of spontaneous reporting. A probabilistic approach. *J Clin Epidemiol* **45**: 283–6.

Tubert-Bitter P, Bégaud B (1993) Comparing safety of drugs. *Post Marketing Surveillance* **7**: 119–37.

Tubert-Bitter P, Bégaud B, Moride Y, Chaslerie A, Haramburu F (1996) Comparing the toxicity of two drugs in the framework of spontaneous reporting. A confidence interval approach. *J Clin Epidemiol* **49**: 121–3.

Tubert-Bitter P, Haramburu F, Bégaud B, Chaslerie A, Abraham E, Hagry C (1998) Spontaneous reporting of adverse drug reactions: who reports and what? *Pharmacoepidemiology and Drug Safety* **7**: 323–9.

Turner WM (1984) The Food and Drug Administration algorithm. Special workshop–regulatory. *Drug Inf J* **118**: 259–66.

Venulet J (1973) Adverse reactions to drugs. *Int J Clin Pharmacol* **7**: 253–64.

Venulet J (1988) Possible strategies for early recognition of potential drug safety problems. *Adv Drug React Ac Pois Rev* **1**: 39–42.

Venulet J (1992) Role and place of causality assessment. *Pharmacoepidemiology and Drug Safety* **1**: 225–34.

Waller PC, Lee EH (1999) Responding to drug safety issues. *Pharmacoepidemiology and Drug Safety* **8**: 535–52.

Wartenberg D, Greenberg M (1993) Solving the cluster puzzle: clues to follow and pitfalls to avoid. *Stat Med* **12**: 1763–70.

Wechsler ME, Garpestad E, Flier SR, Kocher O, Weiland DA, Polito AJ, Klinek MM, Bigby TD, Wong GA, Helmers RA, Drazen JM (1998) Pulmonary infiltrates, eosinophilia, and cardiomyopathy following corticosteroid withdrawal in patients with asthma receiving zafirlukast. *J Am Med Assoc* **279**: 455–7.

Wysowski DK, Green L (1995) Serious adverse events in Norplant users reported to the Food and Drug Administration's MedWatch Spontaneous Reporting System. *Obstet Gynecol* **85**: 538–42.

Wysowski D, Fourcroy JL (1996) Flutamide hepatotoxicity. *J Urology* **155**: 209–12.

20

Statistical Methods of Signal Detection

London School of Hygiene and Tropical Medicine, London, UK

INTRODUCTION

The term "Signal Recognition" arises from electronic engineering, where with radio or radar waves there is a real signal that exists but it is accompanied by "noise" in the background, and there is a need to detect the signal, distinguishing it from the background. This terminology has been used in other contexts, notably in medical diagnosis where similarities to the problems in electronics can also be seen. The terminology of electronics has been continued with "Receiver-Operating-Characteristic" curves. These illustrate that with a given amount of information there must always be a trade-off between the risk of the two different errors of classification; calling noise a signal (a false positive) and calling a true signal noise (a false negative). The sensitivity of a diagnostic test is high when there is a low false negative rate; the specificity of a diagnostic test is high when there is a low false positive rate.

With adverse drug reactions (ADRs) there are two levels of diagnosis of causality: first, diagnosis at a single case level; secondly, at a public health or epidemiological level. ADR causality in an individual patient is not the subject of this chapter, but statistical approaches may help with single cases. The public health and epidemiological perspective is of greatest importance and statistical methods can be of some help. The objective is to find those signals that are indicative of causal effects, and to reject those signals of effects that are not caused by a particular drug. Where they are of public health significance they will either affect large numbers of individuals or have extremely serious effects in smaller numbers. In these circumstances, the public health view requires that true reactions caused by a medicine be recognised as early as possible. At the same time, those suspected reactions that are not caused by a medicine should be recognised as such and minimal resource should be spent on investigating them.

Signals of potential harmful effects may arise from literature reports, observational epidemiological studies, randomised trials and spontaneous reports of suspected ADRs. In some countries the emphasis is on suspected reactions but in others the emphasis is on adverse events. This chapter will concentrate on the analysis of large volumes of these spontaneous reports. Their source will usually be health professionals but may also

Pharmacovigilance. Edited by R.D. Mann and E.B. Andrews

include patients. The early evidence from sponta-neous reports can be regarded as a potential "signal". This has been defined as showing a "... possible causal relationship between an ad-verse event and a drug. Unknown ... previously" (Wood *et al.*, 1994). The object is to distinguish the real signals from "noise" precisely.

The details of spontaneous reporting will not be covered here. The salient feature is that health professionals, particularly doctors, report sus-pected ADRs centrally; this can be to a regulatory authority or to a company. These reports are processed and entered on to a database. Whether they are reported as suspected ADRs or as adverse events there will inevitably be some background reports that are not caused by the drug. There will often be a very large number of reports and an essential task is to prioritise those that should be investigated first. The purpose of collecting these reports is to detect signals. Even in countries where reporting of ADRs is supposed to be compulsory, reporting rates will usually be much less than 100%. A typical figure is said to be 10%, but it depends very much on the seriousness and newness of the ADR. In the case of fibrosing colonopathy caused by high-strength pancreatic enzymes the rate was shown to be 100%.

WHAT CONSTITUTES A SIGNAL?

If resources were available, then every single report would constitute a signal, but in practice, some have used simply the number of reports for a particular reaction/drug combination as a cut-off. This cut-off has been, for example, two or more, or three or more reports. This is a reasonably sensitive but a very non-specific test. The number of reports, whether the signal is a causative effect or not, will depend on the number of patients exposed to the drug. The first step in the process is to attempt to estimate incidence. The number of reports is taken as the numerator but a question exists as to what is the correct denominator. Possible alternatives are:

- Sales
- Prescriptions written
- Prescriptions dispensed

Even if the data on prescriptions dispensed are available, they do not necessarily relate to the important factors related to a causal effect. If it is simply patient-years of exposure, then the total number of prescriptions dispensed is a reasonable measure. However, this assumes that the risk of having the ADR is constant over time. If this is not so, then we need patient-years grouped by dura-tion of treatment. This requires individual patient-based data or at least the distribution of the number of prescriptions per patient.

A cut-off for a signal could then be an incidence rate that is greater than background. This is the basis of the Poisson method of examining signals. This has utility in some specific areas where the background rate is well known and rare, and where the reporting rate is known to be reasonably high or at least well known. It can be used to compare reporting rates of two drugs using sales data as a denominator.

CLASSIFICATION OF ADR REPORTS

Each report must be assigned to one or more drugs and to one or more medical terms describing the reaction. There is a need for a distinction between a drug reported as being suspected of causing the adverse effect and one that is simply co-medica-tion. This distinction made by the reporter of the reaction may not be made correctly, especially when it is an interaction between drugs that is causing the effect.

For the value of the report to be optimal, both the trade name and the drug substance name may need to be recorded separately. For initial statistical approaches to signal detection then the drug substance name is the one that is used.

The minimum information for a valid report is usually an identifiable (but not necessarily identi-fied) patient, a drug and a reaction. The reaction must be classified using some form of medical dictionary. There are several different dictionaries in wide use, including those from the Food and Drug Administration (FDA) (COSTART) and the World Health Organisation (WHO) (WHO-ART). In the United Kingdom, the Medicines Control Agency (MCA) use their own ADROIT dictionary and a project to unify these dictionaries, based partly on the ADROIT dictionary has been carried out, resulting in the internationally (International Conference on Harmonisation (ICH)) agreed MedDRA.

Most of the dictionaries have a form of hierarchy from the widest grouping—"System Order Class"—e.g. cardiovascular, through "High Level Terms" to "Preferred Term", e.g. myocardial infarction. A second type of classification relates to the public health impact of a reaction classed as fatal, serious or non-serious. The definition of "serious" is not always consistent between countries or dictionaries but within a particular database it will (or should) be consistent.

CHARACTERISTICS OF SPONTANEOUS REPORTS

It is well known that reporting is biased: severe ADRs are more likely to be reported; known reactions are less likely to be reported. In the United Kingdom, there is a tendency for reporting rates to be higher when a drug is newly introduced to the market, but the effect of media or regulatory action may distort this pattern. The consequence is that reporting rates cannot be relied upon as estimates of the incidence of adverse reactions. This situation will always apply, and although there may be calls from those unfamiliar with pharmacovigilance to improve reporting rates so that spontaneous reports do reflect true incidence, this is not their purpose. They can be used to detect signals, and they are certainly capable of doing this.

Given the biases in reporting rates, one obvious way to assess the strength of a signal is to study the spontaneous reports alone without an external comparison group. This means that many of the biases that apply to reporting rates will apply to all reports and within the database an increased validity of comparison may be made.

PROPORTIONAL REPORTING RATIOS

Proportional reporting ratios (PRRs) compare the proportion of reports for a specific ADR reported for a drug with the proportion for that ADR in all other drugs (Evans et al., 1998, 2001). The principles are not new, but were set out in a similar way by Patwary (1969) and Finney (1974) for ADR reporting with WHO data. The methods were not fully used subsequently, either in WHO or in the United Kingdom, and were effectively reinvented in 1995 at the UK MCA, where they have been used routinely since 1997. The PRR can also be seen as a numerical version of the ADR profile; this simply uses a bar chart for a particular drug giving the numbers in each system organ class (SOC). An implicit comparison is made with a bar chart derived from another group of drugs. A similar approach is used in classical epidemiology with death data—the "Proportional Mortality Ratio" (see, for example, Rothman and Greenland, 1998).

The calculation of the PRR is very simple in principle as shown in Table 20.1:

$$PRR = [a/(a + b)]/[c/(c + d)].$$

This is analogous to a relative risk. An obvious alternative is to use an odds ratio (ad/bc) that may be regarded as a "Proportional odds ratio" (POR). This has slightly more desirable statistical properties than a PRR, but will be very similar in magnitude since in most circumstances $b \geqslant a$ and $d \geqslant c$.

When a reaction is new and rare then a (in the 2×2 table, Table 20.1) can be one or a very small number, and it is possible that there are no other drugs with that exact reaction. This means that b is zero and the PRR or POR is not calculable. However, it is possible to use the table for practical purposes in a way that is not exactly statistically rigorous. The second row can refer to all drugs rather than "all other drugs". This means that c is never zero and the POR or PRR is always able to be calculated, and the estimated values are less

Table 20.1.

	Specific ADR	All other reactions
Specific drug	a	b
All other drugs	c	d

than they would be otherwise. This conservatism applies when the numbers are small and does no harm when using the PRR or POR for prioritisation.

A more general approach is to ask, "What is the expected number of reports for this ADR and this drug?" and then to compare the observed number with the expected number. A first attempt to obtain the expected number is to assume that the proportion of reports for this ADR with this drug will be the same as the proportion for this ADR in the database as a whole, P_{ADR}. The expected number can then be obtained using the total reports for this drug, N_{drug}:

$$E_{ADR,drug} = P_{ADR} * N_{drug}.$$

The deviation of the observed number from the expected number can be expressed as a ratio, that is, the *PRR*

$$PRR = O_{ADR,drug}/E_{ADR,drug}.$$

This approach can more easily be seen to be generalisable to allow the expected number to be calculated in a less crude way. It can be modified to allow for age and sex to be taken into account. This is equivalent to having a set of 2×2 tables stratified by age and sex, where a POR can be derived using a general Mantel–Haenszel estimator from several 2×2 tables (Rothman and Greenland, 1998). It is also possible to use logistic regression to obtain such an estimate.

These measures have allowed for the *magnitude* of the effect to be assessed; they have not made any allowance for chance variation. The simplest way to make such allowances is to calculate statistical significance tests of the hypothesis that the PRR or POR is one. It is also possible to use the equivalent confidence intervals Tubert-Bitter *et al.* (1996). The usual chi-square test (corrected using Yates' method to be conservative), or for stratified tables using the Mantel–Haenszel method, can be calculated. This chi-square value indicates the contribution of chance to the magnitude of the PRR. Table 20.2 gives an example of an extreme PRR. The proportion of reports of uveitis with the drug rifabutin is

Table 20.2. Example calculation of PRR.

	Uveitis	All other reports	Total
Rifabutin	41	14	55
All other drugs	754	591 958	592 712
Total	795	591 972	592 767

$(41/55) = 0.75$, while the proportion for all drugs is $754/591\,958 = 0.0013$: PRR = 586, chi-square $= 22\,736$, $p \ll 0.00001$.

It should be realised that all of this process should be used for the purpose of signal detection, and even more importantly, for prioritisation of the detected signals to help decide which ones require most urgent further investigation. The basic data are still subject to biases; they are at very best observational data and to use a high value of a PRR or POR as the sole convincing evidence of causation is unwarranted. They raise a serious question that merits further study. At the same time, it should be remembered that where the reports are of suspected ADRs, then the reporter suspected a causal relationship and the fear that raised PRRs or PORs will generate too many false positive signals is probably also unjustified.

RATIONALE FOR PROPORTIONAL METHODS

A basic question to be asked is whether the use of the proportion of reports for a particular reaction (compared with all reports) is sensible. As a first step, it is reasonable to examine the trends in proportions of reports over time within a major database. The figure below gives the cumulative total number of reports and the cumulative number of reactions reported as suspected ADRs in the UK MCA database (Waller *et al.*, 1996). This database, called Adverse Drug Reactions Online Information and Tracking (ADROIT), has suspected ADRs reported on Yellow Cards since 1964. Over this period, the number of reports in the database has risen dramatically but the pattern in proportions in different SOCs has remained relatively stable.

Figure 20.1 shows the cumulative numbers of reports and reactions by year. Figure 20.2 shows

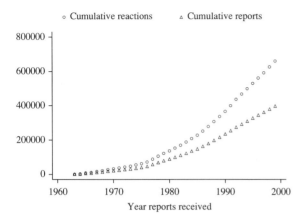

Figure 20.1. The cumulative number of reports and reactions in the UK ADROIT database.

the cumulative proportion (on a log scale) of reactions reported for a cross-section of the SOCs. These show that cardiovascular reports are stable at a high level, while "ear" reports are fairly stable at a low level. Eye reactions show a notable rise in 1974—a result of practolol; skin reactions are stable at a high level with a peak in 1982 (benoxaprofen).

THE USE OF PRRS IN MONITORING DRUGS

One method of screening for signals for drugs in the United Kingdom that are under intensive monitoring ("Black Triangle" drugs) is to use both the PRR and the chi-square statistic. A cut-off for each can be used; for example, a PRR > 2 and chi-squared > 4 and the number of reports > 2. When this method is first used with these criteria on an existing database, many of the signals generated will already be known problems. In the first usage at the UK MCA slightly more than 60% were known; e.g. uveitis with rifabutin. About 15% were not believed to be caused by the drug but were events—effects of disease or a function of the patient population being treated, e.g. haemoptysis with dornase alpha. About 25% were new signals that required more detailed evaluation, e.g. renal failure with losartan.

In general, the method is used for continuing monitoring so that known problems will not

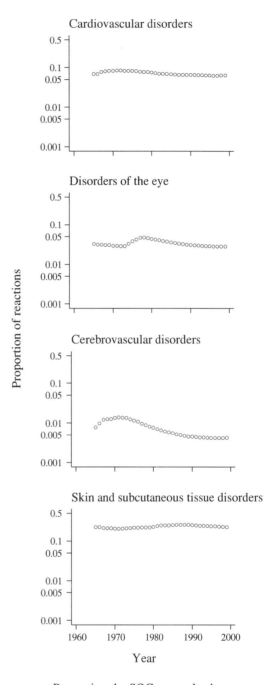

Proportions by SOC over calendar year

Figure 20.2. The proportions of reactions in some SOCs over time.

constitute a new signal. The triggers that constitute a signal will then be a change in PRR to raise it above the threshold or a 30% increase in PRR previously above threshold, but where the previous judgement was that the (small) raised PRR was not sufficient evidence of a signal.

FURTHER DEVELOPMENTS AND KEY ISSUES

Further improvements to the sensitivity and specificity of the method include stratifying by age and sex; examining serious or fatal reactions only. (The proportion of reactions that are fatal, stratified by age is itself a potential signalling method.) Where a drug has a well-known ADR that is reported very frequently, such as gastrointestinal (GI) bleeding with non-steroidal anti-inflammatory drugs (NSAIDs), this will distort the PRR for other reactions with that drug. The best approach is then to remove the known reactions from the totals for that drug and the database as a whole and recalculate the PRR for all other reactions with that drug. This is simple to do on an *ad hoc* basis but is more difficult to implement in an automated way.

The comparison used need not be the entire database. It is possible to use PRRs within drug classes or indications so that the comparator is all drugs in that class or those used for a particular indication.

The expected number of reactions could also incorporate prior beliefs about the ADR profile, using a fully Bayesian method. (The approaches used at the FDA and WHO do not incorporate prior beliefs.)

The grouping of terms used in the medical dictionary for the database is an important feature. Little empirical study of the effect of choosing different levels in the hierarchy of terms has been done. In most instances, the grouping is at "Preferred Term" (PT), which is a relatively low level. There are a large number of medical terms at this level, so that the numbers for any particular combination of drug and reaction can be small. This can lead both to the general statistical problem of multiplicity, with many possibilities

for signals, and to instability in the PRR based on small expected numbers.

It is possible to use a two-stage process—using, say, SOC to screen for raised PRRs, then to re-examine the PRRs using PTs within the SOC where the PRR was raised. The automation of this process is possible in principle, but has not been done yet. An alternative is to use an intermediate level within the hierarchy—a "High Level Term" (HLT), for example. This has the advantage of being a single stage process and avoids the use of too many terms, reducing the problems of multiplicity and small expected numbers.

The use of the method in general is easiest within a large database that contains a wide range of drugs, but it can be used within a pharmaceutical company database. Here, the potential for incorporating prior beliefs is at its greatest. A further possibility for companies is to use the proportions of reactions from the FDA database, which is publicly available, to calculate expected numbers for their own drugs. Other regulatory databases are not yet publicly available but increasing transparency may change this in the future.

CONCLUSIONS

The validity of the method has been demonstrated. It detects existing problems; it finds new signals and prioritises them for the benefit of assessors; it is very simple, transparent, and objective; and it can be automated very easily indeed.

The "Bayesian Data Mining" approach used by the FDA (DuMouchel, 1999) is very similar, but offers a better statistical analysis when very small numbers are involved. It emphasises ranking of the equivalent of the logarithm of PRR. It uses an "Empirical Bayes" method, which shrinks log (O/E) towards zero, and the shrinkage is important if E is small, but gives very similar results when observed or expected numbers of reactions are reasonably large. It is slightly more complex in the calculations, and consequently less transparent.

The WHO has a new approach (Bate *et al.*, 1998) based on a Bayesian confidence propagation neural network, but again is very similar to a PRR. It uses the log (to the base 2) of the PRR based on the same 2×2 table as used with PRRs. Its use of Bayes' theorem in a 2×2 table is not controversial and does not incorporate prior belief. The cut-off for a signal is based on the confidence interval around their statistic. The method has the ability to scan the whole database relatively rapidly, forming all tables for combinations of drugs and reactions that occur together and is used routinely.

The major issues are the potential for misinterpretation of the signals and over-reliance on automation. The statistical methods are a first stage of assessment and careful evaluation using medical scientific knowledge is still required. At the same time, the potential contributions of statistical methods and of statisticians have not been fully realised. The advances in the past few years seem to have been greater than in the previous 20 years, although it is recognised that there has been some re-invention. Further statistical creativity is possible, particularly in integrating spontaneous reporting with epidemiological methods and randomised trial data.

ACKNOWLEDGEMENTS

The late Dr Susan Wood and many of her colleagues at the MCA and on the UK Committee on Safety of Medicines encouraged this type of approach. I am grateful to them for the opportunity to apply some statistical thinking to problems in the safety of medicines.

REFERENCES

Bate A, Lindquist M, Edwards IR, Olsson S, Orre R, Lansner A, De Freitas RM (1998) A Bayesian neural network method for adverse drug reaction signal generation. *Eur J Clin Pharmacol* **54**: 315–21.

DuMouchel W (1999) Bayesian data mining in large frequency tables, with an application to the FDA Spontaneous Reporting System. *Am Stat* **53**: 177–90.

Evans SJW, Waller P, Davis S (1998) Proportional reporting ratios: the uses of epidemiological methods for signal generation. *Pharmacoepidemiology and Drug Safety* **7**: S 102.

Evans SJW, Waller PC, Davis S (2001) Use of proportional reporting ratios (PRRs) for signal generation from spontaneous adverse drug reaction reports. *Pharmacoepidemiology and Drug Safety* **10**: 483–6.

Finney DJ (1974) Systematic signalling of adverse reactions to drugs. *Meth Inf Med* **13**: 1–10.

Patwary KW (1969) *Report on Statistical Aspects of the Pilot Research Project for International Drug Monitoring*. Geneva: WHO.

Rothman KJ, Greenland S (1998) *Modern Epidemiology*. Philadelphia: Lippincott-Raven, pp. 76, 270.

Tubert-Bitter P, Bégaud B, Motide Y, Chaslerie A, Haramburu F (1996) Comparing the toxicity of two drugs in the framework of spontaneous reporting: a confidence interval approach. *J Clin Epidemiol* **49**: 121–3.

Waller PC, Coulson RA, Wood SM (1996) Regulatory pharmacovigilance in the United Kingdom: current principles and practice. *Pharmacoepidemiology and Drug Safety* **5**: 363–75.

Wood SM, Coulson R, Eccles S. (1994) Signal generation in the UK. In: Fracchia GN, ed., *European Medicines Research*. Amsterdam: IOS Press, pp. 360–3.

21

Statistical Methods of Evaluating Pharmacovigilance Data

BERNARD BÉGAUD

Département de Pharmacologie Clinique—Unité de Pharmaco-épidémiologie, ARME-Pharmacovigilance,
Université Victor Segalen, Bordeaux, France

INTRODUCTION

The three main challenges of pharmacovigilance, i.e. to detect, to assess and to prevent risks associated with medicines (Bégaud, 2000), may concern both the patient level and the populational level. Similarly, the latter may rely on classical epidemiological studies, e.g. cohort or case–control, or on cases-only analyses, which is the scope of spontaneous reporting (SR).

In cohort studies (Kramer, 1988), subjects are followed in a forward direction from exposure to outcome (e.g. the occurrence of a given disease), and inferential reasoning is from cause to effect. For example, in the case of a cohort study with a reference group, the subjects can be split, at the end of the follow-up, among the four cells of the following classical two-by-two table:

	Diseased	Not diseased
N_1 (exposed)	a	b
N_2 (not exposed)	c	d
t_0	follow-up	t_1

In case–control studies, subjects are investigated in a backward direction, from outcome (disease) to exposure and inference is from effect to cause:

Exposed	Not exposed	
a	b	N_1 diseased (cases)
c	d	N_2 not diseased (controls)
past exposure ascertainment		← index date

In both designs, the compared groups are generally drawn from a larger source population, which raises the problem of possible selection biases; however, the subjects are generally exhaustively classified according to a binary variable: to present or not to present the considered disease in cohort studies, or to have been or not to have been exposed to the studied factor in case–control studies. SR, *per se*, is a passive surveillance method involving the whole source-population, e.g. all subjects of a given country treated with a given medicine; however, SR

Pharmacovigilance. Edited by R.D. Mann and E.B. Andrews
© 2002 John Wiley & Sons, Ltd

suffers two major limitations (Bégaud, 2000):

- it does not provide any direct and reliable information on the size, characteristics and exposure patterns of the source population;
- the term *spontaneous* refers to the random character of the case collection from the exposed population; indeed, reporting assumes that the observer (i) identifies the adverse event, (ii) imputes its occurrence to a drug exposure, (iii) is aware of the existence of a pharmacovigilance system, and (iv) is convinced of the need to report the case if relevant, e.g. new and/or serious adverse drug reactions (ADRs).

This results in the major plague of this surveillance method: an inescapable *under-reporting*, the magnitude and selectivity of which are unknown and extremely difficult to assess. Indeed, if a number a of cases of a given event have occurred in a population during the "follow-up" period, then it is likely that only a part $k = a/U$ of these cases will be reported, U being the *under-reporting coefficient* varying from 1 to infinity, e.g. $U = 4$ if 25% of cases have been reported.

Moreover, it is hard to believe that each of the a cases that have occurred have an identical probability $1/U$ to be reported. Many factors have been shown to influence reporting (Pierfitte *et al.*, 1999) such as the age of the patient, the seriousness of the event and its onset delay. Thus, because of a selection bias, k could be a non-representative sample of the source population of cases.

From a biostatistical point of view, the rather bizzare design of SR could be compared to a cohort study without reference group in which:

- the "followed" population is extremely large, i.e. the whole population of the surveyed territory treated with drugs;
- the characteristics of this population, e.g. age and gender distributions, concomitant diseases, are unknown as are its characteristics of exposure (indications, dose, duration, co-medications, etc.);
- the number of "investigators" is extremely large, i.e., all health professionals in the territory;

- the case collection does not rely on a precise protocol and is thus non-systematic and may be subjective.

Moreover, because of the open character of this method of surveillance (any type of drug, any type of event), there is in fact a quasi infinite number of sub-cohorts, one for each type of drug exposure:

	Diseased	Not diseased	Total
Exposed	a	b	N_1

t_0 Cohort study t

	Diseased	Not diseased	Total
Exposed	k	?	?

t_0 Spontaneous reporting t

While the cohort study can estimate the risk associated with a given drug exposure by calculation of the incidence rate a/N_{1t} (number of new occurrences of the disease produced by the surveyed population during the period t), to estimate risks from SRs requires rather complex assumptions and calculations.

RISK ESTIMATON FROM SR

ESTIMATION OF THE NUMERATOR

As previously mentioned, the actual number a of cases that have occurred during the surveillance period t could theoretically be estimated by

$$a = k \cdot U,$$

where k is the number of reports during the surveillance period and U is the under-reporting coefficient varying from one (exhaustive reporting) to infinite (i.e. the reporting rate is null).

Unfortunately, it is extremely difficult and/or hazardous to estimate the magnitude of this under-reporting, even if in most cases it can be thought to be huge, even for serious cases (Alvarez-Requejo *et al.*, 1998; Eland *et al.*, 1999).

For example, in 1998 a nation-wide prospective study conducted in a representative sample of French public hospitals estimated that 128 768 patients (95% CI: 100 916–156 620) were admitted that year in these hospitals because of an ADR (Pouyanne *et al.*, 2000). This study did not consider other aspects of seriousness such as death, nor admissions to private hospitals. Nevertheless, the obtained figure (128 768) was far larger than the number of serious reactions (about 15 000) reported during the same period to the French pharmacovigilance system still considered as particularly efficient.

The *capture–recapture* approach, when applicable, could appear appealing to estimate the total number of cases of a given effect that have occurred in the surveyed population (Jeeger *et al.*, 1996). This approach derives the size of the source-population from the number of individuals both "captured" by two independent samplings from this population (a more accurate estimate would be obtained by a greater number of samplings, e.g. three or four). To apply this method to pharmacovigilance consists in considering two or more independent sources of reports in the same territory. For instance, if k_1 and k_2 reports have been collected, respectively, during the same period, through two independent sources, e.g. the regional pharmacovigilance centres network and the concerned manufacturer and if c was the number of duplicates (i.e. cases identified by both sources 1 and 2), then the total number of cases would be

$$a = \frac{k_1 \cdot k_2}{c}.$$

If k_1 and k_2 were large enough (e.g. $\geqslant 15$), the normal approximation can be used to calculate the $1 - \alpha$ confidence interval (CI) for a:

$$\text{CI}_{1-\alpha} = a \pm Z_{1-\alpha}\sqrt{\frac{k_1 \cdot k_2 \cdot (k_1 - c) \cdot (k_2 - c)}{c^3}}.$$

Example: During a one-year surveillance period, 127 cases were reported to the first system and 42 to the second; 12 duplicates were identified. The estimate for the total number of cases is

$$a = \frac{127 \times 42}{12} = 444,$$

and its two-sided 95% CI is:

$$444 \pm 1.96\sqrt{\frac{127 \times 42 \times (127 - 12) \times (42 - 12)}{12^3}}$$

$$= [242; 646].$$

One can deduce that the actual number of cases has 95 chances in a hundred of being between 242 and 646. The number of cases identified by SR being $(127 + 42) - 12 = 157$, the reporting ranges between 24% and 65%.

However, the validity of such an estimate requires that reporting to one system or the other be a truly random and independent phenomenon which could be an unverified assumption. For this reason, the safest way is probably to cease to estimate the actual number of cases and to deal with *reporting rates* instead of *incidence rates*!

ESTIMATION OF THE DENOMINATOR

In some countries, the size N and characteristics of the exposed population and its conditions of exposure can be precisely derived from health insurance databases. In this case, except for the poor quality of case collection (i.e. under-reporting), SR approaches the cohort design.

Unfortunately, in most cases, it is necessary to estimate these parameters from sales statistics and/or drug prescription on drug utilization panels (Bégaud *et al.*, 1993). The use of such agregated data precludes any possibility of considering some individual or sub-group characteristics in the analysis.

The necessary "ingredients" for computation are: the number of exposure units, e.g. tablets, capsules, injection doses sold in the territory during the relevant period of time, and the average daily dose (ADD) of the considered drug used in this population, the latter being estimated from prescription panels or other sources. By default, the defined daily dose (DDD) or the recommended daily dose (RDD) can be used as proxy.

Example: 780 000 packages of 20 capsules have been sold in a one-year period, the used daily dose is 2.1 capsules. This corresponds to the quantity necessary for a cumulative duration of treatment of: $(780\,000 \times 20)/2.1 = 2\,666\,667$ days, or 87 719 months. In a more epidemiological parlance, the exposure level in the source-population is 87 719 person-months.

As for incidence density calculations, this total probably sums individual exposure periods which are extremely different. Moreover, because of its ecological character, this approach precludes any risk analysis based on the duration of exposure.

To estimate the number of treatments or the number of subjects treated would require knowing the average duration of a treatment (ADT) with the considered drug. In the previous example, if the ADT was 23 days, the number of treatments for the considered period would be: $2\,666\,667/23 = 115\,942$.

However, in the absence of direct information from a health insurance database, the use of measurements made on panels or relatively small samples, both for the average daily dose and duration of treatment, will greatly increase the statistical instability of the estimate. In the previous example, if the 95% CIs were [1.6; 2.7] and [16; 31] for the ADD and ADT, respectively, then the CI for the number of treatments would range from 31 860 to 104 167. For this reason, it is often preferable to keep person-time estimates for further calculations.

ESTIMATION OF REPORTING RATES

As for incidence rates, the number of cases reported during a given period of time is standardized for the corresponding person-time denominator. For example, if 18 cases of severe neutropenia have been reported for a cumulative exposure time (estimated from sales statistics) of 87 719 months, the reporting rate is: $18/87\,719 = 2.05$ for 10 000 person-months

Table 21.1. 95% confidence limits, two-sided, left and right one-sided, for m according to the Poisson distribution. To estimate the CI of a proportion p, bounds are divided by N. For a left one-sided interval, the upper bound of np is $+\infty$ and of p is 1. For a right one-sided interval, the lower bound of np is $-\infty$ and that of p is 0 (computations made by the author by using a HP 49G calculator).

m	Two-sided	Left one-sided	Right one-sided
0	—	—	3
1	0.03–5.57	0.05	4.74
2	0.24–7.23	0.35	6.29
3	0.62–8.77	0.82	7.75
4	1.09–10.24	1.37	9.15
5	1.62–11.67	1.97	10.51
6	2.20–13.06	2.61	11.84
7	2.81–14.42	3.28	13.15
8	3.45–15.76	3.98	14.43
9	4.12–17.08	4.69	15.71
10	4.80–18.39	5.42	16.96
11	5.49–19.68	6.17	18.21
12	6.20–20.96	6.92	19.44
13	6.92–22.23	7.69	20.67
14	7.65–23.49	8.46	21.89
15	8.40–24.74	9.25	23.10
16	9.15–25.98	10.03	24.30
17	9.90–27.22	10.83	25.50
18	10.67–28.45	11.63	26.69
19	11.44–29.67	12.44	27.88
20	12.22–30.89	13.25	29.06
21	13.00–32.10	14.07	30.24
22	13.79–33.31	14.89	31.41
23	14.58–34.51	15.72	32.58
24	15.38–35.71	16.55	33.75
25	16.18–36.91	17.38	34.92
26	16.98–38.09	18.22	36.08
27	17.79–39.28	19.06	37.23
28	18.61–40.47	19.90	38.39
29	19.42–41.65	20.75	39.54
30	20.24–42.83	21.59	40.69
31	21.06–44.00	22.44	41.84
32	21.89–45.17	23.30	42.98
33	22.71–46.34	24.15	44.13
34	23.54–47.51	25.01	45.27
35	24.38–48.68	25.87	46.40
36	25.21–49.84	26.73	47.54
37	26.05–51.00	27.59	48.68
38	26.89–52.16	28.46	49.81
39	27.73–53.31	29.33	50.94

of exposure. It is sensible to consider that the occurrence of cases in the exposed population and their reporting, both correspond to a pseudo-random process which can be described by an *ad hoc* probability model. Given that, in pharmaco-vigilance, the source population is generally extremely large and the probability of occurrence very low, the Poisson distribution is expected to be quite a satisfactory model (Snedecor and Cochran, 1989). In these conditions, the calculation of the 95% two-sided CI for the reporting rate consists of considering the lower and upper limits for the Poisson parameter read in a table such as Table 21.1.

In the above example, the 95% Poisson CI for the observed number 18 is [10.67; 28.45]. The CI for the reporting rate is thus: 10.67 to 28.45 for 87 719 months, i.e. 1.2 to 3.2 per 10 000 person-months of exposure. When the number k of reports is large enough, i.e. 15 or preferably 30, the CI can be calculated by using the normal approximation for a Poisson count (Daly *et al.*, 1991):

$$CI = k \pm Z_{1-\alpha}\sqrt{k}.$$

In both cases, this CI defines the set of values which could be observed because of the sampling variation, all parameters remaining identical.

STATISTICAL MODELING OF SR

If N is the size of the exposed population, i.e. the number of subjects treated or having been treated with the considered drug during the surveillance period, and p is the reference risk of a given event, i.e. the risk in this population if not exposed, then the number of fortuitous (i.e. non-causal) occurrences of this event expected during the period is $N \cdot p$.

If RR is the relative risk associated with drug exposure and U the under-reporting coefficient, then the expected number of reports is (Tubert-Bitter *et al.*, 1992):

$$m = \frac{N \cdot p \cdot RR}{U}.$$

Referring to the classical Poisson formula, the probability of receiving x reports is:

$$Pr(k = x) = \frac{e^{-m} \cdot m^x}{x!},$$

and the cumulative probability of receiving at least x reports is:

$$Pr(k \geqslant x) = 1 - \sum_{x=0}^{x-1} \frac{e^{-m} \cdot m^x}{x!}.$$

Table 21.2 gives the probability of receiving at least one report according to the value of m. One can see that to have a good chance of detecting an adverse event requires m to be greater than one, i.e. 1.61 for an 80% chance, 2.30 for 90% and 3 for 95%, respectively.

It should be kept in mind that for serious conditions, the baseline incidence p is usually extremely low, therefore m remains markedly below one, except if N is extremely large and RR/U greater than one, i.e. if the association between drug exposure and the considered event is strong and the reporting is reasonably good.

Let us take the example of a non-steroidal anti-inflammatory drug for which the average duration of use is two weeks. In a given country, 2.5 million two-week treatments have been made in one year, corresponding to a cumulative time of exposure of 5 millions weeks, i.e. 96 154 years. Considering the generally recognized value of 7 per million for the annual incidence of agranulocytosis in the general

Table 21.2. Value of the expected number m necessary to have a given probability $Pr(k \geqslant 1)$ of observing at least one case of an event (calculations made by using the Poisson formula).

m	$Pr(k \geqslant 1)$	m	$Pr(k \geqslant 1)$
0.1	0.095	0.9	0.593
0.2	0.181	1	0.632
0.3	0.259	2	0.865
0.4	0.330	3	0.950
0.5	0.393	4	0.982
0.6	0.451	5	0.993
0.7	0.503	6	0.998
0.8	0.551	7	0.999

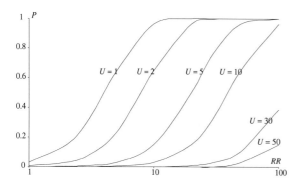

Figure 21.1. Probability P of receiving at least three case-reports according to several theoretical values of RR and under-reporting coefficient U (see text).

population, the expected number of fortuitous, i.e. non-causal, associations is: $0.0961 \times 7 = 0.67$. According to the Poisson formula (cumulative probabilities), there is only 48% chance that one case or more really occurs by chance in this population. Considering a probable under-reporting, it becomes highly improbable that one or more of such a non-causal association will be reported. For example, if $U = 4$ (25% of cases which have occurred were reported), $m = 0.67/4 = 0.17$. The probability of receiving one report or more under these conditions is 16%. This probability falls to 0.07% for three reports or more, which allows us to exclude the possibility of a non-causal association (Bégaud et al., 1994). This simulation explains the well recognized value of SR for signal generation (Fletcher, 1991; Tubert-Bitter et al., 1992): for rare events, only causal associations (characterized by a RR far greater than one) have a good chance of being reported, even if the reporting approaches 100%. This is illustrated by Figure 21.1 which plots, for different theoretical values of under-reporting and RR, the probability of receiving three reports or more when the expected number of fortuitous associations is, as above, 0.67.

COMPARING TOXICITY BETWEEN DRUGS

Despite the fact that population databases and health insurance databases are increasingly used for designing comparative pharmacoepidemiological studies, SRs remain the main source for pharmacovigilance decisions. In a classical study, e.g. a comparative cohort, the incidence rates a_1/N_1 and a_2/N_2 measured in each group (exposed and not exposed to the studied drug, respectively) are compared. In the framework of SR, the validity of such a comparison is jeopardized (i) because of the absence of information on the actual number of cases which have occurred during the considered period of time, and (ii) because of the questionable character of the estimates of the denominators N_1 and N_2. We will address both issues separately.

THE PROBLEM OF UNDER-REPORTING

As discussed above, it is highly probable that the number of reports involving Drug 1 (k_1) and Drug 2 (k_2), respectively, are only a part of the numbers a_1 and a_2 of cases which have occurred. The issue is that the magnitude of this under-reporting may differ across the two drugs compared (Bégaud et al., 1991). If the respective values of under-reporting coefficients, U_1 and U_2, were assessable, one could write:

$$a_1 = U_1 \cdot k_i \qquad \text{and} \qquad a_2 = U_2 \cdot k_2.$$

Therefore, the relative risk for Drug 1 compared with Drug 2 would be:

$$RR = \frac{U_1 \cdot k_1/N_1}{U_2 \cdot k_2/N_2} = \frac{U_1 \cdot k_1 N_2}{U_2 \cdot k_2 N_1}.$$

Let us note that if $U_1 = U_2$, then the estimate of the RR remains identical, whatever the magnitude of under-reporting. Thus, a comparison based upon the number of reports would lead to the same estimate as if based on the actual number of cases. The only consequence would be a dramatic decrease in the statistical power of the comparison test because it was computed on smaller samples.

This is illustrated by Table 21.3 showing the values of the statistic of a chi-square test performed on the basis of a theoretical number of 120 cases for Drug 1 and 60 for Drug 2, respectively; the number of patients treated being chosen identical ($N_1 = N_2 = 300\,000$) for simplification purposes. One can see that a complete

Table 21.3. Values for the chi-square statistic computed on the basis of 120 cases for Drug 1, and 60 cases for Drug 2, respectively (the exposed population size being the same for both drugs: 300 000 patients) according to several theoretical values of the under-reporting coefficient U (bold figures correspond to differences which are significant at the 0.05 level).

		U_1				
		1	2	5	10	20
U_2	1	20	0	15.4	32	44.2
	2	54	10	0.67	7.7	16
	5	88.3	32	4	0	2
	10	103	44.2	10.8	2	0

reporting leads to a χ^2 statistic of 20 which allows one to conclude that Drug 1 is more toxic than Drug 2 with a high confidence level ($p < 10^{-4}$). This conclusion would be reversed if the under-reporting affected Drug 1 predominantly, e.g. if $U_1 = 10$ and $U_2 = 2$. In this case, one would conclude that there was a significantly higher toxicity of Drug 2 ($p = 0.006$).

Moreover, for an equal but more marked under-reporting, e.g. $U_1 = U_2 = 10$, a statistical comparison based on the numbers of reports would not allow one to conclude there was a significant difference (χ^2 statistic = 2; $p = 0.16$).

An elegant approach for "neutralizing" the effect of an unbalanced under-reporting has been proposed by Tubert-Bitter et al. (1996). It consists in expressing the CI for RR as a function of $U = U_1/U_2$:

$$\text{CI}_{RR} = \left[U \times \frac{N_2}{N_1} \times \frac{k_1 - Z_{\alpha/2}\sqrt{\dfrac{k_1 k_2}{k_1 + k_2}}}{k_2 + Z_{\alpha/2}\sqrt{\dfrac{k_1 k_2}{k_1 + k_2}}}; \right.$$

$$\left. U \times \frac{N_2}{N_1} \times \frac{k_1 + Z_{\alpha/2}\sqrt{\dfrac{k_1 k_2}{k_1 + k_2}}}{k_2 - Z_{\alpha/2}\sqrt{\dfrac{k_1 k_2}{k_1 + k_2}}} \right].$$

Example: The Committee on Safety of Medicines (CSM) (1990) has published complete data on post-marketing surveillance of non-steroidal anti-inflamatory drugs (NSAIDs) in the United Kingdom, for two drugs launched approximately at the same date, piroxicam (1980) and diclofenac (1979). The number of serious gastrointestinal reactions reported to the CSM during the same time interval (five years) was 538 for 9.16 million prescriptions for piroxicam versus 68 for 3.25 million prescriptions for diclofenac. The RR estimated from these data is $U \times [(538 \times 3.25)/(68 \times 9.16)] = 2.81 U$ and the corresponding 95% two-sided CI is calculated as:

$$\left[U \times \frac{3.25}{9.16} \times \frac{538 - 1.96\sqrt{\dfrac{538 \times 68}{606}}}{68 + 1.96\sqrt{\dfrac{538 \times 68}{606}}}; \right.$$

$$\left. U \times \frac{3.25}{9.16} \times \frac{538 + 1.96\sqrt{\dfrac{538 \times 68}{606}}}{68 - 1.96\sqrt{\dfrac{538 \times 68}{606}}} \right]$$

$$= [2.23 U;\ 3.72 U].$$

Assuming that the reporting ratios were the same for both drugs ($U = U_1/U_2 = 1$), the 95% CI for RR [2.23; 3.72] does not include one. Therefore, the null hypothesis H_0: ($RR = 1$) will be rejected and piroxicam considered more gastro-toxic than diclofenac as long as $U > 1/2.23$. Reporting 2.23 times lower for diclofenac than for piroxicam would have precluded this conclusion, while it would have been reversed (diclofenac more gastrotoxic than piroxicam) by a reporting 3.72 times lower for diclofenac.

The calculation process does not impose assignment of a priori values for U_1 and U_2. The only assumption required is the order of magnitude of the ratio $U = U_1/U_2$, regardless of the individual and unknown values of U_1 and U_2.

As to the context, the concern is to know whether it is plausible to consider a marked difference in reporting across the two compared drugs. It is generally acknowledged that under-reporting is roughly of the same order of magnitude provided that the two drugs belong to the same therapeutic class, have been launched approximately at the same date, are compared for the same type of events and do not differ with regard to the information provided for the potential reporters (Griffin, 1984 ; Haramburu *et al.*, 1997; Pierfitte *et al.*, 1999). For instance, in the CSM (1990) data, benoxaprofen was launched in the United Kingdom approximately at the same time (1980) as diclofenac (1979), the number of serious reactions (of any type) involving benoxaprofen was 332 over 1.47 million prescriptions versus 128 over 3.25 million prescriptions for diclofenac, which leads to a *RR* value of 5.73*U* (95% CI: 4.72*U*–7.11*U*). This gives some credibility to the decision to withdraw benoxaprofen from the UK market in 1984 because of unacceptable excess toxicity.

COMPARABILITY OF DENOMINATORS

Another source of bias when comparing the toxicity of drugs is the non-coherence of denominators. It is therefore crucial to ensure that under the null hypothesis of a non-difference in toxicity, the risk of an adverse event is expected to be the same for the two drugs compared.

A typical example relies on different durations of exposure. Let us take the example of anaphylactic reactions which, by definition, are expected to occur at initiation of the treatment. Ninety-two reactions were reported for drug A and 242 for drug B. On the basis of a total exposure (estimated from sales statistics) of 2.8 million months and 1.9 million months, respectively, the risk appears to be 3.9 times greater for drug B. However, this conclusion could be reversed if the number of first users was much greater for this drug because of shorter duration of treatment. It could happen, even if the two drugs belong to the same pharmacological and/or therapeutic class. For instance, such differences are observed with analgesics or NSAIDs: for more or less obscure

reasons, some are used chronically when others are preferred for the treatment of acute pain. Therefore, it is a safe practice, before any decision-making, to try to obtain relevant informations on the utilization patterns of the drugs compared in order to avoid gross misinterpretation errors.

CONCLUSION

Despite the relatively soft character of the data analyzed, simple statistical calculations may apply to SR. Their main interest is to make SR more reliable for alert processes. Moreover, they can avoid major biases and misinterpretation especially when comparing the toxicity across drugs.

REFERENCES

Alvarez-Requejo A, Carvajal A, Bégaud B, Moride Y, Vega T, Arias LH (1998) Under-reporting of adverse drug reactions. Estimate based on a spontaneous reporting scheme and a sentinel system. *Eur J Clin Pharmacol* **54**: 483–8.

Bégaud B (2000) *Dictionary of Pharmacoepidemiology*. Chichester: Wiley.

Bégaud B, Moride Y, Tubert-Bitter P, Chaslerie A, Haramburu F (1994) False-positives in spontaneous reporting: should we worry about them? *Br J Clin Pharmacol* **38**(4): 401–4.

Bégaud B, Péré JC, Miremont G (1993) Estimation of the denominator in spontaneous reporting. In: *Methodological Approaches in Pharmacoepidemiology*. ARME-P Editions. Amsterdam: Elsevier, pp. 51–70.

Bégaud B, Tubert P, Haramburu F, Moride Y, Salamé G, Péré JC (1991) Comparing toxicity of drugs: use and misuse of spontaneous reporting. *Post Marketing Surveillance* **5**(1): 59–67.

Committee on Safety of Medicines (1990) Non-steroidal anti-inflammatory drugs and serious adverse drug reactions—2. *Br Med J* **300**: 22–3.

Daly LE, Bourke GJ, McGilvray J (1991) *Interpretation and Uses of Medical Statistics*. London: Blackwell Scientific.

Eland IA, Belton KJ, van Grootherest AC, Meiners AP, Rawlins MD, Stricker BH (1999) Attitudinal survey of voluntary reporting of adverse drug reactions. *Br J Clin Pharmacol* **48**(4): 623–7.

Fletcher AP (1991) Spontaneous adverse drug reaction reporting versus event monitoring: a comparison. *J R Soc Med* **84**: 341–4.

Griffin JP (1984) Is better feedback a major stimulus to

spontaneous adverse drug reaction monitoring? *Lancet* **ii**: 1098.

Haramburu F, Bégaud B, Moride Y (1997) Temporal trends in spontaneous reporting of unlabelled adverse drug reactions. *Br J Clin Pharmacol* **44**(3): 299–301.

Jeeger JD, Schumock GT, Kong SX (1996) Estimating the rate of adverse drug reactions with capture–recapture analysis. *Am J Health Syst Pharm* **53**(2): 178–81.

Kramer MS (1988) *Clinical Epidemiology and Biostatistics. A Primer for Clinical Investigators and Decision-Makers*. Berlin: Springer-Verlag.

Pierfitte C, Bégaud B, Lagnaoui R, Moore ND (1999) Is reporting rate a good predictor of risks associated with drugs? *Br J Clin Pharmacol* **47**(3): 329–1.

Pouyanne P, Haramburu F, Imbs JL, Bégaud B (2000) Admissions to hospital caused by adverse drug reactions: cross-sectional incidence study. French Pharmacovigilance Centres. *Br Med J* **320**(15): 1036.

Snedecor GW, Cochran WG (1989) *Statistical Methods*, 8th edn. Ames: Iowa State University Press.

Tubert-Bitter P, Bégaud B, Péré JC, Haramburu F, Lellouch J (1992) Power and weakness of spontaneous reporting: a probabilistic approach. *J Clin Epidemiol* **45**(3): 283–6.

Tubert-Bitter P, Bégaud B, Moride Y, Chaslerie A, Haramburu F (1996) Comparing the toxicity of two drugs in the framework of spontaneous reporting: a confidence interval approach. *J Clin Epidemiol* **49**(1): 121–3.

22

Data Mining

I. RALPH EDWARDS, MARIE LINDQUIST AND ANDREW BATE
Uppsala Monitoring Centre, Stora Torget 3, Uppsala, Sweden

ROLAND ORRE
Department of Mathematical Statistics, Stockholm University, Stockholm, Sweden

BACKGROUND

The WHO has defined a signal as: "Reported information on a possible causal relationship between an adverse event and a drug, the relationship being unknown or incompletely documented previously." An additional note says: "Usually more than one report is required to generate a signal, depending on the seriousness of the event and the quality of the information" (Edwards and Biriell, 1994).

A signal is therefore very tentative in nature; the first expression that something might be wrong with a medicinal product, or a hint given by new information that might support or explain a medicinal product/adverse reaction relationship already known.

Both quantitative and qualitative factors come into the decision of whether something is a signal or not (Edwards et al., 1990). Many algorithms have been proposed for determining causality between a signal and an adverse reaction, but there is no perfect way of doing this that fits all possible situations. Perhaps the use of the Bayesian approach proposed and developed by Auriche (1985) and Naranjo and Lancetôt (1991) is the most attractive, since Bayesian logic allows one to build up a pattern of probability that changes according to the addition of new information. This intuitively fits the clinical diagnostic approach, and is transparent.

Apparent causality in a single case, or even a series, is not the only issue in comprehensive early signal detection. One might exclude many of the case reports with limited information, yet, because a case record does not allow for remote assessment of the case, this does not mean that the original observer was incorrect, only that one cannot confirm the observation. Thus, the quantity as well as the quality of reports of associations is valuable.

The use of "poor quality" reports as a trigger for a signal should be considered more carefully if the clinical event is serious. Early warning is more important, and a signal based on doubtful evidence should promote the search for better.

There may be certain items of information within a set of reports that trigger consideration of a signal other than just the medicinal product and clinical event. It might be the apparent over-representation of higher doses of the relevant drug, concomitant treatment, or certain patient characteristics.

Pharmacovigilance. Edited by R.D. Mann and E.B. Andrews

The above are just some of the common reasons for someone to consider during the evaluation of an early signal. There are many others, such as the finding of a problem with one medicinal product that triggers a search into products with similar effects. What is clear is that there are very complex interacting patterns of information that may trigger ideas.

Apart from the complexity of possible important patterns in data, the volume of case reports on suspected medicinal product adverse reactions is massive. The WHO Programme for International Drug Monitoring database holds nearly 3 million case reports. There is more in the published literature and even more from varieties of clinical studies. One begins to see the problem as looking for the proverbial "needle in a haystack" (Edwards, 1997).

If the above does not make the problems daunting enough, we must see medicinal product safety in the context of the use of those products. We need to know not only the numbers of people exposed to the products, but also why they were used, in what kind of patients, for what reason, and with what outcome.

The human brain is excellent at finding significant patterns in data: humans would not have survived if that were not so! On the other hand, the vast quantities referred to above cannot be usefully observed, let alone held in the memory for a person to analyse. Many people are involved in pharmacovigilance, but we are not yet wise enough to divide up the great task we have. Even if we did, there would still be a place for bringing the data we have to us for analysis in ways that allow us to see patterns more easily, and without our preconceptions blinding us to see things only in a certain way, conditioned by our experience.

It is true that in looking for significant patterns by sifting through data, one will eventually come up with something that *looks* significantly probable by chance: data "dredging" or "trawling" or a "fishing expedition" is bound to catch something, but not much that is useful. In trying to find signals, this view is too rigid; first, since one acknowledges that an early signal is tentative, that simply urges further work to be performed on that hypothesis. Secondly, from experience, a principal

argument has evolved in drug safety, namely if important signals are not to be missed, the first analysis of information should be untrammelled by prejudice and rigid protocols. Thirdly, and notwithstanding the second point, data mining is not necessarily a random rummaging through data in an aimless fashion, which is what the term "dredging" implies. It is certainly true that the involvement of objects and the characterisation of any relationships in advanced pattern recognition is largely unsupervised, but the level of supervision and the kind of logic that is applied to data is flexible and transparent: this can be compared with the conventional use of "mining", which is defined as "a *system* of excavations made for the extraction of minerals". In essence we consider that data dredging should be used as a pejorative term for unstructured fiddling about with data, or worse, the application of a structure to data to make it fit a biased hypothesis in a way to give added credibility to the result. Data mining, on the other hand, should be considered as a term for the application of a tool or tools to analyse large amounts of data in a transparent and unbiased fashion, with the aim of highlighting information worth closer consideration.

DATA MINING

In this chapter we use the term "data mining" for any computer method of automatic and continuous analysis of data, which turns it into useful information. Data mining can clearly be used on any data set, but the approach seems particularly valuable when the amount of data is large and the possible relationships within the data set numerous and complex. Although data mining of drug utilisation information, and other relevant data sets such as those relating to poisoning, will add greatly to pharmacovigilance, this has not yet been done to our knowledge. Our work in this area is preliminary and will not be referred to here.

In principle the Uppsala Monitoring Centre (UMC) has been doing data mining since the mid 1970s, using an early relational database. As with many automated systems, the relational database to a very large extent replicated a manual approach. In this instance it was the Canadian "pigeon hole" system (Napke, 1977), where reports were physically assigned a slot, which encouraged visual inspection. Thus, observation could be made of when certain categories of report were unexpectedly high.

From the UMC database, countries in the WHO Programme for International Drug Monitoring have been provided with information, reworked by the UMC, on the summarised case data that is submitted from each national centre. This information has been presented to them according to agreed categories and classifications as determined among Programme members from time to time. This kind of system suffers from the following limitations:

- It is prescriptive, the groupings being determined on what is found broadly useful by experience.
- Each category is relatively simple, but the information beneath each heading is complex, and formatted rigidly.
- There is no indication of the probability of any relationship other than the incident numbers in each time period.

This system does not even have all the user friendliness of the pigeon hole system, which allowed a user to visually scan the amount of reports as they were filed to see the rate of build up in each pigeon hole. Admittedly, the sorting was relatively coarse, but the continuous visual cue given by the accumulation of case reports was very useful.

In improving on the pigeon hole system one can imagine a computer program being able to survey all data fields looking for patterns, really just any relationships that stand out as being more frequent than normal between any number of data fields. This ambitious goal might also be linked with some probability of the link(s) not being present by chance, given the background of the total data set.

At the other end of the spectrum one might merely ask the question: "Are there any drugs which seem to be more or less probably linked to a reported adverse reaction term in this data set?" This latter question may be tackled in an automated way by calculating the proportional

reporting ratio (PRR), which is akin to a relative risk, a reporting odds ratio (OR) or the Yules Q, for all medicinal products and adverse drug reaction (ADR) terms. These are point estimates giving the relativity of reporting of a particular drug and ADR to all the ADRs for that drug, compared with similar considerations for all drugs and the target ADR and all ADRs. This can be done without the use of neural networks and using the χ^2 test for probability and other methods of precision estimation.

Bayesian logic may also be used, finding the prior probability of an occurrence of the drug amongst the case data and then the posterior probability of the drug linked with the specific ADR. Bayesian logic is intuitively correct for a situation where there is a need continuously to reassess the probability of relationships with the acquisition of new data and over time. Bayesian logic does not impose any rigidity other than deciding on the initial a priori level of probability, and then allows the acquisition of data to modify to a posterior probability. This process can be iterated continuously.

The next level of complexity is to consider the effects of adding other objects as variables. Stratification or the use of Bayesian complex variable analysis complicates the calculations and the computational complexity to a level that makes a neural network architecture an advantage. A neural network is a matrix of interconnected nodes. Each node is connected to all other nodes, and represents one data field of specified type. A neural network learns according to the data provided to it and according to its predetermined logic. For evaluating complexity in a very large data set, the WHO Collaborating Centre for International Drug Monitoring (the UMC) has chosen a Bayesian confidence propagation neural network (BCPNN) as the most favourable platform for development in this area. The use of Bayesian logic seems natural where the relationship between each node will alter as more data are added. The neural network "learns" the new probabilities between nodes, and can be asked how much those probabilities are changed by the addition of new case data or by the consideration of multiples rather than singlets or duplets.

DESCRIPTION OF DATA MINING METHODOLOGY USED BY THE UMC

The UMC's main purpose is to find novel drug safety signals: new information. From experience a principal argument has evolved in drug safety, that, if important signals are not to be missed, the first analysis of information should be free from prejudice and a priori thinking (Hand, 1999). Quantitative filtering of the data focuses clinical review on the most potentially important ADR combinations (Bate *et al.*, 1998; Hand, 1999; Lindquist *et al.*, 1999, 2000; Orre *et al.*, 2000). Human intelligence and experience are able to operate better with a transparent filtering method in the generation of hypotheses.

The BCPNN is a feed-forward neural network where learning and inference are done using the principles of Bayes' law. For regular routine output we use it as a one-layer model (Lansner and Ekeberg, 1989), although it has been extended to a multilayer network (Holst, 1997). Such a multilayer network can be used in further investigations of combinations of several variables in the WHO database and has already been successfully applied to areas like diagnosis (Holst and Lansner, 1996), expert systems (Holst and Lansner, 1993) and data analysis in pulp and paper manufacturing (Orre and Lansner, 1996).

Estimates of precision (standard deviation) are provided for each point estimate of the information component (IC); thus both the point estimate of unexpectedness as well as the certainty associated with it can be examined. Despite the presence of missing data, the IC and its standard deviation can be calculated for any combination of variable values; additionally, the interpretation of the probability distributions is intuitive.

The network is transparent, in that it is easy to see what has been calculated and robust, and that valid, relevant results can still be generated despite missing data. This is advantageous as most reports in the database contain some empty fields. The results are reproducible, making validation and checking simple. The network is easy to train; it only takes one pass across the data, which makes it highly time efficient. A small proportion of all possible drug–adverse reaction combinations are

actually non-zero in the database, thus use of a sparse matrix method makes searches through the database quick and efficient.

The neural network provides an efficient computational model for the analysis of large amounts of data and combinations of variables, whether real, discrete or binary. The efficiency is enhanced by the IC being the weight in the neural network. The neural network architecture allows the same framework to be used both for data analysis/data mining as well as prediction, as used for pattern recognition and classification. Bayesian statistics fits intuitively into the framework of a neural network approach as both build on the concept of adapting on the basis of new data. The method has also been extended to detect dependencies between several variables and is robust in handling missing data. Pattern recognition by the BCPNN does not depend upon any a priori hypothesis since an unsupervised learning approach is used. This is useful in new syndrome detection, finding age profiles of ADRs, determining at-risk groups and dose relationships, and can thus be used to find complex dependencies that have not necessarily been considered before. Naturally, changes in patterns may also be important (Hand, 1999).

The BCPNN methodology thus uses a neural network architecture to identify unexpectedly strong dependencies between variables (e.g. drugs and adverse reactions) within the WHO database, and how dependencies change after the addition of new data. The dependencies are selected using a measure of disproportionality called the information component (*IC*):

$$IC = \log_2 \frac{p(x, y)}{p(x)p(y)},$$

where

p_x = the probability of a specific drug being listed on a case report;
p_y = the probability of a specific ADR being listed on a case report; and
p_{xy} = the probability that a specific drug–adverse reaction combination is listed on a case report.

Thus the *IC* value is based on:

- the number of case reports with drug X (c_x);
- the number of case reports with ADR Y (c_y);
- the number of reports with the specific combination (c_{xy}); and
- the total number of reports (C).

Positive *IC* values indicate that the particular combination of variables is reported to the database more often than statistically expected from reports already in the database. The higher value of the *IC*, the more the combination stands out from the background.

From the distribution of the *IC*, expectation and variance values are calculated using Bayesian statistics. The standard deviation for each *IC* provides a measure of the robustness of the value. The higher the C_x, C_y and C_{xy} levels are, the narrower the confidence interval becomes. If a positive *IC* value increases over time and the confidence interval narrows, then this shows a likelihood of a positive quantitative association between the studied variables. The UMC, as the WHO Collaborating Centre for International Drug Monitoring, is responsible for the technical and scientific maintenance and development of the WHO International Drug Monitoring Programme. The Programme now has more than 60 member countries, annually contributing around 150 000 suspected ADR reports to the WHO database in Uppsala.

One of the main aims of the international pharmacovigilance programme is to identify early signals of safety problems related to medicines. To aid this, a new ADR signalling system has been provided for national monitoring centres and authorities, using the BCPNN. It complements the previous signal generation procedure that involved the examination of unwieldy, large amounts of sorted and tabulated material by an expert panel. An overview of the new signalling approach, including results from the first part of an evaluation including a comparison against another signalling system, has been published (Lindquist *et al.*, 2000).

The new system is based using the BCPNN to scan incoming ADR reports and compare them statistically with what is already stored in the database.

A new quarterly output to national centres contains statistical information from the BCPNN scan. It also contains frequency counts for each drug and ADR listed, both individually and occurring together. The figures from the previous quarter are also included and the data are provided in computerised format.

Drug–adverse reaction combinations that are statistically significantly different from the background of reports ("associations") are sent to a panel of reviewers for evaluation and expert opinion. Within the WHO Programme a "signal" concerns "information regarding a possible relationship between a drug and an adverse event or interaction". As previously, signals of possible safety problems are circulated to all national centres participating in the international pharmacovigilance programme for consideration of public health implications.

"VALIDATION" OF THE DATA MINING APPROACH

Critics of data mining can reasonably suggest that, with all the possible relationships in a huge data base, many medicine/adverse reaction associations will occur by chance, even though they seem to be significantly associated. The Bayesian methodology used by the UMC does take account of the size of the database in assigning probabilities; on the other hand, one must be as sure as possible that national centres and reviewers are not provided with what amounts to a huge amount of useless probabilistic information. However, it is clear that finding signals early will entail some false positives.

Determining the performance of the BCPNN is a difficult task because there is no "gold standard" for comparison. Also there are different definitions of the term signal. According to the definition used in the WHO Programme a signal is essentially a hypothesis together with data and arguments, and it is not only uncertain but also preliminary in nature: the situation may change substantially over time (Edwards and Biriell, 1994; Meyboom *et al.*, 1997).

For the purpose of a study (Lindquist *et al.*, 2000) we felt we would achieve a reasonable estimate of the predictive power of the BCPNN tool by checking historical associations identified by the BCPNN against standard reference sources. *Martindale* has worldwide coverage, recognition and wide availability and was used as a standard for well-known, recognised ADRs. The US *Physicians Desk Reference* (*PDR*), though not international, gives very recent information on drugs. It has a comprehensive ADR listing, generally more inclusive than that of *Martindale*. However, *PDR* includes suspected adverse reactions, whether substantiated or not. We considered an ADR listed in *PDR* an indication of a possible drug–adverse reaction relationship.

Two main studies of the performance of the BCPNN have been reported in a single paper (Lindquist *et al.*, 2000). One study concerned a test of the BCPNN predictive value in new signal detection as compared with reference literature sources (*Martindale's Extra Pharmacopoeia* from 1993; 2000; the *Physicians Desk Reference* from 2000). In the study period (the first quarter year 1993) 107 drug–adverse reaction combinations were highlighted as new positive associations by the BCPNN, and referred to new drugs. Fifteen drug–adverse reaction combinations on new drugs became negative BCPNN associations in the study period.

The BCPNN method detecting signals with a positive predictive value was 44% and the negative predictive value was 85%. Seventeen as yet unconfirmed positive associations could not be dismissed with certainty as false positive. The second study was a comparison of the new BCPNN with the results of the former signalling procedure.

Of the 10 drug–adverse reaction signals produced by the former signal detection system from data sent out for review during the study period, six were also identified by the BCPNN. These six associations have all had a more than 10-fold increase in reports and four of them have been included in the reference sources. The remaining four signals that were not identified by the BCPNN had a small, or no increase in the number of reports, and are not listed in the reference sources.

The length of time chosen for the retrospective check against the literature was not arbitrary, but based on the assumption that seven years would be enough for ADRs to be included in the reference sources, allowing for the maximum reporting for new drugs to have taken place (the Weber effect). We know, however, that one new association appeared in *Martindale* between 1999 and 2000, and seven years still may not be long enough. Publishing delay must be considered in the use of these reference sources, but this is minimised now by their availability on-line using an Internet browser.

The use of our selected literature sources as a "gold standard" is open to debate. The literature is not intended as an early signalling system, and uses many sources for its information other than the WHO database: the biases affecting inclusion and exclusion of ADR information therefore may be very different. Factors, such as those affecting the differential reporting to WHO and the inclusion of new information in the reference sources, will have an effect which is independent of the performance of the BCPNN. The BCPNN is run every quarter, and we selected just one quarter: since the BCPNN is used in continuous analysis, the specificity and sensitivity are subject to necessary time-dependant changes in classification of "positives" and "negatives". It is difficult to consider something as a "non-association" because of this time dependency, and it is clear that there is an asymmetry in the effect of time on our results. This is explicable using the following logic.

Exceptionally high reporting of an ADR-to-product combination, which causes the combination to stand out from the background of the whole database, will cause any other product-to-ADR combination containing the product *or* ADR to stand out slightly less. It is not common for alterations in the background to significantly alter the status of an association.

On the other hand, it is more common for the reporting of a particular ADR and medicinal product to increase at a rate that is broadly related to the incidence of the ADR to the point where it becomes an association. Publicity about an ADR may affect this rate dramatically, but this by no means invalidates the association, only complicates its interpretation. Another asymmetry is that the negative associations are a selection of all non-associations. This assumes that definite negative associations represent all non-associations, though it is clear that some non-associations will became positive associations in time. Thus, a non-association can be either a combination of an ADR term with a medicinal product that is not a positive association and remains stable, or one that is statistically a negative association at a high probability of becoming positive. Considering all this, we have in this study defined the inverse of a positive association as a definite negative association, i.e. one that is statistically not associated. This again shows the difficulty in evaluating a signalling system.

An assumption was made that a substantial increase in the number of reports of an association over the period indicated ongoing clinical interest in an association. More reports may be seen as support for the validity of the associations, though there is often a tendency for ADRs that are becoming well known to be reported more anyway.

Another obvious limitation is that the BCPNN method for signal generation is dependent on the terminology used for recording adverse reactions. Very little work has been done on any of the medical terminologies in use or proposed to determine their relative value in searching for new drug signals.

Although we found that the our use of the BCPNN gave a 44% positive predictive value, and a high negative predictive value of 84%, the normal methods for assessing the power of a method are difficult to apply to the BCPNN, because of the reasons above. It is for this reason that "validation" is placed in quotation marks in the title of this section. The BCPNN is not a panacea for drug safety monitoring. The drug–adverse reaction combinations that reach significance do so only in comparison with the background experience of 2+ million case reports. This is particularly important for commonly reported ADRs, which, however serious, would not reach significance until the quantitative experience for a drug and such an ADR is excessive. We have stressed (Lindquist et al., 2000) that the BCPNN has its limitations, is not a substitute for expert review, but has a place particularly where large volumes of data are involved. It is reassuring, however, that all signals identified in the previous system that went on to become frequently reported in the WHO database were also identified in the retrospective BCPNN analysis.

On the other hand, the BCPNN has the power to analyse signals further. We are developing its use to look at complex variables and, in unsupervised pattern recognition, to see whether parameters such as gender, age, and other drug use increase the strength of association, and whether "syndromes" of reported terms are present. However, as with any subdivision of data, a very large amount is necessary initially in order to attain statistical significance in sub-sets. This is a major advantage of using the large pooled WHO database, and we are trying to maximise this potential.

COMPARISON OF METHODS

In this chapter we have concentrated on the use of the BCPNN, partly because it is the most examined system used at present. There has, however, been one study (van Puijenbroek et al., 2002) comparing the BCPNN with other methods. As mentioned above, in various centres, different measures are used to quantify the extent to which a certain ADR is reported in a disproportionate relationship to a certain drug compared with the generality of the database, i.e. standing out from the background of all reports. In this comparative study the level of concordance was measured of the various estimates to the measures of the IC and IC-2std produced from the BCPNN.

The investigation was performed on the data set of the Netherlands Pharmacovigilance Foundation (Lareb), which maintains the spontaneous ADR reporting system in the Netherlands on behalf of the Dutch Medicines Evaluation Board.

In essence all the other methods could pick up the signals which the BCPNN could, and indeed more with a lower number of cases. When the "disproportionality" was based on relationships with four or more reports (about 11% of the Lareb database), all the methods were comparable. It was only at low count values where any difference could be detected.

The above finding is significant. The precise method used for data mining should be based upon the benefits and drawbacks of each. Crucial to the Bayesian method is the initial setting of the a priori probability. How this is set determines the performance of the BCPNN at low counter values. At the UMC we chose an a priori probability of independence that is consistent with the WHO definition of a signal and the previous publication (Edwards *et al.*, 1990), suggesting that normally

more than one report would be needed to trigger an expert to think that he/she had found a signal, unless there was something exceptional *qualitatively* about a report (such as a case with proven, true re-challenge). Moreover, the WHO database has many more incident reports than the Lareb data base so that as greater numbers of reports are submitted, little time will be lost in finding the signal even though the BCPNN requires about three more to trigger.

It is clear that the other methods may be just as suitable as the BCPNN for routine use to identify

Table 22.1. Conditions, advantages and disadvantages of different measures of disproportionality.

Measure of disproportionality	Expected "null value"	Conditions	Advantages	Disadvantagess
ROR – 1.96 SE	1	Cells a, b, c and d have to contain reports	• Easily applicable • Different adjustments possible in logistic regression analysis • In logistic regression analysis, interaction terms can be used for the analysis of drug interactions and syndromes	• Odds ratio and standard error cannot be calculated if denominator is zero (specific ADRs) • Interpretation difficult • Results not always reliable in the event of small numbers in cells a, b, c and d of the contingency table
PRR – 1.96 SE	1	Cells a and c have to contain reports	• Easy interpretation	• Standard error cannot always be calculated
Yule's Q – 1.96 SE	0	Cells a, b, c and d have to contain reports		• Standard error cannot always be calculated • Difficult to interpret
IC – 2 SD	0	None	• Always applicable • Large numbers of calculations can be made efficiently • Can be used for pattern recognition in higher dimensions	• Relatively non-transparent for people not familiar with Bayesian statistics
Poisson		Only for rare events	• Correction for different covariates can be easily established in Poisson regression	• Only *P*-value provided
Chi-square (Yates correction)			• Always applicable	• Difficult to interpret

Reproduced from van Puijenbroek *et al.* (2002) by permission of John Wiley & Sons, Ltd.

cases on a continuous basis which deserve follow-up for more information. The higher sensitivity of the other methods needs to be investigated further for predictive value at a practical signal detection level. Table 22.1, taken from the comparisons paper, gives a very good idea of some of the comparative benefits of the methods

THE LIMITATIONS AND USE OF DATA MINING

Data mining is intended to alert the observer to unusual relationships within a data set. It is essential to understand that in pharmacovigilance, what is reported and contained within the data set does not represent the true epidemiology of adverse reactions to medicines. There is the very well-known problem of under-reporting, but more than that, many countries ask health professionals to be selective in their reporting to cut down the "noise". One problem with data mining is the temptation to turn it into data dredging. There is a difference: data mining uses objectively predeter-mined (if flexible) logic to examine relationships in data transparently. Data dredging is based upon a series of prejudiced queries which might imbue chance relationships with plausibility, and in which a strict logic or strategy is not followed.

In the past, it has seemed reasonable for pharmacovigilance experts to reduce their work load and avoid having to see multitudes of reports of more trivial or well-known adverse reactions, but this has both health and methodological consequences. It is often forgotten that "serious adverse and unexpected" reactions can be pre-ceded by less serious phenomena. The best known is the xerophthalmia related to practolol being the harbinger of sclerosing peritonitis. Also, the persistent reporting of a well-known (to experts) adverse reaction–product combination can be important since it may indicate that practitioners in the field are concerned about it for some practical reason. The reasons may be that they see the reaction more frequently than they think they should, that there is something unusual about the duration or severity, or that there are systematic errors associated with the use of the product which

lead to problems (similar confusing labelling of different products, for example).

Data mining should allow for much easier and useful handling of large amounts of information. Since the "triaging" of information is done automatically, there is no longer any need to specify that only serious and unexpected reactions need be reported. Indeed, data mining in pharma-covigilance will function better for us if there is a large amount of "ordinary" adverse reaction in formation to serve as the background. If we just record the serious and unexpected, only the more serious and unexpected will stand out, progres-sively. This slow shift of emphasis would be deleterious for public health.

Data mining has its main future in the detection of complex patterns in the data. It is possible that, if doctors reported all the medicinal product safety issues that concern them, we would be able to identify some issues of use and poor use of medicines that could be addressed (Edwards and Aronson, 2000).

Data mining, then, is proving to be a useful tool. Its full potential has not yet been reached, and it may be that some of the current drug regulations and attitudes may need to be reconsidered as its use becomes more widespread. In spite of its potential as the primary search tool in pharmacovigilance, it is clear that its use must be accompanied by the wise interpretation of the information. Since no database is representative of what truly happens, other observations, monitoring and epidemiology must continue to be used in a complementary way. Only by the interactive interpretation of findings using different observational methodology are we likely to even approach the truth.

REFERENCES

Auriche M (1985) Bayesian approach to the imputability of undesirable phenomena to drugs. *Therapie* **40**(5): 301–6.
Bate A, Lindquist M, Edwards IR, Olsson S, Orre R, Lansner A, *et al.* (1998) A Bayesian neural network method for adverse drug reaction signal generation. *Eur J Clin Pharmacol* **54**: 315–21.
Edwards IR (1997) Adverse drug reactions: finding the needle in the haystack (Editorial). *Br Med J* **315**: 500.

Edwards IR, Aronson JK (2000) Adverse drug reactions: definitions, diagnosis, and management. *Lancet* **356**: 1255–9.

Edwards IR, Biriell C (1994) Harmonisation in pharmacovigilance. *Drug Safety* **10**: 93–102.

Edwards IR, *et al.* (1990) Quality criteria for early signals of possible adverse drug reactions. *Lancet* **336**: 156–8.

Hand DJ (1999) Statistics and data mining: intersecting disciplines. *SIGKDD Expl* **1**: 16–19.

Holst A (1997) The use of a Bayesian neural network model for classification tasks. Thesis dissertation. Royal Institute of Technology, Stockholm.

Holst A, Lansner A (1993) A flexible and fault tolerant query-reply system based on a Bayesian neural network. *Int J Neural Syst* **4**: 257–67.

Holst A, Lansner A (1996) A higher order neural network for classification and diagnosis. In: Gammerman A, ed., *Computational Learning and Probabilistic Reasoning*. Chichester: Wiley, pp. 199–209.

Lansner A, Ekeberg O (1989) A one layer feedback artificial neural network with a Bayesian learning rule. *Int J Neural Syst* **1**: 77–87.

Lindquist M, Edwards IR, Bate A, Fucik H, Nunes AM, Ståhl M. (1999) From association to alert—a revised approach to international signal analysis. *Pharmacoepidemiology and Drug Safety* **8**: S15–S25.

Lindquist M, Ståhl M, Bate A, Edwards IR, Meyboom RHB (2000) A retrospective evaluation of a data mining approach to aid finding new adverse drug reaction signals in the WHO international database. *Drug Safety* **23**(6): 533–42.

Meyboom, RHB, *et al.* (1997) Principles of signal detection in pharmacovigilance. *Drug Safety* **16**(6): 355–65.

Napke E (1977) Present ADR monitoring methods. In: Gross TP, Inman WHW, eds, *Drug Monitoring*. London: Academic Press, pp. 1–10.

Naranjo CAL, Lanctôt KL (1991) Microcomputer-assisted Bayesian differential diagnosis of severe adverse reactions to new drugs. A 4-year experience. *Drug Inf J* **25**(6): 243–50.

Orre R, Lansner A (1996) Pulp quality modelling using Bayesian mixture density neural networks. *J Syst Eng* **6**: 128–36.

Orre R, Lansner A, Bate A, Lindquist M. (2000) Bayesian neural networks with confidence estimations applied to data mining. *Comput Stat Data Anal* **34**(8): 473–93.

van Puijenbroek EP, Bate A, Leufkens HG, Lindquist M, Orre R, Egberts AC (2002) A comparison of measures of disproportionality for signal detection in spontaneous reporting systems for adverse drug reactions. *Pharmacoepidemiology and Drug Safety* **11**(1): 3–10.

23

Epidemiology of Adverse Events Associated with Epilepsy and Use of Lamotrigine

PATRICIA TENNIS

Worldwide Epidemiology, GlaxoSmithKline, Research Triangle Park, NC, USA

INTRODUCTION

Epidemiology within Glaxo Wellcome (GW) has been used for quantifying medication safety issues for over a decade. Clearly, the collection and review of spontaneous reports from throughout the world is an important component of generating new safety signals. In this chapter we focus on the use of pharmacoepidemiology to address safety issues recognized during clinical development and through spontaneous reporting. Some issues addressed include:

- quantifying the expected background risk of adverse events related to an indicated condition for a new medication,
- quantifying the frequency of a serious adverse event known to be related to a new medication,
- assessing one component of the benefit–risk relationship by quantifying the frequency of a serious adverse event known to be related to some of the alternative therapies for a new medication,

- monitoring for the possibility of a new and unknown risk in pregnancies exposed to a new medication.

We illustrate these issues by describing the program of studies performed to quantify safety outcomes observed in people using lamotrigine in epilepsy. Lamotrigine was first available for epilepsy in the Republic of Ireland in 1991, and it was approved soon after within the United Kingdom. Its use spread throughout Europe shortly thereafter, and it was first available in the United States in 1995.

QUANITIFYING RISK AND RISK FACTORS FOR SERIOUS EVENTS ASSOCIATED WITH THE INDICATED CONDITION

Prior to the development and introduction of lamotrigine, there were case reports and a case series describing sudden death (SUD) in epilepsy.

Pharmacovigilance. Edited by R.D. Mann and E.B. Andrews

Following the observation of a small number of cases of SUD co-occurring with lamotrigine therapy during the clinical development (Leestma et al., 1997), GW sponsored several cohort studies of the incidence of SUD in epilepsy. At the time, a literature search showed that there was little quantification of the frequency of these events in epilepsy. However, there were a number of case series from autopsies describing SUD in epilepsy. The new observational studies initiated by GW consisted of cohort studies of people with epilepsy and were performed in the large multipurpose administrative health care databases of Saskatch-ewan Health (Tennis et al., 1995), Group Health Cooperative (Jick et al., 1992), and General Practitioners Research Database (GPRD) (Derby et al., 1996). In all these studies, people with epilepsy were identified through their anticonvul-sant prescriptions, and diagnoses or patterns of medication use were used to exclude people without epilepsy. The incidence of SUD ranged from 0.5 to 1.3 per 1000 person-years in all subjects with epilepsy. By stratifying on surrogate markers for refractory epilepsy, e.g. number of concomitant antiepileptic drugs, the Saskatchewan study showed that risk increased with the number of concomitant anticonvulsant medications, sug-gesting that people with refractory epilepsy had a higher incidence of SUD. Subsequent literature has confirmed the relatively high rate of SUD in people with refractory epilepsy (Nashef et al., 1995a; 1995b; Annegers et al., 1998).

To classify deaths, multiple types of records, including hospital discharge summaries, death certificates, and autopsy reports were requested so that the investigators could rule out explanatory causes of death However, these records were inconsistently available and deaths could not always be well categorized. Therefore, deaths were classified as possible, probable or definite, and by including and excluding the less definite categories in the numerators, a range of rates could be calculated.

Another rare event spontaneously reported in patients on lamotrigine is multi-organ failure (MOF). These events occur so rarely that a study could not be designed to quantify the frequency of this event. MOF does not occur in isolation but represents a non-specific process associated with a number of severe illnesses including sepsis and status epilepticus. In addition, MOF may occur in the setting of severe allergic or hypersensitivity reactions to some drugs, including lamotrigine. Descriptions of MOF have been reported sponta-neously for lamotrigine and are described in the product label. A literature review showed that such events were known to occur very rarely in people with seizures (Yuen and Bihari, 1992).

Because there were no databases judged to be large enough to quantify the frequency of this event in people with epilepsy, a case–control study of MOF and multi-organ dysfunction (MOD) following status epilepticus or aborted status epilepticus was initiated. This study was designed to better understand the risk factors for MOF following uninterrupted seizures. Ramesh Sach-deva and J.F. Annegers conducted this case–control study, and cases and controls were identified from two hospital admissions databases in a large US city. Controls were also identified from these databases and these had experienced status epilepticus or aborted status epilepticus but had not experienced MOF or MOD. The strongest and most consistent risk factor was the duration of status epilepticus (Sachdeva, 1996). These obser-vations were consistent with the hypothesis that most cases of MOF in patients on lamotrigine were likely to be related to rare sequelae of seizures. Although the numbers of cases exposed to individual antiepileptic drugs (AEDs) were small, there was no indication that MOF or dysfunction were related to any specific AEDs.

QUANTIFYING THE RISK OF AND RISK FACTORS FOR SERIOUS ADVERSE EVENTS ASSOCIATED WITH A MEDICATION

Early in the postmarketing phase of lamotrigine development, it was evident that some patients using lamotrigine developed serious cutaneous reactions. As almost all of these reactions occurred during the first eight weeks of therapy, the at-risk period was limited to the initiation of lamotrigine. Lamotrigine is initiated through a dose escalation phase which lasts a minimum of six weeks. A program of epidemiologic studies was launched in order to ask the following:

1. What is the risk of serious cutaneous reactions in patients initiating lamotrigine?
2. What is the risk of serious cutaneous reactions during initiation of alternative anticonvulsant therapies?
3. Are there factors that increase the risk of having a serious cutaneous reaction in patients initiating lamotrigine therapy?

The classification of cutaneous reactions can be problematic without photographic evidence. Therefore, most of the epidemologic studies of rash in lamotrigine focused on rash associated with hospitalization during therapy initiation. Use of this definition may overestimate the seriousness of rash since some patients with epilepsy are hospitalized for seizure control when an anticonvulsant medication is withdrawn. By including all serious rash, however, the full impact of cutaneous adverse events could be assessed.

In most European countries and in the United States the first approved indication for lamotrigine was adjunctive therapy in adults with partial seizures, with or without secondary generalization. Since the initial approval of use in adults, lamotrigine has become available in >50 countries for children with epilepsy. At the time of first availability of lamotrigine, two cohort studies were initiated to quantify the adverse event profile in general clinical practice: Prescription–Event Monitoring (PEM) was initiated in the United Kingdom in 1991 and a large prospective US cohort study was initiated in 1995. In addition a retrospective cohort study was performed in the GPRD.

Over time, experienced clinicians found that the frequency of common, non-serious rash associated with lamotrigine could be reduced by slowing the dose escalation schedule, and dose escalation packs were developed by the manufacturer to facilitate appropriate dosing. Pediatric approvals came later to most countries, and in some countries children were initially prescribed lamotrigine without availability of pediatric formulations. Epidemiologic observational studies were initiated to quantify the safety profile of lamotrigine, and

results suggested that children experienced higher rates of serious rash than adults. One hypothesis generated to explain this observation involved higher than recommended dosing in children because of lack of an available pediatric formulation. There was also some evidence that comedication with valproic acid, which inhibits the metabolism of lamotrigine, might be a risk factor for serious rash in people using lamotrigine, and children could be using valproic acid more often. The recommended dosing escalation for lamotrigine in children was slowed in 1998, and lamotrigine was subsequently initiated at lower doses than originally recommended. As dose escalation practices changed, observational data could provide some indication of the role of lamotrigine dose as a risk factor for serious cutaneous reactions.

The PEM study of lamotrigine users was conducted by the Drug Safety Research Unit (DSRU) at the University of Southampton, UK (Mackay et al., 1997). All first-time users of lamotrigine between December 1991 and February 1995 were identified through General Practitioner (GP) prescriptions from the national British Prescription Pricing Authority. Six months after the first lamotrigine prescription, a follow-up form was sent to each prescribing GP. On this form the GP listed any adverse event, regardless of cause, occurring since the first lamotrigine prescription. For any significant medical event, such as hospitalization for rash or reported Stevens–Johnson Syndrome (SJS), the DSRU followed up for more information. Lamotrigine was not licensed for use in pediatric patients in the United Kingdom before May 1994, and neither pediatric dosing guidelines nor the formulation (5 mg tablets) of lamotrigine needed to dose many children accurately were available prior to licensing for use in pediatric patients. If serious rash is associated with dosing in children, then it is likely that the frequency of serious rash observed in this study was higher than that for children who use the currently recommended slower dose escalation schedule.

Of 19 448 six-month green forms posted during this study, follow-up data on 11 316 patients were collected. There were 12 events reported as SJS and 10 involved hospitalization. There were an additional two hospitalizations for cutaneous reactions not reported as SJS (personal communication). In adults, the observed risk was seven events in 10 741 adults (1.1 per 1000), and in children < 12 years of age the observed risk was five in 1598 children (3.1 per 1000).

These rates are consistent with those observed during the early clinical development program, including the higher rate of reported SJS in children (Messenheimer *et al.*, 1998, 2000). All clinical and observational data on adults and on children have consistently shown that the frequency of serious rash in children initiating lamotrigine is three times higher than in adults.

Valproic acid is known to be a risk factor for common *non-serious* rash in people initiating lamotrigine therapy. However, because of the small numbers of events in any individual study, the relationship between lamotrigine serious rash and valproic acid use is difficult to assess. In this study, four of the seven adult cases and five of the five of the pediatric cases were on valproic acid. Data from the GPRD have shown that concomitant valproic acid use was ~40% in lamotrigine users in the United Kingdom (Drug Research Unit, Lexington MA, USA, personal communication). Although these data are consistent with the hypothesis that valproic acid is a risk factor for serious rash in patients initiating lamotrigine, the number of cases is too small to assess this relationship.

The GPRD was used to supplement the time period covered by the PEM study. All individuals receiving lamotrigine prescriptions were identified, and hospitalizations for possibly drug-related events and all deaths within 60 days of a lamotrigine prescription were identified. Each prescribing GP was contacted to confirm the event, to obtain anonymized medical records about a possibly drug-related serious adverse event for review, and to obtain information on whether the GP was the first prescriber of lamotrigine for that individual. A total of 1722 individuals were identified, 279 were aged 12 years or younger, and 117 were aged 60 years or older. On the basis of earlier surveys of GPs listed in the GPRD about lamotrigine prescribing, it was estimated that 150 of the 279 children initiated their lamotrigine therapy through the GP. In these children, there

were two mentions of rash, and none was associated with hospitalization.

In the United Kingdom, patients frequently start lamotrigine through a specialist and prescribing is then transferred to the GP. Because PEM and GPRD are GP-based, these studies cannot capture the initial period of drug exposure for some patients and may not capture some adverse events occurring prior to the transfer of prescribing to the GP. Unpublished GPRD data have shown that 31%–38% of GPRD lamotrigine users in 1993–1994 (predominantly adults) initiated lamotrigine therapy through non-GPs (Drug Research Unit, personal communication). Given the durations of non-GP prescribing, it was estimated that PEM or GPRD might not include up to 20%–27% of events leading to discontinuation within seven days of therapy in new lamotrigine users of all ages. A more recent analysis showed that 61% of children aged ≤12 years initiated lamotrigine therapy through a non-GP (Drug Research Unit, personal communication) in 1995.

Of the 876 adults in the GPRD estimated to have gotten their first prescription through the GP, none had a rash involving hospitalization and discontinuation. There was one patient with an unknown source of first lamotrigine prescription who had SJS while taking concomitant sodium valproate and had a gradual recovery.

These results on risk of serious rash were similar to what was observed in a US observational study of adults initiating lamotrigine therapy before starter packs were available (Tennis *et al.*, 1996). In this study, there were two cases of rash (one also on valproic acid) associated with hospitalization and without sequelae in 767 adults. Because of the small number of cases, risk factors for serious cutaneous reactions could not be evaluated. Although all of the risk estimates for serious rash are based on small numerators, and the issue of neurologist prescribing in the United Kingdom generates some questions about underestimation of serious rash, the risk of serious rash in adults was consistently close to 1/1000. Because of the recent revision of the dosing recommendations in children, it is not yet feasible to quantify the risk of serious rash in children initiating lamotrigine under current prescribing conditions in general clinical practice.

AT-RISK PERIOD FOR SERIOUS RASH

Without knowledge of the risk associated with the initiation of alternative anticonvulsant therapies, the benefit–risk assessment for lamotrigine was not definable. National registries had published rates of SJS and toxic epidermal necrolysis (TEN) associated with alternative therapies. However, these estimates were based on total defined daily doses in the denominator (Roujeau *et al.*, 1990; Schöpf *et al.*, 1991). Given that the at-risk period was likely to be limited to the first few weeks, it seemed likely that denominators based on the total population exposed to an individual therapy would underestimate those at risk by using a denominator which was too large. Therefore, several retrospective cohort studies were initiated to measure the risk of serious cutaneous reactions in new users of older alternative antiepileptic medications associated with serious cutaneous reactions.

RECORD LINKAGE STUDIES OF ADVERSE EVENTS RISK ASSOCIATED WITH ALTERNATIVE THERAPIES

In two North American databases (Saskatchewan Health and Medicaid), studies were initiated by different investigators. New users were identified as anyone with at least a two-year history in the insurance plan at the time of the first prescription of one of three anticonvulsant drugs. Hospitalizations for *cutaneous* conditions during the first 60 days of drug exposure were identified, and anonymized medical records were reviewed by dermatologic experts to substantiate the discharge diagnosis. The specific case definitions were left to the discretion of each investigator, but the basic study designs were similar. The Saskatchewan study showed that the risk associated with phenytoin initiation was 1/1000 (Tennis and Stern, 1997) and the risk associated with initiation of carbamazepine was 0.6 per 1000. In the two Medicaid states (US), the risks associated with two alternative therapies ranged from 0.3 to 1.6 per 1000 (Judith Jones, personal communication). Although based on small numbers of cases, these results suggested that the overall risk of serious cutaneous reactions in patients initiating lamotrigine was not dissimilar from that in patients initiating some alternative therapies. However, because of the very small numbers of events, the real-world risk of serious rash in children has not yet been well defined for these other anticonvulsant therapies.

When the International Case–Control Study on Severe Cutaneous Adverse Reactions published data on the association of anticonvulsant therapies with SJS and TEN (Rzany *et al.*, 1999) it appeared that the risk associated with lamotrigine was similar to that of other anticonvulsants (Table 23.1). However, the number of cases using lamotrigine was small.

This study shows how case–control studies can be useful for detecting the role of medications as risk factors for an outcome. However, case–control studies alone cannot quantify the frequency of an event.

The German population-based registry of severe skin reactions was extremely useful for understanding SJS or TEN associated with lamotrigine.

Table 23.1. Relative risks associated with initiation (<8 weeks of use) of anticonvulsant medications reported by the International Case–Control Study of SJS and TEN (Rzany *et al.*, 1999).

Anticonvulsant and duration of use (weeks)	No. of cases exposed to anticonvulsant (total no. of cases = 73)	No. of controls exposed to anticonvulsant (total no. of controls = 28)	Relative risk for new user of specific anticonvulsant, compared with population risk	Relative risk 95% confidence intervals
Phenobarbital, <8 wks	23	2	57	16–360
Phenytoin, <8 wks	14	0	91	26–∞
Carbamazepine, <8 wks	18	0	120	34–∞
Lamotrigine, <8 wks	3	0	25	5.6–∞

This registry is an observational registry collecting information on cases of SJS, TEN, and erythema multiforme with mucosal involvement throughout Germany. They make every effort to identify all hospitalized cases of SJS and TEN within the country, and they collect information on drug exposures prior to the event. Each possible case is reviewed by an expert group to assign a diagnosis. For estimation of rates, they utilize prescription data (defined daily doses, or DDDs) as a surrogate for the number of people exposed to each medication, and initially when lamotrigine was first marketed in Germany their data seemed to demonstrate that the rate based on DDD denominators for SJS or TEN in lamotrigine was substantially higher than other anticonvulsants. However, as the market matured and the percentage of total use which was new use declined, the ratio of the number of cases to the number of DDDs declined (Schlingmann, 2000). This observation is consistent with the concept that for mature medications the rates of SJS and TEN are substantially underestimated because the denominators are overestimated with the inclusion of long-term use. Nevertheless, given that the numbers of SJS or TEN cases failed to increase while the use of lamotrigine was increasing, it is likely that other factors, such as the reduction of the lamotrigine starting dose, may have also contributed to this decline in rate.

LAMOTRIGINE PREGNANCY REGISTRY

Pregnancy exposure registries, which are simple cohort studies, are useful for monitoring and quantifying the impact of medications on birth defect frequency. There are several factors which contribute to the decision to develop a pregnancy registry. These factors include the need for treatment of the indicated condition during pregnancy, a medication indication associated with birth defects, alternative therapies associated with birth defects, and background information about the medication itself (e.g. animal data).

As with many chronic conditions, epilepsy is treated chronically. Pregnancies in women with epilepsy are exposed to anticonvulsant medications from conception and throughout pregnancy. The literature shows that women with epilepsy and using anticonvulsant medications during pregnancy have an elevated risk of major birth defects compared with the general population (Samren, 1997; Canger et al., 1999), and some anticonvulsants have been associated with an elevated frequency of specific major malformations (Omtzigt et al., 1992; Dravet, 1992; Arpino et al., 2000). Although there was no pre-clinical evidence of teratogenicity for lamotrigine, the Lamotrigine Pregnancy Registry was initiated to monitor for the possible elevated risk of birth defects. With the entry of a number of new medications into the armamentarium for treating epilepsy, anticonvulsant exposure in pregnancy has become a growing issue. Prospective pregnancy exposure registries focusing on anticonvulsant exposures have been initiated in North America and in Europe with support from a number of pharmaceutical sponsors. Each registry enrolls exposures and follows the pregnancies prospectively to evaluate the pregnancy outcome, specifically major structural birth defects. Each registry is based on a different methodologic model. The North American Pregnancy Registry invites women with ongoing pregnancies to enroll themselves, and the European Anticonvulsant Registry works with epilepsy centers within multiple countries where clinicians enroll exposed pregnancies.

The Lamotrigine Pregnancy Registry, initiated in 1992, invites physicians throughout the world to enroll pregnancies exposed to lamotrigine. Physicians enroll exposed pregnancies anonymously before the outcome of the pregnancy is known. After the expected date of delivery, a follow-up form is sent to the physician requesting information on the pregnancy outcome. Birth defects are included if they meet the criteria for birth defects established by the Centre for Disease Control (CDC) in their birth defects monitoring program. An advisory committee consisting of independent experts in teratology, epidemiology and epilepsy semiannually review the data. As of September 2000, outcome data on 243 first-trimester exposures, 100 involving monotherapy, have been identified. The number of exposures is too small to make definitive conclusions about the risk of birth defects following lamotrigine exposure during pregnancy. However, to date the frequency of birth defects following monotherapy exposures, 3.0% (95% confidence interval 0.8%–9.2%), does not suggest a signal for concern.

CONCLUSIONS

In summary, pharmacoepidemiology is uniquely useful for quantifying the risks of adverse events and risk factors for adverse events within populations larger and more diverse than those exposed during clinical development. It is also useful for obtaining essential data to assess whether adverse events may be related to the background condition being treated. To be more specific, the data on the incidence of SUD in epilepsy were instrumental in addressing regulatory questions regarding the rate of this event during clinical trials and, during the early postmarketing phase, regarding reported deaths in people taking lamotrigine. These data, along with the demonstration that length of status epilepticus was a major risk factor for MOF, confirmed that serious events occurring in people with epilepsy can be related to seizures.

Serious rash in association with lamotrigine use has been of interest to GW and to regulatory bodies throughout the world. The first observation that the risk of serious rash was higher in children taking lamotrigine than in adults arose during the PEM study, and these results triggered hypothesis-generating to explain this pattern. Possible explanations included high dosing in children related to lack of available pediatric formulations. The PEM Study, the GPRD Study, the German Registry, and the International Case–Control Study consistently suggested together that the absolute risk to children in general clinical practice was not as high as that observed in the early clinical trials. These observational data were crucial for assessing the risk–benefit of lamotrigine when an early pediatric clinical trial yielded a single case of serious rash within a small number of children. The Saskatchewan and Medicaid studies, although sometimes criticized because of the difficulty of classifying serious rash without photographs, demonstrated that the risk associated with the initiation of older

anticonvulsant therapies was not as low as that previously estimated. In addition, these observational record linkage studies were consistent with the case–control study which demonstrated that the principal at-risk period for these medications is during the first eight weeks of therapy.

Clinicians and patients have been keenly interested in any information which can provide a perspective on expected risks in pregnancies involving lamotrigine exposures. The literature shows that women with epilepsy and using anticonvulsant medications during pregnancy have elevated risk of major birth defects compared with the general population (Samren, 1997; Canger et al., 1999), and some anticonvulsants have been associated with an elevated frequency of specific major malformations (DiLiberti et al., 1984; Ardinger et al., 1988; Dravet, 1992; Lindhout et al., 1992; Omtzigt et al., 1992; Arpino et al., 2000). Even without statistical power to compare medications, results have been crucial for providing to patients and clinicians information key to the management of pregnancies in women using this chronic medication. In addition, the results of other pregnancy registries will provide important information on all new anticonvulsant medications and updated information on older anticonvulsants.

In summary, pharmacoepidemologic studies have been instrumental in addressing questions posed by regulatory bodies and clinicians. The funding of pharmacoepidemiologic efforts has been an integral part of the overall cost of drug development and continued safety surveillance. By providing quantitative real-world data on some risks related to epilepsy and the frequency of serious rash related to lamotrigine treatment and to some alternative treatments, the approach has provided regulatory bodies, clinicians and patients with the information needed to understand lamotrigine treatment in the world of diverse patients and clinician approaches.

ADDENDUM

Recently the risk of hospitalization with SJS or TEN in patients initiating lamotrigine was estimated. Sales of low-dose lamotrigine for initiation of treatment were used to estimate numbers of new adult and pediatric users of lamotrigine in Germany. Numbers of cases identified by the German Registry of Severe Cutaneous Reactions were used as the numerator. Based on 1 pediatric case and 9 adult cases during 1998–2000, the risk was estimated as 1.5 in 10 000 adults and 2.1 in 10 000 children.

REFERENCES

Annegers JF, Coan SP, Hauser WA, Leestma J, Duffell W, Tarver B (1998) Epilepsy, vagal nerve stimulation by the NCP system, mortality, and sudden unexpected, unexplained death. *Epilepsia* **39**(2): 206–12.

Ardinger HH, Blackston JF, Elsas LJ, Clarren SK, Livingstone S, Flannery DB, Pellock JM, Garrod MJ, Lammer EJ, *et al.* (1988) Verification of the fetal valproate syndrome phenotype. *Am J Med Gen* **29**(1): 171–85.

Arpino C, Brescianini S, Robert E, Castilla EE, Cocchi YG, Cornel MC, *et al.* (2000) Teratogenic effects of antiepileptic drugs: use of an international database on malformations and drug exposure (MADRE). *Epilepsia* **41**(11): 1436–43.

Canger R, *et al.* (1999). Malformations in offspring of women with epilepsy: a prospective study. *Epilepsia* **40**(9): 1231–6.

Derby LE, Tennis P, Jick H (1996) Sudden unexplained death among subjects with refractory epilepsy. *Epilepsia* **37**(10): 931–5.

DiLiberti JG, Frandon PA, Dennis NR, Curry CJ (1984) The fetal valproate syndrome. *Am J Med Gen* **19**(33): 473–81.

Dravet C, Julian C, Legras C, *et al.* (1992) Epilepsy, antiepileptic drugs, and malformations in children of women with epilepsy. A French prospective cohort study. *Neurology* **42** (Suppl 5): 75–82.

Jick SS, Cole TB, Mesher RA, Tennis P, Jick H (1992) Idiopathic epilepsy and sudden unexplained death. *Pharmacoepidemiology and Drug Safety* **1**: 59–64.

Leestma JE, Annegers JF, Brodie M, Brown S, Schraeder P, Siscovick D, Wannamaker BB, Tennis P, Cierpial M, Earl N (1997) Sudden unexplained death in epilepsy: observations from a large clinical development program. *Epilepsia* **38**(1): 47–55.

Lindhout D, Meinardi H, Meijer JWA, Nau H (1992) Antiepileptic drugs and teratogenesis in two consecutive cohorts. *Neurology* **42** (Suppl 5): 94–110.

Mackay FJ, Wilton LV, Pearce GL, Freemangle SN, Mann RD (1997) Safety of long-term lamotrigine in epilepsy. *Epilepsia* **38**(8): 881–6.

Messenheimer, J, Mullens IL, Giorgi L, Young F (1998) Safety review of adult clinical trial experience with lamotrigine. *Drug Safety* **18**(4): 281–90.

Messenheimer, JA, Giorgi L, Risner ME (2000) The tolerability of lamotrigine in children. *Drug Safety* **22**(4): 303–12.

Nashef L, Fish, DR, Garner S, Sander JWAS, Shorvon SD (1995a). Sudden death in epilepsy: a study of incidence in a young cohort with epilepsy and learning difficulty. *Epilepsia* **36**(2): 1187–94)

Nashef L, Fish DR, Sander JWAS, Shorvon SD (1995b). Incdence of sudden unexpected death in an adult outpatient cohort with epilepsy at a tertiary centre. *J Neurol Neurosurg Psychiatry* **58**: 462–4.

Omtzigt JGC, Los JF, Grobbee DE, *et al.* (1992) The risk of spina bifida aperta after first-trimester exposure to valproate in a prenatal cohort. *Neurology* **42** (Suppl 5): 119–25.

Roujeau JC, Guillaume MC, Fabre JP, Penso D, Flechet ML, Girre JP (1990) Toxic epidermal necorlysis (Lyell syndrome) incidence and drug etiology in France, 1981–1985. *Arch Dermatol* **126**: 37–42.

Rzany B, Correla O, Kelly J, Naldi L, Auquier A, Stern R (1999) Risk of Stevens–Johnson-Syndrome and toxic epidermal necrolysis during first weeks of antiepileptic therapy: a case control study. *Lancet* **353**: 2190–4.

Sachdeva R (1996) Status epilepticus and multiple organ system dysfunction. Ph.D. Dissertation. University of Texas Health Science Center at Houston, School of Public Health.

Samren EB, *et al.* (1997) Maternal use of antiepileptic drugs and the risk of major congenital malformations: a joint European prospective study of human teratogenesis associated with maternal epilepsy. *Epilepsia* **38**(9): 981–90.

Schlingmann J, Mockenhaupt M, Schroeder W, Schlingmann E (2000) Severe cutaneous advsere reactions (SCAR) after the use of anticonvulsants. Poster presented at 16th International Conference on Pharmacoepidemiology. Barcelona, August.

Schöpf E, Stühmer A, Rzany B, Victor N, Zentgraf R, Kapp JF (1991) Toxic epidermal necrolysis and Stevens–Johnson Syndrome. An epidemiologic study from West Germany. *Arch Dermatol* **127**: 839–42.

Tennis P, Cole TB, McNutt M, Annegers JF, Leestma JE, Rajput A (1995) Cohort study of sudden unexplained death in persons with seizure disorder treated with antiepileptic drugs in Saskatchewan, Canada. *Epilepsia* **36**(1): 29–36.

Tennis P, Stern R (1997) Risk of serious cutaneous disorders after initiation of use of phenytoin, carbamazepine, or sodium valproate: a record linkage study. *Neurology* **49**: 542–6.

Tennis, P, Wozniak C, Cosmatos I, Frick M (1996) A large prospective study of lamotrigine safety. *Epilepsia* **37** (Suppl 5): 161.

Yuen AWC, Bihari DJ (1992) Multiorgan failure and disseminated intravascular coagulation in severe convulsive seizures. *Lancet* **Sept 5**: 618.

24

Pharmacovigilance in the Netherlands

A.C. VAN GROOTHEEST AND E.P. VAN PUIJENBROEK
Netherlands Pharmacovigilance Centre Lareb, Goudsbloemvallei 7, 5237 MH 's-Hertogenbosch, The Netherlands

HISTORY AND ORGANIZATION

HISTORY

In the Netherlands, consideration for the surveillance of adverse drug reactions developed at a relatively early stage. In the early 1950s, at a time when international literature had included only incidental reports of "side effects", Leo Meyler laid the basis for paying more systematic attention to adverse drug reactions. In 1951, he published his book (in Dutch) *Schadelijke nevenwerkingen van geneesmiddelen* (literally, *Harmful Effects of Prescription Drugs*). The second edition, fully revised with a number of supplements, appeared in 1954.

In his preface to the first edition, Meyler wrote the following (here in translation):

> The prescribing of drugs will always entail a greater or lesser degree of risk, and in each case the physician must ask himself whether the nature of the condition about which he is being consulted justifies taking such a risk.

Meyler's work was prompted by his own experiences with tuberculostatic preparations. He warned also against the inappropriate use of drugs.

Meyler based much of his work on reports in various medical journals, at a time without the convenience of the Internet or other conveniences of modern times. The first English edition of Meyler's seminal work was published as *The Side Effects of Drugs: An Encyclopaedia of Reactions and Interactions* in 1952. Its fourteenth edition, edited by Graham Dukes, appeared in 2000. Dukes has been the editor since the eighth edition, published in 1978, of what has now become the standard reference work in its field. Dukes' own scientific background was largely gained in the Netherlands.

ORGANIZATION OF PHARMACOVIGILANCE IN THE NETHERLANDS

Following the thalidomide affair of the late 1950s and early 1960s, the Netherlands decided to adopt a more systematic approach to the safety of prescription medicines. The Dutch Medicines Evaluation Board was founded in 1963. Based on the American model of the Food and Drug Administration, this would assess new pharmaceutical preparations for both effectiveness and safety prior to marketing authorization. Also in 1963, the Royal Dutch Medical Association

Pharmacovigilance. Edited by R.D. Mann and E.B. Andrews

(KNMG) joined the government in setting up a reporting system for adverse drug reactions. In 1965, the task of processing reports was taken over by the National Drug Monitoring Centre, which was part of the Public Health Supervisory Service and came to acquire an extremely good reputation. With a relatively small staff, the Centre produced a significant number of publications calling attention to the potential adverse effects of prescription drugs (de Koning, 1984). Each year, the National Drug Monitoring Centre received approximately 1000 reports from interested doctors.

In 1986, a number of pharmacists called for greater attention to be devoted to the potential adverse effects of prescription medicines. These pharmacists were convinced that greater awareness of the possibility of adverse effects would improve the quality of pharmacotherapy as a whole. Their initiative led to the creation of the Lareb Foundation (in full, the Netherlands Pharmacovigilance Foundation Lareb), in 1991. The Lareb Foundation collected reports of adverse effects, mostly made by general practitioners and pharmacists. This information was supplementary to the work done by the National Drug Monitoring Centre (Meyboom *et al.*, 1996), and at times created overlap. A new aspect was that pharmacists felt also their responsibility in the identification of adverse effects and would consider it their task to call attention to such effects (de Koning *et al.*, 1992).

In 1995, European legislation having been made more stringent, the Dutch government decided to restructure the system of pharmacovigilance in the Netherlands. The Lareb Foundation was designated the national centre for all reports of suspected adverse drug reactions concerning registered drugs. Currently, the Health Inspectorate is responsible for monitoring the quality of pharmacovigilance activities and receives reports relating to preparations that have not (yet) been given marketing authorization, especially reports of adverse reactions that are observed during the statutory clinical trials.

The Medicines Evaluation Board Agency plays a central coordinating role. It receives reports from Lareb, as well as those made directly by the pharmaceutical industry, and it advises the Medicines Evaluation Board. The Medicines Evaluation Board makes the final decision regarding marketing authorization for the Netherlands. Where deemed necessary, it is empowered to require amendments to a drug's "Summary of Product Characteristics", and in serious cases may revoke a drug's marketing authorization altogether. The Medicines Evaluation Board includes a pharmacovigilance department primarily concerned with adverse drug reactions and with maintaining international contacts in this field. Many decisions are taken at European level by the European Medicines Evaluation Agency (EMEA).

SPONTANEOUS REPORTING IN THE NETHERLANDS: THE LAREB FOUNDATION

DIRECT RESPONSIBILITY OF DOCTORS AND PHARMACISTS

The Lareb Foundation is an organization which was founded by doctors and pharmacists and which is still run by doctors and pharmacists today. All large medical and pharmacists' associations are represented on its administrative board. The Lareb Foundation maintains the national "spontaneous" reporting system for the Netherlands. That this task falls to an independent foundation rather than the government sets the Netherlands apart from most other countries. Although some (such as Germany, Switzerland, New Zealand and Great Britain with its Drug Safety Research Unit) have organizations investigating adverse drug reactions that are allied to universities or professional organizations, the role of professional practitioners is particularly prominent in the Netherlands. The government restricts itself to a supervisory and coordinating role, while also providing funding for the Lareb Foundation's activities.

The Dutch model has a significant number of advantages and works very well in practice. It is doctors and pharmacists who see the occurrence of adverse drug reactions in day-to-day practice. If given co-responsibility for the proper monitoring of drug safety, they will be more inclined to contribute. This enhances the premise that doctors and pharmacists are themselves responsible for the safe and responsible use of prescription drugs. The barriers to reporting suspected adverse reactions would be significantly lowered if those reports were made to a peer group organization. After all, the occurrence of an adverse reaction may cause the doctor or pharmacist to ask himself (or herself) whether he should assume partial responsibility for this reaction. It is possible that some would be less eager to report an adverse drug reaction to a "higher authority" such as the government.

REGIONAL ORGANIZATION

For an organization such as the Lareb Foundation, in which several professions meet, it is relatively easy to maintain an extensive network of doctors and pharmacists. This is indeed facilitated by the Foundation's regional organization under which the Netherlands is divided into five regions. The Foundation's headquarters in 's-Hertogenbosch acts as one regional office, with the other four in university hospitals throughout the country. Each regional office has a regional coordinator, responsible for maintaining contact with the doctors and pharmacists in that region. Such contact is both individual (through personal visits) and collective, involving presentations in hospitals and to groups of invited general practitioners and pharmacists. Wherever possible, education and "refresher" courses are offered.

The regional coordinator also personally assesses some of the incoming reports in order to remain involved in the Lareb Foundation's "core business" and will contribute to relevant publications wherever possible. A meeting of all the Lareb's scientific staff is held monthly at the head office, providing an opportunity for consultation and further "in-service" training. The Lareb Foundation is a small organization, with a staff of only 18. Some work part-time. There are four supportive (administrative) staff members, the remainder are all doctors, pharmacists or medical biologists by profession. Details are to be found on the foundation's website at www.lareb.nl.

MARKED INVOLVEMENT OF PHARMACISTS

In the context of pharmaceutical patient care, pharmacists in the Netherlands are very much involved in ensuring the safe and responsible use of medicines. Pharmacists played an important part in setting up the Lareb Foundation. Today, pharmacists (see Table 24.1) provide about 40% of the reports the Foundation receives.

Most reports are made by community pharmacists, which is perhaps to be expected given the Foundation's background. Hospital pharmacists lag somewhat behind in this respect. Accordingly, the Lareb Foundation has joined forces with the Netherlands Society of Hospital Pharmacists in attempting to encourage greater involvement on the part of its members. One objective is to establish a protocol in hospitals whereby house pharmacists are not only expected to provide effective pharmacotherapy, but will also play a coordinating and facilitating role in terms of the collation and forwarding of adverse drug reaction reports. A survey held in early 2001 indicated that 97% of hospital pharmacists are eager to report any adverse reactions; they know what must be reported and in what way. The complaint that pharmacists are themselves able to provide little or no clinical information in a report has been shown to present no great problem in practice. Often, the good cooperation between doctors and pharmacists will ensure that adequate information can be given, particularly if the relevant report is being made from a hospital situation. If necessary, it is possible to contact the prescribing doctor to obtain further information. That pharmacists are able to provide a complete picture of a patient's prescription history is a significant advantage.

Table 24.1. Sources of reports.

Year	Pharmacists	Doctors
1996	46.3	53.7
1997	44.9	55.1
1998	44.5	55.5
1999	41.6	58.4
2000	41.1	58.9

THE GENERATION OF SIGNALS

The primary objective of any reporting system is to generate a "signal": an early indicator or warning of a potential problem. It may be compared to the task of a fire-watcher, who looks for smoke and, if he thinks he spots it, must then determine whether there is indeed a fire and where that fire is located. In pharmacovigilance, it falls to the Medicines Evaluation Board to determine whether there are sufficient arguments to shout "fire!", whereupon it will take the necessary measures.

The reports received by the Lareb Foundation are first assessed by one of its staff doctors or pharmacists. They examine the probability of a causal link, and will use the current literature, previous reports and the description of the drug's pharmacological mechanism to assist them. The results of their assessment are notified to the reporter as well as to the government.

A weekly assessment meeting involves all scientific staff. The reports and their subsequent assessments are discussed to determine whether further action is necessary. Such further action may entail more detailed analysis of the relationship between the reported reaction and the suspect drug. Research within Lareb has revealed a number of factors that can play a significant role in the decision to conduct further analysis. These include the seriousness of the reported reaction, the number of reports related to similar reports on other drugs received by the Foundation, and whether existing literature has devoted attention to the suspected reaction.

During the weekly assessment meeting, all new reports are discussed and further action is scheduled if there seems to be sufficient justification. As a general rule, such action will entail notifying the Medicines Evaluation Board, and in many cases an article will be published.

Computer automation now plays an important role in the internal report assessment process, with all incoming reports undergoing a set sequence of events. The information on the report forms themselves, together with that in any other relevant documentation, is stored in digital form. The weekly assessment meeting also makes use of information obtained through automated quantitative signal generation. The "Reporting Odds Ratio" is calculated for all reports, providing a statistical indication of the reporting frequency of each of the suspected reactions compared with other reports in the Lareb Foundation's database. The results of the Bayesian Confidence Propagation Neural Network analysis, submitted quarterly by the World Health Organization (WHO) Monitoring Centre in Uppsala are also automatically linked to each report.

At the time of writing (early 2001) the Lareb Foundation's database contained over 30 000 reports. Besides providing a valuable aid to case-by-case analysis, quantitative information can also be used to distil useful information from a large collection of data. Such information will not be provided by a single case analysis. The Lareb Foundation is particularly interested in the possibilities for identifying specific syndromes and in detecting *interactions* between drugs (van Puijenbroek *et al.*, 1999, 2000). Ongoing research is being conducted into whether certain risk factors for drug reactions can be identified using the information now filed in the database.

COMMUNICATION

The Lareb Foundation is a small organization in a big world. Its most important contacts are the professional organizations, the government and the pharmaceutical industry.

Doctors and Pharmacists

Because the Foundation is itself an organization of doctors and pharmacists, it has ready access to practitioners in the field. Current European legislation does not permit direct reporting by patients themselves, although the Lareb Foundation would not be opposed to its future introduction. Partly in view of the fact that doctors and pharmacists report suspected adverse drug reactions on a purely voluntary basis, it is important to inform them of the importance of reporting. In addition to the feedback it provides, both direct and in the form of publications, the Foundation offers targeted information to potential reporters in the form of mailings and presentations. The report form itself has a carefully designed layout and is distributed in various ways, such as inclusion with the regular *Drug Bulletin* and the annual *Parmacotherapeutisch Kompas*, the pharmacopoeia which forms a standard desk reference book for 90% of Dutch doctors. It is important that the reporter can rely on respect to privacy and confidentiality. Lareb does not receive any information about the identity of the patient and no information about the reporter will be given to third parties. The Dutch law is also strict on privacy.

An important means of communication with the reporting parties is the "feedback report". Not only is receipt of each report acknowledged, but the assessment made by the Lareb and the conclusions drawn with regard to the reported adverse drug reaction are notified to the person making the report.

Besides wishing to encourage reporting, the Lareb Foundation believes that it is important to raise the level of awareness among doctors and pharmacists with regard to adverse drug reactions. This will not only lead to a better standard of reporting but will serve to reduce significantly the harmful effects of prescription medicines as well. Doctors will prescribe more critically and will be more inclined to consider adverse drug reactions as the cause of complaints at an earlier stage in their differential diagnosis, whereupon they will become able to discontinue use of the drug or to adapt the dosage to avoid both unnecessary costs and unnecessary impact in terms of patient health.

The Government

Because the Lareb Foundation is an independent organization working on behalf of the government, good communication with that government is very important. Reports are forwarded to the Medicines Evaluation Board Agency weekly. Every six weeks, a meeting is held between the Lareb Foundation, the Agency and the Health Inspectorate. Besides possible "signals", these meetings also discuss international developments.

Marketing Authorization Holders

Needless to say, the Lareb Foundation maintains close contact with the pharmaceutical industry, which also has a vested interest in effective pharmacovigilance. All serious ("15-day") reports are forwarded to the relevant Marketing Authorization Holder, as required by international legislation. These reports are anonymous, neither the patient nor the reporter can be traced. Similarly, all such reports made directly by the pharmaceutical industry to the government are entered into the Lareb Foundation's database. In the short term, the Foundation aims to achieve a free exchange of less serious reports as well. All articles concerning a specific preparation are submitted for comment to the relevant Marketing Authorization Holder prior to publication.

RESULTS

The "output" of the Lareb Foundation can be assessed by looking at both the quantity and quality of incoming reports, aspects that owe much to the efforts of the Foundation. Other criteria include the number of publications for which the Foundation has been responsible and the number of notifications of possible signals it has made.

Reports: Quantity

The number of incoming reports continues to increase each year. The development in the number of reports included in the database is shown in Table 24.2. Lareb sees under-reporting

Table 24.2. Total reports and percentage of serious reports according to the criteria of the WHO or CIOMS.

Year	Reports total	WHO criteria % reports serious	CIOMS criteria % reports serious
1996	3042	10.6	3.6
1997	3649	12.1	4.7
1998	3434	14.5	11.5
1999	3686	17.1	14.1
2000	3702	19.9	18.1

as an inherent characteristic of a spontaneous reporting system and not necessarily as a drawback.

Reports: Quality

Although an adequate number of reports are necessary to ensure a reliable reporting system, the Lareb Foundation attaches greater importance to the *quality* of those reports.

The quality of reports can also be seen to have risen each year. Quality is continuously assessed according to a number of criteria, one of which is the extent to which the report is documented. In an increasing number of cases, reports are accompanied by adequate clinical information, including the specialists' clinical notes to the patient's family practitioner. The fact that more complete information is now available may be attributed in part to the greater number of reports being made by hospital practitioners. The increase in the number of reports adjudged to be of a serious nature is shown in Table 24.2.

Although preparations which have been on the market for some time may occasionally reveal new adverse reactions (as in the case of vigabatrine, which had been available for over 10 years before a link with patients' restricted field of vision was made), the Lareb Foundation is particularly interested in new medicines. Table 24.3 shows the percentage of reports relating to preparations that have been on the market for less than five years.

Publications and Presentations

Having adopted a scientific and academic level as the basis for its working methods, the Lareb

Table 24.3. Total reports and percentage of reports on drugs marketed less than five years.

Year	Reports	<5 years (%)
1996	3042	22.3
1997	3649	23.7
1998	3434	29.6
1999	3686	28.3
2000	3702	35.6

Foundation is regarded as a serious partner by others, particularly the professional organizations. The scientific quality of the Foundation's work is monitored by a Scientific Advisory Board, comprising experts in various disciplines. Each year, the Lareb Foundation publishes over 30 articles in international or national journals, among which is the Dutch *Drug Bulletin*. It also makes more than 30 presentations to groups of doctors and/or pharmacists and is frequently represented at international scientific conferences.

FURTHER INITIATIVES IN PHARMACOVIGILANCE IN THE NETHERLANDS

Besides the spontaneous reporting system and the activities undertaken by, or under the auspices of, the government, there are various other pharmacovigilance initiatives in the Netherlands. Of these, the most notable are those undertaken by the marketing authorization holders and universities.

MARKETING AUTHORIZATION HOLDERS

Needless to say, pharmaceutical companies in the Netherlands must comply with international legislation relating to pharmacovigilance. Reports that meet the Council for International Organizations of Medical Sciences (CIOMS) criteria must be made to the Medicines Evaluation Board within 15 days and will also be included in the Lareb Foundation's database. In addition, Marketing Authorization Holders are required to submit periodic safety update reports, to include all information known to them concerning the safety of the preparations for which they hold marketing authorization. The Netherlands does not have a tradition of reports being made directly to the pharmaceutical industry by doctors or pharmacists; the vast majority of reports concerning suspected adverse drug reactions pass through the Lareb Foundation.

UNIVERSITIES

Three Dutch universities have departments of pharmacoepidemiology. These devote considerable attention to the occurrence of adverse drug reactions at group level. A number of initiatives have been developed whereby these can be studied more closely in the context of day-to-day medical and pharmacological practice. The resulting systems are more suitable for the assessment of signals than for their generation.

The Department of Pharmacoepidemiology of the University of Utrecht developed the "PHARMO" system (which is now operated independently). It is a record-linkage system that uses information provided by a number of pharmacists in combination with hospital clinical records. The department of Epidemiology and Biostatistics of Rotterdam's Erasmus University is responsible for the Integrated Primary Care Information (IPCI) system. It relies on digital information recorded by general practitioners. The Department of Social Pharmacy and Pharmacoepidemiology of the University of Groningen has joined forces with the Lareb Foundation in developing an intensive monitoring system which will use the initial signals notified by pharmacists as well as responses to surveys conducted among general practitioners. It is believed that such a system will result in a first impression of possible adverse reactions in the case of newly authorized preparations.

SUMMARY AND FUTURE DEVELOPMENTS

The Netherlands can now look back on 50 years of systematic attention for adverse drug reactions. This began with the first edition of the book now popularly known simply as "Meyler's", and has developed to a stage at which the emphasis is on effective pharmacovigilance and at which "Meyler's" is now the work of several different authors. On behalf of and in co-operation with the government, the Lareb Foundation maintains the spontaneous reporting system for the Netherlands. A notable characteristic of the Dutch situation is that doctors and pharmacists are themselves responsible for this system, with pharmacists taking a significant role.

Besides continued consideration for both the quantity and quality of reports, the future is likely to see further development of automatic signal generation and even greater concern for good communication with potential reporters, in order to increase awareness of adverse drug reactions. Developments at the European level are certain to have a significant influence in this regard.

REFERENCES

de Koning GPH (1984) A regionalized spontaneous surveillance programme for adverse drug reactions as a tool to improve pharmacotherapy. *Academic thesis* produced for the Utrecht University Faculty of Pharmaceutical Sciences.

de Koning GPH, Bakker A, Leufkens HGM (1992) Postmarketing surveillance in pharmacy: an orientation. *Pharmaceutisch Weekblad* **127**: 76–9.

Dukes MNG, Aronson JK, eds (2001) *Meyler's Side Effects of Drugs*, 14th edn. Amsterdam.

Meyboom RHB, Gribnau FWJ, Hekster YA, de Koning GHP, Egberts ACG (1996) Characteristics of topics in pharmacovigilance in the Netherlands. *Clin Drug Invest* **4**: 207–19.

van Puijenbroek EP, Egberts ACG, Meyboom RHB, Leufkens HGM (1999) Signaling possible drug–drug interactions in a spontaneous reporting system: delay of withdrawal bleeding during concomitant use of oral contraceptives and itraconazole. *Br J Clin Pharmacol* **47**: 689–93.

van Puijenbroek EP, Egberts ACG, Heerdink ER, Leufkens HGM (2000) Detecting drug–drug interactions using a database for spontaneous adverse drug reactions: an example with diuretics and non-steroidal anti-inflammatory drugs. *Eur J Clin Pharmacol* **56**: 733–8.

25

CIOMS Working Groups and their Contribution to Pharmacovigilance

SUE RODEN

GlaxoSmithKline Research & Development Ltd, Greenford, Middlesex, UK

INTRODUCTION

The term "CIOMS" is in daily use in international pharmacovigilance departments. For example, CIOMS forms are used for expedited case reporting, CIOMS line listings are used for presenting groups of cases, and CIOMS frequency definitions are used in product information labelling. The aim of this chapter is to describe who or what CIOMS is and to examine the contributions that the individual working groups have made to present-day pharmacovigilance practice.

The Council for International Organisations of Medical Sciences (CIOMS) is an international, non-governmental, non-profit organisation which was established in 1949 under the auspices of the World Health Organisation (WHO) and the United Nations Educational, Scientific and Cultural Organisation (UNESCO). It is responsible for the collection and dissemination of informed opinion on new developments in biology and medicine, and exploring their social, moral, administrative and legal implications. In 1977 it was recommended that CIOMS should facilitate discussions between national regulatory authorities and pharmaceutical companies on policy matters by providing an independent forum. It also convenes groups of experts to make recommendations on specific topics when appropriate.

In 1986, CIOMS set up the first pharmacovigilance working group to discuss international reporting of adverse drug reactions (ADRs). Since then, five further working groups have completed recommendations and suggested guidelines for harmonisation of various aspects of pharmacovigilance (Table 25.1).

Table 25.1. The CIOMS initiatives.

Working group	Initiative
CIOMS I	Expedited reporting of individual ADRs (1990)
CIOMS IA	Harmonisation of data elements and fields for electronic reporting of individual ADRs (1995)
CIOMS II	Periodic safety updates (1992)
CIOMS III	Core clinical-safety information (1995; 1999)
CIOMS IV	Benefit–risk evaluation (1998)
CIOMS V	Good case management and reporting practices (2001)

Pharmacovigilance. Edited by R.D. Mann and E.B. Andrews
© 2002 John Wiley & Sons, Ltd

CIOMS drug safety working groups are composed of pharmacovigilance specialists from regulatory agencies and pharmaceutical manufacturers principally from North America and Europe. Historically, members were selected for their personal expertise and contributions rather than to represent specific organisations. Observers from organisations such as the WHO and the International Federation of Pharmaceutical Manufacturers Association (IFPMA) are also invited. The size of the groups has usually been restricted to 20–30 members to ensure optimum discussion and completion of tasks. Considerable overlap of membership between consecutive working groups has enhanced productivity. Consultation with various specialists has also occurred when appropriate.

Each working group is co-chaired by a member from a regulatory agency and a pharmaceutical manufacturer. Win Castle deserves particular mention for co-chairing all the working groups until her retirement in 2000. Her enthusiasm, determination and hard work often provided the impetus necessary for the successful completion of each initiative.

As the CIOMS working groups have no legal jurisdiction, reliance is placed on other bodies to incorporate the CIOMS recommendations and guidelines into a regulatory or legislative framework. For example, the International Conference on Harmonisation (ICH) has progressed the CIOMS initiatives on expedited and electronic reporting as well as having used the CIOMS II recommendations as the basis for the requirements for periodic safety update reports (Table 25.2). The ICH process is based on five steps:

- Step 1—Technical discussion by the Expert Working Group who produce a preliminary draft document
- Step 2—The consensus text is released for a six-month period of consultation
- Step 3—Formal consultation outside ICH
- Step 4—Sign off of finalised text
- Step 5—Implementation

Therefore, Step 4 is the stage at which the document is finalised and released with the intention that the countries represented by the ICH

Table 25.2. Uptake of CIOMS initiatives by ICH.

Working group	Initiative	Uptake
CIOMS I	Expedited reporting	ICH E2A October 1994
CIOMS IA	Data elements for electronic reporting	ICH E2B July 1997 ICH M2 November 2000
CIOMS II	Periodic safety update reports	ICH E2C November 1996

(Europe, the United States and Japan) will incorporate the requirements into their local legislation and regulations.

The acceptance, adaptation and utilisation of CIOMS principles by other bodies will be discussed later in this chapter.

CIOMS I—EXPEDITED REPORTING OF INDIVIDUAL ADRS

RATIONALE

It is well established that continuous ADR surveillance is critical to assuring the safety of approved drugs in clinical practice. Prior to 1984, regulatory authorities restricted their requirements for the receipt of individual ADRs to domestic reports only. However, between 1984 and 1987 the United Kingdom, France, the United States, Italy and Germany introduced regulatory requirements for the submission of foreign reports. That is, manufacturers were required to report ADRs occurring in one country to the regulatory authorities in other countries where the drug was also marketed. As each regulatory authority had different requirements regarding time frames, formats and definitions, and were concerned about different types of ADRs, manufacturers were confronted with many problems.

The purpose of the CIOMS I working group was, therefore, to develop an internationally acceptable reporting method so that manufacturers could report post-marketing ADRs rapidly, efficiently and effectively to regulators.

PROCESS

On the understanding that the CIOMS members would modify their own international reporting procedures accordingly, the working group set out to define what constituted a reportable individual reaction, the elements of a report and the procedure and format for submitting individual reports. As most reporting depends on legal requirements, it became clear that the regulators needed to reach consensus. When this had been achieved a pilot test was undertaken to demonstrate the feasibility and utility of standardised reporting. The effort was geared towards the international exchange of post-approval reports of suspected, unexpected (unlabelled) serious ADRs. The manufacturers in the working group reported local cases according to the domestic requirements in that country and then entered the cases on to single common forms and submitted them to the other regulatory authorities represented on the CIOMS working group. Reports received from a country outside the participating six were entered on a single report and submitted to all six regulators.

The advantages of standardisation to the manufacturers were that it avoided a multitude of different requirements from different regulators, eased communication of reports between international corporate affiliates, and lessened regulatory ambiguities. From the regulatory perspective, standardisation could improve standards and reporting compliance by manufacturers and facilitate the exchange of information between regulators.

RECOMMENDATIONS

The CIOMS recommendations for the case criteria for expedited reporting of a foreign ADR were defined as follows:

- Serious
- Medically substantiated
- Unlabelled (unexpected)
- Suspected to be product related
- Occurring with a marketed product
- In an identifiable patient

Such reports were to be submitted in English on the prescribed CIOMS form within 15 working days of receipt. The subsequent amendments to these recommendations are mentioned later in this chapter.

CIOMS reports were, and still are, restricted to ADRs and not "events". This implies that a physician or other professional healthcare worker has judged it a reasonable possibility that the observed clinical occurrence was caused by the drug. In addition, it was emphasised that manufacturers should not select cases for reporting based on their own causality assessment. All spontaneous reports of serious unlabelled reactions made by a medical professional should be considered as CIOMS reports. Submission of such a report does not necessarily constitute acceptance of causality by the manufacturer.

As product labelling differs from country to country it was suggested that manufacturers should review all serious reports and then decide on a country-by-country basis, either centrally or at affiliate level, whether the reported ADR is labelled or not. It was also agreed that there should be a minimum of four pieces of information before a report is considered to have reached the standard threshold for reporting. These are an identifiable report source; a patient (even if not precisely identified by name and date of birth); a suspect drug; and a suspect reaction.

CIOMS reports should be submitted to regulatory authorities as soon as they are received and in no case later than 15 working days after receipt. The 15-day period begins as soon as a company, or any employee in any part or affiliate of a company, receives the report.

The CIOMS I report was published in 1990 (CIOMS, 1990).

INCORPORATION IN REGULATION

Many of the CIOMS I criteria for expedited reporting were incorporated into ICH E2A, *Clinical Safety Data Management: Definitions and Standards for Expedited Reporting*, which reached final agreement in October 1994 (ICH, 1994). This document expanded on the CIOMS I definitions and terminology. In particular, it introduced the concept of the "medical" seriousness category that recognised that events may not be immediately life threatening, or result in death or hospitalisation, but may jeopardise the patient or require intervention to prevent such outcomes. Although ICH E2A focused on pre-approval clinical trials, its definitions and other criteria have been applied by regulators to expedited reporting of both pre- and post-marketed products. The reporting time frame was reduced from 15 working days to 15 calendar days, with seven days for the initial report on fatal or life-threatening suspected adverse reaction cases from clinical trials.

the specifications for the standard units for laboratory data. Many of these definitions and recommendations were incorporated into the similar project initiated under ICH around the same time as CIOMS IA was active; the former reached final agreement in July 1997 as ICH E2B (ICH, 1977). The document was subsequently revised in November 2000 to clarify some of the issues raised during pilot feasibility studies and became ICH E2B (M) (ICH, 2000).

Although the single database envisioned by COMS IA does not exist, pilot studies of electronic expedited reporting are in progress in Europe, Japan and the United States.

CIOMS 1A—HARMONISATION OF DATA ELEMENTS AND FIELDS FOR ELECTRONIC REPORTING OF INDIVIDUAL ADRS

CIOMS IA was completed in 1995 but the final report was never formally published by CIOMS. The initiative was run in parallel with the CIOMS III working group but is presented here, out of chronological order, because it was an extension of the CIOMS I initiative.

The vision of CIOMS IA was for the more efficient and rational exchange of safety information by electronic rather than paper submission of expedited reports. Ideally, submission would be to a single shared database accessed by all regulatory authorities and with appropriately restricted access for manufacturers. This would enable the entry of individual cases only once by either a manufacturer or regulatory authority, facilitate the entry and speed of availability of follow-up information, ensure that everyone had access to the same data at the same time and reduce the administrative processes associated with hard copy reports. Increasing the efficiency of the process and standardisation of the data elements and fields would theoretically increase the time available for signal detection and evaluation activities.

CIOMS IA produced detailed definitions of the data structure required for both administrative and case details for electronic reporting of individual expedited ADRs. This even included

CIOMS II—PERIODIC SAFETY UPDATES

RATIONALE

This initiative was started in November 1989 at a time when several countries had requirements for periodic safety updates; however, individual local regulatory authorities were requesting that data (both foreign and domestic) be presented according to different inclusion criteria, formats and time intervals. Due dates were often determined by the national licensing approval date and therefore varied between individual formulations of the same drug substance. Preparation of these summarised safety updates had become a significant administrative burden for manufacturers. Figure 25.1 shows the report preparation schedule for a fictitious drug with different due dates and periods for review.

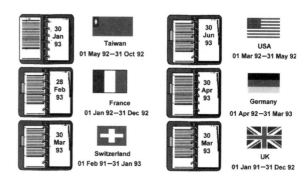

Figure 25.1. Report schedule for Qweasytrol.

The purpose of the CIOMS II working group was to explore the possibility of developing a harmonised approach to preparing periodic safety updates that would meet most existing needs and forestall any diversity in future requirements. It was also hoped that if the guidelines on this approach were adequate and reasonable other regulatory authorities would adopt them in the future. Standardisation would also enable pharmacovigilance staff to focus on reviewing the data rather than generating a battery of different reports.

PROCESS

The working group undertook a survey of the currently existing requirements for periodic safety updates, noting the diversity and identifying the questions which needed to be addressed in defining the content and format, and what might be considered to be the essential elements. After considerable debate and compromise on several controversial issues relating to scope and content, a series of proposals was then drafted in preparation for the pilot phase. Each manufacturer representative undertook to draft a single prototype summary-report on one of their own drugs using the proposed guidelines. Each report was then sent personally to each regulator in the working group and a "sanitised" version was sent to the other manufacturer representatives. All members of the working group took part in the critical evaluation of each pilot report to examine the feasibility (data availability), resources required in compilation and utility to the regulators of the information provided. On the basis of the experiences gained in the pilot study, the guidelines were refined and used to produce a model report on a fictitious drug (Qweasytrol) for inclusion in the final report.

RECOMMENDATIONS

The underlying principles of CIOMS II periodic safety updates were that they should be prepared to standard criteria that are practical and achievable, while containing sufficient information to reassure regulators that the data are regularly reviewed. They should be as brief as possible; it was recommended that the narrative content should not exceed about 10 pages. Data for all formulations of the same drug (including combination products) should be included in one report and the same report should be submitted at the same time to all regulatory authorities with a requirement for safety updates.

Scope

The proposal was that the guidelines should be applied to safety summaries produced for all new chemical entities licensed for the first time in 1992. Subsequent updates would be based on six-month interval data with cumulative data only included where it gave a perspective on safety issues. Each subject drug would have an international birth date (IBD), the first approval date for the first formulation of the drug anywhere in the world, that would determine the date at which six-monthly reports commenced. A data-lock point (DLP) six months after the IBD would be used to "freeze" the database. Normally, the manufacturer should make the report available within 45 calendar days of the DLP.

It should be emphasised that periodic safety summaries were not intended for the first communication of urgent safety information. This should be reported separately in the usual expedited manner.

Content

The working group proposed that the periodic safety update was presented in nine sections as follows:

1. Introduction
2. Core data sheet—the reference document for determining "expectedness"
3. The drug's licensed status
4. Update on regulatory or manufacturer actions taken for safety reasons
5. Patient exposure
6. Individual case histories (CIOMS line listing)
7. Studies
   — newly analysed studies containing important safety information

— targeted new safety studies
— published safety studies

8. Overall safety evaluation
9. Important information received after the DLP

It was proposed that the individual case histories received during the six-month period of review, and meeting specified criteria, should be presented in body system order of the most serious presenting sign or symptom, in a CIOMS line-listing format. The criteria for case inclusion were as follows:

● Unlabelled, serious attributable cases from studies (published or unpublished)
● All serious and non-serious unlabelled spontaneous reports (including relevant medically unconfirmed consumer reports)
● Serious published case histories
● Serious cases from other sources (e.g. from regulatory authorities)

The CIOMS line listing should consist of:

● Company reference number
● Country of origin of report
● Source of report (e.g. physician, literature)
● Age of patient
● Sex of patient
● Dose of drug
● Duration of treatment prior to event (time to onset)
● Description of reaction (as reported)
● Outcome

A comment column was also suggested for use by the manufacturer to highlight important case information such as concurrent medication or underlying disease. It could also be used for the causality assessments (imputability) required by the French regulatory authority.

The overall safety evaluation should be a concise critical analysis and opinion explicitly including:

● Increased frequency of known toxicity
● Drug interactions
● Overdose and its treatment

● Drug abuse
● Positive and negative experiences during pregnancy and lactation
● Effects of long-term treatment
● Any specific safety issues relating to the treatment of special patient groups (e.g. elderly, children)

Finally, the evaluation should indicate whether the interim safety data remained in line with the cumulative experience to date or whether any modifications were necessary to the company's core safety information.

The CIOMS II report was published in 1992 (CIOMS, 1992).

INCORPORATION IN REGULATIONS

The CIOMS II proposals for periodic safety updates were rapidly incorporated into the European Draft *Notice to Applicants* but with a few significant modifications, including the concept of a European rather than an international birth date. This effectively implied that periodic safety reports currently scheduled to the IBD had to be rescheduled to the first European approval date—a step away from the vision of harmonisation. A European schedule for the frequency of submission was also included which stated that six-monthly reports were required for the first two years after approval, followed by annual reports for three years and then five-yearly thereafter. As individual countries began to implement their own periodic safety update requirements they requested this schedule based on their own local approvals. The scope of CIOMS II was also expanded to include all marketed products, not just those approved in or after 1992.

Before the European requirements could be finalised, ICH E2C adopted many of the CIOMS II principles in the *Clinical Safety Data Management: Periodic Safety Update Reports for Marketed Drugs* document that reached Step 4 in November 1996 (ICH, 1996). This included further modifications to the CIOMS II scope and format, including some reordering of the sections and introduction of new materials such as the summary tabulations to complement the line listing in section 6. Figure 25.2 shows the ICH E2C table of contents and highlights the changes from CIOMS II. There was also an additional requirement to explain to local regulators any differences between the local product information and the company core safety information.

Fortunately, ICH E2C reverted to the IBD for scheduling reports and the time for submission after the DLP was increased to 60 days. However, while this may be achievable for six-monthly reports, there is concern because the ICH E2C format is now being requested for periodic safety updates covering longer periods (including the five-year reports for local product renewals in Europe).

Currently, ICH E2C has been implemented in Japan and included in Volume IX of the *Rules Governing Medicinal Products in the European Union—Notice to Marketing Authorisation Holders: Pharmacovigilance Guidelines*. It is expected that the US Food and Drug Administration (FDA) will soon be introducing periodic reporting requirements based on ICH E2C.

In summary, the principles and guidelines proposed by CIOMS II achieved a harmonised approach to preparing periodic safety updates that

1. Introduction

2.* World-wide Market Authorisation Status

3.* Update on RA or MAH actions for safety reasons

4. Changes to reference safety information (new)

5. Exposure data

6.* Individual case histories (summary tabulations)

7.* Studies

8.* Other information

9.* Overall safety evaluation

10. Conclusion

Appendices–including CCSI

* ICH E2C amendments to CIOMS II

Figure 25.2. ICH E2C—Table of contents.

met most existing requirements in 1992. However, they were unable to forestall the diversity of future requirements following their incorporation into regulatory requirements around the world.

CIOMS III—CORE CLINICAL-SAFETY INFORMATION

RATIONALE

CIOMS II introduced the concept of the core data sheet. It is a document prepared by the pharmaceutical manufacturer, containing the minimum essential safety information, such as ADRs, which the manufacturer stipulates should be listed in all countries where the drug is marketed (see Figure 25.3). It is also the reference document by which "labelled" and "unlabelled" (or listedness and unlistedness for ICH E2C) are determined. Thus, it should focus on the important information required for rational clinical decision making and harmonise safety statements world-wide for public health and regulatory purposes.

The CIOMS III working group set out to propose principles and guidelines for consistent decision-rules on the content of the Core Safety Information (CSI), standard terms and definitions, and a standard format. One of the major concerns was to minimise confusion among prescribers and other healthcare professionals due to inconsistencies between the safety information presented in different countries and by different manufacturers.

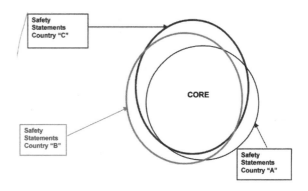

Figure 25.3. CIOMS III—The vision.

It was therefore hoped that regulatory authorities would harmonise their basic requirements for safety information in their local data sheets. However, the working group acknowledged the possible need for cultural differences due to medical and legal differences.

The first edition of the CIOMS III report published in 1995 (CIOMS, 1995) focused on CSI for marketed products, including the initial CSI that is prepared in conjunction with the first market authorisation submission, review and approval. During CIOMS V discussions it was proposed that the same basic philosophy and practices be applied to the safety information provided to clinical investigators during a development programme. The concept of development core safety information (DCSI) as a discrete, focused section of the Investigator's Brochures, which would have the same format as, and would evolve into, the CSI at initial marketing of the product, was therefore agreed. A second edition of the CIOMS III report was issued in 1999 (CIOMS, 1999) including the new proposals for Investigator's Brochures.

PROCESS

The task of the working group was to develop proposals for standard principles and guidelines addressing the what, when, how and where of CSI. The summary of product characteristics (SPC), the official document of the European Union, was used as a model to try to answer the following general questions:

- What evidence is needed, and how should it be used, to influence a decision on whether an adverse experience should be included, excluded or removed from the CSI?
- At what point in the accumulation and interpretation of information is the threshold crossed for inclusion or change in the CSI?
- What "good safety-labelling practices" can be specified concerning the clinical relevance of information, how it is expressed and the appropriateness of "class-labelling"?
- What should the sections of the CSI be called, how should they be defined and where should specific information be located?

At the beginning of the process the group hoped to develop specific threshold criteria, or an algorithm, for determining when information should be included in the CSI. However, this was not possible and it became necessary to rely on collective judgement to reach consensus. A series of case scenarios was created from real-life examples for which the decision to amend a data sheet was equivocal. Each member of the group was asked individually to make decisions on the available data. In addition, each person was asked to list the factors taken into consideration when reaching their conclusions. A total of 39 factors were identified and each member of the working group was asked to rank the factors in order of importance. As expected, there was a considerable divergence of opinion but overall the mostly highly ranked criterion for a positive decision was the presence of positive rechallenge information. The reader is referred to the original report for the remaining factors and their respective rankings.

RECOMMENDATIONS

The working group formulated a total of 65 proposals relating to general principles of good safety information and the what, when, how, where and who (responsibilities) for CSIs. A selection of the most useful principles is given below.

What?

- The CSI should be determined by the needs of healthcare professionals in the context of a regulatory and legal environment.
- Include what is practical and important to enable the prescriber to balance risks against benefit and to act accordingly.
- Avoid including events, especially minor events, that have no well-established relationship to therapy.
- There is a legal duty to warn but this must be balanced against the need to include only substantiated conclusions in the CSI.
- The CSI should include important information which physicians are not generally expected to know. (The converse is also true.)

When?

- As soon as relevant safety information becomes sufficiently well established it should be included in the CSI.

It was not possible to define this more precisely but the working group introduced the concept of "threshold". This is dependent on the quality of information available and the body and strength of the evidence according to the 39 criteria (plus two additional ones subsequently identified) in the ranking exercise described above. Situations in which the threshold should be lowered were identified. In general, information should be added sooner whenever it is likely to help the physician make a differential diagnosis related to an adverse event, spare extra tests, lead to the use of a specific targeted test or facilitate early recognition of an event. Similarly, the threshold should also be lowered if the ADR is medically serious or irreversible, if good alternative drugs are available, a relatively trivial condition is being treated, or the drug is being used for prophylaxis.

How?

- Keep ADRs identified in the initial CSI (premarketing experience) separate from those identified subsequently.
- ADRs should be listed by frequency in body system order.
- Whenever possible, an estimate of frequency should be provided, expressed in a standard category of frequency.

While the working group recognised that precise frequency rates can only be obtained from studies and are limited to the more common reactions, it was agreed that estimates of frequency in a standard format should be provided whenever possible. Although it is difficult to estimate incidence on the basis of spontaneous reports due to the uncertainties in estimating denominator and the degree of under-reporting, the group recommended the standard frequencies shown in Table 25.3.

Table 25.3. CIOMS III standard frequencies.

Incidence	Standard frequencies
Very common[a]	>1/10 (10%)
Common (frequent)	>1/100 and <1/10 (1%–10%)
Uncommon (infrequent)	>1/1000 and <1/100 (0.1%–1%)
Rare	>1/10 000 and <1/1000 (0.01%–0.1%)
Very rare[a]	<1/10 000 (<0.01%)

[a] Optional categories

Finally, the working group defined the safety sections of the CSI, providing guidance on the information which should be included in each section and outlined the responsibilities of the company for remaining diligent and pro-active, including undertaking the scientific investigation of signals. The shared responsibility of healthcare providers, patients, editors of medical journals and regulators is also addressed.

INCORPORATION IN REGULATION

Since the standards proposed by the CIOMS III working group would require continuous evaluation, updating and refinement, it was suggested that they be retained as guidelines and not adopted as regulations. They have been used as the basis of the European Labelling Guidelines and most regulatory authorities have adopted the standard categories of frequency.

CIOMS IV—BENEFIT–RISK EVALUATION

RATIONALE

CIOMS IV can be regarded as a logical progression from both CIOMS II and III. The aim of the working group was to develop guidance for regulators and manufacturers on assessing the balance between benefits and risks of marketed products with a newly established or suspected major safety problem. It would also provide guidance for deciding what options for action

should be considered and on the decision-making
process should such action be required. Pragmatic approaches to re-assessing the benefit–risk
relationship, producing a standard report and
good decision-making practices are highly desirable, but no standard existed. Although most
signals will not warrant formal benefit–risk
evaluation, it was recognised that any concepts
proposed by the working group would be useful
in any periodic or special evaluation of relative
benefits and risks.

PROCESS

In formulating its proposals the working group
developed, reviewed and made use of actual case
histories taken from the experience of companies
and regulators in several countries. These examples were used to illustrate basic principles and
methodologies as well as to suggest ways of
displaying data in connection with benefit estimation, risk estimation and benefit–risk evaluation.

Guidance on the decision-making process and
the use of outside experts was supported by
information from a survey of regulators and
companies in which details of recent significant
safety issues and the decision-making process were
requested.

RECOMMENDATIONS

The proposals are very different from the usual
case-specific ADR evaluations undertaken in
pharmacovigilance departments. Convention-
ally, these reports focus on the ADR of concern
and provide relevant details of pre-clinical,
clinical trial and post-marketing experience.
The benefit–risk assessment proposed by
CIOMS IV takes into account not only the new
signal but also the overall safety profile of the
product relative to that of an appropriate
comparator. It examines not only the benefits
and risks to the individual being treated but also
the net benefits across individuals being treated
or, as with the case of vaccines, the net benefit to
society.

The outline for the recommended standard
format and content of a benefit–risk evaluation
report is as follows.

Introduction

- Brief description of the drug and where marketed
- Indications for use, by country if there are
differences
- Alternative therapies, including surgery
- Very brief description of the major safety
problem

Benefit Evaluation

- Epidemiology and natural history of the target
disease(s)
- Purpose of treatment (e.g. cure, prophylaxis)
- Summary of efficacy and general toleration
data compared with other treatments or no
treatment

Note that benefit does not equate only with
clinical trial efficacy data. It also includes additional measures such as quality of life, compliance
with therapy, outcomes and experience in the "real
world".

Risk Evaluation

- Introduction
- Weight of evidence for the suspected risk
- Detailed presentations and analyses of data on
the new suspected risk
- Probable and possible explanations
- Preventability, predictability and reversibility of
the new risk
- The issue as it relates to alternative therapies
and no therapy
- Review of the complete safety profile of the
drug, using diagrammatic representations when
possible ("risk profiles"); when appropriate
focus on, for example, the three most common
and the three most medically serious ADRs
- Provide similar profiles for alternative drugs
- When possible, estimate the excess incidence of
any adverse reactions known to be common to
the alternatives

- When there are significant adverse reactions that are not common to the drugs compared, highlight important differences between the drugs

Benefit—Risk Evaluation

- Summarise the benefits as related to the seriousness of the target disease and the purpose and effectiveness of treatment
- Summarise the dominant risks (seriousness/severity, duration, incidence)
- Summarise the benefit–risk relationship, quantitatively and diagrammatically if possible, taking into account the alternative therapies or no treatment
- Provide a summary assessment and conclusion

Options Analysis

- List all appropriate options for action
- Describe the pros and cons and likely consequences (impact analysis) of each option under consideration, taking alternative therapies into account
- If relevant, outline plans or suggestions for a study that could provide timely and important additional information
- If feasible, indicate the quality and quantity of any future evidence which would signal the need for a re-evaluation of the benefit–risk relationship
- Suggest how the consequences of the recommended action should be monitored and assessed

It will be noted that the emphasis of the benefit–risk evaluation is on quantification wherever possible and an example of a report prepared to CIOMS IV specifications would have been useful. There are examples of previous benefit–risk evaluations that illustrate the various methodologies that have been used but they are not necessarily directly applicable to a manufacturer faced with a request for an urgent assessment. In particular, it would have been valuable to include some guidance on how to create summary metrics that combine benefit and risk data to allow straightforward quantitative comparisons of different treatment options. An example is given in terms of potential lives saved as the result of treatment versus potential lives lost as a result of adverse reactions. The CIOMS IV report calls for additional research and development of appropriate methodologies and metrics to introduce more science and less art to this important area.

While the logic behind the inclusion of most of these points is self-evident, it is recognised that obtaining the necessary information, especially on the risks and benefits of other manufacturers' new products as comparators, is either very difficult, or impossible, in practice. For older, but not new, products this information may be found in the literature (see dipyrone example).

The CIOMS IV report was published in 1998 (CIOMS, 1998). There has been no official regulatory uptake of the recommendations although it is known that at least one regulatory authority has requested a benefit–risk evaluation report from a manufacturer using this format.

CIOMS V—GOOD CASE MANAGEMENT AND REPORTING PRACTICES

RATIONALE

This is the most ambitious of the CIOMS initiatives to date. It addresses many of the new challenges faced in pharmacovigilance, such as the internet as a source of individual case reports, together with many of the older unresolved issues from previous CIOMS initiatives (e.g. reporting and labelling of deaths). The completed report is intended as a handbook for pharmacovigilance departments and offers many pragmatic solutions to a number of issues. The title, *Current Challenges in Pharmacovigilance: Pragmatic Approaches* (CIOMS, 2001) is, therefore, an apt one.

OVERVIEW

The report is divided into the following five main subject areas:

- Sources of individual case reports
- Good case management practices

- Good summary reporting practices: periodic safety update reports (PSURs) reconsidered
- Population exposure data
- World-wide clinical safety reporting regulations

It is not the intention to review the details of all the topics in this chapter but some of the recommendations and guidelines are of particular interest and will be highlighted for the reader.

Sources of Individual Case Reports

Consumer Reports

The value of consumer reports has always been a point of issue between Europe and North America. The CIOMS V consensus was that it is the quality of the report and not the quality of the reporter that is important. It was agreed that medical confirmation should be sought for consumer reports and that it is important to distinguish between verification (i.e. that the events as related by the consumer occurred) and confirmation of a suspected ADR (i.e. attribution). It may even be appropriate to submit a consumer report to the regulatory authorities as an expedited report when medical confirmation is not obtainable if the case might influence the benefit–risk relationship or has implications for labelling changes.

Literature

Companies should routinely search at least two internationally recognised databases for case reports not less frequently than monthly. The clock-start date for reporting is the date the reference was identified. If the paper is not in English it may be appropriate to translate the abstract or relevant sections only. Automated searches should be supplemented to include publications relevant to the drug or circumstances. That is, it is not adequate to search only for references specific to a particular drug (e.g. salbutamol) when class review may be appropriate (e.g. beta2 agonists). It was not considered necessary to monitor the lay media but if information is made available on a case, then attempts should be made to ascertain details.

Internet

It was not considered necessary to surf the internet beyond the company's own site(s) but it is advisable to screen the latter daily for ADR reports. There was also a suggestion that it may be useful to visit known sites from which patients may obtain information on specific drugs and diseases. There was some concern over the validity of case reports posted here, since the reporter may not always be identifiable. It was agreed that if the site is secure the company could encourage ADR reporting via its "home page". This could be used to advantage in gathering good quality data by ensuring that some fields were made mandatory for completion.

Solicited Reports

Patient support programmes are frequently being used by pharmaceutical companies to obtain follow-up data on product use (e.g. smoking cessation help lines). During the course of conversation the patient may mention the occurrence of an adverse event. It was agreed that the source of this report is neither truly spontaneous nor from a clinical trial. An additional case source, the solicited report, was proposed. It was suggested that these cases be collected and processed separately and that a company causality assessment is required before expedited reporting of serious solicited reports.

Disease-Specific Registries and Other Databases

As there are a large number of external databases it is unreasonable to expect companies to review them for ad hoc signals. However, they should be pro-actively monitored when there are known specific problems (i.e. when there is a hypothesis). As databases are used to generate signals there is no need to report individual cases on an expedited basis. However, if an increased frequency of a serious ADR was determined in an epidemiology study it may be appropriate to notify the regulatory authority. Since individual case report forms are not always appropriate, CIOMS V introduced the concept of a "15-day letter of prompt notification".

Good Case Management Practices

Clinical Evaluation

This is important for determining any further action required to characterise a case, in particular to establish the accuracy of the diagnosis and appropriate coding. It also enables the case to be suitably prioritised for follow-up and/or expedited reporting. It was recognised that many companies are coding every event of which they become aware, even if not causally related to the drug. The concept of an "incidental event" was introduced. This is an event which, although it occurs in reasonable temporal association with the use of a drug, is not the intended subject of a spontaneous report and there is no implicit or explicit expression of possible drug causality by the reporter or the company. Cases in which only the incidental events are serious should not be submitted as expedited reports.

Seriousness

CIOMS V recommended the universal adoption of the ICH E2A definition of seriousness, including medically important events. For consistency it was suggested that all companies maintain a list of terms which should always be considered serious. However, it was recognised that this could never be fully comprehensive and that it does not replace medical judgement.

Cases with a fatal outcome are only serious when the ADR is a direct or indirect cause of death.

Expectedness

Events are only expected when they are included in the ADR section of the reference safety information (RSI). If they differ in nature, severity, specificity or outcome, then they are unexpected. Class labelling and statements such as "relationship not established" or "observed with similar frequency to placebo" do not imply expectedness.

Principles of Reporting Deaths

This was perhaps the most contentious of all the discussions. Some regulators considered that they needed to know about all reports of deaths, while manufacturers generally maintained that they would be swamped with reports, especially for drugs used in serious medical conditions. It was upheld that cases with a fatal outcome were only serious when the drug caused or contributed to death but there was general disagreement about whether this could always be determined from individual case details, or implied if the case was a spontaneous report. Further discussion centred on whether death was considered expected or unexpected if it was not specifically mentioned in the label (e.g. "anaphylaxis" versus "anaphylaxis, sometimes fatal"). It was agreed that physicians should be aware of medical conditions frequently associated with a fatal outcome and therefore the working group decided actively to discourage indiscriminate labelling of deaths. The final outcome of this discussion was to recommend that fatal reports should be expedited until labelled and that all reports with a fatal outcome should undergo special medical review.

Follow-up

Guidance is given on prioritising cases for follow-up, the highest priority being given to all serious cases; unexpected cases; special interest cases and those which are uninterpretable in order to seek clarification. As always, the topic of whether cases should be followed to resolution was raised as there was concern that a non-serious rash, for example, may become Stevens–Johnson Syndrome. It was suggested that when a letter of acknowledgement was sent, as is good practice, the reporter should be asked to notify the company if any further information becomes available on the case.

Good Summary Reporting Practices: PSURs

Whilst agreeing that the full ICH E2C format PSUR should be produced every six months for most drugs, the working group recognised that this presents a number of practical difficulties in terms of format and content. At one extreme, there are high volume reports that may contain thousands of ADR case reports or an unmanageable volume of publications. At the other extreme, there are older drugs with a well-established profile for which there is little or no new information to report. Modifications to PSUR content are proposed for the former high volume reports and recommendations for simplifying reports, with an example, are given for the latter. It is emphasised that the working group is not suggesting new format reports but simply offering pragmatic suggestions for adapting the ICH E2C content and format in certain circumstances.

One of the greatest dilemmas in producing PSURs is fulfilling the different frequency and periodicity requirements for different regulatory authorities in different countries. For example, in Europe, the schedule for submission changes to annual after two years and then five-yearly after the first renewal. Under ICH E2C provisions, regulators who do not wish to receive six-monthly reports are expected to accept two six-monthly reports as an annual report or the appropriate series of reports as a five-year report. The working group therefore proposed the use of the *summary bridging report* to facilitate the review of a series of reports. The summary bridging report is a concise document integrating the information presented in two or more PSURs that is submitted to a regulatory authority to cover a specified period over which a single report is required. An example is presented in the final report.

The concept and use of the IBD for PSURs have not been fully accepted by all regulators. Some require that PSURs are scheduled according to the local approval date and, in addition, not all companies will have synchronised their renewal dates by bringing them forward to the IBD in those countries where this is permissible. To avoid producing additional reports for those countries perceiving that any report with a DLP more than 60 days before submission is out of date, the working group recommended the use of an *addendum report*. This is an update to the most recently completed scheduled PSUR when a regulatory authority (or the company) requires a

safety update outside the usual reporting cycle, and more than a brief amount of time has elapsed since the most recent PSUR. The working group proposed the minimum information for inclusion in the addendum report.

Finally, other issues of practical importance in managing the preparation of PSURs that are not directly related to format and frequency are discussed. Many of these topics were issues raised in a survey undertaken by the working group to identify the current PSUR burden to industry.

WORLD-WIDE CLINICAL SAFETY REPORTING REGULATIONS

This chapter summarises the diversity of current regulatory reporting requirements, pre- and post-marketing, for expedited and periodic safety update reporting, many of which purport to be based on existing harmonisation initiatives. It is hoped that the plea for improved harmonisation will be heeded.

The CIOMS V report was published during the second quarter of 2001 (CIOMS, 2001). It is of note that in February 2002 the ICH Steering Committee agreed to launch two new topics: the development of a further guidance on PSURs which will be an addendum to the existing E2C guideline, and a guidance on Good Case Management Practices which will be a follow-up of the E2A guideline. Both will consider the CIOMS V recommendations for incorporation and are expected to reach Step 2 in September 2002.

CIOMS VI—THE FUTURE

The first five CIOMS initiatives focused primarily on post-marketing safety surveillance. In contrast, the sixth CIOMS working group is currently addressing the collection, monitoring, assessment and reporting of safety data during clinical trials. Their recommendations on such issues as blinding versus unblinding and communications with investigators, ethics committees, and data/safety management boards are awaited with interest. Progress on this topic can be monitored on the new CIOMS web site (www.cioms.ch).

CONCLUSION

From the scope of work presented in this chapter it is very evident that the CIOMS working groups have made significant contributions to present-day pharmacovigilance practice, especially in their attempts towards achieving harmonisation. They have frequently focused on areas for simplification, clarification and harmonisation of practices on topics that are rarely or never addressed by regulations or guidelines. Much of the success of the working groups was due to the realisation of the vision of Zbigniew Bankowski, the Secretary General of CIOMS until his retirement at the end of 1999. This vision was that problems could best be solved by small working groups of constructive individuals gathered together to represent different aspects of a shared problem in an unofficial environment.

The work of safety surveillance and public health protection is never completed because regulations and requirements are constantly changing. Innovations and improvements will always be needed and, with finite pharmacovigilance resources in both industry and regulatory authorities, we must all do our outmost to maintain the vision that pharmacovigilance is about promoting public health and not bureaucracy.

REFERENCES

CIOMS (1990) *International Reporting of Adverse Drug Reactions: Final Report of CIOMS Working Group*. Geneva: Council for International Organisations of Medical Sciences.

CIOMS (1992) *International Reporting of Periodic Drug-Safety Update Summaries: Final Report of CIOMS Working Group II*. Geneva: Council for International Organisations of Medical Sciences.

CIOMS (1995) *Guidelines for Preparing Core Clinical-Safety Information on Drugs: Report of CIOMS Working Group III*. Geneva: Council for International Organisations of Medical Sciences.

CIOMS (1998) *Benefit–Risk Balance for Marketed Drugs: Evaluating Safety Signals: Report of CIOMS Working Group IV*. Geneva: Council for International Organisations of Medical Sciences.

CIOMS (1999) *Guidelines for Preparing Core Clinical-Safety Information on Drugs*, 2nd edn. *Report of CIOMS Working Groups III and V*. Geneva: Council for International Organisations of Medical Sciences.

CIOMS (2001) *Current Challenges in Pharmacovigilance: Pragmatic Approaches: Report of CIOMS Working Group V*. Geneva: Council for International Organisations of Medical Sciences.

ICH (1994) *E2A: Clinical Safety Data Management: Definitions and Standards for Expedited Reporting* (Step 4; October)

ICH (1997) *E2B: Clinical Safety Data Management: Data Elements for Transmission of ADR Reports* (Step 4; July)

ICH (2000) *E2B (M): Maintenance of the ICH Guideline on Clinical Safety Data Management Including the Maintenance of the Electronic Transmission of Individual Case Safety Reports Message Specification* (ICH ICSR DTD Version 2.1) (Step 4; July 1997, amended November).

ICH (1996) *E2C: Clinical Safety Data Management: Periodic Safety Update Reports for Marketed Drugs* (Step 4; November).

A guideline on the summary of product characteristics (1999) In: *The Rules Governing Medicinal Products in the European Union*, Vol. 2A, and *The Notice to Applicants*, Vol. 2B. December.

Notice to Marketing Authorisation Holders: Pharmacovigilance Guidelines (January 1999).

26

PEM in the UK

SAAD A.W. SHAKIR

Drug Safety Research Unit, Southampton, UK

BACKGROUND

As early as 1965, L.J. Witts wrote that "the final test of the safety of a drug is in fact its release for general use". The recognition that not all hazards could be known before a drug was marketed and that spontaneous adverse drug reaction reporting systems may fail to identify all hazards, led to several proposals for schemes based on the identification of patients by means of prescription data. These schemes were largely intended to provide information on populations of known size so that the incidence of adverse reactions could be estimated with reasonable accuracy. The proposals included "Recorded Release", Registered Release", "Retrospective Assessment of Drug Safety" and a number of variants (Inman, 1978a).

One of the limitations of spontaneous reporting is that doctors may fail to identify and report illnesses which they do not suspect to be due to a drug. This realisation led to the development of systems based upon "event" reporting in which the doctor did not need to diagnose or suspect the true cause but was asked merely to record events. To this thinking the distinguished statistician, D.J. Finney, made a fundamental contribution in a paper in 1965 in which an event was defined as "a particular untoward happening experienced by a patient, undesirable either generally or in the context of his disease" (Finney, 1965).

These ideas—published only four years after the original announcements of Lenz regarding thalidomide and congenital abnormalities (Lenz, 1961, 1962)—came together in the founding by W.H.W. Inman of prescription–event monitoring (PEM). The establishment of PEM at the University of Southampton in 1980 and Inman's early experience with this technique have been recorded in publications (Inman, 1981, 1981b; Inman et al., 1981) which established that the key objective was to recruit the first 10 000 patients who received a new drug of interest so that any adverse event that occurred in more than one in 1000 patients would be reliably identified.

METHOD

PEM is a non-interventional, observational cohort form of post-marketing surveillance. It is non-interventional because nothing happens to interfere with the doctor's decision regarding which drug to prescribe for each individual patient. Thus, the method provides "real-world" clinical data involving neither inclusion nor exclusion criteria: the patients studied are those who receive the drug

Pharmacovigilance. Edited by R.D. Mann and E.B. Andrews
© 2002 John Wiley & Sons, Ltd

in everyday medical practice. This ensures that the data are generalisable.

In the United Kingdom virtually all persons are registered with a general practitioner (GP) who provides primary health care and issues prescriptions (FP10s) for the medicines medically necessary. The patient takes the prescription to a pharmacist who dispenses the medication and then sends the FP10 to a central Prescription Pricing Authority (PPA) which arranges the pharmacist's reimbursement. The Drug Safety Research Unit (DSRU) is, by virtue of a long-standing and confidential arrangement, provided with electronic copies of all those prescriptions issued nationally for the drugs being monitored by PEM. These arrangements continue for a collection period which allows exposure data to be collected for 20 000–30 000 patients. For each of these patients the DSRU prepares a computerised longitudinal record comprising, in date order, all of the prescriptions for the monitored drug. Thus, in PEM, the exposure data are national in scope throughout the collection period and unaffected by the kind of selection and exclusion criteria that characterise clinical trials. The exposure data are of drugs dispensed and provided to the patient but there is no method of measuring compliance or the use of non-prescription medication.

After an interval of 3–12 (usually 6) months from the first prescription for each individual patient the DSRU sends to the prescriber a "green form" questionnaire seeking information on any events that may have occurred since the drug was first prescribed. An event is defined as any new diagnosis, any reason for referral to a consultant or admission to hospital, any unexplained deterioration (or improvement) in a concurrent illness, any suspected drug reaction, any alteration of clinical importance in laboratory values, or any other complaint which was considered of sufficient importance to enter in the patient's notes.

Information which identifies the patient is deleted from the database when the green form is received from the doctor. The doctor enters any number or code used in the practice to identify the patient. This ensures that the clinical information received by the DSRU is anonymised. The practice code or number is used if follow-up information is sought from the doctor. In order to avoid placing an unreasonable demand on GPs no more than four green forms are sent to each doctor in any one month. The green form is illustrated in Figure 26.1, which shows the other information requested of the doctor.

The green form has been modified for certain studies with a small number of additional questions (with yes, no, don't know answers). These questions focus on issues specific to the drug under study, for example the green form for the PEM study on the NSAID meloxicam included questions about previous history of gastrointestinal conditions and intolerance to NSAIDs to identify possible confounding by indication.

GPs are not paid to fill in green forms. The arrangements allow good contact between the doctor and the DSRU and this facilitates the collection of any follow-up data that may be considered necessary by the research physicians monitoring each study and working within the DSRU. One of the strengths of PEM is follow-up with the GP or the health service to obtain further information from the doctor for a large number of reports. A list of reports for which additional information is sought is included in Table 26.1.

Over the 78 studies listed in Table 26.2, an average of 58% of the green forms sent out have been returned by the GPs to the DSRU. The cohort sizes, with an average of 10 613 patients, as

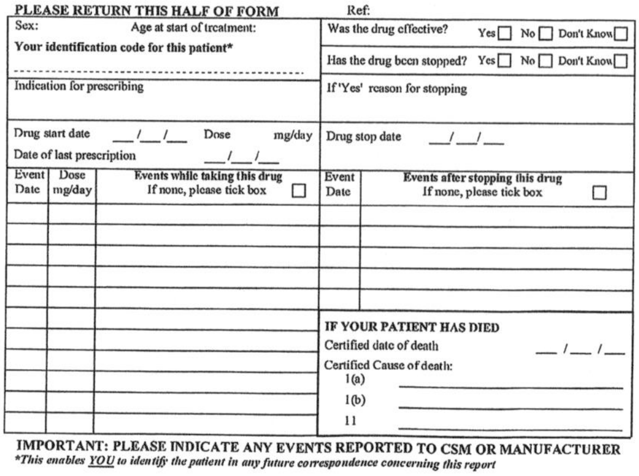

PLEASE RETURN THIS HALF OF FORM   Ref:

Sex: Age at start of treatment:
Your identification code for this patient*

Was the drug effective? Yes ☐ No ☐ Don't Know ☐
Has the drug been stopped? Yes ☐ No ☐ Don't Know ☐

Indication for prescribing
If 'Yes' reason for stopping

Drug start date __/__/__ Dose mg/day
Date of last prescription __/__/__
Drug stop date __/__/__

Event Date	Dose mg/day	Events while taking this drug If none, please tick box ☐	Event Date	Events after stopping this drug If none, please tick box ☐

IF YOUR PATIENT HAS DIED
Certified date of death __/__/__
Certified Cause of death:
1(a)
1(b)
11

IMPORTANT: PLEASE INDICATE ANY EVENTS REPORTED TO CSM OR MANUFACTURER
This enables YOU to identify the patient in any future correspondence concerning this report

Figure 26.1 Green form.

Table 26.1. Reports for which additional information is sought.

- Medically important adverse events reported during pre-marketing development
- Medically important events reported during post-marketing in other countries (for products launched elsewhere before the UK)
- Events considered to be possibly associated with the product during the PEM
- All pregnancies
- Any deaths for which the cause is not known or which may be related to the medication
- Reports of overdose and suicide

given in Table 26.2, are derived from the mean 52% of returned green forms which provide clinically useful data.

PEM collects event data and does not ask the doctor to determine if any particular event is due to an adverse drug reaction (ADR). If, however, the doctor does consider the event to be an ADR or he has completed a yellow card (a spontaneous ADR report) regarding the event, then he is asked to indicate this on the green form.

Further details of the methodology of PEM, including the methods of data coding, computerisation, and analysis, have been provided in a number of publications (Inman, 1978b; Freemantle *et al.*, 1997; Mann *et al.*, 1997).

Table 26.2. List of 78 completed studies.

	Generic name	Drug name	Group	% returned	Cohort
1	Cisapride	PREPULSID	Antispasmodic	62.4%	13 234
2	Femotidine	PEPCID	H$_2$-antagonist	51.8%	9500
3	Nizatidine	AXID	H$_2$-antagonist	44.7%	7782
4	Misoprostol	CYTOTEC	Prostaglandin analogue	67.3%	13 775
5	Lansoprazole	ZOTON	Proton pump inhibitor	51.0%	17 329
6	Omeprazole	LOSEC	Proton pump inhibitor	62.4%	16 204
7	Pantoprazole	PROTIUM	Proton pump inhibitor	44.5%	11 541
8	Betaxolol	KERLONE	Beta-blocker	54.7%	1531
9	Doxazosin	CARDURA	Alpha-blocker	60.1%	8482
10	Enalapril	INNOVACE	ACE-inhibitor	68.3%	15 361
11	Lisinopril	ZESTRIL + CARACE	ACE-inhibitor	63.5%	12 438
12	Perindopril	COVERSYL	ACE-inhibitor	53.4%	9089
13	Ramipril	TRITACE	ACE-inhibitor	47.3%	1371
14	Irbesartan	APROVEL	Antihypertensive	59.4%	14 397
15	Losartan	COZAAR	Antihypertensive	59.9%	14 522
16	Valsartan	DIOVAN	Antihypertensive	54.7%	12 881
17	Amlodipine	ISTIN	Ca-antagonist	58.7%	12 969
18	Diltiazem	TILDIEM	Ca-antagonist	67.3%	10 112
19	Isradipine	PRESCAL	Ca-antagonist	51.3%	3679
20	Mibefradil	POSICOR	Ca-antagonist	54.1%	3085
21	Nicardipine	CARDENE	Ca-antagonist	62.6%	10 910
22	Nicorandil	IKOREL	K-channel activator	58.3%	13 620
23	Xamoterol	CORWIN	Inotropic	68.7%	5373
24	Fluvastatin	LESCOL	Lipid-lowering	63.2%	7542
25	Bambuterol	BAMBEC	Beta$_2$ agonist	50.8%	8098
26	Eformoterol	FORADIL	Beta$_2$ agonist	52.9%	5777
27	Salmeterol	SEREVENT	Beta$_2$ agonist	61.9%	15 407
28	Nedocromil	TILADE	Asthma prophylaxis	68.1%	12 294
29	Montelukast	SINGULAIR	Leukotriene antagonist	53.6%	15 612

(continued)

Table 26.2. *Continued.*

	Generic name	Drug name	Group	% returned	Cohort
30	Acrivastine	SEMPREX	Antihistamine	56.5%	7863
31	Cetirizine	ZIRTEK	Antihistamine	57.4%	9554
32	Fexofenadine	TELFAST	Antihistamine	50.9%	16 638
33	Loratadine	CLARITYN	Antihistamine	50.7%	9308
34	Zolpidem	STILNOCT	Hypnotic	49.0%	13 460
35	Zopiclone	ZIMOVANE	Hypnotic	54.8%	11 543
36	Buspirone	BUSPAR	Anxiolytic	54.1%	11 113
37	Olanzapine	ZYPREXA	Antipsychotic	68.9%	8858
38	Quetiapine	SEROQUEL	Antipsychotic	58.9%	1725
39	Risperidone	RISPERDAL	Antipsychotic	64.7%	7684
40	Sertindole	SERDOLECT	Antipsychotic	78.2%	436
41	Moclobemide	MANERIX	MAOI	58.8%	10 835
42	Fluoxetine	PROZAC	SSRI	58.4%	12 692
43	Fluvoxamine	FAVERIN	SSRI	59.9%	10 983
44	Paroxetine	SEROXAT	SSRI	61.6%	13 741
45	Sertraline	LUSTRAL	SSRI	60.2%	12 734
46	Mirtazapine	ZISPIN	Antidepressant	56.0%	13 554
47	Nefazodone	DUTONIN	Antidepressant	54.9%	11 834
48	Venlafaxine	EFEXOR	Antidepressant	54.6%	12 642
49	Tramadol	ZYDOL	Analgesic	55.8%	10 532
50	Sumatriptan	IMIGRAN	Antimigraine	70.8%	14 928
51	Lamotrigine	LAMICTAL	Anti-epileptic	67.9%	11 316
52	Vigabatrin	SABRIL	Anti-epileptic	69.2%	10 178
53	Gabapentin	NEURONTIN	Anti-epileptic	66.4%	3100
54	Donepezil	ARICEPT	Alzheimer's treatment	58.9%	1762
55	Cefixime	SUPRAX	Cephalosporin	39.6%	11 250
56	Azithromycin	ZITHROMAX	Macrolide	52.4%	11 275
57	Ciprofloxacin	CIPROXIN	Quinolone	60.0%	11 477
58	Enoxacin	COMPRECIN	Quinolone	44.5%	2790
59	Norfloxacin	UTINOR	Quinolone	50.0%	11 110
60	Ofloxacin	TARIVID	Quinolone	45.7%	11 033
61	Fosfomycin	MONURIL	Antibacterial	45.6%	3363
62	Fluconazole	DIFLUCAN	Antifungal	68.6%	15 015
63	Itraconazole	SPORANOX	Antifungal	63.5%	13 645
64	Aciclovir	ZOVIRAX	Antiviral	74.1%	11 051
65	Famciclovir	FAMVIR	Antiviral	65.4%	14 169
66	Valaciclovir	VALTREX	Antiviral	64.1%	12 804
67	Acarbose	GLUCOBAY	Antidiabetic	62.8%	13 655
68	Troglitazone	ROMOZIN	Antidiabetic	60.3%	1344
69	Finasteride	PROSCAR	Prostate treatment	63.0%	14 772
70	Alendronate	FOSAMAX	Biphosphonate	59.4%	11 916
71	Tamsulosin	FLOMAX MR	Alpha-blocker	57.4%	12 484
72	Terodiline	TEROLIN	Anticholinergic	69.6%	12 444
73	Tolterodine	DETRUSITOL	Anticholinergic	59.0%	14 526
74	Etodolac	LODINE	NSAID	49.9%	9091
75	Meloxicam	MOBIC	NSAID	52.0%	19 087
76	Nabumetone	RELIFEX	NSAID	54.9%	10 444
77	Rofecoxib	VIOXX	NSAID	38.9%	15 268
78	Tenoxicam	MOBIFLEX	NSAID	44.5%	10 882
			Mean response rate	57.9%	10 613

Each PEM study starts as soon as possible after the new drug has been marketed in England. Each study aims to collect exposure and outcome data on approximately 10 000 patients. Some studies have included almost double that number and attempts are now being made, when PEM is an ideal method for studying the early experience with an important new drug, to maximise the size of the cohort. The drugs included in the system are (as advocated by the Second Grahame–Smith Working Party of the Committee on Safety of Medicines) those intended for widespread, long-term use, special emphasis being given to drugs for which treatment is likely to be both initiated and continued by the GP (Secretary of State, 1986; BMA, 1996). In addition to drugs that are taken

regularly, also it has been possible to study products that are not used daily, such as sildenafil for erectile dysfunction (Shakir *et al.*, 2001).

In summary, the exposure data in PEM are derived from the prescriptions written by GPs attending the individual patients; the outcome data are derived from the green forms completed by those same GPs.

Within the DSRU each green form questionnaire is scanned into the system and the image is reviewed by a medical member of the DSRU staff so that important events can be investigated. In addition to important events (Table 26.1), pregnancies and deaths of uncertain cause are further investigated by the DSRU Research Fellows who can, with the permission of the GP, access the patient's life-time medical records, death certificates etc.

Interim reports are written to summarise the data on each study with every 2500 patients entered to the database. These reports include a listing, by month since the beginning of treatment, of all events reported. They are, if possible, discussed with the Product Licence holder so that reporting obligations to the regulatory bodies can be fulfilled. Wherever possible PEM is undertaken in a collaborative but always independent relationship with the drug originator. The methodology of PEM is summarised in Figure 26.2

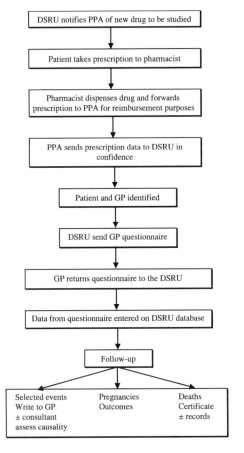

Figure 26.2. Prescription event monitoring in England, DSRU = the Drug Safety Research Unit; PPA = Prescription Pricing Authority.

RESULTS

Data analysis in PEM utilises several approaches which combine the application of epidemiological methods with medical evaluation.

INCIDENCE DENSITIES

Since most adverse drug reactions are the so-called "type A" reactions, which are caused by the pharmacological effects of the product, and commonly occur within a short period after exposure, comparing the rates of events occurring soon after exposure with subsequent periods provides a useful means to generate possible drug safety signals.

PEM provides a numerator (the number of reports) and a denominator (the number of patient-months or patient-weeks of exposure), both collected within a known time frame (the difference, for each patient, between the start and stop dates of the drug being monitored).

The incidence density (ID) for a given time period, t, for each of the event terms in the DSRU dictionary is calculated as follows:

$$ID_t \frac{\text{number of events during treatment for period } t}{\text{number of patient-months (weeks) of treatment for period } t} \times 1000.$$

The IDs per 1000 patient-months (or patient-weeks) of treatment are then ranked to give estimates of the "real-world" frequency of reported events.

While events with higher incidence densities in the period after exposure compared with subsequent periods are considered safety signals for the product under study, such events may be due to the effects of a product taken before the drug under study was started. For example, cough occurring soon after starting an angiotensin-II (A-II) receptor antagonist (e.g. losartan) may have been caused by an angiotensin converting enzyme inhibitor taken before starting the A-II antagonist.

REASONS FOR STOPPING

The green form asks the doctor to specify the "Reason for stopping" the drug being monitored if treatment was stopped. Thus, the ranked "Reasons for stopping" (in terms of the number of reports of each event) is another source for generating signals and can be compared with the ranked IDs for the first month of therapy in each individual patient. As examples, data for the most frequently reported events with the two anti-epileptic drugs, lamotrigine and vigabatrin, are given in Table 26.3.

In general, there appears to be a high degree of correlation between these two sets of values. These values can be used to compare drugs within one therapeutic class: for example with anti-epileptic drugs it shows that rash is the most frequently reported event likely to be a drug side effect with lamotrigine, whereas rash is far less common with vigabatrin; similarly, respiratory tract infection (which occurs month in and month out in all cohorts and which is, with many drugs, unlikely to be related to either the drug or disease being treated) is fairly common among the ID values but

Table 26.3. Most frequently reported events during first month of treatment with the two anti-epileptic drugs, lamotrigine and vigabatrin.

Rank	Lamotrigine Cohort: 11 316 Event	Number	Vigabatrin Cohort: 10 178 Event	Number
1	Convulsion, epilepsy	217	Convulsion, epilepsy	118
2	Rash	212	Drowsiness, sedation	116
3	Respiratory tract infection	110	Respiratory tract infection	116
4	Nausea, vomiting	94	Nausea, vomiting	49
5	Headache, migraine	82	Headache, migraine	44
6	Drowsiness, sedation	68	Malaise, lassitude	36
7	Malaise, lassitude	61	Dizziness	35
8	Dizziness	51	Visual defect	28
9	Visual defect	35	Aggression	25
10	Cough	25	Confusion	25
11	Pain, abdomen	24	Depression	19
12	Injury	11	Behaviour abnormal	18

virtually never appears among the common reasons for drug withdrawal.

GENERATION AND EXPLORATION OF SIGNALS

Signals are generated by an event having an unusually high ID or ranking in the list of "Reasons for stopping" the drug being monitored or being considered medically important by the Research Fellow. While comparisons of incidence densities nearly always utilise the differences between the incidence density in the first month and subsequent months, it has been possible to use the difference between incidence densities in month 6 with months 1–5 in a 6-month study to generate signals for delayed adverse reactions such as gynaecomastia with finasteride (Wilton *et al.*, 1996), a product used for benign prostatic hypertrophy.

Many signals have been generated in PEM, examples include visual field defects in patients taking vigabatrin (Wilton *et al.*, 1999), gastrointestinal intolerance due to acarbose (Mackay *et al.*, 1997a), oesophageal reactions with alendronate (Mackay *et al.*, 1997b), aggression, agitation and abnormal dreams with donepezil (Dunn *et al.*, 2000), diarrhoea in the elderly with lansoprazole (Martin *et al.*, 2000), and serotonin syndrome with antidepressants (Mackay *et al.*, 1999).

FOLLOW-UP OF IMPORTANT EVENTS

Analysis and evaluation of pharmacoepidemiological data should include medical assessment, both to improve the understanding of signals raised by epidemiological techniques and to raise (and evaluate) new signals or hypotheses by using medical judgement with appropriate systems for causal inference.

Medical evaluation of individual case reports and clusters of reports is an important part of PEM. Important safety signals have been generated in this way. In the PEM study of the antiepileptic drug vigabatrin, following published case reports of visual field defects associated with the use of the product, four cases of visual field defects were identified initially in the PEM cohort. In view of the importance of the signal, 7228 patients who were reported to be taking the product by the end of the study were followed up by sending a simple questionnaire to the GP to ask whether any serious adverse events or changes in vision had been reported since the initial green form had been returned. In addition, if the patient has been seen by an ophthalmologist for visual problems, the ophthalmologist was asked to complete a questionnaire giving details of visual field testing before and during treatment with vigabatrin. The follow-up information revealed an additional 29 cases of visual field defects which were considered by the ophthalmologist to be probably or possibly related to vigabatrin, giving an incidence of risk of 7.00 per 1000 patients (Wilton *et al.*, 1999). The follow-up exercise in the PEM study of vigabatrin contributed to the understanding of this important adverse reaction and provided a method to compute the reported rate of the adverse reaction in real clinical use which was not possible with spontaneous reporting or in clinical trials.

THE OUTCOME OF EXPOSED PREGNANCIES

All pregnancies reported during PEM studies are followed up by the medical and scientific staff of the DSRU in order to determine the outcome in those babies exposed during pregnancy to the drugs being monitored.

A review (Wilton *et al.*, 1997) showed that 2508 pregnancies have been followed up in 34 PEM studies. The study drug was known to have been dispensed during 904 of these pregnancies (839 during the first trimester and 65 during the second/third trimesters). The first trimester pregnancies produced 553 live births among which 20 (3.6%) abnormalities were reported. The findings are little different from the proportion of abnormalities reported in the general population in the United Kingdom. Thus, these observational data may be of value to those who need to advise pregnant women exposed to newly marketed medicines. The pregnancy database of PEM is expanding. Moreover, the DSRU currently is analysing the pregnancy exposure data with the application of comparative statistical methods between products in the PEM database or with external data, e.g. national statistics of congenital abnormalities, and the results will be published in due course.

LONG LATENCY ADVERSE REACTIONS

Delayed reactions can be investigated by sending out further green forms relating to those patients shown in the initial PEM survey to be receiving long-term medication. One such study has provided reassuring data on the safety of long-term use of lamotrigine in epilepsy (MacKay *et al.*, 1997).

COMPARING DRUGS IN THE SAME THERAPEUTIC CLASS

The size of the PEM database (78 completed studies with a total of one million patients) and advances in information technology are providing increasing opportunities to compare the safety profiles of products in the same therapeutic class. In the last few years many comparative studies (Table 26.4) have been conducted using PEM data which contributed to the understanding of the safety of many products.

Comparisons in PEM have included the application of nested case–control methodology (Dunn *et al.*, 1999). Nested case–control design appears

Table 26.4. Comparative studies using the PEM data.

1. The safety profiles of antibiotics, ciprofloxacin, norfloxacin, ofloxacin, azithromycin and cefixime
2. Calcium channel blockers and other cardiovascular agents and the prevalence of depression
3. The tolerability of newer antidepressants, fluoxetine, sertraline, paroxetine, moclobemide, venlafaxine and nefazodone
4. The rates of sedation with four new "non-sedating" antihistamines, loratadine, fexofenadine, cetirizine and acrivastine
5. The rates of common adverse events with three proton pump inhibitors, omeprazole, lansoprazole and pantoprazole

to have useful applications to PEM and will be applied increasingly in the future. Another method that is currently being developed for signal generation in PEM is the routine application of comparative reporting rates for reported events in PEM.

INVESTIGATION OF SAFETY SIGNALS FROM OTHER SOURCES

The DSRU monitors the literature and the worldwide web for important drug safety signals generated elsewhere, particularly those that cause public health or regulatory concerns. The Unit also receives requests from regulatory authorities and manufacturers to investigate drug safety signals in the PEM database. Whenever possible the DSRU conducts retrospective analyses (which usually include follow up of reports for the drug in question and comparator drugs). Such analyses contribute to the debates on these signals and to regulatory and public health decisions.

One example is the study on sertindole (Wilton *et al.*, 2001). Sertindole is an atypical antipsychotic known to be associated with prolongation of the QTc interval. The product was withdrawn from markets in the European Union following reports of sudden death and serious cardiac arrhythmias. The comparative analyses of the PEM studies of sertindole and two other atypical antipsychotics, risperidone and olanzapine, studied cardiovascular events, deaths from cardiovascular events as well as deaths from other causes such as suicide. The report of the comparative analysis was considered to be a very important source of information for the regulatory decision on the matter.

Another example of a retrospective analysis of a PEM study is the analysis conducted on the association between selective serotonin re-uptake inhibitors (SSRIs) and bleeding, which showed a possible weak association (Layton *et al.*, 2001).

While such comparisons produce valuable additions to the understanding of the safety of medicines, it is important to emphasise that comparisons of independent cohorts are subject to bias and confounding, which must be taken into consideration in the analysis and evaluation process. However, the paucity of post-marketing safety studies in large populations makes the information provided by these comparative studies very useful. Real benefit can only be achieved when not only the limitations of any post-marketing safety study are taken into consideration but when its results are considered in relation to other studies that had been conducted on the same product.

COMPARISON WITH NATIONAL DATA

Where appropriate, comparisons are made between event rates in PEM studies and other data resources, e.g. national statistics. An example is the analysis of cardiovascular events of the PEM study on sildenafil (Shakir *et al.*, 2001) (the product used for erectile dysfunction). Reported deaths from myocardial infarction and ischaemic heart disease in users of sildenafil in the PEM study were found to be no higher than expected according to national mortality statistics. The precautions with regard to possible sources of bias and confounding also apply to external comparisons.

DISCUSSION

PEM is best regarded as a hypothesis-generating method of pharmacovigilance. However, provided appropriate care is taken, the kind of hypotheses it provides can be further explored, or tested, by validation of selected cases, the study of age- and sex-adjusted relative risks, comparing products in the same therapeutic class, comparing reported events with national statistics, and conducting nested case–control studies. Hypothesis-testing methods, such as randomised controlled clinical trials, can only be satisfactorily undertaken when a hypothesis is already available.

The disadvantages and limitation of PEM, like those of most of the available techniques of pharmacovigilance, are however real. They include the following:

1. An average of only 58% of the green forms sent out are returned and an average of only 52%

contain clinically useful data. This is significantly higher than the reporting rate in the yellow card and similar schemes (Martin *et al.*, 1998; Wilton *et al.*, 1998) but could conceal biases as it cannot be established in each PEM study whether the patients whose doctors return the green forms are in any way different from those whose doctors fail to complete and return the questionnaire. We already know (MacKay, 1998) that the responding and non-responding GPs differ very little in the distribution of ages in which they became principals or in their geographical distribution. Recently, second green forms were sent to doctors who did not return the first green form, the data will be analysed to see whether there are differences in the safety profile between these patients and those reported initially.

2. PEM does not yet extend into hospital monitoring, although pilot studies have been conducted. Thus, for drugs started in hospital it is important to follow up reports of interest in order to identify the first prescriptions because a "survivor bias" can operate for patients who both started and stopped a drug under hospital care and may never receive a GP prescription and may, therefore, be undetected by PEM. None of the current methods of pharmacovigilance is ideal in respect of this problem— hence the importance of extending PEM into hospital practice.

3. PEM data include confounders, for example the highest value for ID_1 with the anti-epileptic drugs lamotrigine and vigabatrin for convulsions. Medical evaluation and relating the various finding in PEM to each other is an essential part of the analysis. However, even without analysis, lists of reported events are useful to prescribing doctors for they show which events are reported in everyday clinical practice and the relative frequency with which these events will be seen. They are perhaps more useful than the unquantified long lists of possible side-effects given in the standard prescribing information.

4. It is a further limitation that statistical comparisons between drugs need to be undertaken with great care. Each PEM study begins as soon as

the drug is launched and the "trade-off" is between capturing the real-world and generalisable data from PEM and randomisation in clinical trials, which have many logistical and even ethical difficulties as well as limited external validity caused by exclusion criteria and other restrictions.

5. While one of the strengths of PEM is that it collects dispensed rather than prescribed data, compliance is not examined routinely in PEM studies. However, it is possible, if necessary, to monitor repeated dispensing for the same patient as an indicator of compliance.

In essence, PEM can be as good but can be no better than the clinical case notes of the GPs or their precision in completing event forms for their patients.

The advantages of PEM are:

1. It is non-interventional and thereby minimises the selection biases that occur when the study design interferes with the doctor's choice of drug for the individual patient.

2. It is national in scale and the cohort comprises all patients given the drug immediately after its launch into general practice. In Europe it is the only database that can identify cohorts of more than 10 000 patients for newly introduced medicines soon after launch.

3. The system prompts all prescribers who automatically receive a green form for each patient prescribed the drug being monitored. It is probably this prompting function that is responsible for the success of the method: it does not rely on the doctor taking the initiative to report happenings. These features ensure that the studies are population based and that they disclose the real-life clinical experience with the drug: there are no exclusions and all patients prescribed the drug are recruited even if they are very old, very young, or receiving several drugs concurrently for multiple illnesses.

4. Because the data are concerned with events, the system could detect side-effects which none of the doctors has suspected to be due to the drug. The information provided by event reporting does not require the doctor to decide whether or not an individual event in a single patient is drug related. It thereby avoids a very difficult clinical decision for, as most reactions resemble fairly common clinical events, avoiding the doctor having to decide on causation may well encourage reporting.

5. The system allows direct contact between the doctors working in the DSRU and GPs so that follow-up surveillance of individual cases or deaths and all pregnancies is facilitated.

6. PEM can explore the possibility of long-latency adverse reactions and cohorts can be tagged on the NHS Central Register so that very long-term or lifetime follow-up can be undertaken.

7. Additional advantages accrue from the increasing size of the PEM database which has been built up since 1984. The database now contains information on 78 completed PEM studies and one million patients. This has started to provide opportunities for comparing products and patient groups in the database. As time passes and more studies are completed the value of the database as a research tool increases progressively.

Future plans include hospital monitoring, establishing registries of iatrogenic diseases, monitoring by community pharmacists, monitoring the safety of herbal products, and the establishment of an investigational unit in which the mechanisms of some of uncommon ADRs identified by PEM can be explored by pharmacological and pharmacogenetic techniques.

CONCLUSION

Prescription–event monitoring (PEM) is a valuable and well-established method of hypothesis-generating pharmacovigilance. Its use since 1984 has produced a substantial database which itself forms an important research tool. PEM has found its own place in pharmacovigilance and is at its best in monitoring drugs receiving wide-spread, long-term GP use. The method lends itself to validation of individual case reports and allows the data to be explored by well-established epidemiological and clinical research techniques.

ACKNOWLEDGEMENTS

PEM is the product of a unique partnership between the DSRU and thousands of GPs in England, to whom we are most grateful. The DSRU thanks the PPA for providing exposure data for PEM and for their continuous support.

I am most grateful to Professor Ron Mann, the previous director of the DSRU and Emeritus Professor at Southampton University, for providing me with material without which it would not have been possible to write this chapter. My thanks also go to Gill Pearce, Georgina Spragg and Lesley Flowers.

REFERENCES

BMA (1996) *Reporting Adverse Drug Reactions*. A BMA policy document. London: BMA.

Dunn NR, Freemantle S, Mann RD (1999) Nicorandil and diabetes: a nested case–control study to examine a signal generated by prescription–event monitoring. *Eur J Clin Pharmacol* **55**: 159–62.

Dunn NR, Pearce GL, Shakir SAW (2000) Adverse effects associated with the use of donepezil in general practice in England. *J Psychopharmacol* **14**: 406–8.

Finney DJ (1965) The design and logic of a monitor of drug use. *J Chron Dis* **18**: 77–98.

Freemantle SN, Pearce GL, Wilton LV, *et al.* (1997) The incidence of the most commonly reported events with 40 newly marketed drugs—a study by Prescription-Event Monitoring. *Pharmacoepidemiology and Drug Safety* **6** (Suppl 1): 1–62.

Inman WHW (1978a) Detection and investigation of drug safety problems. In: Gent M, Shigematsu I, eds., *Epidemiological Issues in Reported Drug-Induced Illnesses*. Hamilton, Ontario: McMaster University Library Press.

Inman WHW (1978b) An introduction to Prescription-Event Monitoring. In: Mann RD, ed., *Adverse Drug Reactions*. Carnforth, UK: Parthenon Publishing, pp. 177–99.

Inman, WHW (1981a) Postmarketing surveillance of adverse drug reactions in general practice. I: Search for new methods. *Br Med J* **282**: 1131–2.

Inman, WHW (1981b) Postmarketing surveillance of adverse drug reactions in general practice. II: Prescription-event monitoring at the University of Southampton. *Br Med J* **282**: 1216–7.

Inman WHW, Rawson NSB, Wilton LV (1981) Prescription-event monitoring. In: Inman WHW,

ed., *Monitoring for Drug Safety*, 2nd edn. Lancaster UK: MTP Press, pp. 213–35.

Layton D, Clark D, Pearce G, Shakir SAW (2001) Association between Selective Serotonin Reuptake Inhibitors (SSRI) and the risk of abnormal bleeding. *Eur J Clin Pharmacol*, in press.

Lenz, W (1961) Kindliche Missbildungen nach Medikament—Einnahme Während der Graviditat? *Dtsch med Wschr* **86**: 2555.

Lenz, W. (1962) Thalidomide and congenital abnormalities. *Lancet* **1**, 45.

MacKay F (1998) Postmarketing studies: the value of the work of the Drug Safety Research Unit. *Drug Safety* **19**: 343–53.

MacKay F, Wilton LV, Pearce G, *et al.* (1997) Acarbose and gastrointestinal intolerance. *Pharmacoepidemiology and Drug Safety* **6** (Suppl 2): Abstract 044.

MacKay FJ, Wilton LV, Pearce G, *et al.* (1997) Alendronate and oesophageal reactions. *Pharmacoepidemiology and Drug Safety* **6** (Suppl 2): Abstract 045.

MacKay FJ, Wilton LV, Pearce GL, *et al.* (1997) Safety of long-term lamotrigine in epilepsy. *Epilepsia* **38**(8): 881–6.

Mackay FJ, Dunn NR, Mann RD (1999) Antidepressants and the serotonin syndrome in general practice. *Br J Gen Pract* **49**: 871–4.

Mann RD, Wilton LV, Pearce GL, *et al.* (1997) Prescription-event monitoring (PEM) in 1996. A method of non-interventional observational cohort pharmacovigilance. *Pharmacoepidemiology and Drug Safety* **6** (Suppl 3): S5–S11.

Martin RM, Dunn NR, Freemantle S, Shakir S (2000) The rates of common adverse events reported with treatment with proton pump inhibitors used in general practice in England: cohort studies. *Br J Clin Pharmacol* **11**: 67–73.

Martin RM, Kapoor KV, Wilton LV, Mann RD (1998) Underreporting of suspected adverse drug reactions to newly marketed, black triangle drugs in general practice. *Br Med J* **317**: 119–20.

Secretary of State for Social Services Medicines (adverse reactions) (1986) *Hansard (Commons)* (30 Jan.). Col. 622

Shakir S, Wilton LV, Heeley E, Layton D (2001) Cardiovascular events in users of sildenafil: results from first phase of prescription-event monitoring in England. *Br Med J* **322**: 651–2.

Wilton LV, Freemantle S, Martin RM, Mann RD (1998) Is the incidence of upper respiratory infections independent of drug treatment in large cohort studies? Proceedings of the European Society of Pharmacovigilance, Berlin. *Pharmacoepidemiology and Drug Safety* **7** (Suppl 1): S4–10.

Wilton LV, Heeley E, Pickering RM, Shakir SA (2001) Comparative study of mortality rates and cardiac arrhythmias in post marketing surveillance studies of sertindole and two other atypical antipsychotic drugs. *J Psychopharmacol*, in press.

Wilton LV, MacKay FJ, Pearce GL, Mann RD (1997) The outcomes of pregnancy in women prescribed newly marketed drugs in 34 studies conducted by Prescription-Event Monitoring (PEM). *Pharmacoepidemiology and Drug Safety* **6**(2): Abstract 072.

Wilton LV, Pearce GL, Edet E, *et al.* (1996) The safety of finasteride used in benign prostatic hypertrophy a non-interventional observational cohort study in 14 772 patients. *Brit J Urol* **78**: 379–84.

Wilton LV, Stephens MDB, Mann RD (1999) Visual field defects association with Vigabatrin. *Br Med J* **319**: 1165–6.

Witts, LJ (1965) Adverse reactions to drugs. *Br Med J* **ii**: 1081.

27

PEM in New Zealand

DAVID M. COULTER

Intensive Medicines Monitoring Programme, Department of Preventive and Social Medicine, University of Otago, Dunedin, New Zealand

BACKGROUND

Prescription–event monitoring (PEM) is a term applied to a method of post-marketing surveillance using prospective observational cohort studies of selected individual drugs. The cohorts are established using prescribing data and adverse events are solicited from the prescribers using standard questionnaires. This chapter describes how the method has been developed in New Zealand (NZ) as the main tool of the Intensive Medicines Monitoring Programme (IMMP).

In 1976 the national Committee on Adverse Drug Reactions, advisory to the then Department of Health, recommended supplementing the NZ pharmacovigilance system's spontaneous reporting activities ("yellow card" scheme) with a new early post-marketing surveillance programme. The purpose was to speed up the identification of previously unrecognised adverse drug reactions (ADRs) and to provide better information about risk (McQueen, 1977). The stimulus for this was the international recognition that spontaneous reporting had proved inadequate in recognising the serious oculomucocutaneous syndrome with the new beta-blocker practolol, even though the early symptoms were quite common (Skegg and

Doll, 1977). The new programme, which commenced in 1977, was called the "Intensified Adverse Drug Reaction Reporting Scheme" and was aimed at selected new drugs. It was to function by establishing patient cohorts from prescription information provided by dispensing pharmacists and "intensified" spontaneous reporting. For the drugs selected for study, this intensified reporting was an attempt to change the nature of reporting from that of suspected adverse reactions of recognisable clinical significance, to that of reporting all adverse events of any type or severity and without any judgement on causality. Thus a high rate of reporting of all types of events was expected to provide greater opportunity for identifying signals of previously unrecognised adverse reactions, and the cohorts of identifiable patients would allow the estimation of rates or incidence of adverse events and thus provide a measure of risk.

The first drugs monitored in this way were metoprolol, atenolol, acebutolol, labetalol, perhexiline, sodium valproate and cimetidine. Although the reporting rates for these drugs were much higher than rates in the standard spontaneous reporting programme (Coulter and McQueen, 1982), it was decided to send questionnaires to the

Pharmacovigilance. Edited by R.D. Mann and E.B. Andrews

prescribers after the drugs had been on the market for at least six months requesting information on any adverse events noted in the patients' records. These were called "event recording surveys" and their use was aimed at enhancing the reporting rate still further. In addition, it was possible to identify when patients were no longer having their drug dispensed and specific questionnaires were then sent out asking why treatment had ceased. The use of these two questionnaires was the first endeavour at what has since been called PEM (Inman, 1981b) and the first publication resulting from the use of this methodology was the report and investigation of a new signal with labetalol (Coulter, 1979). Other findings published in this very early period concerned perhexiline (Department of Health, 1979, 1980), reasons for cessation of therapy with perhexiline, sodium valproate and labetalol (Coulter, 1981) and sodium valproate (McQueen, 1982). The early stages of the scheme were reviewed after five years' activity (Coulter and McQueen, 1982).

PEM methodology in NZ has since developed considerably and has become much more comprehensive. The scheme has also been given a more appropriate name, the Intensive Medicines Monitoring Programme (IMMP) and recent reviews of the IMMP have been published (Coulter, 1998, 2000). The IMMP is a national post-marketing surveillance scheme and is part of the Centre for Adverse Reactions Monitoring (CARM) along with the Spontaneous Reporting Programme. Both activities of CARM are undertaken under contract to the Ministry of Health and report to the Ministry and its expert advisory group the Medicines Adverse Reactions Committee (MARC). CARM functions within the Department of Preventive and Social Medicine of the Dunedin School of Medicine, University of Otago, together with the National Poisons Centre.

The basic methodology of the IMMP is that of long-term prospective observational cohort studies on selected new drugs, aiming for cohorts of around 10 000 patients. Throughout the monitoring period regular questionnaires for each patient are sent to prescribers in hospital and/or private practice for as long as prescriptions continue. Intensified spontaneous reporting continues to be available and supplements significantly the PEM

acquired events. Participation by pharmacists and doctors is voluntary and unpaid. This chapter describes and illustrates the methodology in some detail, particularly those features that are unique to the NZ IMMP.

SELECTION OF MEDICINES FOR MONITORING

THE PRINCIPLES

New drug applications are considered by the Medicines Assessment Advisory Committee (MAAC) which is advisory to the Ministry of Health. The MAAC has traditionally made the recommendations for which drugs should be monitored. Changes in the process were instituted in the year 2000. The first three medicines of a new class are now, by default, recommended to be considered for monitoring based on the premise that clinical trials alone produce inadequate safety data and therefore intensive monitoring is important in the early post-marketing period.

THE PROCESS

For each drug recommended, the Director of the IMMP undertakes a feasibility study to examine and report on potential usage, sponsor company interest and/or concerns, methodology, special requirements and the resources required to undertake the monitoring. An important consideration is the demand being made on practitioners who must complete the questionnaires. Should this become too onerous, then compliance is likely to drop. The feasibility studies are then considered by an expert panel of four and a final recommendation is made to the Ministry of Health. The panel gives priority to monitoring those drugs where the following conditions apply:

- use is expected to be widespread and/or long term;
- safety issues have been raised from clinical trials or post-marketing experience and further evaluation is needed;

Table 27.1. Completed monitoring studies.

Drug	Monitoring commenced	Period (months)	Patient numbers	Prescription numbers	Adverse events
Acebutolol	Apr 77	36	2019	4864	141
Atenolol	Apr 77	36	2837	6559	299
Metoprolol	Apr 77	36	9719	28 038	403
Perhexiline	Apr 77	52	5052	16 309	195
Sodium valproate	Apr 77	72	19 310	56 746	167
Cimetidine	Nov 77	45	10 526	17 270	130
Labetalol	Nov 77	28	3143	7635	99
Nifedipine	Oct 80	52	10 575	62 771	443
Captopril	Apr 81	68	16 342	68 901	1395
Amiodarone	Jul 82	67	6939	23 059	403
Aciclovir (oral)[a]	Jan 83	86	6052	8665	192
Mianserin	Apr 83	58	10 899	43 377	321
Enalapril	Jun 84	55	25 686	90 028	1535
Lisinopril	Feb 88	38	12 132	41 777	903
Fluoxetine	Feb 88	60	6616	15 458	524
Bezafibrate	Feb 89	61	10 226	46 769	776
Gemfibrozil	Feb 89	61	4541	18 650	411
Simvastatin	Feb 89	61	7588	32 177	477
Moclobemide	Mar 90	73	17 322	52 026	1191
Omeprazole	Mar 90	78	22 702	131 972	1684
Sumatriptan[a]	Apr 91	92	14 964	107 646	3997

[a] Nationwide PEM.

- there are related drugs with significant problems;
- the target disease is of low risk and any increased risk arising from therapy would adversely affect the benefit–risk balance;
- safe treatment options are already available and any increase in risk would be unacceptable;
- another drug of the same class is being monitored or considered, which provides the added value of a comparator and also raises the question of equity for the sponsors.

COMPARATORS

For about 50% of the drugs it has been possible to monitor more than one of the same class, or for a similar indication (beta-blockers, ACE inhibitors, lipid lowering agents and antidepressants), although not always concurrently (Table 27.1). Having comparators has obvious advantages, but unlike a clinical trial, there are frequent confounders that can make interpretation of differences difficult (Beggs *et al.*, 1998). It is not always

possible to provide a suitable comparator and it is not always desirable from the point of view of cost and the demands being made of practitioners. Even with comparators, it may be necessary to set up a specific study designed to elucidate a signal (Beggs *et al.*, 1998). It is probably more cost effective to monitor two different types of drug than to monitor one and select another for the sole purpose of being a comparator.

THE COHORTS

SOURCE

Pharmacies

The cohorts are established using identifiable patients from prescription records supplied by community and hospital pharmacists. All pharmacies in NZ maintain prescription records on computer. Suppliers of computer software for pharmacies flag IMMP medicines and provide a program for producing a printout of all prescriptions dispensed for IMMP medicines. These are sent to the IMMP at regular intervals on request with Freepost envelopes supplied. All prescriptions for the monitored medicine during the period of monitoring (historical mean 58 months) are recorded. These provide a prescribing history for each patient for as long as treatment continues. Pharmacy compliance with returning the prescription reports is currently 86%.

Intra-Uterine Devices

By agreement with the sponsors of Multiload Cu375 and Mirena these cohorts have been established with the use of registration forms supplied in each pack containing the device. The pre-addressed form is completed at the time of insertion and posted to the IMMP (Figure 27.1).

Lack of Central Data

In NZ to date, it has been essential to use dispensing pharmacists as the source of drug usage. There is a central agency which collects prescription information, but only when there is reimbursement being paid by the government for the cost of prescriptions. It is now unusual for a new drug to be subsidised at the time of its market launch and so pharmacies are the only source of prescription data for these drugs until such time as subsidy is introduced. Delay in subsidy usually results in low usage and slows the growth of the cohort as do some other policies aimed at restricting the use of new medicines in order to contain the national pharmaceutical budget. The involvement of pharmacists in the IMMP however has distinct advantages. Many provide professional input by way of noting adverse events and particularly death, or may comment on usage trends, which alert to problems of tolerance, inefficacy, medication error, misuse or abuse.

Intensive Medicines Monitoring Programme | **MIRENA** (levonorgestrel IUS)

Doctor - Please fill in particulars and return this form | **Batch No:**

Patient Registration Form

Please note: this form must only be used for MIRENA users.

Patient's surname: | First Names:

Address

Date of birth: | National Patient No:

Inserting Doctor's name: | Registration No.:

Address:

General Practitioner's name: | Registration No.:

(if different from inserting doctor)

Address:

Indication for use: Contraception [ ] Menorrhagia [ ] Other (please specify)

Is the patient considering hysterectomy as an alternative option? Yes [ ] No [ ]

Is the patient currently on a waiting list for a hysterectomy? Yes [ ] No [ ]

Parity: Gravida: Mirena Renewal?: Yes [ ] No [ ]

Problems with insertion or other problems noted:

Timing of insertion: within 7 days of onset of menstruation [ ] post first trimester abortion [ ]
6 weeks postpartum [ ] Other (please specify) [ ]

Date of insertion: | Doctor's signature:

Fold | Fold | Fold | Fold

Figure 27.1. Registration form for intra-uterine device.

PATIENT IDENTIFICATION

Details of each patient recorded include first and last names, address, date of birth and the prescribing doctor's name with specific worksite address. The type of doctor is also recorded—general practitioner or specialist type. National health identification (NHI) numbers have been introduced but are not yet complete and are insufficiently reliable for accurate statistics. In addition, many practices cannot identify patients by the NHI number and so it is essential when sending questionnaires to continue to use personal information to identify patients.

MANUAL DATA ENTRY

Prescription and patient records are entered into the computer database manually. It would be possible to receive electronic data from pharmacists, but this has been evaluated and at this stage would have no advantage in the IMMP. For privacy reasons it would be necessary to obtain the data on floppy disk rather than by direct electronic transmission. Handling data in this way from multiple sources (currently 983 pharmacies) immediately decreases the convenience. In addition, electronic entry would have disadvantages in the context of the entry of multiple prescriptions per patient over time. With manual entry, the previous data screen for each patient is easily replicated for new prescription entries and the data are immediately checked for inconsistencies. This provides for easy, continuous validation of the data. The checking of new prescription entries against older ones using electronic submission would be less convenient.

COHORT SIZE

The medicines monitored are listed in Tables 27.1 and 27.2. Monitoring has been completed for 22 and 16 are currently undergoing monitoring. Enrolling of new patients has ceased for three of the latter, Multiload Cu375, salmeterol and eformoterol, but follow-up work is still continuing. The mean cohort size was 10 964 patients for drugs where monitoring has been completed and the mean duration of monitoring was 58 months. The desirable size for a cohort is around 10 000 patients (Inman, 1981a). The medicines ranged from those with regular long-term use (e.g. lipid lowering agents) to those used intermittently (e.g. sumatriptan) and intra-uterine devices. Prescription returns are received from pharmacies throughout the whole country for all the monitored medicines. Thus the cohorts consist of

virtually the total population of patients prescribed each monitored drug.

LONGITUDINAL MONITORING

The long period usually taken to achieve a substantial cohort is a disadvantage in terms of producing quick results and is due to the small NZ population (3.8 million) and restrictions on reimbursement for most new medicines, which slows market uptake. However, the necessity to undertake a longitudinal approach to monitoring has advantages as follows: a proportion of patients are monitored for several years and this provides greater opportunity for identifying (a) delayed effects; (b) use in pregnancy or lactation; (c) death rates and causes of death; (d) reasons for cessation of therapy; (e) changed indications (these frequently broaden over time); (f) evidence of tolerance or dependence; (g) changes in prescribing practice which for new medicines takes time to be established; and (h) changes in patient characteristics which in the early post-marketing phase of a drug frequently differ from later use. Patients with severe disease who have failed other therapy are often tried on a new drug as a last resort and in the early months of use, this group is over-represented

Table 27.2. Current monitoring studies.

	Monitoring commenced	Patient numbers	Prescription numbers	Adverse events
Multiload Cu375[a]	Jul 91	16 159	17 468	7559
Salmeterol[a]	Mar 92	9974	70 377	1499
Eformoterol[a]	Mar 92	2107	14 885	371
Mirena[a]	Mar 98	5880	5991	927
Montelukast[a]	Dec 98	1202	5334	39
Nefazodone	Dec 98	3506	24 612	224
Olanzapine	Apr 99	2754	23 161	109
Quetiapine	Apr 99	96	828	20
Tolcapone[a]	Apr 99	429	6071	172
Clozapine	Dec 00	91	328	239
Risperidone	Dec 00	267	650	70
Zafirlukast[a]	Dec 00	nil	nil	nil
Entacapone[a]	Dec 00	7	17	2
Celecoxib[a]	Dec 00	7649	23 221	291
Rofecoxib[a]	Dec 00	5949	12 009	149
Sibutramine[a]	Dec 00	992	2104	8

[a] Nationwide PEM.

compared with later use. An extreme example of this in the IMMP was a death rate of 25% in the first year of marketing of captopril. It is desirable both to be able to achieve the target cohort rapidly, and to monitor longitudinally.

In an evaluation of angioedema and urticaria with angiotensin converting enzyme (ACE) inhibitors, longitudinal monitoring was able to demonstrate that 40% of the reports of angioedema were of delayed onset occurring weeks or months after the commencement of treatment. It was also seen that patients might have multiple episodes with long symptom free intervals, creating diagnostic difficulty (Pillans et al., 1996).

PRESCRIPTION DATA

The data elements captured from the prescription information are listed in Table 27.3. Each has a particular use.

DRUG NAME AND FORMULATION

The brand name is coded as well as the generic name. Where more than one brand is being monitored, this provides the opportunity to compare differences between brands. The formulation is also recorded because a reaction may be caused by an excipient or propellant rather than the drug. With salmeterol (Serevent), for example, three formulations are in use, Serevent Accuhaler,

Table 27.3. data elements recorded from prescriptions.

Patients
- Name including first name
- Title; gender
- Address
- Date of birth

Doctor
- Name
- Specific worksite address

Drug
- Drug name and formulation
- Dose
- Date of dispensing
- Quantity dispensed

Rotadisk and Aerosol inhaler. The reaction "paradoxical bronchospasm", which is an immediate response, has occurred only with the aerosol inhaler and is presumably due to the propellant.

DOSE

Doses are recorded as daily doses. Over time, changes in dose for individual patients can be observed, but also changes in prescribing patterns overall. With captopril, the mean daily dose for each patient's first prescription in the first five years after release was 121 mg, 91 mg, 78 mg, 63 mg and 54 mg, respectively, reflecting changes in dosage recommendations and clinical practice. Changes like this are relevant to the incidence of ADRs that are dose related.

DISPENSING DATES AND QUANTITY

It is well recognised that a proportion of prescriptions given to patients is not submitted for dispensing. Records of dispensing are therefore a more reliable indicator of drug use than prescriptions, although uncertainty remains as to the compliance of patients in using the medicines dispensed. With the continuous records of dispensings in the IMMP, patients who have ceased therapy can be identified when prescription records stop being received. The prescriber is then sent a questionnaire asking the reason for cessation. This provides important information, which is discussed below.

The monitoring of omeprazole demonstrated another use of continuous recording of prescriptions. Some patients had relatively short courses and others remained on treatment long term. In understanding the use of the drug it was useful to be able to identify how many courses of treatment patients were having and how long these were. Patients who had been on continuous therapy for a year or longer were followed up annually for evidence of the development of reactions of long latency. This questionnaire included questions about endoscopic examinations of the upper gastrointestinal tract and any evidence of the development of malignancy or carcinoid tumours.

These have been considered as a potential risk of prolonged reduction of gastric acid. This long-term follow-up is as yet incomplete, but benign, multiple, gastric polyps have been identified in two patients. This problem has been attributed by others as a reaction to prolonged achlorhydria with omeprazole (Graham, 1992; Schenk *et al.*, 1997).

CONCOMITANT THERAPY

Information on concomitant therapy is not routinely requested during the primary stage of monitoring because this is time consuming for practitioners and compliance with completing the questionnaires would fall. Should this information be required at a secondary stage during the evaluation of a problem, it is requested then (Beggs *et al.*, 1999). However, when it is clear that knowledge of concomitant therapy is going to be essential, it is requested on the primary questionnaires, e.g. corticosteroid use with montelukast and anti-ulcer therapy with the COX-2 inhibitors.

EVENT REPORTING/RECORDING

DEFINITION AND ADVICE

Adverse events are described as any untoward experience whether or not the event is thought to be drug related. All new events should be reported and also adverse changes in a pre-existing condition, abnormally changed laboratory values, pregnancy, unexpected failure of therapeutic effect, any possible interactions, accidents and all deaths. From time to time all doctors are sent "desk reminder cards", which list the medicines being monitored and describe the type of reporting required. This latter advice is shown in Figure 27.2. Because the IMMP is primarily a method of drug surveillance designed to detect new adverse reactions early in the post-marketing phase, emphasis is given to the reporting of *adverse* events. However, doctors are also encouraged to report unexpected favourable events and, to this end, promotion of reporting usually refers to "events", omitting the adjective "adverse".

Intensive Medicines Monitoring Programme

The Intensive Medicines Monitoring Programme is aimed at the early identification of unexpected adverse reactions with selected new medicines. To enable this practitioners are requested to report all adverse events occurring in patients on these medicines.

Events are not reactions only, but include any and all random clinical incidents. Unknown reactions cannot be identified if only recognised reactions are reported and an assessment of the significance of events can only be performed effectively on a large aggregation of reports.

Please report:
- all new events, including common minor ones
- change in a pre-existing condition
- abnormal changes in laboratory tests
- accidents
- **all deaths** and the cause
- possible interactions – remember alcohol and the "pill"

To enable accurate identification and careful epidemiological assessment please include on prescriptions:
- date of birth
- first name

Figure 27.2. Advice to prescribers.

SOURCING THE EVENTS

Doctors record any events manually. They may be reported by any one of three methods: (1) systematic follow-up using questionnaires (PEM); (2) on duplicate prescriptions; or (3) by intensified spontaneous reporting.

Questionnaires

Following receipt of the pharmacy printouts of prescription records, questionnaires are sent to the prescribers at regular intervals. For a new patient, information is requested on any adverse events from the commencement of therapy. If questionnaires have been sent previously, doctors are requested to record events from the date of the most recent questionnaire and this date is given to facilitate record searching. The questionnaires are computer generated and include all prescribing and patient data and the first and most recent dispensing dates for reference. Searching and recording by the doctor is therefore kept to a minimum. The doctor is requested to check the printed data for accuracy and add any missing details, e.g. date of birth. Thus, with each questionnaire for a patient, the data are being validated and updated (e.g. change of dose or correction of name spelling), resulting in patient and prescribing data of high quality. Doctors record descriptively with dates any events noted in their patient's file over the period indicated. For drugs used intermittently, e.g. sumatriptan, where the doctor has no follow-up information, he/she is asked to contact the patient. This may be by phone, or the questionnaire is frequently sent to the patient to complete. It is suggested as an alternative that the questionnaire is filed in the patient's record for completion at the next attendance. The compliance rate of returning the questionnaires is seldom less than 80%.

Duplicate Prescriptions

There is also regional use in 25% ($n = 950\ 000$) of the population of special IMMP duplicate prescription pads, which were developed to enhance event reporting. Personalised pads are given to private practitioners and pads for hospitals are printed with the name of the hospital. The prescription forms request the date of birth (not a requirement on regular prescriptions except for children). Doctors give the original and copy of the prescription to the patient who takes both to the pharmacist. The accumulated copies are then sent to the IMMP along with the pharmacist's printout of IMMP prescriptions.

A pilot study of the use of IMMP duplicate prescription forms was undertaken in 1984. This compared the event reporting rate in a region using duplicate prescriptions with a comparable region using intensified spontaneous reporting. Both regions had the same promotion of monitoring activities. The event reporting rate in the duplicate prescription region was 14 times greater than that of the control region (Coulter, 1986). In using these forms prescribers are asked to tick a box to indicate whether or not any adverse events have occurred since the previous prescription, or if it is the first prescription (Coulter, 1998). If the "yes" event box is marked, the doctor may record the event on the prescription copy. If not, a questionnaire is sent out within two months for the

event to be recorded. The use of the IMMP duplicate prescriptions frequently obviates the need to send questionnaires and means events are reported more quickly. Not only is this method much more successful at eliciting event reports than intensified spontaneous reporting, but it is more efficient than using questionnaires alone. Their use is restricted due to lack of resources, although the method is gradually extending on a national basis without additional cost to the IMMP through the developing use of computerised clinical records in general practice.

Intensified Spontaneous Reporting

In an early review, the rate of intensified spontaneous reporting of adverse events in the IMMP was shown to be much higher than the reporting rate for the standard spontaneous adverse reaction reporting programme. Using drug sales figures as a denominator, the rate of reporting for acebutolol, atenolol and metoprolol ranged between 16 and 61 times higher than that for propranolol, which was not being monitored (Coulter and McQueen, 1982). Even so, IMMP intensified spontaneous reporting achieves a much lower rate of reporting than the use of the questionnaires and/or duplicate prescriptions (PEM). For some drugs it has been necessary to restrict PEM methodology to certain regions because of lack of resources and reliance has been placed on intensified spontaneous reporting in the other regions (Tables 27.1 and 27.2). Spontaneous reporting, however, always remains an option and is frequently of particular value. Spontaneous reports usually arise from specific clinical concerns and contain greater detail than is provided on most of the questionnaires returned. They often form the index case report(s) for a series being considered as a signal. Over the last five years spontaneous reports have comprised 4.8% of the total reports received for IMMP medicines.

QUESTIONNAIRE TYPES

Basic

Doctors are asked to record "any events—clinical incidents and/or reactions including possible interactions, accidents or death (give cause)—since the first prescription or last questionnaire". Dates of onset are requested. The date of the previous questionnaire is given together with the first and latest dispensing dates for ease of reference.

Pregnancy and Lactation

In women of child-bearing age, questions on pregnancy and outcome are incorporated into the questionnaires. The estimated date of conception or last menstrual period or expected date of delivery is requested so that the times of drug exposure during the pregnancy can be identified. If the mother was breast feeding while taking the drug, then any adverse events occurring in the infant are requested together with the age of the infant at the time.

Cessation of Therapy

When prescription records for patients stop coming, the General Practitioner (GP), who is the preferred contact, or other prescriber, is sent a questionnaire requesting the reason for cessation of therapy. They are asked to indicate with appropriate detail which of the following is applicable: lost to follow-up; poor compliance; inadequate therapeutic response; no longer necessary; change of therapy for reasons unrelated to the drug (e.g. change of diagnosis); patient death; possible adverse reaction.

Special Requirements

It is sometimes necessary to specify the need for particular information. This may be added to the standard questionnaire or an additional form is designed for the purpose. For the monitoring of salmeterol and eformoterol a "severity questionnaire" was developed which asked questions about hospital admissions, admissions to an intensive care unit, urgent non-inpatient treatment, and use of oral corticosteroids for asthma. It was felt that death rates would need to be stratified by severity of asthma. For the monitoring of the intra-uterine devices, specific questions were added about expulsion, unintended pregnancy with outcome,

pelvic inflammatory disease and device removals for this and other problems. For the follow-up of long-term omeprazole use questions were asked about the results of any endoscopy checks. Baseline and serial liver function tests were requested for the monitoring of tolcapone. For the COX-2 inhibitors questions related to a previous history of peptic ulcer disease were asked.

COHORT STUDY FOR REACTIONS OF LONG LATENCY

This refers to the use of the prescription database for studies several years after the official monitoring period has been completed, aiming to establish rates of mortality, carcinogenesis and other selected morbidity. A pilot trial of record linkage using GP records, hospital discharge summaries and national registers of mortality, cancer and morbidity has been commenced with data collection undertaken for 200 patients from each of the metoprolol and captopril cohorts. The results from matching with national mortality, cancer and morbidity data have not yet been analysed. The combined results of record linkage with hospital and GP records resulted in useful data being received for 50% of patients whose treatment had commenced 10–16 years previously. This percentage should increase with the addition of the data from national registers.

DEATHS

Source

Death rates are calculated and attempts are made to identify any significant differences in death rates between comparator drugs or changes in death rate over time and any differences from standardised population rates from national health statistics. Deaths are very poorly reported spontaneously. Most are obtained from the questionnaire on reasons for cessation of therapy.

Follow-up

If the data concerning death are incomplete, then a letter is sent to the doctor requesting the missing details. These may include the date and cause of death and confirmation that the patient was using the drug at or near the time of death. If the drug was not being used at the time of death, then the reason for cessation of therapy is requested. Copies of autopsy and/or coroners' reports are requested if these are available. It is sometimes helpful to ask if death was expected or unexpected. If death rates are particularly important, then record linkage is undertaken with the NZ Health Information Service, which maintains the national database of deaths, to identify any deaths that may have been missed by the routine follow-up procedures.

Assessment of Deaths

Death was the most common event recorded for omeprazole and the apparent high death rate was cause for concern. Over the monitoring period there were 407 deaths (18.5 per 1000 patients) compared with 140 (8.1 per 1000) for moclobemide being monitored at the same time. However, the omeprazole group was significantly older (mean 60 years) than the moclobemide cohort (mean 49 years) and when age-specific rates were examined there were no statistically significant differences. Death rates are particularly important in the study of drugs used in the treatment of asthma, as was revealed in the experience with fenoterol (Crane et al., 1989). At the time of writing they were being studied with particular care with the long acting beta agonists eformoterol and salmeterol (Castellsague et al., 1999). Data are also being collected on the severity of disease with the objective of stratifying the results according to severity.

PATIENT INVOLVEMENT

In the monitoring of sumatriptan it is estimated that 50% of the forms were completed by telephone interview ($n = 10\,918$) and 15% ($n = 3950$) were completed by patients (see above). Patients completed the questionnaires carefully and competently and, in general, have described events in better detail than the doctors.

Two surveys of patients have been undertaken in order to investigate signals. The first was a comparative study of labetalol and metoprolol involving 593 patients to investigate signals of scalp tingling, polyuria and polydipsia with labetalol (Coulter, 1979). The second was a comparative study of nifedipine and captopril in order to validate a signal of eye pain with nifedipine and to characterise the reaction of taste disturbance with captopril (Coulter, 1988). A total of 1265 patients were involved in this study. Compliance with returning questionnaires was high: 87%, 77%, 84% and 86% for labetalol, metoprolol, nifedipine and captopril, respectively. The questionnaires were completed with care and both studies produced rational results with no evidence of spurious responses. Patients were willing to give personal information such as date of birth.

PROCESSING OF EVENTS

REVIEW OF REPORTS

All events are assessed by a physician using the same process as for reviewing ADR reports in the spontaneous reporting programme. A "relationship" is established between the drug and the event following the protocol for causality assessment recommended by the World Health Organisation Collaborating Centre for International Drug Monitoring (WHO) (Meyboom and Royer, 1992). The events are classified according to system–organ class using the IMMP events dictionary which is a hierarchical terminology based on the WHO adverse reactions terminology (WHOART). The hierarchy has five levels and events can be sorted at each level into their clinically related groupings or individually. There are approximately 2600 event terms in the dictionary.

DRUG–EVENT RELATIONSHIP ASSESSMENT

Each drug–event relationship is coded as one of the following: definite, probable, possible or unlikely. These assessments are based mainly on duration to onset of the event and the response to withdrawal and/or rechallenge. They are not regarded as "causality" assessments and are made without prejudice. Judgements on causality for many of the events can only come later when epidemiological evidence using aggregated IMMP and other available data can be considered along with biases and confounders and pharmacological plausibility. With this background thinking, and to facilitate further evaluation, the assessed events are divided into two categories: those events with a relationship of certain, probable or possible are classified as "reactions" and those with a relationship of unlikely are called "incidents" (because they are likely to be incidental to the use of the drug and represent the background noise of the condition being treated, or community morbidity). These two groups are then evaluated for signals of previously unidentified adverse reactions. This is largely undertaken by observation of the nature and pattern of events being reported, examining comparative rates controlled for age, gender, indication and severity of disease as appropriate, and differences in profiles. Signals arising from this process may be investigated further by special studies.

INCIDENTS AS CONTROLS

Unless the incident group contains unrecognised adverse reactions, it should represent the background noise and this should be generally similar for drugs of similar indication. If the incident rates are similar for comparator drugs, then it can be assumed that reporting bias is not present. If there are statistically significant differences between the incident profiles of comparator drugs, then this may be due to the presence of an unrecognised adverse reaction or confounding, e.g. by indication or reporting bias. Any such differences are therefore investigated. There is no automated process of signal identification.

Incidents are also used as within-drug controls for characterising adverse reactions. The variables associated with, respectively, the reactions and incidents for a drug are compared and also the patient characteristics, and should there be differences these may indicate risk factors for the reaction under study, e.g. a gender or dose difference. An example of the use of incidents as

Table 27.4. Comparison of prescription event monitoring rates (% of cohort who sustained an event).

Drug	Reactions (%)	Incidents (%)	Total events (%)
Omeprazole	2.0	10.2	12.2
Moclobemide	9.8	7.5	17.3
Fluoxetine	12.6	6.9	19.5
Bezafibrate	12.4	9.5	21.8
Gemfibrozil	10.8	8.4	19.3
Simvastatin	7.7	9.1	16.8

within-drug controls is as follows. The rates of adverse reactions were higher in women than men for moclobemide (relative risk (RR) 1.7; 95% confidence interval (CI) 1.4–2.0) and fluoxetine (RR 1.7; 95% CI 1.3–2.2). There was no significant gender difference seen in the incident rates. It would appear therefore that the gender difference seen for the reactions is a true risk factor and not due to reporting bias.

For these two drugs, which were monitored concurrently, the incidents were also used as between-drug controls. The reaction rate for fluoxetine was 50% higher than for moclobemide (RR 1.5; 95% CI 1.2–1.7). There was no significant difference between the incident rates, suggesting an absence of reporting bias and strengthening the finding of greater risk with fluoxetine (Coulter, 1996). The monitoring of omeprazole provides another example. The results for this drug showed a very low rate of reactions. However, the incident rate was slightly higher than for other drugs monitored concurrently, suggesting once again an absence of reporting bias and a strengthening of the finding (Table 27.4).

SIGNAL GENERATION

SIGNAL DEFINITION

In practice, events are treated as signals if they arouse strong suspicion of a hitherto unrecognised adverse reaction. This may be the result of a single case report of high quality with a positive dechallenge and rechallenge ("definite" relationship), regarded as an index case, or a cluster of cases where the relationship that can be established may be of lesser strength. The number of reports and the strength of the relationship may be such that causality can be confirmed with the data on hand (Coulter and Edwards, 1987).

In order to demonstrate the hypothesis-generating activity of the IMMP, signals generated in 11 drugs over the last 10 years were searched from the agenda material and minutes of the MARC (see above) meetings and from publications. For the purposes of this evaluation a signal was recorded as such if the MARC was alerted prior to the date of the second non-IMMP publication. The date that the MARC was alerted to each signal was recorded and this date was compared with the date of the first two publications (if any) found by Medline and AdisBase searches of the international literature (all languages with an English abstract). Medline was searched from 1985 and AdisBase from 1989. Case reports and clinical trials were included in the searches. AdisBase searches included publications from regulatory authorities internationally. Data sheets were not searched. The dates of any IMMP publications were also recorded. Any recommendations of the MARC as a result of considering the signals were noted. Events that are expected as a result of known pharmacological action (e.g. tremor with beta-agonists) were not recorded as signals.

SIGNALS GENERATED

These results of the analysis of signals generated by the IMMP are preliminary. There were 153 signals recorded from the 10-year period. Of these, 132 (86%) were notified to the MARC prior to any publication found in the international literature. Eighty-six (56%) of the signals have since been strengthened or confirmed by at least one non-IMMP publication. In 72 (47%) instances the IMMP publication was the first report of the signal identified and in 23 (18%) it was the second. On 39 (25%) occasions the MARC recommended action after considering the signals. These included articles in *Prescriber Update* (a Ministry of Health bulletin), writing to pharmaceutical companies for further information, changes to data sheets, and further investigation.

Many of the signals were first published in articles in *Prescriber Update* or the *NZ Family Physician* published by the Royal NZ College of General Practitioners. The topics of these articles are listed in Tables 27.5 and 27.6. An example of the signals generated from the IMMP is given in Table 27.7 for sumatriptan. Signals published in the wider medical literature include ACE inhibitors and anaemia (Edwards and Coulter, 1989), the intestinal effects of captopril (Edwards *et al.*, 1992), psoriasis with ACE inhibitors (Coulter and Pillans, 1993), hypertension with moclobemide (Coulter and Pillans, 1995b) and fluoxetine and extrapyramidal effects (Coulter and Pillans, 1995a).

THE VALUE OF CLINICAL APPRAISAL

Personal examination of all events resulted in the identification of a new adverse reaction to sumatriptan. Aggravation or activation of pain was noted at sites of trauma or inflammation in 22 reports. The varied descriptions did not link them with any particular body system or organ and there was no reaction or event term in use which could be used to identify these events. Recall of the various events by the reviewer resulted in linking

Table 27.5. Titles of articles in *Prescriber Update* (First issue 1993).

Adverse respiratory reactions to long-acting beta-agonists. 1999
Top 10 adverse events to sumatriptan in the IMMP. 1998
Top 10 adverse reactions with Multiload Cu375 in the IMMP. 1997
Top 10 adverse reactions to omeprazole in the IMMP. 1997
Interactions with fluoxetine and other SSRIs. 1997
Top 10 adverse reactions to fluoxetine in the IMMP. 1996
Top 10 adverse reactions to moclobemide in the IMMP. 1996
Sumatriptan in the media. 1996
Interactions with moclobemide and serotonergic antidepressants. 1996
Omeprazole and bacterial overgrowth in the gut. 1995
Selective serotonin reuptake inhibitors and hyponatraemia. 1994
Chest pain and sumatriptan in the IMMP. 1994
Adverse effects of omeprazole. 1993

Table 27.6. Titles of recent articles in the *New Zealand Family Physician*.

Specialist only drug snags may present to GPs first (nefazodone, olanzapine, tolcapone and Mirena). 1999
Salmeterol and eformoterol monitoring: progress report. 1999
Reactions to omeprazole obscured by ageing process. 1998
Psychiatric and behavioural responses to sumatriptan (Imigran). 1997
Interim results of Multiload Cu375 monitoring reassuring. 1997
Moclobemide and fluoxetine compared. 1996
Beta2 agonists under scrutiny. 1996
Sumatriptan and possible autonomic imbalance. 1995
Monitoring of omeprazole. 1995
Further experience with monitoring sumatriptan (Imigran). 1995
Lipid lowering agents and reasons for cessation of therapy. 1994
Fluoxetine interactions. 1993
Early experience with sumatriptan. 1993
Bezafibrate, gemfibrozil and simvastatin. 1992
Early results from moclobemide. 1991
A review of reactions to ACE inhibitors. 1990
ACE inhibitors and pancreatitis. 1990
Experience with aciclovir. 1990

Table 27.7. Signals arising from the sumatriptan cohort.

Amnesia	Muscle weakness
Angioedema	Myalgia
Anxiety	Pain inflammation
Apnoea	activated
Autonomic disturbance	Pain trauma activated
Chest pain	Panic
Confusion/disorientation	Rebound headache
Depersonalisation	Rigors
Depression	Sensory disturbance
Dry mouth	Somnolence
"Flight or fight" reaction	Sweating
Hallucinations	Tachycardia
Ischaemic optic	Tachyphylaxis/tolerance
neuropathy	Throat tightness

them to a common syndrome which was named "pain activation syndrome" (Coulter, DM, presentation at the 19th Annual Meeting of National Centres Participating in the WHO International Drug Monitoring Programme, Switzerland, 1997). "Pain trauma activated" and "pain inflammation activated" were terms adopted in **WHOART**. With the varied presentation and absence of specific terms for the events, it is unlikely that this syndrome could have been identified by automated signal generation.

VALIDATION OF SIGNALS

Investigating Signals by Survey of Cohort Sample

When comparing the incident profile of bezafibrate, gemfibrozil and simvastatin, bezafibrate was found to have a statistically significant excess of cardio-vascular incidents (Coulter, 1992). This was due mainly to a greater rate of angina. A special study was undertaken to evaluate this signal by means of detailed questionnaires to the doctors of a random sample of patients from each cohort. The results confirmed an excess of angina in patients on bezafibrate but showed that this was due to confounding by indication. Bezafibrate had been prescribed preferentially for patients with diabetes mellitus and the number of patients with diabetes mellitus and also hypertension was significantly higher than for the other two drugs (Beggs *et al.*, 1999). These two conditions are risk factors for ischaemic heart disease and increase the likelihood of angina. Another example concerned neurological problems with amiodarone (Coulter, 1990).

Use of Prescription History

The evaluation of 50 reports coded as "tolerance" with sumatriptan was facilitated by having a longitudinal record of prescription data with the numbers of tablets or injections dispensed recorded for many patients over a period of several years. The reports described patients who claimed that over a period of months or years the drug did not work as well as it did initially and they required higher or more doses to relieve an attack of migraine, or the drug did not work at all. In the natural history of the disease there are fluctuations in frequency and severity of attacks and so these reports were difficult to interpret. It was felt that if there was any general trend to tolerance, then mean usage per patient over time would increase.

Table 27.8. Sumatriptan: mean numbers of injections (0.6 mg) dispensed per patient per six-month intervals.

Interval	Patients	Mean
2	1765	5.23
3	1372	5.87
4	1031	6.67
5	750	8.76
6	494	10.34
7	300	13.49
8	135	18.61
9	41	26.46

The prescription data were therefore analysed and the mean number of injections or tablets (100 mg equivalent) per patient per six-month interval was calculated. The results for those patients who had used injections only are shown in Table 27.8 over a period of eight intervals and an increase was demonstrated at each interval. The first interval was omitted because it would be a trial period of use and for many patients may not be typical of later use. The latest interval was also excluded because it may not have been complete. The slope of the changes was statistically significant for both the injections and the tablets, but the changes were more marked for the injections. There were no identifiable confounders (Coulter, DM, presentation at the 18th Annual Meeting of National Centres Participating in the WHO International Drug Monitoring Programme, Portugal, 1996).

OTHER USE OF DATA

REASSURANCE

IMMP data were used to reassure the Ministry of Health and the public following media scares related to suicidal ideation with fluoxetine (rates were compared with moclobemide) (MARC minutes 12 November 1991, 71st meeting) and death from sumatriptan as a result of myocardial infarction or stroke (Medsafe, 1996). IMMP data were found to be reassuring concerning a signal generated elsewhere of acute arthritis with omeprazole. Of the six drugs listed in Table 27.4, omeprazole had the second lowest rate of acute arthritis and the related events of arthralgia and synovitis (0.7 per 1000 patients). The rate for the other drugs ranged from 0.6 to 1.5 per 1000. These findings suggested that acute arthritis was no more common with omeprazole than with most other drugs and that the events recorded may represent the background incidence, or that along with the other drugs omeprazole may provoke the onset of acute arthritis uncommonly, but to no greater extent.

CONFIRMATION OF SIGNALS AND RISK COMPARISON

IMMP data were also used to confirm and further describe other signals generated elsewhere, e.g. fluoxetine and hyponatraemia (Pillans and Coulter, 1994) and urticaria with Multiload Cu375 (Coulter, 1997). Comparative risks, which are an aid to prescribing choice, have also been described (Coulter, 1992, 1996).

STUDIES USING IMMP DATA

Both the cohorts and the events data are available for special studies. One such study used patients from the IMMP with adverse reactions in a pharmacogenetic study. This was a pilot trial of methodology for genotyping patients with reactions and comparing them with a control group from a population of blood donors from the general population (Clark et al., 2000). An epidemiological study of the respiratory effects of ACE inhibitors was also undertaken (Wood, 1995).

PREGNANCY AND LACTATION

As a result of pro-active monitoring for foetal defects following maternal drug exposure to sumatriptan, the IMMP has records of outcomes in 26 pregnancies from 31 pregnancy exposures. This compares with 223 pregnancy outcomes in the international sumatriptan pregnancy registry managed by GlaxoWellcome (Eldridge and Ephross, 1999). There is no evidence that sumatriptan causes foetal defects. There are also 30 reports of outcome following lactation exposure. Again there is no evidence of a problem.

ROUTINE ANALYSIS OF DATA

Standard reports are prepared as follows for each drug studied:

- *Reporting rates*. For each drug monitored, rates per 1000 patients are calculated for the numbers of (1) reports, (2) all events, (3) reactions and (4) incidents, respectively, in total and by gender. If PEM is not conducted nation-wide, rates are also calculated by spontaneous and PEM regions. The overall reaction and incident rates are useful for comparing sub-groups and for between-drug comparisons, but in contrast to rates for individual events, do not provide a specific measure of risk because some patients have several events associated with the one report.
- *Age and gender distribution*. This is presented in tabular format with numbers and percentages and as a histogram.
- *Regional distribution*. This analysis demonstrates any differences in prescribing of the drug between administrative regions.
- *Dose distribution*. This provides a distribution table for the different common doses used at the time of the first and latest prescription. Dose analyses on latest prescriptions are performed only if there have been more than three prescriptions in order to assess the doses being prescribed at a time when treatment is likely to be stabilised. The mean doses are calculated for the first, latest and all prescriptions.
- *Duration of exposure*. The total exposure of the cohort is calculated in patient-years. The mean duration of exposure per patient is also calculated. This may be in terms of completed courses of therapy.
- *Indications for treatment*. These are presented for the whole cohort as numbers and percentages.
- *Reaction rates by dose*. The data are sorted by the standard dosages used and the overall reaction rates are presented for each dosage level.
- *Profile of adverse events*. This provides a table and histogram showing numbers and rates by system/organ class of reactions, incidents and all events, respectively.

- *Reasons for cessation of therapy*. This shows the frequency, proportion of total withdrawals and the rate for each category recorded (see above).
- *Most frequent events*. These are shown (usually the top 10) with numbers and rates together with the numbers and rates of withdrawals and deaths for these events.
- *Reactions with rates*. This provides a listing of all events assessed as reactions, showing the percentage of each within each system/organ class, the percentage of each reaction amongst all reports and the rate of occurrence of each reaction. These are sorted into clinical groupings within each class.
- *Table of all events*. This listing of all the individual events is presented by system/organ class and within the classes the events are sorted into clinically related groupings. This allows a clinically orientated visual assessment of the events reported and is useful in signal detection. It shows, for every event, the age and gender of the patient, the dose, the duration to onset and the relationship that was established at the time of the review of the report. It also shows deaths and withdrawals. The individual events can be cross referenced with the table of reports, which presents the events in the context of the whole reaction.
- *Table of reports*. This is a listing by report and shows all the events associated with each report, e.g. one report describing eosinophilia, arthralgia, malaise and rash with omeprazole, thus presenting the events in the context of the whole reaction. The age and gender for each patient is shown along with the dose, severity, relationship and outcome of each event.

THE IMPORTANCE OF QUOTING REPORTING RATES

The profiles of adverse events for a drug are different at high and low reporting rates. At specific rates of reporting, some events are more likely to be reported than others and, equally important, some are less likely to be reported. The IMMP provides a unique opportunity for comparing the rates of IMMP (intensified) spontaneous reporting of specific events with the rates from using PEM questionnaires. Angioedema/urticaria, extrapyramidal effects and blood dyscrasias were as likely to be reported spontaneously as with PEM. Conversely, cardiac dysrythmias, dry mouth, dyspepsia, constipation, death and events suggesting immunological disorders were, by comparison, very unlikely to be reported spontaneously. Other events ranged between these two extremes. It needs to be emphasised that this refers to IMMP "intensified" spontaneous reporting which has a higher rate of reporting than the standard spontaneous reporting programme in NZ. It follows therefore that studies on specific drugs are not comparable unless the reporting rates are similar. Similarly, rates of reporting may provide a guide as to what types of reactions may have been missed.

CONCLUSIONS

The IMMP is both pro-active and non-interventional, which offers a number of advantages. It is best suited for drugs newly released in order to gain early information, but can be used for the study of signals generated by spontaneous reporting (Coulter and Edwards, 1990). In the context of the IMMP, a much higher reporting rate is achieved with PEM methodology than with intensified spontaneous reporting. At times PEM is used only in certain regions and the programme then relies on intensified spontaneous reporting for the other regions. The information is gained in the "real world" of normal clinical practice where the use of drugs is subject to many influences not present in the artificial world of controlled clinical trials, e.g. the presence of diseases other than the one under study with the trial drug and the use of multiple drugs concurrently. It provides data that are not collected in the standard spontaneous reporting schemes, e.g. rates, but the two methods are complementary in pharmacovigilance. When a drug has more than one indication, this information is collected for the whole cohort and rates are calculated for each indication. The demographics of the cohort of patients prescribed the drugs are

routinely established, as are the doses used. Risk can be measured and risk factors identified. Observations can be made on the full range of patients, some not usually included in clinical trials—the young, the old, the pregnant. Some of these patients may be outside the age range for approved use. With longitudinal monitoring, trends in prescribing can be seen and there is a greater chance of identifying longer term outcomes or events such as pregnancy or death. Reasons for cessation of therapy provide information routinely on deaths, compliance and efficacy. Death rates can be calculated.

The IMMP is also highly adaptable. It has been used successfully to study drugs used long term for the treatment of chronic diseases and for drugs used intermittently, e.g. for the relief of migraine. It has also proved to be a good method for the study of the adverse effects of intra-uterine devices. The questionnaires can incorporate requests for specific information for particular drugs, e.g. severity of asthma, tests of liver function. The cohorts can be used for investigation of signals and there is potential for their use in the identification of reactions of long latency using record linkage.

The IMMP is not suitable for the study of rare reactions where very large cohorts are required to provide adequate statistical power. In these circumstances the method is not cost effective. Neither is it suited for drugs that are unlikely to be used widely, particularly if their use is restricted to small specialist groups or hospital inpatients.

The full safety profile of new drugs just released is unknown and it is to the benefit of all concerned to get good information on safety as quickly as possible. There is scope for PEM methodology to be used much more widely and pooled information from several centres would provide added value. Countries with a large population who feel unable to mount a national scheme, could use the method regionally. NZ has a population of only 3.8 million, but the IMMP has been able to produce results that have made a significant contribution to pharmacovigilance. Countries struggling to obtain a "worthwhile" number of reports from their spontaneous reporting programmes could switch resources to PEM studies of a few selected drugs.

Experience in NZ has shown that PEM stimulates awareness and interest in drug safety. An immediate effect of the IMMP was a doubling of the number of reports in the spontaneous reporting programme. The cost–benefit ratio of getting very good information on a small number of drugs important in a particular society would seem to be more favourable than getting very little information on a wide range of drugs. The cost of doing this is not high. Most of the IMMP work has been done on a budget of less than US$150 000 per annum providing for a half time physician and a small group of support staff. The use of modern information technology and simple epidemiological methods facilitates this cost effectiveness.

REFERENCES

Beggs PW, Clarke DWJ, Williams SM, Coulter DM (1999) A comparison of the use, effectiveness and safety of bezafibrate, gemfibrozil and simvastatin in normal clinical practice using the New Zealand Intensive Medicines Monitoring Programme (IMMP). *Br J Clin Pharmacol* **47**: 99–104.

Castellsague, Ashton J, Pethica D, Coulter DM (1999) Mortality among users of formoterol in the New Zealand Intensive Medicines Monitoring Programme [abstract]. *Am J Resp Crit Care Med* **159**(2): A136.

Clark D, Morgan A, Hananeia L, Coulter D, Olds R (2000) Drug metabolism genotypes and their association with adverse drug reactions in selected populations: a pilot study of methodology. *Pharmacoepidemiology and Drug Safety* **9**: 393–400.

Coulter DM (1979) A comparison of scalp tingling, thirst and polyuria in patients on labetalol and metoprolol. *NZ Med J* **90**: 397.

Coulter DM (1981) Study of reasons for cessation of therapy with perhexiline maleate, sodium valproate and labetalol in the intensified adverse drug reaction reporting scheme. *NZ Med J* **93**: 81–4.

Coulter DM (1986) Pilot trial in the use of duplicate prescription pads for the Intensified Adverse Drug Reaction Reporting Scheme. In: *Research Review*. Auckland: The Medical Research Council of New Zealand, pp. 180–1.

Coulter DM (1988) Eye pain with nifedipine and disturbance of taste with captopril: a mutually controlled study showing a method of postmarketing surveillance. *Br Med J* **296**: 1086–8.

Coulter DM (1990) Survey of neurological problems with amiodarone in the New Zealand Intensive Medicines Monitoring Programme. *NZ Med J* **103**: 98–100.

Coulter DM (1992) Intensive Medicines Monitoring Programme: bezafibrate, gemfibrozil and simvastatin. *NZ Family Physician* **19**(1): 30.

Coulter DM (1996) Moclobemide and fluoxetine compared. *NZ Family Physician* **23**(6): 39–40.

Coulter DM (1997) Top ten adverse reactions with Multiload Cu375 in the IMMP. *Prescriber Update* **Aug**(15): 37–40.

Coulter DM (1998) The New Zealand Intensive Medicines Monitoring Programme. *Pharmacoepidemiology and Drug Safety* **7**: 79–90.

Coulter DM (2000) The New Zealand Intensive Medicines Monitoring Programme in pro-active safety surveillance. *Pharmacoepidemiology and Drug Safety* **9**: 273–80.

Coulter DM, Edwards IR (1987) Cough associated with captopril and enalapril. *Br Med J* **294**: 1521–3.

Coulter DM, Edwards IR (1990) Mianserin and agranulocytosis in New Zealand. *Lancet* **336**: 785–7.

Coulter DM, McQueen EG (1982) Post marketing surveillance: achievements and problems in the Intensified Adverse Drug Reaction Reporting Scheme. *NZ Family Physician* **1**: 13–7.

Coulter DM, Pillans P (1993) Angiotensin-converting enzyme inhibitors and psoriasis [letter]. *NZ Med J* **106**: 392–3.

Coulter DM, Pillans P (1995a) Fluoxetine and extrapyramidal side effects. *Am J Psychiatry* **152**: 122–5.

Coulter DM, Pillans PI (1995b) Hypertension with moclobemide [letter]. *Lancet* **346**: 1032.

Crane J, Flatt A, Jackson R, Ball M, Pearce N, Burgess C, *et al.* (1989) Prescribed fenoterol and death from asthma in New Zealand 1981–83: case–control study. *Lancet* **i**: 917–22.

Department of Health (1979) Perhexiline maleate (Pexid). *Clinical Services Letter*, No. 190, 12 November, p. 3.

Department of Health (1980) Perhexiline maleate (Pexid). *Clinical Services Letter*, No. 192, 11 March, p. 2.

Edwards IR, Coulter DM (1989) ACE inhibitors and anaemia [letter]. *NZ Med J* **102**: 325.

Edwards IR, Coulter DM, Macintosh D (1992) Intestinal effects of captopril. *Br Med J* **304**: 359–60.

Eldridge RR, Ephross SA (1999) International sumatriptan pregnancy registry: interim results. *Cephalalgia* **19**: 420.

Graham JR (1992) Gastric polyposis: onset during long-term therapy with omeprazole. *Med J Aust* **157**: 287–8.

Inman WH (1981a) Postmarketing surveillance of adverse drug reactions in general practice I. Search for new methods. *Br Med J* **282**: 1131–2.

Inman WH (1981b) Postmarketing surveillance of adverse drug reactions in general practice II.

Prescription-event monitoring at the University of Southampton. *Br Med J* **282**: 1216–7.

McQueen EG (1977) Intensified adverse drug reaction reporting scheme [letter]. *NZ Med J* **85**: 296–7.

McQueen EG (1982) Drug safety monitoring using recorded release and results with sodium valproate. *Adv Pharmacol Therapeutics II* **6**: 79–89.

Medsafe (1996) Sumatriptan in the media. *Prescriber Update* **July** (12): 7.

Meyboom RHB, Royer RJ (1992) Causality classification at pharmacovigilance centres in the European Community. *Pharmacoepidemiology and Drug Safety* **1**: 87–97.

Pillans PI, Coulter DM (1994) Fluoxetine and hyponatraemia—a potential hazard in the elderly. *NZ Med J* **107**: 85–6.

Pillans PI, Coulter DM, Black P (1996) Angioedema and urticaria with angiotensin converting enzyme inhibitors. *Eur J Clin Pharmacol* **51**: 123–6.

Schenk BE, Kuiipers EJ, Klinkenberg-Knol EC, Eskes SA, Bloemena E, *et al.* (1997) Gastric polyps during long-term omeprazole treatment for gastro-oesophageal reflux disease. *Eur J Gastro Hepatol* **9**(12): A2–A3.

Skegg DCG, Doll R (1977) Frequency of eye complaints and rashes among patients receiving practolol and propranolol. *Lancet* **ii**: 475–8.

Wood R (1995) Bronchospasm and cough as adverse reactions to the ACE inhibitors captopril, enalapril and lisinopril. A controlled retrospective cohort study. *Br J Clin Pharmacol* **39**: 265–70.

Woods DJ, Coulter DM, Pillans P (1994) Interaction of phenytoin and fluoxetine [letter]. *NZ Med J* **107**: 19.

28

MEMO in the UK

DOUGLAS STEINKE
Primary Care Information Group, Information and Statistics Division, Edinburgh, UK
JOSIE M.M. EVANS AND THOMAS M. MACDONALD
Medicines Monitoring Unit, University of Dundee, Ninewells Hospital and Medical School, Dundee, UK

INTRODUCTION

The Medicines Monitoring Unit (MEMO) is a University-based organisation that has access to data generated within the UK National Health Service (NHS). MEMO uses record-linkage techniques to carry out studies to detect and quantify adverse effects of drugs in the community. Currently, MEMO utilises data from the Tayside region of Scotland, which is geographically compact and serves over 400 000 patients. A computerised record of all patients registered with a general practitioner and inpatient hospital morbidity and mortality data are available to MEMO and form the backbone of the record-linkage system.

Although MEMO was originally set up for pharmacoepidemiologic research and this is still the main focus of its research activities, recent advances mean that studies in outcomes research, general epidemiology and health economics are also possible.

DESCRIPTION OF THE DATABASE

Every person who is registered with a General Practitioner (GP) in Scotland is allocated a 10-digit unique patient identifying number called a Community Health Index (CHI) number. The CHI database contains additional demographic information such as patient's address (including postal code), GP registered with, and date of death (if applicable). For practical purposes, the entire Tayside population is registered with a GP and thus appears in the central computerised records of the Community Health Master Patient Index. Once patients are allocated a CHI number it is never re-allocated so record-linkage of medical data over a large number of years is possible.

The CHI number is used as the patient identifier for all healthcare activities in primary and secondary care in Tayside. The patient-specific number allows for efficient linkage of records of patient activity and outcome.

Pharmacovigilance. Edited by R.D. Mann and E.B. Andrews

PRESCRIPTION DRUG DATA

After a patient receives a prescription from his/her doctor, the patient takes it to the community pharmacy where it is dispensed. Dispensed prescriptions are then sent to the Pharmacy Practice Division (PPD) of the Information and Statistics Division of the Common Services Agency to obtain reimbursement and dispensing fees. After paying the pharmacists and dealing with any appeals, PPD sends the cashed prescription forms to MEMO. GP prescribing information is captured by MEMO by a unique menu driven computer system, which links the prescribing information with the CHI number database (Figure 28.1). Using this system, it is possible to allocate the CHI number from the patient details on the prescription.

All items from the prescription are entered and stored on a database for research purposes. The date the prescription was written as well as the GP that prescribed the medication is recorded. The drug prescribed is entered via a "drop-down menu" to ensure product availability and to avoid miscoding of preparation and spelling errors.

Both generic and proprietary names are used so the ability to differentiate between product types is available. The total amount of drug dispensed is also entered together with the dosing instructions, thus allowing the duration of any prescription to be calculated. Community prescribing data have been entered for selected medications from January 1989 (notably non-steroidal anti-inflammatory drugs, ulcer healing drugs, lipid-lowering drugs and hormone replacement therapy) and all prescribed medications from January 1993. MEMO now has records of 15 million prescriptions dispensed in Tayside up to December 1996.

HOSPITAL DATA

Since 1961, all hospitals in Scotland have been required to compile and return coded information on all acute inpatient admissions, forming the basis of the Scottish Morbidity Record 1 (SMR1), which contains administrative, demographic and diagnostic information. In Tayside this is coded by medical clerks before being entered onto computer and subjected to quality control. The data are then sent to the Information and Statistics Division (ISD) of the Common Services Agency of the National Health Service. Each SMR1 record has one principal and five other diagnostic fields coded according to the International Classification of Diseases 9th Revision (ICD9) (World Health Organisation, 1977). In 1996, the NHS introduced the 10th Revision of the ICD codes (World Health Organisation, 1992). There is also one main operation or procedure field and three others coded according to the Office of Population and Census Surveys 4th Revision (OPCS4) classification (HMSO, 1990). In Tayside, there are approximately 63 000 hospital discharges per year available as a CHI number specific record. MEMO holds historical SMR1 data from 1980 allowing for a past medical history of hospitalisation for a condition to be controlled (Figure 28.1).

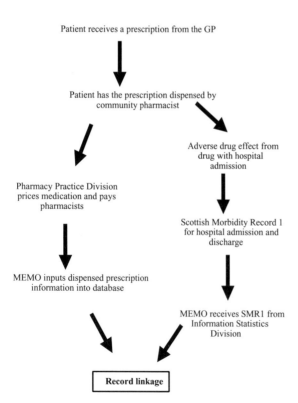

Figure 28.1. Schematic of record-linkage of data.

OTHER IN-HOSPITAL AND OUTCOME DATA SETS

Any healthcare data set that is indexed by the CHI number can be linked to MEMO's record-linkage database, including other Scottish Morbidity Record returns supplied by the ISD. In MEMO, commonly used data sets are the cancer registration database (SMR6), child development records, maternity records (SMR2), psychiatric records (SMR4), and neonatal discharges (SMR11).

RECORD-LINKAGE OF OTHER DATABASES

Most of primary and secondary care use the CHI number as the patient identifier; however, if data do not have CHI numbers, these can be allocated from patient demographic details, such as name, date of birth and postcode. MEMO can identify the correct CHI number for a very high proportion of patients in the database. This is the same method as is employed to allocate CHI numbers to prescription data. MEMO has constructed a database of 100 000 endoscopy and colonoscopy procedures, and, in collaboration with Tayside Police, subjects involved in 22 000 road traffic accidents in Tayside using this allocation procedure.

CLINICAL LABORATORY DATA

Clinical laboratory investigations for the Tayside region since 1989 are held on a computerised archive in the Department of Biochemical Medicine in Ninewells Hospital. The database has CHI-specific biochemical, haematology, microbiology, virology and serology laboratory results and reports. CHI-specific results from all pathology investigations since 1990 for Tayside are electronically stored in MEMO. These data can be record-linked to the MEMO database to complete the clinical characteristics of disease or hospital admission.

PRIMARY CARE DATA

Progressively more GPs are using computerised systems to aid in patient management, although at present they are not available to MEMO for record-linkage. However, it is possible to abstract written records in primary care manually and research nurses in MEMO have been granted access to primary care records for specific studies (Morris et al., 1997a; Evans et al., 1998).

OTHER INFORMATION

Since all patients and their addresses are known, including postcode, and information is available from the decennial census regarding the relative deprivation levels of postcode areas, the so-called Carstairs deprivation score can be used as a relatively crude indicator of the socioeconomic status of patients (Carstairs, 1990; Evans et al., 1997a). The deprivation category component variables are the percentage of people in a postcode sector with no car, the percentage living in overcrowded housing, the percentage with the household head in semi- or unskilled occupations, and the percentage of men unemployed.

Details of all deaths in Tayside since 1989 are electronically recorded through a copy of the General Registers Office—Death Certification Database and held within MEMO. The date and underlying cause of death can be identified and linked to the MEMO database using the CHI number of the patient.

CURRENT AREAS OF INVESTIGATION

DRUG SAFETY RESEARCH

Numerous drug safety studies have been completed in MEMO. For example, the cohort study design has been used to evaluate the risk profile of non-steroidal anti-inflammatory drugs (NSAIDs). Although the increased risk of upper gastrointestinal complications associated with NSAID use is well-established (Hawkey, 1990), the large number of study subjects and the additional information available in MEMO has allowed more detailed investigations. For example, a cohort study among 78 191 patients newly exposed to NSAIDs and 78 207 unexposed comparators, showed that there was an increased risk only among patients without a history of upper gastrointestinal events (McMahon et al., 1997). Another study in 50 000 subjects investigated the risk with duration of use, and found that it remained constant with continuous exposure (MacDonald et al., 1997) in contrast to previous findings (Carson et al., 1987).

The case–control method is an efficient study design requiring fewer subjects than cohort studies. This is an important consideration when a study involves validating information by checking the original medical notes of patients. The case–control design has been used in a range of studies investigating the adverse effect profile of topical NSAIDs. These studies found that oral NSAIDs, but not topical NSAIDs, are implicated in hospitalisation for upper gastrointestinal haemorrhage and perforation (Evans et al., 1995a), acute renal failure (Evans et al., 1995b) and acute colitis (Evans et al., 1997b), but that they are unlikely to be associated with acute appendicitis (Evans et al., 1997c).

The case–crossover design was employed in a study examining the risks of road traffic accidents associated with benzodiazepine use (Barbone et al., 1998). This design is suitable for the evaluation of transient risks, and because cases are used as their own controls, problems of confounding can be dealt with neatly.

DRUG UTILISATION RESEARCH

MEMO is able to produce detailed drug utilisation data, broken down by age, sex, date, day of week prescribed, prescriber, generic or proprietary dispensing, co-prescribing, acute prescribing and/or repeat prescribing, dose, and duration. One important dimension is the audit of GP prescribing in the population, although GP-specific data are analysed anonymously and individual GPs are never identified. For example, one study identified rare instances of potentially hazardous co-prescribing of β-antagonists and β-agonists to patients in Tayside likely to have asthma or chronic obstructive airways disease, by linking the dispensed prescribing database to hospital admission records (Hayes et al., 1996). The processing of prescribing data according to the demographic characteristics of prescribing GPs

has also yielded some useful insights into the characteristics of "good" prescribers. For example, a difference in the prescribing of antibiotics was seen between GP registrar training and non-training practices (Steinke et al., 2000).

VARIATION IN PRESCRIBING AND MEDICATION COMPLIANCE

Prescribing may vary by patient factors that are independent of need or disease severity. For example, the variation of use of hormone replacement therapy by socio-economic status independent of need (Evans et al., 1997a). Compliance to labelled medication direction or therapy is a related issue. By assessing how patients collect dispensed medication, in terms of numbers of prescriptions dispensed and intervals between them, and linking to outcome data sets, patient compliance or non-compliance to medication can be studied. For example, a study in diabetes showed that adolescents in Tayside who have "brittle" diabetes are often non-compliant with insulin (Morris et al., 1997b).

PHARMACOECONOMICS AND HEALTH RESOURCE USE

Pharmacoepidemiology studies often have a pharmacoeconomic analysis "attached" to the protocol. Both methods have specific objectives that are clearly defined and apparently independent. Pharmacoeconomic analyses have become more widely used over the past 10 years. Their primary use is for selecting more efficient drugs; in other words, those exhibiting a better relationship between acquisition cost and therapeutic effects and/or economic benefits. Pharmacoeconomic studies use the tools of clinical pharmacology, epidemiology and economics to obtain data on the effects (beneficial or harmful) of drugs and the costs of treatment alternatives.

MEMO has the ability to identify the drug, type of medication (either generic or proprietary), strength, amount and directions for use and therefore can accurately cost the medication for cost analyses. For example, a comparison of the use and cost of self-monitoring reagent strips and patterns of drug use by type 1 and type 2 diabetics was investigated by Evans et al. (1999, 2000). Both studies found a difference between the diabetes type and the cost of medication and health resource use.

CHRONIC DISEASES EPIDEMIOLOGY AND AUDIT

Diabetes Audit and Research in Tayside, Scotland (DARTS)

The MEMO/DARTS collaboration is a joint initiative of the Department of Medicine and MEMO at the University of Dundee, together with the Diabetes Units at three Tayside Health Care Trusts (Ninewells Hospital and Medical School, Dundee; Perth Royal Infirmary and Stracathro Hospital, Brechin) and all Tayside GPs with an interest in diabetes care. They have combined their expertise to create the Diabetes Audit and Research in Tayside, Scotland (DARTS) initiative (Morris et al., 1997a). It has been in operation since 1995, continually developing and gathering data from the population base of Tayside.

The MEMO/DARTS collaboration has used electronic record-linkage of information to create a robust clinical information system of all patients with type 1 and type 2 diabetes in Tayside whether they attend primary or secondary care. The DARTS database has information from many different sources including: patients attending hospital diabetes clinics, dispensed prescriptions for diabetes-related medication and monitoring equipment, patients discharged from hospital, patients attending a community-based mobile diabetic eye screening facility, glycosylated haemoglobin and plasma glucose results from the regional biochemistry database, and information collected from case records of patients in every general practice in Tayside. The register has been used for pharmaco-epidemiologic research (Morris et al., 1997b, 1997c).

Epidemiology of Liver Disease in Tayside (ELDIT)

The Epidemiology of Liver Disease in Tayside (ELDIT) study group has registered and validated a group of patients with potential and definite liver

disease in Tayside for research purposes only. This disease register has a range of liver diseases that affect the whole organ including viral hepatitis (A, B and C) (Steinke et al., 2000b), autoimmune hepatitis, alcoholic liver disease (Steinke et al., 2000c), primary biliary cirrhosis and hepatocellular carcinoma (Weston et al., 2000) and complications of liver disease like ascites. The ascertainment of liver disease by electronic record-linkage was maximised because of the unique integration of multiple sources of data to create a patient-specific information system. The specificity of virology, immunology and biochemistry tests increase the completeness of the data. Accurate incidence and prevalence rates of liver disease and its complications are used to ensure that hepatology services run effectively and efficiently.

Heart-disease, Evidence-based Audit and Research in Tayside, Scotland (HEARTS)

The latest addition to MEMO's disease management databases is the HEARTS database of cardiovascular disease in Tayside. This is a regional collaborative effort to support improvements in clinical care, education and research in cardiovascular disease and to provide GPs with information that will be useful for audit and clinical governance purposes. The database contains information on high-risk patient populations like those who have suffered a myocardial infarction (MI) and those who have undergone coronary angioplasty or artery bypass grafting (CABG). The database includes a variety of other cardiovascular diseases. For example, those with angina pectoris, peripheral vascular disease, ischaemic stroke, cardiac failure, hypertension and those undergoing primary prevention for cardiovascular disease. The aims of HEARTS are to identify and determine the risk factors of cardiovascular disease from a population base and to evaluate and determine whether medications are optimised in these patients. This information is fed back in various ways to GP practices in an effort to support them in improving care. HEARTS also provides high quality epidemiological data for research, understanding and care of similar patients and their families.

CONFIDENTIALITY AND ETHICS IN MEMO

Studies in MEMO use highly confidential, although anonymised, medical data. MEMO has an agreement with the Local Medical Committee of the British Medical Association never to divulge person-specific or GP-specific data, unless it is to a doctor requesting information on one of his or her own patients. All staff in MEMO sign confidentiality agreements and all databases are registered for research purposes with the Data Protection Officer. All studies in MEMO use de-identified data. The anonymisation process uses a randomly selected number mapped to the CHI number. The random number then becomes the link between databases. The Data Protection Officer is the only person that holds the mapping key. Ethics committees and Caldicott Guardians must approve study protocols before each study begins. Approved studies are logged in MEMO and may be audited by Caldicott Guardians at anytime. Any changes to a study protocol require resubmission to the ethics and Caldicott Guardians for approval of the change. As data protection and ethical issues continue to evolve, MEMO will ensure that it meets the standards in both these areas (Data Protection Act, 1998).

STRENGTHS

PATIENT IDENTIFICATION

One of the greatest advantages with using data from Tayside is the unique patient identifier. This allows for relative ease of record-linkage and generation of comparator groups from the population. Selection of patients for both cohort and case–control studies is efficient.

POPULATION-BASED DATA

MEMO is regularly supplied with updated copies of the Community Health Master Patient Index from the Tayside Health Board, and uses this to track the population of patients alive and resident in Tayside to define study populations for drug safety studies. Such population-based data allow the calculation of incidence rates, excess risk, and attributable risk.

DRUG EXPOSURE DATA

The data captured at MEMO represent prescriptions that have been dispensed at a pharmacy and so primary non-compliance is eliminated. In a study carried out to assess the extent of primary non-compliance in Tayside, a large family practice (11 500 patients) wrote all prescriptions in duplicate (carbon copy) form over a three-month period (Beardon et al., 1993). The copies were sent to MEMO. The original top-copy forms that were redeemed by the patients at community pharmacies were also returned to MEMO by PPD. Duplicate forms for which no original was present represented the prescriptions that were not redeemed.

A further advantage of Tayside is that there is currently no structure to inhibit the prescribing of newly marketed drugs. Thus, studies of new agents that penetrate the market at a high rate are possible.

ACCESSIBILITY TO MEDICAL RECORDS

A major strength of MEMO is the ability to examine original hospital records where necessary. Several studies validating the computerised diagnostic data with the case records have been carried out, with variable results depending on the criteria used (Kohli and Knill-Jones, 1992; Park et al., 1992; Pears et al., 1992). Within the National Health Service, such case record searching for the purposes of drug safety evaluation is ethically permissible once Medical Ethics Committee approval from the Caldicott guardians has been obtained (HMSO, 1992).

WEAKNESSES

The current population of Tayside is approximately 400 000 people and is comparatively small, even for the study of commonly prescribed drugs. However, drug exposure data in Tayside are only available from 1989 and cover only a limited set of drugs until January 1993 from when all dispensed prescriptions have been collected. Scottish doctors are conservative prescribers of new drugs, so new agents tend to penetrate the market a few years after their launch. This limits the ability to study new chemical entities, arguably the most important and interesting drug group to study. Offsetting these disadvantages, the profile of certain diseases, for example cardiovascular disease, is higher in Scotland than in other populations and consequently the prescribing of drugs used in the prevention and treatment of these diseases is proportionately higher.

Another weakness, but one that is common to many drug safety databases, is the inability to capture directly exposure to over-the-counter drugs or drugs prescribed in hospital. Perhaps more importantly, the diagnostic indication for prescribing is not available to the researcher. In some cases, the indication for drug use may be clear; for example, glyceryl trinitrate is used primarily for angina. However, difficulties arise when a drug has more than one indication for use, leading to misclassification of exposure or outcome. For example, beta andreoceptor blocking drugs can be given for indications varying from anxiety to hypertophic cardiomyopathy. This may be a potential source of error called confounding-by-indication that is difficult to adjust for in pharmacoepidemiologic research if the information is not available.

MEMO cannot contact patients directly to elicit information on possible confounding factors. However, with Ethical Committee approval GPs can do this in a collaborative manner. Primary care and hospital records can also be checked and some data on smoking and alcohol can be retrieved from them, although the quality does vary (Evans *et al.*, 1998). This is also a method to identify outpatient diagnoses, which are not available electronically for record-linkage in MEMO. MEMO is therefore currently best suited for the study of serious drug toxicity that requires hospital admission.

One of the criticisms levelled at record-linkage studies is the inaccuracy of computerised medical diagnoses. The discharge diagnoses for SMR1 are abstracted from the clinical discharge summaries by specially trained coding clerks. These clerks on occasions have to interpret the "soft diagnoses", such as symptoms, for which no cause can be found. In addition, non-standard terminology may be employed to describe an illness, for example eponymous terms, and so the coding of diagnoses may be imprecise. Computerised algorithms exist to detect and reject the most glaring errors, but errors of interpretation persist within any database. Several validation studies of the accuracy of hospital discharge data in Scotland have been performed comparing the coded diagnoses with diagnoses inferred by one or more senior doctors who have reviewed the original case records (Kohli and Knill-Jones, 1992; Park *et al.*, 1992; Pears *et al.*, 1992). The most pertinent of those studies carried out on Tayside data found 18% of internal medicine diagnoses to be clinically unacceptable (Pears *et al.*, 1992). Since the publication of this study, steps have been taken, mainly for resource management reasons, to improve the diagnostic accuracy of computerised data by involving clinicians in quality control. This initiative has substantially improved the diagnostic accuracy of records.

FUTURE DEVELOPMENTS IN MEMO

Dispensed prescribing data collection in MEMO is labour-intensive and expensive. The automated capture of computerised dispensed prescribing data has been investigated in five test pharmacies, a method that could eventually become Tayside wide or Scottish wide (McGilchrist and MacDonald, 1996). Of 200 000 prescription items from which data were collected using this methodology, a comparison with a sample of duplicate data collected by MEMO in the usual way showed that there was agreement for 98% of the items.

CONCLUSION

In conclusion, MEMO is a comprehensive record-linkage system that can be used for the detection and quantification of serious drug toxicity, outcomes research and pharmacoeconomic studies.

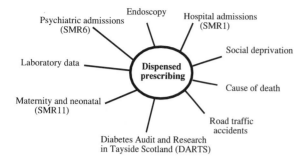

Figure 28.2. Data available to MEMO for record-linking.

The realisation of disease management also strengthens the capabilities of MEMO. Figure 28.2 summarises the record-linked data sets that are available in MEMO.

REFERENCES

Barbone F, McMahon AD, Davey PG, Morris AD, Reid IC, McDevitt DG, MacDonald TM (1998) Association of road-traffic accidents with benzodiazepine use. *Lancet* **352**: 1331–6.

Beardon PHG, McGilchrist MM, McKendrick AD, McDevitt DG, MacDonald TM (1993) Primary non-compliance with prescribed medication in general practice. *Br Med J* **307**: 846–8.

Carson JL, Stron BL, Soper KA, West SL, Morse L (1987) The association of non-steroids anti-inflammatory drugs with upper gastrointestinal tract bleeding. *Arch Intern Med* **147**: 85–8.

Carstairs V (1990) Deprivation and health in Scotland. *Health Bull (Edinburgh)* **8**: 162–75.

Data Protection Act (1998) *Chapter 29*. London: The Stationery Office Limited.

Evans JMM, McMahon AD, McGilchrist MM, White G, Murray FE, McDevitt DG, MacDonald TM (1995a) Topical non-steroids anti-inflammatory drugs and admission to hospital for upper gastrointestinal bleeding and perforation: a record-linkage case–control study. *Br Med J* **311**: 22–6.

Evans JMM, McGregor E, McMahon AD, McGilchrist MM, Jones MC, White G, McDevitt DG, MacDonald TM (1995b) Non-steroids anti-inflammatory drugs and hospitalisation for acute renal failure. *Q J Med* **88**: 551–7.

Evans JMM, Orr C, Duncan ID, MacDonald TMM (1997) Use of hormone replacement therapy in the community. Could this be improved? *Pharmacoepidemiology and Drug Safety* **6**: S81.

Evans JMM, McMahon AD, Murray FE, McDevitt DG, MacDonald TM (1997b) Non-steroids anti-inflammatory drugs are associated with emergency hospitalisation for colitis due to inflammatory bowel disease. *Gut* **40**: 619–22.

Evans JMM, MacGregor A, Murray FE, Vaidya K, Morris AD, MacDonald TM (1997c) No association between non-steroids anti-inflammatory drugs and acute appendicitis: a case–control study. *Br J Surgery* **84**: 372–4.

Evans JMM, McMahon AD, Steinke DT, McAlpine RR, MacDonald TM (1998) Do H_2-receptor antagonists cause acute pancreatitis? *Pharmacoepidemiology and Drug Safety* **7**: 383–8.

Evans JMM, Newton RW, Ruta DA, MacDonald TM, Stevenson RJ, Morris AD (1999) Frequency of blood glucose monitoring in relation to glycaemic control: observational study with diabetes database. *Br Med J* **319**: 83–6.

Evans JMM, Ruta DA, MacDonald TM, Leese G, Morris AD (2000) Impact of type 1 and type 2 diabetes on patterns and costs of drug prescribing. *Diabetes Care* **23**: 770–4.

Hawkey CJ (1990) Non-steroids anti-inflammatory drugs and peptic ulcers. Facts and figures multiply, but do they add up? *Br Med J* **300**: 278–84.

Hayes JL, Evans JMM, Lipworth BP, MacDonald TM (1996) Potentially hazardous co-prescribing of β-adrenoceptor antagonists and agonists in the community. *Br J Gen Practice* **46**: 423–5.

HMSO (1990) *Office of Population Censuses and Surveys. Tabular List of the Classification of Surgical Operations and Procedures, Fourth Revision.* London: HMSO.

HMSO (1992) *The Scottish Office, Home and Health Department. Local Research Ethics Committees*, Vol. 9: Edinburgh. London: HMSO.

Kohli HS, Knill-Jones RP (1992) How accurate are SMR1 (Scottish Morbidity Record 1) data? *Health Bull* **50**: 14–23.

MacDonald TM, Morant SV, Robinson GC, Shield MJ, McGilchrist MM, White G, Murray FE, McDevitt DG (1997) The upper gastrointestinal toxicity of non-steroids anti-inflammatory drugs is constant with continued exposure. *Br Med J* **315**: 1333–7.

McGilchrist MM, MacDonald TM (1996) Automatic capture of community prescribing. *Pharmacoepidemiology and Drug Safety* **5**: S37.

McMahon AD, Evans JMM, White G Murray FE, McGilchrist MM, McDevitt DG, MacDonald TM (1997) A cohort study (with re-sampled comparator groups) to measure the association between new NSAID prescribing and upper gastrointestinal haemorrhage and perforation. *J Clin Epidemiol* **50**: 351–6.

Morris AD, Boyle DIR, MacAlpine R, Emslie-Smith A, Jung RT, Newton RW, MacDonald TM (1997a) The diabetes audit and research in Tayside Scotland (DARTS) study: electronic record-linkage to create a diabetes register. *Br Med J* **315**: 524–8.

Morris AD, Boyle DIR, McMahon AD, Greene SA, MacDonald TM, Newton RW (1997b) Adherence to insulin treatment, glycaemic control and ketoacidosis in insulin dependent diabetes mellitus. *Lancet* **350**: 1505–10.

Morris AD, Boyle DIR, McMahon AD, Pearce H, Evans JMM, Newton RW, Jung RT, MacDonald TM (1997c) ACE inhibitor use is associated with hospitalisation for severe hypoglycemia in patients with diabetes. *Diabetes Care* **20**: 1363–7.

Park RHR, McCabe P, Russell RI (1992) Who should log the Ships? The accuracy of Scottish Hospital Morbidity Data for Wilson's Disease. *Health Bull* **50**: 24–8.

Pears J, Alexander V, Alexander GF, Waugh NR (1992) Audit of the quality of hospital discharge data. *Health Bull* **50**: 356–61.

Steinke DT, Bain DJD, MacDonald TM, Davey PG (2000a) Practice factors that influence antibiotic prescribing in general practice in Tayside. *J Antimicrob Chemother* **46**: 509–12.

Steinke DT, Weston T, Morris A, MacDonald TM, Dillon JF (2000b) Population-based epidemiology of vial hepatitis. *Gut* **46** (Suppl II): A60.

Steinke DT, Weston T, Morris A, MacDonald TM, Dillon JF (2000c) Population-based epidemiology of alcoholic liver disease. *Gut* **46** (Suppl II): W54.

Weston T, Steinke D, MacDonald T, Morris A, Dillon J (2000) The incidence of liver and intrahepatic bile duct cancer in Tayside, Scotland: a population-based cohort study. *Gut* **46** (Suppl II): A62.

World Health Organisation (1977) *International Classification of Diseases. Manual of the International Statistical Classification of Diseases, Injuries and Causes of Death, Ninth Revision*, Vol. 1. Geneva: WHO.

World Health Organisation (1992) *ICD-10. International Statistical Classification of Diseases and Related Health Problems, Tenth Revision*. Geneva: WHO.

29

GPRD in the UK

LOUISE WOOD

General Practice Research Database Division, Medicines Control Agency, London, UK

INTRODUCTION

The General Practice Research Database (GPRD) is the world's largest computerised database of anonymised longitudinal patient records from general practice and a unique public health research tool, which has been used widely for pharmacoepidemiological studies. Several issues have threatened the viability of the database in recent years and in April 1999 responsibility for its management and financial control was transferred to the UK Medicines Control Agency (MCA). An overview of the database, the MCA's new services and future vision for the GPRD are presented in this chapter.

HISTORICAL OVERVIEW

The GPRD was created in June 1987 as the Value Added Medical Products (VAMP) Research Databank. VAMP provided computerised general practitioner (GP) software and enabled GPs to contribute anonymised data to a central database for subsequent use in public health research. Subsequent to acquiring VAMP in 1993, Reuters Health Information donated the research database to the UK Department of Health in 1994 stipulating that the database be used exclusively for medical and public health research on a non-profit-making basis. It was at this stage that the database was renamed GPRD. UK Health Ministers decided that the database should be self-financing and a licensing system was introduced whereby licencees paid a fee of £500 000 per annum. From 1994 until October 1999, the database was managed by the Department's Statistics Division and operated by the Office for National Statistics (ONS) (Lawson et al., 1998).

Data for the GPRD are collected from GPs using practice software supplied by In Practice Systems® (InPS) formally known as VAMP. Initially, this was restricted to the DOS VAMP Medical software but in 1995 the Microsoft Windows-based Vision software was introduced. The GPRD which researchers are familiar with comprises data solely from GPs using the VAMP Medical software. Although software was developed for collecting data from practices using Vision software, the licence fees did not generate sufficient revenues to allow modification of the GPRD to load and integrate data from these practices. Hence, several years of data were collected but not made available to researchers. The situation was exacerbated as the millennium approached and many practices began upgrading to Vision or other non In Practice Systems GP software. Doubts were cast on the future viability of the database.

Management responsibility for the database was transferred to the MCA in April 1999. The existing VAMP Medical GPRD database and its operating staff were transferred to the MCA in October 1999 when work commenced on developing the new "Full Feature" GPRD. The MCA has invested £3 million in the GPRD to secure its future viability and utility, with an initial priority of making the data collected from Vision practices available to researchers. It recognises the GPRD as a critical resource to support drug development and post-licensing activities and a superb public health research tool, which it wishes to see used more widely.

CURRENT USAGE OF GPRD

At present, data are collected from 3 million patients from practices throughout the United Kingdom, representing approximately 5% of the UK population. More than 35 million patient-years worth of data are available to researchers, and this will increase when the totality of data collected to date are aggregated.

Contributing GPs are provided with guidelines that define what information should be recorded electronically for GPRD purposes:

- Demographics, including age and sex of patient
- Medical diagnosis, including comments
- All prescriptions
- Events leading to withdrawal of a drug or treatment
- Referrals to hospitals or specialists
- Treatment outcomes, including hospital discharge reports where patients are referred to hospital for treatment
- Miscellaneous patient care information, e.g. smoking status, height, weight, immunisations, lab results
- Date and cause of death
- Pregnancy-related information.

It should be recognised, however, that GPs are using their computers primarily to create electronic medical records for the purpose of managing their patients. GPRD is a "spin-off" and the completeness of data recording by practices is variable. Nevertheless, several published studies have demonstrated a high degree of data completeness.

The GPRD is used by researchers internationally in academia, the pharmaceutical industry, regulatory authorities, the National Health Service and UK Government Departments. The GPRD Scientific and Ethical Advisory Group (SEAG) reviews protocols to ensure protection of patient confidentiality and to determine whether the researchers have a well-defined hypothesis, will be using appropriate methodology for the proposed study, and have taken into consideration possible bias and confounding. The membership and terms of reference for SEAG are currently under review.

An analysis of the 350 protocols submitted to SEAG by the end of 2000 revealed that the GPRD was being used for the following types of studies: pharmacoepidemiology 49%; disease epidemiology 32%; drug utilisation 11%; pharmacoeconomics 7%; and environmental hazards 1%. The GPRD is also being used to support delivery of the UK National Health Service Plan, e.g. by identifying inequalities in treated heart disease and mental health (Moser, 2001) and to examine time trends in outpatient referrals (Hodgson and Ellis, 2001) to assess likely future demand for hospital services. Consideration is being given to how it can support clinical and genomic/pharmacogenomic research in the United Kingdom. Over 200 papers have been published in peer reviewed journals testifying to the quality of the data. A bibliography can be found on the GPRD website (www.gprd.com).

USE OF THE GPRD FOR PHARMACOVIGILANCE

To date, use of the GPRD in pharmacovigilance has focused on hypothesis testing (see García Rodriguez and Gutthann, 1998, for review). Hershel Jick and his colleagues at the Boston Collaborative Drug Surveillance Programme pioneered the use of the GPRD for pharmacoepidemiology over a decade ago. Today, regulatory authorities and the research-based pharmaceutical industry in Europe and the United States rely on data from GPRD to strengthen or refute signals of safety hazards, to quantify risk, and identify risk factors. Consequently, studies in GPRD have been instrumental in influencing regulatory action to restrict the use of medicines or to provide reassurance about their safety in the face of spurious signals.

There is heightened awareness of the promise which resources such as GPRD offer for signal generation. The implementation of powerful databases and application of pattern recognition techniques developed in other spheres, e.g. banking and defence, mean that investigation of the utility of GPRD in this area is now possible.

DEVELOPMENT OF THE FULL FEATURE GPRD

Researchers have provided critical input to help the MCA develop the Full Feature GPRD. Some indicated that, in the past, they had been precluded from using the GPRD or using it as extensively as they might. The cost of access, requirement for extensive software and hardware to store the data, and the need for sophisticated programs to extract and analyse the data were cited as rate limiting factors in its use, and this has informed the development approach adopted for the new database and services offered from it. The approach has focused on:

- *Development of a robust data model.* GP computer systems will continue to evolve to support GPs in managing their practices more efficiently, while the nature of the diagnostic and treatment data will remain relatively static. Hence, the data model that has been developed is based on the elements of a patient record rather than on the data structures required by the GP computer software. This will facilitate future collection and storage of additional data from practices using both InPS software and from other potential data sources.
- *Availability to researchers of the raw data collected from GPs.* Researchers will continue

to have access to the anonymised data as they were recorded in the GPs' practices.
- *Provision of "value added" information to researchers,* e.g. *on data quality, which is clearly distinguished from the raw data.*
- *Access to data subsets (data marts), a frozen dataset and to a continuously updated database.*
- *Provision of hierarchical dictionaries to support data retrieval.* Historically, InPS practices used *OXMIS* medical terms. Currently they use *Read Clinical Terms* as mandated by the UK Department of Health. It is likely that *SNOMED Clinical Terms* will be adopted as the UK National Health Service standard in the future. Similarly, various drugs dictionaries are used by GPs in the United Kingdom. Researchers using GPRD will be able to analyse the data using *Read Clinical Terms* or the *Medical Dictionary for Regulatory Activities (MedDRA)* terminology and the ATC or *GPRD Drugs/ Product* dictionary to support comprehensive data retrieval. For example, a search on fluoxetine will retrieve all information on the drug substance, drug substance variants, formulations and licensed products via one query.
- *Reducing the opportunity costs of using GPRD.* The total size of the new database is in the range of one terabyte. To date, GPRD data have been distributed as flat files to users. The MCA is offering on-line access to the Full Feature GPRD which:
  — reduces the cost of accessing the database since researchers will no longer require extensive hardware and software on site;
  — enables a wider range of services to be provided by the MCA in keeping with the MCA's vision for increasing GPRD use; and
  — ensures that all users have access to the same base data.

The technical architecture for the Full Feature GPRD is summarised in Figure 29.1. All GPRD data are stored in an Informix database called the Operational Data Store, an area which also includes medical and drugs terminology information and operational data to support the GPRD Data Collection and Processing Management

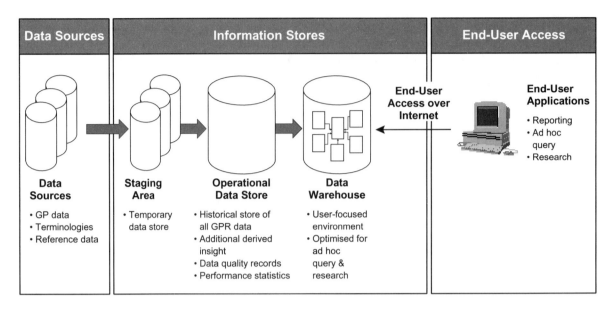

Figure 29.1. The Full Feature GPRD.

System. It provides a transactional system for data management, access to which is restricted to the GPRD Group. Once validated, data are loaded into a Redbrick data warehouse which has been optimised to support data analysis. This is the environment that researchers access via the internet, with querying via "Set Analyzer and Business Objects" analytical tools.

OPERATIONAL FRAMEWORK

The GPRD is operated by a self-financing Division of the MCA, which is separate from the Agency's medicines regulatory functions. The Manager is directly accountable to the MCA's Chief Executive. The database is run on a non-profit-making basis and in accordance with the terms by which it was donated to the Department. Other Divisions of the MCA that wish to access the database are subject to the same fees and access conditions as non-MCA users.

The GPRD Division's five-year vision statement is "to promote and protect public health by establishing the GPRD as the premier source of longitudinal patient data and to be recognised internationally as an innovative public sector enterprise which sets the standard in information management and customer service". The operating model for the GPRD Division is represented diagrammatically in Figure 29.2. In summary, GPRD staff are responsible for:

● Data collection—ensuring that the data collected from contributing GPs are of appropriate quality, quantity, representativeness and timeliness. In addition, staff distribute feedback reports to GPs which inform them about the completeness of recorded data and that seek corrective action when necessary. They also liaise frequently with practice managers to provide guidance in specific data-recording issues. Additional "value added" services for contributors are being developed in association with GP representatives.
● Database management—implementing best practices in information management, enhancing the efficiency of operations (e.g. the introduction of electronic data capture) and compliance with relevant data protection legislation and patient confidentiality guidance.
● Provision of data access and research services to customers, which include: those who wish to have continuous access to the database for their

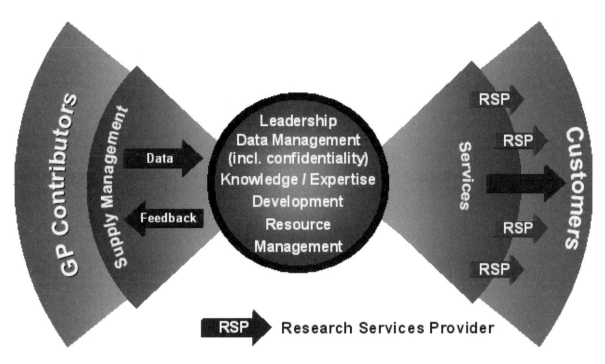

Figure 29.2. GPRD: operating model.

own research purposes; those who want *ad hoc* access; and those who will act as Research Service Providers by offering services to third parties. The GPRD Division has also established its own research team.

LAUNCH OF NEW GPRD SERVICES

The new Full Feature database was implemented in October 2000 and an Introductory Launch phase, in which the new system was piloted by 22 organisations internationally, was held between November 2000 and April 2001.

Since April 2001 the GPRD Division has offered data access services which include on-line access to the total raw dataset and query tools, and access to standard research queries which can be parameterised by drug and medical conditions. It also provides training in the use of GPRD which covers the characteristics of the data collected from the GPs, the UK primary care system, the data model and practical use of the query tools in

an interactive learning environment. Research services include feasibility studies, guidance with protocol development and partial or complete conduct of commissioned studies. Services will evolve in response to user feedback. Details are posted on the GPRD website.

SUMMARY

Over the past 10 years the GPRD has proven to be a unique research tool contributing to the understanding of public health issues, including drug safety, internationally. Implementation of the new Full Feature GPRD will allow researchers access to all the data collected and has enabled the introduction of new services to facilitate wider usage of the database in a more resource-effective manner. Whilst technology can dramatically enhance the efficiency of the research process, GPRD will never be a "plug in and play" application. Scientific and clinical expertise and understanding of the limitations of the data collected and of the UK primary care environment are critical to conducting high quality research on the GPRD.

ACKNOWLEDGEMENT

This chapter is adapted from Wood, L and Coulson, R (2001) Revitalizing the General Practice Research Database: Plans, challenges and opportunities. *Pharmacoepidemiology and Drug Safety* **10**: 379–383.

REFERENCES

García Rodriguez LA, Pérez Gutthann S (1998) Use of the UK General Practice Research Database for pharmacoepidemiology. *Br J Pharmacol* **45**: 419–25.

Hodgson C, Ellis C (2001) Time trends in GP outpatient referrals. *Health Stat Q* **10**: 14–9.

Lawson DH, Sherman V, Hollowell J (1998) The General Practice Research Database. *Q J Med* **91**: 445–52.

Moser K (2001) Inequalities in treated heart disease and mental illness in England and Wales, 1994–1998. *Br J Gen Practice* **51**: 438–44.

30

Overview of North American Databases

BRIAN L. STROM AND JUDITH L. KINMAN

Center for Clinical Epidemiology and Biostatistics, University of Pennsylvania School of Medicine, Philadelphia, PA, USA

THE CHALLENGE

Once hypotheses are generated by pharmacovigilance, techniques are needed to test these hypotheses. Large electronic databases can often meet the need for a cost-effective and efficient means of conducting post-marketing surveillance studies (Strom and Carson, 1990). In North America, such databases are primarily administrative in origin, generated by the request for payments, or claims, for clinical services and therapies. To meet the needs of drug surveillance, the ideal generic database would include records from inpatient and outpatient care, emergency care, mental health care, all laboratory and radiological tests, and all prescribed and over-the-counter medications, as well as alternative therapies. The population covered by the database would be large enough to permit discovery of rare events for the drug(s) in question, and the population would be stable over its lifetime. Although it is generally preferable for the population included in the database to be representative of the general population from which it is drawn, it may sometimes be advantageous to emphasize the more disadvantaged groups that may have been absent from pre-marketing testing. The drug(s) under investigation must of course be present in the formulary and be prescribed in sufficient quantity to provide adequate power for analyses.

Other requirements of an ideal database are that all parts are easily linked by means of a patient's unique identifier, that the records are updated on a regular basis, and that the records are verifiable and are reliable. The ability to conduct chart review to confirm outcomes is also a necessity for most studies (Strom and Carson, 1990), as diagnoses entered into an electronic database may include interim diagnoses and recurrent/chronic, as opposed to acute, events. Information on potential confounders, such as smoking and alcohol consumption, may only be available through chart review or, more consistently, through patient interviews. With appropriate permissions and confidentiality safeguards in place, access to patients is sometimes possible and useful for assessing compliance with the medication regimen as well as obtaining information on other factors that may relate to drug effects. Information on drugs taken intermittently for symptom relief, over-the-counter drugs, and drugs not on the formulary must also be obtained directly from the patient. The advantage of a claims database remains, i.e. data do not have to

Pharmacovigilance. Edited by R.D. Mann and E.B. Andrews
© 2002 John Wiley & Sons, Ltd

be collected *de novo*, investigations can be completed more efficiently and more economically, and data on exposures are not subject to recall or interviewer bias. With the caveat of the need to confirm outcomes, the availability of such databases is an important asset for post-marketing surveillance.

In the United States, health insurance is typically covered through one's place of employment, and may not include coverage for prescription drugs. A major disadvantage of this system for use in drug surveillance includes the instability of the population due to job changes, employers' changes of health plans, and changes in coverage for specific employees and their family members. The opportunity for longitudinal analyses is thereby hindered by the continual enrollment and dis-enrollment of plan members. Strategies can be adopted for selecting stable populations within a specific database, and for addressing compliance, such as examining patterns of refills for chronically used medications. Validation analyses and consistency checks must be considered for any surveillance based on claims data.

In the following sections we will discuss five major US health plans and one Canadian health plan and their associated databases.

GROUP HEALTH COOPERATIVE OF PUGET SOUND

Group Health Cooperative of Puget Sound (GHC) is a health maintenance organization (HMO), established in 1947, which provides health care on a prepaid basis to approximately 415 000 persons in western Washington State, located in the northwestern corner of the United States (Saunders *et al.*, 2000). Most of these enrollees receive all their care at Group Health facilities. An additional 47 000 residents of western Washington belong to a subsidiary of GHC, established in 1990, which provides a "point of service" option that permits care from community providers other than Group Health providers. As the point of service coverage is more expensive than that provided by Group Health providers, most of the coverage remains within the Group Health network. Although the

majority of enrollees receive health benefits through their place of employment, coverage has been extended to 54 000 Medicare, 25 000 Medicaid, and 26 000 Washington Basic Health Plan recipients, thereby expanding its membership to include elderly and low-income residents (Saunders *et al.*, 2000).

GHC offers comprehensive health care coverage for outpatient care, inpatient services, emergency care, mental health services, and prescribed drugs, although the latter are not provided to Medicare enrollees new to GHC since 1994. Nearly all benefit plans require small co-payments for services, such as prescriptions, outpatient visits unrelated to preventive care, and emergency treatment. Coverage for outpatient drugs is controlled by GHC's drug formulary.

At GHC, each enrollee is assigned a unique number, which remains with that person even if the individual drops out of the plan and then rejoins the health system at a later date. Multiple databases have been developed from the main database, with an individual's records linked through their unique number.

The socio-demographic profile of GHC enrollees is generally comparable to that of the population of the Seattle–Tacoma area, with the GHC enrollees somewhat better educated. The median income of both groups is similar, although the GHC membership is less representative of the highest income category.

Multiple database files exist, and date from varying time-points. The current enrollment file consists of some 460 000 individuals; historical files contain records for some 2 million persons ever enrolled in GHC; 1.5 million persons have been enrolled since 1980 (Saunders *et al.*, 2000). The Pharmacy file, dating from 1977, includes records generated when prescriptions are filled. The drug data include drug number, therapeutic class, drug form and strength, date dispensed, quantity dispensed, cost to GHC, and refill indicator. The file currently includes a field for number of days the medication should last. The hospital database, dating back to the early 1970s, includes diagnoses, procedures, diagnostic-related group (DRG) and discharge disposition. Laboratory data are available since 1986, and specify the test ordered, the date ordered, specimen source, results, and date of the results. All radiographic studies performed at GHC facilities, including MRI and CT scans, are now available in the outpatient visits file. Beginning in the early 1990s, diagnosis and procedure data were incorporated into the outpatient registration database, which also includes date of visit, the provider seen, the provider's specialty, and the location of care.

As a longtime participant in the National Cancer Institute's SEER program (Cancer Surveillance, Epidemiology, and End Results), GHC receives a data file of all newly diagnosed cancers among its enrollees, including anatomical site, stage of diagnosis, and vital status at follow-up. The Fred Hutchinson Cancer Research Center in Seattle maintains a Cancer Surveillance System, consisting of the 13 contiguous counties of northwest Washington, and is one of the 13 SEER population-based registries in the United States (see http://seer.cancer.gov/AboutSEER.html).

GHC has also developed a death file that covers enrollees between the years 1977 and 1997. Data are also available from the Community Health Services department, an immunizations database, and from claims databases for services purchased from non-GHC providers. Cost information is available through the Utilization Management/Cost Management Information System, developed in 1989.

Turnover in membership at GHC is estimated to be approximately 15% per year (Saunders et al., 2000). Since Group Health has been in existence for more than 50 years, a subset of enrollees can be identified whose tenure spans decades.

Limitations to the GHC databases include its small size, a disadvantage in the study of uncommon outcomes as most drugs are used by only a small percentage of the population; the lack of information on some important confounders, such as smoking and alcohol consumption; loss of drug coverage for its Medicare enrollees; and limitations of the GHC formulary, especially with regard to newly marketed drugs, since GHC may decide not to add a new drug or may delay its adoption until it has been on the market for a while. Drugs that offer little therapeutic or cost advantage over drugs already listed on the formulary may be excluded. Non-formulary drugs,

such as sildenafil, fenfluramine, and phentermine, may be purchased for use outside the GHC pharmacy system, and therefore would not be represented in the database.

KAISER PERMANENTE MEDICAL CARE PROGRAM

The Kaiser Permanente Medical Care Program is the largest group practice HMO in the United States (Friedman et al., 2000). Kaiser Permanente Northern California serves the Oakland–San Francisco Bay Area, Santa Clara and Sacramento Counties, and counties north of San Francisco. Kaiser Permanente Southern California serves residents in seven southern California counties: Los Angeles, Orange, San Bernardino, San Diego, Riverside, Kern, and Imperial. Kaiser Permanente Northwest (KPNW) operates in the Portland, Oregon–Vancouver, Washington area and in two smaller communities, Salem, Oregon and Longview-Kelso, Washington, each about 50 miles distant. Each of these regional entities operates its own health research department and manages its own databases (Friedman et al., 2000; Petitti, 2001).

KAISER PERMANENTE NORTHERN CALIFORNIA

Kaiser Permanente's largest and oldest regional entity is in Northern California, and now serves more than 2.8 million enrollees in a 14-county area that includes the San Francisco Bay and Sacramento metropolitan areas (Friedman et al., 2000). About 30% of the population in the area covered by Kaiser Permanente is enrolled, mainly through employment; about 10% enroll as individuals or families after passing a health examination; and about 12% receive some Medicare coverage. Although all ethnic, age groups, and occupations are represented, the indigent and very wealthy are probably under-represented. After the first year or two of membership, during which there is a relatively high turnover, enrollees tend to stay with the program for relatively long periods of time. A unique medical record number is used for all encounters with the Kaiser Permanente program, making possible the linking of various records. Computerized membership files contain records of all members at a given point in time.

The Pharmacy Information Management System has been operational in all 108 Kaiser pharmacies since 1994, recording information on approximately 15 million prescriptions per year. Information on each prescription is entered into the database prior to its being dispensed, and includes patient and prescribing physician identification numbers, drug name, strength, and route, date dispensed, treatment regimen, and days supply. Most of the enrollees have a pharmacy copayment of up to $10 per prescription per month. Importantly, recent surveys suggest that 15%–20% of enrollees fill at least some of their prescriptions at non-Kaiser pharmacies (Friedman et al., 2000).

Other databases include hospitalizations, available since 1971; laboratory, pathology and radiology/diagnostic imaging data, stored since 1992; and information on outpatient visits, stored since 1994. Review of medical records has not been obviated, however, and is recommended for validation of certain computer data.

KAISER PERMANENTE NORTHWEST

Kaiser Permanente Northwest (KPNW) serves over 430 000 members, approximately 25% of the population of the area (Friedman et al., 2000), mostly in the outpatient setting, with one hospital in Portland and beds contracted in other community hospitals. The distribution of the membership by age, race, and gender proportionately reflects that of the population of the Portland–Vancouver area. Services provided by KPNW include hospital and surgical care, maternity care, X-rays, mammography, laboratory testing, allergy testing, home healthcare, doctor office visits, well-baby care, mental health, and dental care. Most of the members are covered by a prepaid drug benefit; for the less than 10% without the drug benefit, prescriptions are provided at or below prevailing community charges.

Databases available at KPNW include the Outpatient Pharmacy System, which began in 1986 and records all prescriptions dispensed by its outpatient pharmacies, totaling more than two million annually (Friedman et al., 2000). Data include National Drug Code (NDC) number, quantity dispersed, days supplied, refill number, date, and other product information. The automated Inpatient Medication System captures all inpatient medication orders, storing the history of each hospitalization in a unique hospital stay number that is generated on admission.

KPNW also maintains an Adverse and Allergic Drug Event Reporting database, from which it prepares reports for the local KPNW Formulary and Therapeutics Committee, and submits data to the MedWatch system of the US Food and Drug Administration (FDA).

Other data systems include The Inpatient Admission/Discharge/Transfer System, which provides data on hospitalizations in Kaiser and non-Kaiser hospitals, and includes information on ambulatory surgical and other major procedures performed in the hospitals since the mid-1960s. EpicCare is an automated clinical information system useful for clinicians providing direct patient care. Spin-offs of subsets of these files can make these data accessible for research purposes.

Additional databases cover the areas of dental care, emergency psychiatric calls and contacts, emergency department visits, laboratory, cytology and histology procedures and results, patient-specific radiology department data, including radiology, ultrasound, magnetic resonance imaging, nuclear medicine, and computerized tomography, prenatal screening, immunization, and a continuing care service database of home care services for homebound members. A Medicare Plus II Database contains data from questionnaires, distributed annually to participants, which measure with standardized instruments levels of functioning and depression.

Multiple disease registries are maintained by KPNW as well, including cancer, benign breast disease, breast cancer family registry, diabetes, and rheumatology registries. Results of cytogenetic testing of more than 5 million members of the Northwest Division and the Northern and Southern California regions are available from 1986, with Hawaii joining this registry in 1992.

The KPNW Center for Health Research also maintains multiple databases that provide data on outpatient utilization, information on health status and behaviors of members, satisfaction with care provided, and other information obtained from surveys based on a sampling of the KPNW membership. The Common Control Pool database contains basic demographic and eligibility data for virtually all people who have been members of KPNW. A Pregnancy Registry identifies pregnant KPNW members, using laboratory data, ultrasound reports, and clinic visits, enabling the tracking of all pregnancy outcomes.

The KPNW membership mostly reflects the population of the area it serves, although again the poor and the very wealthy are under-represented. The membership is relatively stable after one year; the median length of enrollment retention is more than five years. The use of a unique medical record number allows the linkage of drug dispensing with inpatient and outpatient files, and it is possible to calculate prevalence and incidence rates. Access to primary medical records permits validation of diagnostic information and gathering of information on confounding and demographic variables, which, with the exception of age and gender, are absent from the available databases.

The Kaiser Permanente formularies are limited, with the newest and/or most expensive drugs unlikely to be listed. It is also likely that only one brand of a particular drug is available.

KAISER PERMANENTE SOUTHERN CALIFORNIA

Kaiser Permanente Southern California provides comprehensive health care on a pre-paid basis to 3 million residents of Southern California. The population served by the program is diverse and broadly representative of the population of Southern California in terms of ethnicity, education, and income (Petitti, 2001). Kaiser Permanente owns 11 hospitals and more than 100 medical offices in Southern California. The Southern California Permanente Medical Group is a partnership of more than 3400 physicians, who comprise the entire range of medical specialists and subspecialists (Petitti, 2001).

Each member of Kaiser Permanente is assigned a unique number upon joining the plan, which is retained for life, irrespective of leaving and rejoining the plan. This unique identification number allows for linkage of various computer files containing clinical and administrative information (Petitti, 2001).

A vast array of computer-stored information is maintained on membership, hospital admissions and discharges, pharmacy prescriptions, outpatient appointments, and laboratory and radiologic tests. In addition, several special databases have been created specifically for use in research and epidemiologic analyses: MORTLINK-SC was created by linkage of membership data from 1988 to 1999 with information from the California Death Index for the same period of time. The database, which is updated annually, has information on deaths among members who died in California, regardless of health plan membership at time of death; The Diabetes Research Registry database was created by linking information from the Pharmacy Information Management System, the Laboratory Management System, and the hospital database to identify all members with diabetes mellitus. The database has been evaluated against independent sources of information on diabetes and found to have a sensitivity of 0.93 for the identification of diabetes and a positive predictive value of 0.97. About 148 000 members of the health plan in Southern California were in the registry database in 2000 (Petitti, 2001). The Research Subject Demographic file is used to select subjects for surveys and other studies, and consists of information on age, gender, enrollment history, and most current address and telephone number for all active members of the health plan (Petitti, 2001).

HARVARD PILGRIM HEALTH CARE/HARVARD VANGUARD MEDICAL ASSOCIATES

The Harvard Pilgrim Health Care (HPHC) is a non-profit HMO in New England, the northeastern corner of the United States. It is the largest HMO in New England, with approximately 1.1

million members. The median age of the members is 31 years, with more than a quarter of the membership aged 17 or younger, and 7% aged 65 or older (Chan and Platt, 2000). HPHC includes Medicare and Medicaid populations, as well as members from private corporations, state employees, and individual memberships.

The dis-enrollment rate is approximately 14% a year among all members, but, as with the other databases described, is much lower for members who have been enrolled for longer than three years (Chan and Platt, 2000). The attrition rate is also lower among those with chronic conditions, such as asthma or hypertension.

Approximately 90% of HPHC members have prescription drug benefits, which offer a copayment of up to $10 a prescription for a 30-day supply at member pharmacies. For each prescription dispensed, the following data are recorded: unique patient identifying number, gender, date of birth, dispensing date, prescriber identifier, generic drug name, dosage strength, amount dispensed, route, American Hospital Formulary Service (AHFS) code, NDC code, member's contract number, and dependency code (noting the relationship between family members and contract holders).

The basic membership file includes demographic and health plan coverage information for each member, including date of birth, gender, dates of membership (including all starts, stops and changes in coverage or benefit status during each membership interval), and most recent residential zip code. Also recorded, though less reliably, are race, marital status, education, and occupation. Family membership information is noted, as well as the organization through which membership was obtained (Medicare, Medicaid, private employer, etc.).

Ambulatory visits generate claims with diagnosis and procedure codes, as well as provider identifier and dates of visits. Emergency Department visits and hospitalizations also generate claims, with hospital name, dates, discharge diagnoses and procedures performed. The largest single inpatient facility is Brigham and Women's Hospital, where detailed automated patient records are available. Automated searches can also

be made of long-term care and home care provided by physicians, nurses, or other private vendors.

A subset of the HPHC membership is composed of a multi-specialty group, Harvard Vanguard Medical Associates (HVMA), with a membership of 300 000 (Chan and Platt, 2000). For these members, fully automated medical records are available, which include results of most laboratory tests, diagnostic imaging procedures and other tests performed within and outside HVMA facilities, providers' notes and dictations, patients' vital signs, and an unlimited number of diagnoses per encounter (including telephone calls). Hard copy records must be used for electrocardiogram results and information from prior health care providers. Paper text is also reviewed to confirm coded information and to obtain details on the outcomes of interest and on potential confounders and effect modifiers. Routine record reviews have been performed for research and quality assurance purposes.

The data required for research projects are stored in diverse computer systems. These data must be converted into usable databases for each research project. The pharmacy dispensing and claims data have supported a number of studies using a variety of study designs, including cohort and nested case–control studies.

UNITEDHEALTH GROUP

UnitedHealth Group provides a continuum of health care and specialty services to more than 13 million members throughout the United States through HMOs, point of service arrangements, preferred provider organizations, managed indemnity programs, Medicare and Medicaid managed care programs, and the American Association of Retired Persons (AARP) insurance programs. Specialized services include mental health, substance abuse, utilization management, specialized provider networks, third-party administration services, employee assistance services, managed pharmacy services, and information systems. Although the plan structures vary and range from staff or group models to independent practice associations, affiliated health plans are typically the latter, with open access to a wide network of providers. Membership includes approximately 5 800 000 commercial health plan members, 500 000 Medicaid, and 450 000 Medicare members (Shatin *et al.*, 2000). Unique member identifiers allow for tracking across enrollment periods, so that a member can be followed through disenrollment and re-enrollment. Participating providers include 3050 hospitals and 53 000 retail pharmacies by way of a pharmacy benefits management company (Shatin *et al.*, 2000).

The twelve UnitedHealth Group affiliated health plans in the research databases are geographically diverse, with plans in the Northeastern, Southeastern, Midwestern, and Western regions of the United States. These databases were begun in 1990, with 3.5 million members and 2.6 million member-years accumulated by 1997, representing commercial, Medicaid, and Medicare recipients (Shatin *et al.*, 2000). Most of the members have a drug benefit—93% of commercial members and most Medicaid members. Medicare drug benefits vary depending on the plan, so the pharmacy files may not capture all prescriptions in this age range.

The research databases are compiled from membership data, medical and pharmacy claims, and provider data. Data elements in the membership file include, besides the unique member identifier, date of birth, gender, place and type of employment, benefit package, and links to dates of enrollment and dis-enrollment. Medical claims include outpatient as well as inpatient, emergency room, surgery, specialty, preventive, and office-based treatment. Claim forms must be submitted by a health care provider in order to receive payment for a covered service. Pharmacy claims typically are submitted electronically by the pharmacy at the time a prescription is filled. The data submitted specify the patient's and pharmacy's identifiers, drug name, date dispensed, dosage of medication dispensed, duration of the prescription in days, and quantity dispensed. Provider data include physician specialty, and enable researchers to locate medical records for the collection of detailed information not provided in the claims data. The resulting files have been incorporated into software developed by UnitedHealth to facilitate the investigation of questions such as those regarding drug exposures and adverse drug events. Research capabilities include performing record and file linkages, constructing longitudinal histories, identifying denominators to calculate rates, identifying specific treatments at a particular point in time, and calculating person-time at risk and time of event occurrence.

Given the large size of the databases available to UnitedHealth, it is possible to detect rare exposures and rare outcomes. Feasibility studies have been conducted using these data to evaluate drug usage and to study adverse events that are first identified through the Spontaneous Reporting System of the FDA.

UnitedHealth Group has no data on drugs that cost less than the copayment amount, and inconsistent data on those eligible for Medicare, as noted above. Not all drugs are on the preferred drug list. Medical record retrieval is still necessary for obtaining information such as race/ethnicity, confirming a diagnosis, obtaining information on risk factors and outcomes, or determining whether a member is deceased. Another limitation is the time lag in receiving information from claims data, which can be one month for pharmacy claims but up to six months for physician and facility claims.

MEDICAID DATABASES

The US Medicaid Program is a health insurance system created in 1965 to provide access to medical care for economically disadvantaged and disabled persons. It consists of a series of 54 programs, supported jointly by federal and state funds, and managed independently by states or jurisdictions. The Welfare Reform Act of 1996 defined eligible individuals to include children younger than six; pregnant women whose family income is 133% of the federal poverty level or lower; children younger than 19 in families with incomes at or below the federal poverty level; persons eligible for the Supplemental Security Income Program (SSI) because they are aged, blind, or disabled and have limited income; and other specified needy groups (Carson *et al.*, 2000). Compared with the overall US population, the Medicaid population has a disproportionate number of children, females, and non-whites. Eligibility for these specific programs can vary by year, based on employment and income. Tennessee, for example, has lost a quarter of its enrollment in one year, and retained only half after five years, due to losses in eligibility and deaths (Ray and Griffin, 1989).

Although Medicaid recipient services vary by state, the federal government requires that minimum services include physician and nurse-midwife services, home health care, care in skilled nursing facilities, inpatient and outpatient hospital care, rural health clinics, independent laboratory and radiology services, early and periodic screening of children, family planning services, and transportation to and from medical services. Virtually all states provide for reimbursement of prescribed drugs; the list of drugs eligible for reimbursement also varies by state.

In order to administer this large health care program, the US government developed the Medicaid Management Information System, which laid out a set of specifications for the processing of computerized claims and management information. Minimum standards were established for its six components: recipient; provider; claims processing; reference files; surveillance and utilization review; and management and administrative reporting (Carson et al., 2000).

The claims processing files include information on age, gender, state, inpatient and outpatient diagnoses (using the coding system of the International Classification of Disease Ninth Revision—Clinical Modification (ICD-9-CM)), outpatient drugs (using National Drug Code (NDC)), procedures, such as laboratory and radiographic, and information on deaths, which is available in some states. Pharmacy data include records of all outpatient and nursing home prescriptions filled at the pharmacy for drugs, equipment, and supplies that are on the Medicaid formulary. Each record contains the date filled, the NDC code, quantity of the drug dispensed, the number of days the supply is anticipated to last, and pharmacy and prescribing practitioner identifiers. Most drugs are dispensed for no longer than a 30-day period, although some states permit the dispensing of a larger supply for chronically used drugs.

Diagnosis data contain the records of outpatient claims for care provided, and of hospitalizations, including hospital identifier and admission and discharge dates. Although primary and secondary diagnoses and surgical procedures are available in these files only for non-Medicare recipients, they can be obtained from Medicare files for enrollees over 65 for whom Medicare becomes the primary payer.

There is a lag period of up to 2 months between the time a drug is dispensed and the time it appears on the database; the lag time for diagnoses may be up to 3 months.

Historically, considerable research using Medicaid data has been performed using COMPASS, which stands for the Computerized On-Line Medical Pharmaceutical Analysis and Surveillance System. No longer available as COMPASS, these Medicaid Databases are now owned by Protocare Sciences of Herndon, Virginia, and are now called the Protocare Sciences Proprietary Medicaid Database. The older COMPASS database included billing data from Medicaid patients in 11 states, with a total Medicaid population of over 8 million patients (Strom et al., 1985; Morse et al., 1986). Currently, new data are only available for approximately 1.25 million patients from Ohio. Importantly, although the data available for each patient are identical between the two databases, access to medical records is no longer an option, due to increasing societal concern about confidentiality.

The State of Tennessee has contracted with Vanderbilt School of Medicine to collect the claims files of the state's Medicaid program, analyze the quality of the claims, and perform research of interest to the state. Twenty-seven percent of the state's population, or 1.4 million people, were enrolled as of 1997, of whom 11% were 65 years of age and older. Almost half of all births in Tennessee were to women enrolled in Tennessee Medicaid (Ray, unpublished data, 1999).

The Tennessee Medicaid program changed in 1994 from a fee-for-service program to a capitated model consisting of 12 managed care organizations, each with its own formulary that restricts the list of reimbursable drugs (Ruther et al., 1986;

Mirvis *et al.*, 1995). Although the quality of the database has generally been maintained, effort is ongoing to check the completeness and accuracy of the data since financial incentives for submitting data no longer exist.

The Tennessee system has developed linkages to a number of other database files, including Medicare files, vital statistics files, links of files of mothers to children, public health clinic files, motor vehicle files, and the Tennessee cancer registry, so that research on Medicaid enrollees can be expanded. Medical record abstracting has been possible, with permission of the Tennessee Medicaid Program and its constituent providers.

Medicaid databases contain an over-representation of special populations, with greater numbers of pregnant women, the elderly, nursing home residents, and African Americans than would be expected in a representative sample of the population. These are the populations that are often excluded or under-represented in pre-marketing trials. Although considered a disadvantage when a representative population is required, for analytic studies it controls for variation in socio-economic status.

However, as a claims database (similar to most of the other databases described), information is lacking on some variables often needed to control for confounding, such as smoking, environmental exposures, illicit drug use, alcohol use, occupation, family history, and use of over-the-counter drugs.

Experience suggests that medical records must be obtained in many studies to confirm the diagnosis, to characterize the severity of the disease, and to obtain information on potential confounding variables not found in the computer data. Some states never developed a way to access their medical records, and outpatient records have always been difficult to obtain and often do not have the information necessary for a specific study. Regardless, however, medical records are no longer accessible in most of these databases, because of concerns about confidentiality. Studies where primary record confirmation is less important are those which focus on drug-to-drug relationships, or studies which can use drugs or procedures as markers of diagnoses.

HEALTH DATABASES IN SASKATCHEWAN

Saskatchewan is a province in western Canada with a stable population of about 1 million people, or about 3.4% of the total population of Canada. The province provides a publicly funded health system for its residents, who are each assigned a Health Services Number upon registration that uniquely identifies that person, and which is captured in records of health service utilization, enabling the linkage of computer databases. Only a very small percentage (less than 1%) of the population of Saskatchewan is excluded from the health registry (Downey *et al.*, 2000). Prescription plan coverage excludes about 9% of the population, primarily Indians, who are covered by another government agency. Hospital services and most physician services are available to all persons in the health registry. The population registry captures demographic and coverage data on every member of the eligible population, including gender, marital status, date of birth, and date of death.

Drugs covered by the drug plan are listed in the Saskatchewan formulary; non-formulary drugs are generally not covered. The drugs listed are intended for outpatient use, although the database includes prescriptions to residents of long-term care facilities. The formulary is updated semi-annually; as of July 1998, 2875 drug products were listed (Downey *et al.*, 2000). The drug database contains information from September 1975, with an 18-month hiatus in 1987–88 when data were incomplete. The database includes patient, prescriber, pharmacy, and cost information. Drug information includes pharmacologic-therapeutic classification, using the AHFS classification system, active ingredient, generic and brand names, strength and dosage form, drug manufacturer, date, and quantity dispensed. Unavailable is information on non-formulary drug use, over-the-counter drugs, use of professional samples, and in-hospital drugs. The database also does not provide information about the dosage regimen prescribed, the reason the drug was prescribed, or patient compliance. More than 6.2 million prescription claims were processed by the drug plan in fiscal year 1997–98 (Downey *et al.*, 2000).

Data from hospitalizations, including day surgeries, include up to three discharge diagnoses (ICD-9 codes), up to three procedures, an accident code (ICD-9 external cause code), admission and discharge dates, attending physician, and surgeon (where applicable). Procedures are coded using the Canadian Classification of Diagnostic, Therapeutic, and Surgical Procedures. There is a lag time of about 6 months from date of discharge to the date when hospital data are available electronically. In 1997–98 there were approximately 160 000 separations (discharges, transfers, or deaths of inpatients), and 79 000 day surgery patients. There were also 13 000 records of newborns (Downey *et al.*, 2000).

Physician services data are obtained from claims, and include diagnoses (three-digit ICD-9 codes) and procedures (coded from a fee-for-service payment schedule established by the Health Registry and the provincial medical association). These data are limited, however, in that diagnostic data are given only to support the claim for payment, and only one three-digit ICD-9 code is recorded per visit.

Linkage can be made to the Saskatchewan cancer registry, which is required to record all persons diagnosed with cancer, including non-melanoma skin cancers and *in situ* cancers, and suspected as well as confirmed cancers. A lag time of 6 months exists from date of diagnosis to availability of the data.

Vital statistics data are also maintained by Saskatchewan Health; all birth, death, stillbirth, and marriage data are collected. Although cause of death is initially coded as received on a death registration form, it is updated if an autopsy diagnosis is received. The underlying cause of death is recorded electronically as well, and is defined as the disease or injury that initiated the sequence of events that led to death.

Other information available includes institutional long-term care and home care services, mental health services that cover both inpatient psychiatric care and community-based outpatient care, alcohol and drug abuse treatment data, and microbiologic and biochemical laboratory records.

Hospital medical records are retrievable after the appropriate approvals are obtained, with patient identifiers removed from the record. Hospital record retrieval rates often exceed 95%. Outpatient record retrieval has not approached that level of success. Information on potentially important confounders are only available in patient records or through direct patient contact.

HMO RESEARCH NETWORK

The HMO Research Network is a consortium of 14 HMOs that collaborate to perform public domain research. Each of these HMOs has linkable automated pharmacy, claims and membership data, and so are capable of identifying important safety problems within a reasonable time following the marketing of many new drugs. Some also have automated medical records and laboratory data. Nine of the Network HMOs, with a total population of 7.1 million, have been funded by the US government as a Center for Research and Education in Therapeutics (CERTs), bolstering their efforts to create and maintain the infrastructure needed to support research and education in therapeutics, including the standardization of data, provision of central programming support, and mapping of drugs to a standard formulary. The HMOs participating in this effort are Harvard Pilgrim Health Care, which leads the CERTs, Group Health Cooperative of Puget Sound, Health Partners Research Foundation (Minnesota), Henry Ford Health Systems, Fallon Healthcare System, Kaiser Permanente Northern California, Kaiser Permanente Northwest, Kaiser Permanente Georgia, and Kaiser Permanente Colorado. The populations involved are ethnically and geographically diverse, and represent 2%–3% of the US population. These remain nine separate data resources, however, and each HMO can elect to participate, or not, in any given study (Richard Platt, Harvard Pilgrim Health Care, personal communication).

VACCINE SAFETY DATALINK: A SPECIAL PURPOSE DATABASE

In order to identify rare vaccine adverse events, the US Centers for Disease Control and Prevention

(CDC) funded the Vaccine Safety Datalink (VSD), a large database that brings together computerized information on immunizations, medical outcomes, and potential confounders. Beginning in 1991, CDC joined with four HMOs, GHC, KPNW, Kaiser Permanente Northern California and Kaiser Permanente Southern California, all in the western part of the United States. Initially focusing on children up to 6 years of age, the database now includes adolescents and adults as well. All vaccinations given within the HMO study population, either routinely or for special indications, are computerized, including the vaccine type, date of vaccination, concurrent vaccinations, the manufacturer and lot number, and site of vaccination. Outcome data are collected from various sources at each site, such as hospitalizations, emergency department visits and outpatient clinic visits. To preserve patient confidentiality, each site assigns unique study identifiers to its data before shipping to the CDC annually for merging and analysis (Chen *et al.*, 1997).

VSD currently has more than 1 million children enrolled in its four member HMOs (Kramarz *et al.*, 2000). A quality control analysis of three of the HMOs comparing the automated database with paper records for common childhood vaccines showed that from 83% to 99% of the automated records were present in the paper records, and from 82% to 98% of the paper records were present in the automated database (Mullooly *et al.*, 1999).

WEIGHING THE RELATIVE MERITS AND LIMITATIONS

Selecting an appropriate database for the investigation of drug effects warrants consideration of multiple factors. Once it has been determined that a specific drug or set of drugs under investigation is on the formulary, the relative size of the prospective databases may be an important consideration, as the process of evaluating the occurrence of rare effects requires large numbers of users of the drug(s) in question. UnitedHealth and Medicaid offer the largest databases, although UnitedHealth is not population based, and Medicaid recipients over-represent the poor and disabled. GHC and HPHC are the smallest of these North American databases, but they are the only databases that contain information on inpatient drug exposures. The combined HMO Research Network is an important new option for large-scale post-marketing drug studies.

Saskatchewan contains a stable, representative, population-based database, in which loss to follow-up is minimal, making it more desirable for studying outcomes that have a delayed effect. Among the US databases, Kaiser is the most stable, with 3% loss a year after the first two years of enrollment. HPHC includes a disproportionately young population, while Medicaid includes a disproportionately poor population. GHC, Kaiser, HPHC, and UnitedHealth serve a disproportionately employed population.

Drug data vary in their completeness across the databases. Medicaid data would be the most complete, as the formularies are the least restrictive, and Medicaid patients are unlikely to purchase drugs outside of the insurance plan, as they are economically disadvantaged individuals who can obtain them without charge through Medicaid. Saskatchewan drug data are likely to be complete, if the drug is on the formulary. GHC is missing drug data on Medicare patients, i.e. the elderly. Kaiser membership makes substantial use of non-Kaiser pharmacies, resulting in missing data. UnitedHealth lacks pharmacy benefits for 7% of its population, and Medicare drug benefits vary depending on the specific plan, so the pharmacy files will be incomplete in this age range. Most health plans lack the means of assessing drugs purchased that cost less than the plan's copay, or drugs purchased prior to the patient's meeting the annual deductible (e.g. HMOs) or after the patient has reached the drug benefit limit. This is not a problem for Medicaid data.

GHC has access to outpatient diagnosis data, as do HPHC, UnitedHealth, Medicaid, and Saskatchewan. The Saskatchewan outpatient data are very limited, however, as only one code is provided per visit, and only three digits of the five-digit ICD9-CM code are used.

Access to medical records is often crucial for verifying diagnoses, characterizing the severity of a diagnosis, and for obtaining data on important potential confounding variables not found in the computerized data. This access has been possible with all these databases, but is no longer feasible in Medicaid for reasons of confidentiality; the other databases that rely on claims may begin to suffer from the same problems.

None of these databases can assess the use of over-the-counter drugs, use of complementary/ alternative therapies, or the use of physician or other professional samples. Patient compliance is not directly measurable, although the benefit of a claims database compared with use of physician records is knowing that, not only was a prescription written by the physician, it was also dispensed by the pharmacist. Prescriptions that are renewed suggest that the patient was indeed taking the drug. The extent of use of drugs taken intermittently for symptom relief is difficult to assess.

CONCLUSION

Each of these electronic databases has its advantages and disadvantages, but each can be useful in hypothesis testing of signals from pharmacovigilance. The speed with which data can be accessed and the relatively low cost of their use make these databases excellent resources.

REFERENCES

Carson JL, Ray WA, Strom BL (2000) Medicaid databases. In: Strom BL, ed., *Pharmacoepidemiology*, 3rd edn. New York: Wiley, pp. 307–24.

Chan KA, Platt R (2000) Harvard Pilgrim Health Care/Harvard Vanguard Medical Associates. In: Strom BL, ed., *Pharmacoepidemiology*, 3rd edn. New York: Wiley, pp. 285–94.

Chen RT, Glasser JW, Rhodes PH, Davis RL, Barlow WE, Thompson RS, Mullooly JP, Black SB, Shinefield HR, Vadheim CM, Marcy SM, Ward JI, Wise RP, Wassilak SG, Hadler SC (1997) Vaccine Safety Datalink Project: a new tool for improving vaccine safety monitoring in the United States. *Pediatrics* **99**: 765–73.

Downey W, Beck P, McNutt M, Stang MR, Osei W, Nichol J (2000) Health databases in Saskatchewan. In: Strom BL, ed., *Pharmacoepidemiology*, 3rd edn. New York: Wiley, pp. 325–46.

Friedman GD, Habel LA, Boles M, McFarland B (2000) Kaiser Permanente Medical Care Program: Division of Research, Northern California, and Center for Health Research, Northwest Division. In: Strom BL, ed., *Pharmacoepidemiology*, 3rd edn. New York: Wiley, pp. 263–84.

Kramarz P, DeStefano F, Garguillo PM, Davis RL, Chen RT, Mullooly JP, Black SB, Shinefield HR, Bohlke K, Ward JI, Marcy SM (2000) Does influenza vaccination exacerbate asthma? Analysis of a large cohort of children with asthma. Vaccine Safety Datalink Team. *Arch Family Med* **9**: 617–23.

Mirvis DM, Chang CF, Hall CJ, Zaar GT, Applegate WB (1995) TennCare—health system reform for Tennessee. *J Am Med Assoc* **274**: 1235–41.

Morse ML, LeRoy AA, Strom BL (1986) COMPASS®. A population-based postmarketing drug surveillance system. In: Inman WHW, ed., *Monitoring for Drug Safety*. Philadelphia, PA: Lippincott, pp. 237–54.

Mullooly J, Drew L, DeStefano F, Chen R, Okoro K, Swint E, Immanuel V, Ray P, Lewis N, Vadheim C, Lugg M (1999) Quality of HMO vaccination databases used to monitor childhood vaccine safety. Vaccine Safety DataLink Team. *Am J Epidemiol* **149**: 186–94.

Petitti D (2001) Director, Permanente Research and Evaluation, Kaiser Permanente Southern California. Personal communication. February.

Ray WA, Griffin MR (1989) The use of Medicaid data for pharmacoepidemiology. *Am J Epidemiol* **129**: 837–49.

Ruther M, Pagan BA, Rinkle V, Yanck J (1986) *Program Statistics: Medicare and Medicaid Data Book, 1984*. Health Care Financing Administration, June.

Saunders KW, Davis RL, Stergachis A (2000) Group Health Cooperative of Puget Sound. In: Strom BL, ed., *Pharmacoepidemiology*, 3rd edn. New York: Wiley, pp. 247–62.

Shatin D, Drinkard C, Stergachis A (2000) United-Health Group. In: Strom BL, ed., *Pharmacoepidemiology*, 3rd edn. New York: Wiley, pp. 295–306.

Strom BL, Carson JL (1990) Use of automated databases for pharmacoepidemiology research. *Epidemiol Rev* **12**: 87–107.

Strom BL, Carson JL, Morse ML, LeRoy AA (1985) The Computerized On-Line Medicaid Pharmaceutical Analysis and Surveillance System: a new resource for post-marketing drug surveillance. *Clin Pharmacol Ther* **38**: 359–64

31

Pharmacovigilance in the HMO Research Network

RICHARD PLATT

Department of Ambulatory Care and Prevention, Harvard Medical School and Harvard Pilgrim Health Care, Boston, USA

SUSAN E. ANDRADE

Meyers Primary Care Institute, Fallon Healthcare System and University of Massachusetts, Worcester, USA

ROBERT L. DAVIS

Department of Pediatrics and Epidemiology, University of Washington and Group Health Cooperative Center for Health Studies, Seattle, USA

FRANK DESTEFANO

National Immunization Program, Centers for Disease Control and Prevention, Atlanta, USA

JONATHAN A. FINKELSTEIN

Department of Ambulatory Care and Prevention, Harvard Medical School and Harvard Pilgrim Health Care, Boston, USA

MICHAEL J. GOODMAN

HealthPartners Research Foundation, Minneapolis, USA

JERRY H. GURWITZ

Meyers Primary Care Institute, Fallon Healthcare System, and the University of Massachusetts Medical School, Worcester, USA

ALAN S. GO

Kaiser Foundation Research Institute, Oakland, USA

BRIAN C. MARTINSON

HealthPartners Research Foundation, Minneapolis, USA

MARSHA A. RAEBEL

Kaiser Permanente Colorado, and University of Colorado School of Pharmacy, Denver, USA

DOUGLAS ROBLIN

Kaiser Permanente Georgia, Atlanta, USA

DENNIS ROSS-DEGNAN

Department of Ambulatory Care and Prevention, Harvard Medical School and Harvard Pilgrim Health Care, Boston, USA

Pharmacovigilance. Edited by R.D. Mann and E.B. Andrews
© 2002 John Wiley & Sons, Ltd

STEPHEN B. SOUMERAI
Department of Ambulatory Care and Prevention, Harvard Medical School and Harvard Pilgrim Health Care, Boston, USA

DAVID H. SMITH
Kaiser Permanente Center for Health Research, Portland, USA

MARIANNE ULCICKAS-YOOD
Henry Ford Health Systems, Detroit, USA

K. ARNOLD CHAN
Department of Epidemiology, Harvard School of Public Health, Boston, USA

INTRODUCTION

Managed care organizations' electronic claims files, automated medical records, organizational capabilities, and access to both clinicians and members have provided a great deal of otherwise unobtainable information about the use, efficacy, effectiveness cost-effectiveness, and adverse reaction profile of marketed therapeutic agents. They are also important resources for the evaluation of educational and behavior change interventions directed at providers and patients. The ensemble of different types of information, access to members (with safeguards for privacy) and ability to intervene provide important advantages over large claims datasets, e.g. Health Care Financing Agency (HCFA) or Medicaid files. However, studies in single organizations are inadequate for some purposes. They may be of inadequate power because of either too few exposures to drugs of interest, or outcomes might be too rare. Single organizations may also lack desirable diversity in patient populations, provider mix, medical care practices or delivery systems models; all of these features limit the generalizability of data from single organizations. Additionally, the databases of single organizations are susceptible to systematic errors in coding of care that is delivered, in ascertainment of events of interest or in data integrity that might affect the validity of a study's results.

Multi-center database studies can ameliorate some of these problems. However, they do so at the cost of added complexity, time and cost. We describe below two models for conducting such studies: a distributed system that extracts and assembles data when needed to answer a specific question, and a centralized system that assembles data that can answer subsequent questions. The first system is used by the organizations that comprise the Agency for Healthcare Research and Quality (AHRQ)-sponsored HMO Research Network Center for Education and Research in Therapeutics. The second is used by the health maintenance organizations (HMOs) that are part of the Centers for Disease Control and Prevention (CDC) sponsored Vaccine Safety Datalink (VSD). In both cases, the HMOs and their sponsors are working together to perform such studies and to develop methods to perform them more easily. The HMO Research Network, to which all of these HMOs belong, is a 13-member group that facilitates public domain research in managed care settings. The Network is specifically interested in the evaluation of the effectiveness of available tests and treatments, investigation of new therapies, and in prevention or management strategies for common conditions.

Each HMO has pharmacy dispensing records, automated inpatient and outpatient claims data, plus enrolment files containing demographic data and information on dates of eligibility for various kinds of care, including pharmacy benefit status. Each HMO also has access to ambulatory and hospital records; some of these are automated, most are not. The HMOs in the Vaccine Safety Datalink also have automated vaccine exposure registries.

ORGANIZATIONAL MODELS

THE DISTRIBUTED MODEL—THE HMO RESEARCH NETWORK CENTER FOR EDUCATION AND RESEARCH IN THERAPEUTICS

Description of the System

This group includes nine HMOs with a total population of approximately seven million, plus a coordinating center at the Channing Laboratory, a research unit of Harvard Medical School. Each site has a lead investigator; other HMO based investigators also participate. All centers participate in the development of policies, procedures, infrastructure and core studies. New studies are approved by a steering committee, after which centers decide individually whether to participate. Study leadership is distributed among investigators based in the different HMOs. Investigators at every site participate in protocol development, creation of workplans, and writing of manuscripts. The coordinating center supports all studies, usually by leading the creation of study-specific analysis datasets.

The most important organizational principle is to extract data needed for each study from the HMOs' separate databases as the need for this information becomes clear, rather than to create a single merged dataset to support future, still unspecified, studies. This approach has both advantages and disadvantages. The advantages include the fact that it ensures that investigators and support staff who are knowledgeable about the individual HMOs and data systems use their expertise on an ongoing basis. This is important because administrative data systems are typically unique in a variety of ways. They may use locally modified coding conventions, they often contain discontinuities resulting from the use of different computer systems over time, and they often contain undocumented gaps or varying levels of detail that result from different contractual arrangements with selected providers or vendors. They also evolve rapidly, so that this information must be updated frequently.

Maintaining HMOs' data on their host systems also avoids the very large cost and effort required to build and sustain a merged database. This includes the work of extracting and refreshing very large datasets, converting these to a uniform format, creating stable person-level identifiers that protect the confidentiality of individuals, and reconciling and/or annotating anomalies for the entire dataset. This work is required even though most of the data is never used for a multi-center study.

An additional reason for not creating a single large dataset is that it allows each organization to control access to, and use of, its data at all times. To maximize individual centers' control over their information, we have adopted the principle of having each center provide as little data for each study as possible. A method for minimizing the amount of data required is discussed below.

The principal disadvantages of not creating a single merged dataset are the extra time required to assemble a project-specific dataset, and the effort's dependence on individual HMOs to maintain their data in accessible form. Some organizations archive data after several years in a manner that makes it difficult to use for research purposes.

Several types of data sharing can fit within this distributed model. For simple studies, it may be sufficient for each site to ascertain frequencies or rates that can be combined across sites. In essence, each site creates an agreed-upon set of tables, which are then combined. An example of such a study that included three of this center's sites, plus others, is a recent analysis of contraindicated dispensing of cisapride (Smalley *et al.*, 2000). For more complex studies, we have found it preferable to create a pooled analysis dataset. Doing so is essential for conducting multivariate analyses. It also allows more straightforward creation of derived variables, e.g. time windows of drug exposures, or combinations of diagnosis codes, and it reduces the overall amount of effort on the part of investigators and staff at each site.

Capabilities Required to Support Distributed Multi-center Studies

Several kinds of capabilities are needed to support multi-center studies and to improve the interpretability of the results. Considerable effort is required to create mutually interpretable drug identifiers. Although all of the HMOs in our group use National Drug Codes (NDCs) to identify drugs in their dispensing files, there are important differences in their implementation of these codes. Some of these represent different formatting conventions, others are data entry errors, and some are the result of individual HMOs' creation of new codes for local use. Such codes are more common in older data files, but new codes may still be created; for instance, if a pharmacy repackages a bulk supply of medication into smaller units. For our first joint study, of elderly recipients of alendronate, involving approximately 120 000 person years, we identified approximately 20 000 unique formulary entries, 10% of which required manual coding of drug identity. This experience led us to avoid merging the entire drug exposure lists of all the sites, in favor of incremental additions required by individual studies.

An additional centralized function is maintenance of (NDC) lists that map to disease categories that are used to compute the chronic disease score (Von Korff *et al*., 1992; Putnam *et al*., 2002), a comorbidity index that predicts mortality, hospitalization, and total medical resource utilization. The chronic disease score uses pharmacy dispensing as a surrogate for various chronic diseases by assigning empirically derived weights to classes of drugs that have been dispensed during the prior year. Weights are also assigned for age and gender. We have found the chronic disease score to be a useful case-mix adjuster in multi-center epidemiologic studies. Most drug codes have not yet been assigned to chronic disease categories. Our first attempt to use it required manual assignment of several thousand drug codes to chronic disease score categories.

An important feature of efficient multi-center studies is the creation of computer code that can be used at each site to extract and manipulate data, assign unique, arbitrary (for confidentiality) study identification numbers, and format it so that it can be merged with information from other sites. While such programs must be modified to run on each system, they share the same core.

Typically, such code is developed at the coordinating center for each study. This approach has several advantages. It improves data quality, ensuring that algorithms are implemented in the same way at each site. It also reduces the amount of data that must be submitted to the data center, because it is possible to do more complex data manipulations at each site than would otherwise be desirable. In addition, this approach reduces the total amount of programmer effort, since only one person develops the core code. It improves the quality of the programs, since programmers at each site test the same programs, and it ensures consistent implementation of a protocol's logic at each site.

In the near future, the sites will begin to ascertain the completeness of their dispensing records by directly querying a sample of members about their use of prescription medications. This will allow understanding of the potential impact of "out-of-plan" pharmacy use on ascertainment of drug exposures by HMO members. Such exposures have usually been assumed to be negligible, especially for drugs whose cost is high relative to the required co-payment. Although this rationale is still valid, many new pharmacy benefit variations have been introduced, including higher co-payments for some drugs, and periodic out-of-pocket spending requirements before pharmacy benefits apply. Additionally, pharmacy data systems have no information about drugs dispensed by clinicians as samples, or drugs that some members with dual insurance coverage obtain through their "other" policy. For some studies, it is also important to estimate the amount of out of plan dispensing of inexpensive drugs. It can be important to know about some of these inexpensive drugs because they can be the subject of study; for instance, a characterization of overall antibiotic use, or because of their contribution to the chronic disease score. All of these can cause dispensing files to be incomplete.

Examples of Multi-center Studies Using the Distributed System

Our experience thus far leads us to believe that it is possible to perform multi-center epidemiologic studies reasonably efficiently. We have completed a cohort study to determine whether alendronate is associated with an increased risk of hospitalization for gastrointestinal perforation, ulcer or bleeding (Donahue *et al.*, 2002). This study used pharmacy dispensing and enrolment data to identify eligible, exposed individuals and age, sex, HMO-matched unexposed individuals. Part of the eligibility determination included establishing that the individual had pharmacy benefits; there were more than 70 different pharmacy benefit plans in effect during the time covered by this study. We used ambulatory and inpatient claims to identify a second comparison cohort that had experienced a fracture (a surrogate for osteoporosis, the principal indication for alendronate). Hospital discharge diagnosis codes were used to screen for potential events of interest, then the full text records of these hospitalizations were reviewed to confirm the diagnoses. Approximately 80% of hospital records were retrievable for review. An additional "product" of this study was the determination of the sensitivity and specificity of individual International Classification of Diseases, ninth revision, Clinical Modification (ICD-9-CM) diagnosis codes for identification of these gastrointestinal events. These data also supported a case–control study of the relationship between fracture and prior exposure to statins (Chan *et al.*, 2000).

In addition to studies of drug safety and effectiveness, we are planning descriptive studies of drug use (population based rates and indications for antibiotic use in pediatrics), of the impact of changing co-payment levels on the use of prescription drugs (focus on clinicians' prescribing for diabetes and on patients' adherence to prescribed regimens), of clinicians' adherence to prescribing guidelines (use of angiotensin converting enzyme inhibitors after hospitalization for congestive heart failure), and the impact of programs to influence prescriber and consumer behavior regarding prescription drugs. This ensemble of HMOs is also a promising venue for pharmacoeconomic studies, because cost information is generally available, and for pharmacogenetic studies, because it is possible, with appropriate approval and oversight, to contact individuals with conditions of interest or with specified responses to specific medications. Although it is beyond the scope of this discussion,

this center is also well positioned to work with delivery systems to disseminate information to their clinicians and their members about the appropriate use of medical therapies.

Multi-center studies like the ones described here require additional organizational and logistic capacity compared with single center studies. They are therefore only preferred for questions that cannot be addressed in a single delivery system. We believe there will be a substantial number of these situations for the foreseeable future. Although the efforts described here are a work in progress, we conclude that it is possible to create a durable multi-center organization that facilitates such work.

THE CENTRALIZED MODEL—THE VSD

Description of the System

A contrasting strategy for conducting multi-center studies is to create a large, centralized dataset that supports multiple studies of vaccine use and safety. This approach is used by the VSD, which is sponsored by the CDC to study rare adverse events following vaccination (Chen *et al.*, 1997). From 1991 to 2000 the VSD included the Group Health Cooperative in Washington, the Northwest Kaiser Permanente in Oregon, and the Northern California Kaiser and Southern California Kaiser Permanente health programs. In the fall of 2000, Harvard Pilgrim Health Care and Kaiser Permanente of Colorado were added. All five current VSD members are also part of the HMO Research Network Center for Education and Research in Therapeutics.

The main advantage of the VSD database is the ability to address vaccine safety concerns relatively quickly as they arise. The population provides a large cohort of individuals in which key demographic, enrolment, vaccination and healthcare data from several different health plans are maintained in a standardized, edited database. Thus, data are readily available for designing and conducting studies, or for simply assessing whether a study is feasible.

Even in studies in which additional data collection (e.g. chart abstraction) is required, the centralized automated data provide efficiencies. The availability of automated diagnostic codes allows ready identification of potential cases, and provides a source of control selection for case–control studies. When a chart review is required, as often occurs in case–control studies, the amount of review can be minimized. Since the automated vaccination data are of high quality, frequently only cases need to have their charts abstracted to verify case status, but chart review for exposure (i.e. vaccination) is not necessary and thus chart review for controls is not required.

Capabilities Required to Support Centralized Multi-center Studies

Permanent data files maintained by the VSD include a unique study identification number, age and sex, vaccine records (including date and type of vaccination), diagnoses (including those assigned in hospitals, emergency departments, and outpatient visits), plus selected covariate information, e.g. census block codes. Originally, the VSD intended to rely on centrally maintained data to identify potential study subjects. For investigations of specific events or diseases, e.g. seizures, cases were identified from the automated data files maintained at the CDC. The medical records of potential cases were then reviewed according to the individual study protocol at each HMO by trained abstractors to verify case status, document the disease onset date, collect information on competing causes of illness, and gather covariate data. For many studies, however, it has not been practical to rely solely on the central automated datasets to screen for potential cases. In some instances, because of the rarity of the disease and lack of statistical power, it has been necessary to supplement the study sample with cases and controls from earlier years.

The creation and maintenance of high-quality data in a single centralized location comes at a cost. At each VSD site, the data manager and a team of programmers spend several months planning and creating data files. Considerable attention is needed to account for the constantly changing nature of HMO data systems, data collection procedures, and population (including

changes in coverage plans). Once new coverage plans, data systems, or data dictionary changes are researched, new changes are incorporated into the previous year's data creation programs, and then the modified and updated files are tested using sample program runs. After these file modifications have been completed, at some HMOs more than 50 programs are run to identify the study cohort and enrolment intervals, extract utilization data and create the necessary data files. Discrepancy-check programs are then run, and discrepancies resolved when discovered (including occasionally entirely remaking some data files). Finally, a discrepancy summary report is created, and the files are transmitted electronically to a secure CDC site. This last step is time-consuming because of the number and size of the data files.

Examples of Multi-center Studies Using the Centralized System

As noted above, many studies can be conducted utilizing the centralized automated data files alone. The vaccination data, in particular, are continuously monitored and have been shown to be of high quality. So studies of vaccination coverage (e.g. after introduction of a new vaccine or vaccination schedule, or in special populations) can be conducted quickly and without additional data gathering. In some circumstances, health outcomes can also be reliably ascertained using just the automated data. This is the case for conditions in which well-established validated algorithms already exist for the condition, such as asthma, or in which broader categories of health conditions, such as acute respiratory infections, are being evaluated. The centralized database also provides a sampling frame for selecting controls in nested case–control studies.

Specific examples of studies completed using centrally maintained data include those of immunization levels among premature and low-birth-weight infants and risk factors for delayed up to date immunization status (Davis et al., 1999), the epidemiology of diarrheal disease among children enrolled in four west coast HMOs (Parashar et al., 1998), the impact of influenza on the rates of respiratory disease hospitalizations among young children (Izurieta *et al.*, 2000), the rate of influenza vaccination in children with asthma in HMOs (Kramarz *et al.*, 2000a), the impact of influenza vaccination exacerbations of asthma (Kramarz *et al.*, 2000b), and the incidence of Kawasaki syndrome in west coast HMOs (Belay *et al.*, 2000).

Examples of studies completed using expanded or specialized *ad hoc* datasets from VSD sites include the impact of the sequential inactivated polio vaccine/oral polio vaccine schedule on vaccination coverage levels in the United States (Davis *et al.*, 2001), a comparison of adverse event rates after measles–mumps–rubella2 exposure (Davis *et al.*, 1997), assessment of the risk of chronic arthropathy among women after rubella vaccination (Ray *et al.*, 1997), and assessment of the risk of hospitalization because of aseptic meningitis after measles–mumps–rubella vaccination in one-to-two-year-old children (Black *et al.*, 1997)

CONCLUSION

Multi-center studies are likely to grow in usefulness and importance as our ability increases to link automated data, either in an ongoing manner or on an *ad hoc* basis. The best organizational strategy for such studies depends on several factors, including the resources available, the type and variety of the data that are needed, and the speed with which new questions must be answered.

NOTE ADDED IN PROOF

Heightened concerns about data privacy and proposed regulations concerning the use of medical record information are causing the Vaccine Safety Datalink leadership to consider a data structure that aggregates less information in a central location.

ACKNOWLEDGEMENTS

The HMO Research Network Center for Education and Research in Therapeutics is supported by a cooperative agreement U8HS10391 from the Agency for Healthcare Research and Quality. The Vaccine Safety Datalink is supported by contract 200-95-0957 from the Centers for Disease Control and Prevention.

REFERENCES

Belay ED, Holman RC, Clarke MJ, DeStefano F, Shahriari A, Davis RL, *et al.* (2000) The incidence of Kawasaki syndrome in West Coast health maintenance organizations. *Pediatr Infect Dis J* **19**: 828–32.

Black S, Shinefield H, Ray P, Lewis E, Chen R, Glasser J, Hadler S, Hardy J, Rhodes P, Swint E, Davis RL, Thompson R, Mullooly J, Marcy M, Vadheim C, Ward J, Rastogi S, Wise R, the Vaccine Safety Datalink Workgroup (1997) Risk of hospitalization because of aseptic meningitis after measles–mumps–rubella vaccination in one-to-two-year-old children. *Pediatr InfecT Dis J* **16**: 500–3.

Chan KA, Andrade S, Boles M, Buist D, Chase G, Donahue J, Goodman M, Gurwitz J, LaCroix A, Platt R (2000) Inhibitors of hydroxymethylglutaryl-coenzyme A reductase and risk of fracture among older women. *Lancet* **355**: 2185–88.

Chen RT, Glasser JW, Rhodes PH, Davis RL, Thompson RS, Mullooly JP, Black SB, Shinefield HR, Vadheim CM, Marcy SM, Ward JI, Wise RP, Wassilak SG, Hadler SC, *et al.* (1997) Vaccine Safety Datalink Project: a new tool for improving vaccine safety monitoring in the United States. *Pediatrics* **99**: 765–3.

Davis RL, Lieu TA, Mell LK, Capra AM, Zavitkovsky A, Quesenberry CP, Black SB, Shinefield HR, Thompson RS, Rodewald L (2001) Impact of the sequential IPV/OPV schedule on vaccination coverage levels in the United States. *Pediatrics*, in press.

Davis RL, Marcuse EK, Black S, Shinefield H, *et al.* (1997) MMR2 at 4–6 years and 10–12 years of age. A comparison of adverse event rates in the Vaccine Safety Datalink project *Pediatrics* **100**: 767–1.

Davis RL, Rubanowice D, Shinefield HR, Lewis E, Gu D, Black SB, DeStefano F, Gargiullo P, Mullooly JP, Thompson RS, Chen RT, for the CDC Vaccine Safety Datalink Group (1999) Immunization levels among premature and low birth weight infants and risk factors for delayed up-to-date immunization status. *J Am Med Assoc* **282**: 547–3.

Donahue JG, Chan KA, Andrade SE, Beck A, Boles M, Buist DS, Carey VJ, Chandler J, Chase GA, Ettinger B, Fishman P, Goodman JM, Guess HA, Gurwitz JH, Lacroix AZ, Levin TR, Platt R (2002) Gastric and duodenal safety of daily alendronate. *Arch Intern Med* **162**: 936–42.

Izurieta H, Thompson W, Fukuda K, Kramarz P, Shay D, Davis RL, Kramarz P, DeStefano F, Gargiullo

PM, Davis RL, et al. (2000) Influenza and the rates of hospitalization for respiratory disease among infants and young children. *N Engl J Med* **342**: 232.

Kramarz P, DeStefano F, Gargiullo PM, Davis RL, et al. (2000a) Influenza vaccination in children with asthma in health maintenance organizations. *Vaccine* **18**(21): 2288–94.

Kramarz P, DeStefano F, Gargiullo PM, Davis RL, et al. (2000b) Does influenza vaccination exacerbate asthma? Analysis of a large cohort of children with asthma. *Arch Fam Med* **9**: 617–23.

Parashar U, Holman R, Bresee J, Clarke M, Rhodes P, Davis RL, Thompson RS, Mullooly J, Black S, Shinefield H, Marcy M, Vadheim C, Ward J, Chen R, Glass R, and the Vaccine Safety Datalink Team (1998) Epidemiology of diarrheal disease among children enrolled in four West Coast health maintenance organizations. *Pediatr Infect Dis J* **17**: 605–11.

Putnam KG, Buist DS, Fishman P, Andrade SE, Boles M, Chase GA, Goodman MJ, Gurwitz JH, Platt R, Raebel MA, Chan AK (2002) Chronic disease score as a predictor of hospitalization. *Epidemiology* **13**: 340–6.

Ray P, Black S, Shinefield H, Dillon A, Schwalbe J, Holmes S, Hadler S, Chen R, Cochi S, Wassilak S (1997) Risk of chronic arthropathy among women after rubella vaccination. *J Am Med Assoc* **278**: 551–6.

Smalley W, Shatin D, Wysowski DK, Gurwitz J, Andrade SE, Goodman M, Chan KA, Platt R, Schech SD, Ray WA (2000) Contraindicated use of cisapride: the impact of an FDA regulatory action. *J Am Med Assoc* **284**: 3036–9.

Von Korff M, Wagner EH, Saunders K (1992) A chronic disease score from automated pharmacy data. *J Clin Epidemiol* **45**: 197–203

32

Other Databases in Europe

MIRIAM C.J.M. STURKENBOOM

Department of Epidemiology and Biostatistics, Erasmus University Medical Centre, Rotterdam,
The Netherlands, and International Pharmacoepidemiology and Pharmacoeconomics Research Centre (IPPRC),
Desio (MI), Italy

INTRODUCTION

A systematic review of the 384 abstracts presented at the Sixteenth International Conference on Pharmacoepidemiology in 2000 showed that the majority of European pharmacoepidemiological studies ($n = 160$) were conducted by means of automated general practitioner (GP), pharmacy or insurance data (see Table 32.1). Obviously, the UK (General Practitioners Research database (GPRD)) and Scotland alone (Medicines Monitoring Unit (MEMO)) ranked highest in the percentage of abstracts based on automated databases, but the next three positions were taken by The Netherlands, Denmark and Italy. The Netherlands is well known for its automated pharmacy records, and increasingly for its GP databases. Denmark is well known for its regional and national pharmacy claims databases that may be linked to other registries, and the National Health Service (NHS) system in Italy has allowed for building up large regional databases that contain both pharmacy claims as well as hospitalisation data.

This chapter describes the most important automated GP and record linkage databases from The Netherlands, Denmark and Italy that have been used for pharmacoepidemiological research between 1990 and 2001 and it provides a list of pharmacoepidemiological papers that have resulted from the databases in these countries. Since the quality of databases depends on the particular healthcare systems they are embedded in, a summary of the major healthcare characteristics will be provided for each of these countries. Table 32.2 provides a systematic overview of the major characteristics of the databases.

THE NETHERLANDS

GENERAL PRACTITIONERS (GPS)

The Dutch system of healthcare is based on GPs who practice in the community but not in the hospital, referring ambulatory patients to specialists for outpatient or inpatient care. Specialists report their findings to the GP, who acts as a gatekeeper. Approximately 90% of the patients' presenting problems are addressed by the GP (van der Lei et al., 1993; Leufkens and Urquhart, 1994). Full-time staff physicians who are specialists of

Pharmacovigilance. Edited by R.D. Mann and E.B. Andrews
© 2002 John Wiley & Sons, Ltd

Table 32.1. Sources for European abstracts presented at the Sixteenth International Conference on Pharmaco-epidemiology 2000.

Country	Number of abstracts	Percentage based on automated sources % within country	Drug utilisation		Adverse or beneficial effects of drugs	
			Number of ad hoc studies	Number of studies with automated[a] sources	Number of ad hoc studies	Number of studies with automated sources
Scotland	9	78		4	1	4
UK	44	73	2	9	10	23
The Netherlands	28	71	3	9	5	11
Denmark	10	70		6	2	2
Italy	5	60	1	2	1	1
Hungary	2	50	1	1		
Norway	4	50	2	2		
Sweden	6	50	1	1	2	2
Spain	15	33	5	5	5	
Germany	14	21	4	3	7	
France	17	6	6	1	10	
Belgium	2	0	2			
Portugal	2	0	2			
Switzerland	2	0			2	
Total	160	53.8	29 (18.1%)	43 (26.9%)	45 (28.1%)	43 (26.9%)

[a] Automated sources include: GP records, record linkage systems, insurance claims data or drug sales data.

various kinds provide hospital care. Medical care, including prescription drugs, is essentially paid for by a combination of public and private insurers. The public insurers are regional agencies collectively called the Sickfunds. They provide insurance coverage for 60% of the population, i.e. generally those who fall below an annual income level (25 000 euro). A flat fee per year reimburses the GP for Sickfund patients; for privately insured patients the GP is reimbursed on a fee-for-service basis. Patients should be registered with one GP but are free to change, which happens infrequently and nearly always because the patient moves out of the area. When a patient transfers, so does the record. More than 75% of the patients will visit their GP at least once per year (van der Lei et al., 1993). The high degree of computerisation of GPs has given rise to the birth of several GP networks; most of them are connected to one of the seven University Centres. One of the largest GP databases is the Integrated Primary Care Information Project (IPCI), which has been created with the specific purpose to conduct pharmacoepidemiological and pharmacoeconomic studies (van der Lei et al., 1993; Vlug et al., 1999).

THE IPCI

In 1992 the IPCI was started by the Department of Medical Informatics of the Erasmus University Medical School (MIEUR), initially in collaboration with IMS but independently from 1999 onwards. IPCI is a longitudinal observational database that contains data from computer-based patient records of a selected group of GPs throughout The Netherlands that voluntarily chose to supply data to the database (Vlug et al., 1999). GPs only receive a minimal reimbursement for their data and control usage of their data, through the Steering Committee and through the opportunity to withdraw data for specific studies.

Table 32.2. Characteristics of multi-purpose automated databases in Italy, The Netherlands, and Denmark.

Characteristics	Italy		The Netherlands		Denmark
	Pedianet	ISSR (FVG)	IPCI	PHARMO	OPED/PDNJ
Current source population	90 000 children	1.2 million	500 000	650 000	500 000 each
Demographics					
Unique identifier for linking of files	Yes	Yes	Yes (database specific)		
Registration date	Yes	Yes	Yes	No (based on first prescription)	No (based on first prescription)
Date of transferring out	Yes	Yes	Yes	No (based on last prescription)	Yes (6 months delay)
Date of death	Yes	Yes	Yes	No	Yes (6 months delay)
Insurance type	Yes	NHS only	Yes	Yes	NHS only
Date of birth	Yes	Yes	Yes	Yes	Yes
Gender	Yes	Yes	Yes	Yes	Yes
Race	Yes	No	No	No	No
Socio-economic status	No	No	Yes	No	No
Consent procedures required	Yes (active consent has been obtained for participating children).	Yes (For access of hospital charts)	Confidentiality in line with rules of Dutch Board of Registers. Consent required for interventions and patient questionnaires.	Confidentiality in line with rules of Dutch Board of Registers. Patient consent required for access of hospital charts.	Confidentiality in line with rules of Danish Board of Registers
Prescriptions					
Unique product code	Yes (MINSAN)[a]	Yes (MINSAN)	Yes (HPK)	Yes (HPK)	Yes (Varenummeret)
ATC code	Yes	Yes	Yes	Yes	Yes
Date of Rx	Yes	Yes	Yes	Yes	Yes
Quantity	Yes	Yes	Yes	Yes	Yes
Dosing regimen	Yes	No	Yes	Yes	No
Indication	Yes	No	Yes	No	No
Inpatient use of drugs	No		No (free text if registered)	No	No
Prescription drugs	Yes (independent of reimbursement)	Yes (only reimbursed)	Yes (independent of reimbursement)	Yes (independent of reimbursement)	Yes (only reimbursed)

(continued)

Table 32.2. Continued.

Characteristics	Italy		The Netherlands		Denmark
	Pedianet	ISSR (FVG)	IPCI	PHARMO	OPED/PDNJ
OTC drugs	Not validly	No	Not validly	No	No
Outcomes					
Symptoms	Yes (free text)	No	Yes (free text/ICPC)	No	No
Outpatient diagnoses	Yes (ICD-9)	No	Yes (ICPC)	No	No
Hospitalisations	Yes (not complete)	Yes (ICD-9)	Yes	Yes (ICD-9)	Yes (OPED not routinely)
Outpatient specialist care	Yes	No	Yes	No	No
Value of laboratory measurements	Yes	No	Yes	No	No
Costs	Yes (visits/drugs/lab/referrals/hospitalisation)	Yes (drugs/procedures/hospitalisation)	Yes (visits/drugs/lab/referrals/hospitalisation)	Yes (drugs/hospitalisation/inpatient procedures)	Yes (drugs/hospitalisation)
Potential confounding factors					
Smoking	—	No	Yes	No	Yes (PDNJ)
BMI	Yes	No	Yes	No	No
Cardiovascular risk profile	Yes	No	Yes	No	No
Indication	Yes	No	Yes	No	No
Severity	Not directly	No	Not directly	No	No
Access					
Raw data	Yes (through So.Se.Te)	Currently not	Yes (through MIEUR)	Yes (through PHARMO Institute)	Yes (through OPED or PDNJ research institutes)
Original medical charts	Unknown yet	No	Yes (discharge letters)	Yes (discharge letters)	Unknown
Additional data collection from patient	Yes (possibility to insert software modules for prospective data collection)	No	Yes (through GP)	No	No
Contact person	Sturkenboom@epib.fgg.eur.nl Carlog@child.pedi.unipd.it	Not accessible	Sturkenboom@epib.fgg.eur.nl	Ron.Herings@PHARMO.nl	David Gaist (OPED) HT Sorensen (PDNJ)

[a]MINSAN codes are collected but are not provided as raw data.

The collaborating GPs are comparable to other Dutch GPs regarding age and gender.

As of January 2001 there are 73 practices belonging to 140 general practitioners that are providing ongoing data to the database. The first practice was recruited into the IPCI project in 1994. Practices have therefore been supplying data for varying periods of time (average period of data-supply: four years). The database contains information on 485 000 patients. This is the cumulative amount of patients who have ever been part of the dynamic cohort of registered patients. Turnover occurs as patients move and transfer to new practices. The records of "transferred out" patients remain on the database and are available for retrospective study with the appropriate time periods. As of 1 January 2000 there were more than 300 000 active patients registered with the collaborating GPs, 49.1% were male, 57% were insured through the Sickfund, and the mean age was 37.7 years (sd: 21.9). Over the next years IPCI will be extended to cover a population of one million subjects.

The database contains identification information (date of birth, sex, patient identification, insurance, date of registration and transferring out, date of death), notes (subjective and assessment text), prescriptions, and indications for therapy, physical findings, referrals, hospitalisations and laboratory values (see Figure 32.1 for the database structure).

MIEUR has implemented a research specific module in the software that requires linkage of an indication to each prescription. The International Classification of Primary Care (ICPC) is the coding system for patient complaints and diagnoses, but diagnoses and complaints can also be entered as free text that is available as raw data (Lamberts and Wood, 1987). Prescription data such as product name, quantity dispensed, dosage regimens, strength and indication are entered into the computer to produce printed prescriptions (Vlug et al., 1999). The National Database of drugs, maintained by the Z-index, enables the coding of prescriptions, according to the Anatomical Therapeutic Chemical (ATC) classification scheme recommended by the World Health Organisation (WHO) (de Smet, 1988).

Data are downloaded on a monthly basis and the information is sent to the gatekeeper who anonymises all information before further access is provided. Access to original medical records (discharge letters of hospitals) and administration of questionnaires to GPs is possible through the gatekeeper after the approval of the Steering Committee.

Data accumulated in the IPCI database have proven to be of high quality and suitable for epidemiological and pharmacoepidemiological research (Visser et al., 1996; van der Linden et al., 1998; van der Linden et al., 1999; Vlug et al., 1999;

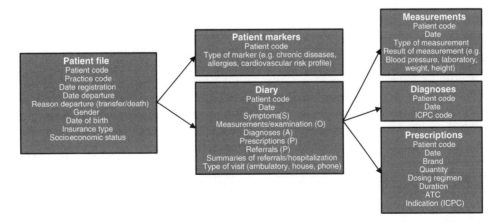

Figure 32.1. IPCI research database structure.

Chapple, 2001; Logie *et al.*, 2001). Data can be used for research purposes but access is possible only through MIEUR and after the approval of the Steering Committee.

COMPUTERISATION OF THE DUTCH COMMUNITY PHARMACY SYSTEM

Computerisation of outpatient pharmacy records in The Netherlands is almost universal, and so is (due to the patient's habit of frequenting only one pharmacy) the compilation of longitudinal prescription drug histories. Although computerisation has started for administrative (reimbursement) purposes, medication surveillance and computerised stock holding and ordering have become important incentives for the optimal registration of drug dispensing. Computerised medication surveillance tracks changes in dosages of chronic medications, correct dosing (especially for the elderly and children), contraindications (deduced from previously prescribed medications) and interactions between concomitant medications. In the case of "abnormal" situations a signal will be generated that needs to be verified by the pharmacist (Herings, 1993; Leufkens and Urquhart, 1994).

All information stored in pharmacy computers, independent of the employed software or hardware, is primarily based on the information written on a prescription order by a GP, dentist or specialist. The information that should be stated on this order is legally regulated and has to comprise the prescribed product, the date of prescription, name and residence of prescriber, a patient identifier (name), and the daily dose regimen. For reimbursement purposes the amount dispensed is also available on each prescription (Herings, 1993).

The longitudinal data collection in pharmacies, the completeness of the data, and the fact that all prescription drugs are recorded (independent of reimbursement) make these data a good source for pharmacoepidemiological research. They have served for national cohort tracking in the case of drug alerts after which outcome data may be either linked or collected by *ad hoc* methods (Stricker *et al.*, 1992). The PHARMO database is based on

pharmacy data and is unique in the Netherlands for its record linkage with national hospitalisation registries.

PHARMO

The PHARMO medical record linkage scheme started in 1985 and includes the drug-dispensing records from community pharmacies and hospital discharge records of all 650 000 community-dwelling inhabitants of nine medium-sized cities in defined demogeographic areas in The Netherlands (Herings, 1993). The underlying population has been defined by using information for each city from the Bureau of Statistics (CBS). Patients that are registered within the pharmacy files are regarded as non-residents and are eliminated from the patient registers if they are not recorded as having a family practitioner residential in one of the cities. Patients are assumed to be present in the source population between the first and last encounter in the pharmacy. For all residents, the drug-dispensing histories are linked on a yearly basis to the national hospital discharge records of the same patient, using a probabilistic algorithm, based on characteristics such as date of birth, gender and a code for the general practitioner since no unique patient identifier is present. Validation showed that these registries are linked with a sensitivity and specificity exceeding 95%, which is comparable to record linkage systems based on unique personal identifiers (Herings *et al.*, 1990, 1992; Herings, 1993). The computerised drug-dispensing histories contain outpatient prescription data concerning the dispensed drug, type of prescriber, dispensing date, dispensed amount, prescribed dose regimens, and the legend duration (prescription length). The hospital records include detailed information concerning the primary and secondary diagnoses, procedures, and dates of hospital admission and discharge. All diagnoses are coded according to the ICD-9-CM. To date, the PHARMO system has provided data for several doctorate theses and pharmacoepidemiological publications in major medical journals (Herings *et al.*, 1993, 1995a, 1995b, 1995c, 1996, 1999, 2000; van der Klaauw *et al.*, 1993, 1999; Herings and Stricker, 1995; Heerdink *et al.*, 1998;

Gerrits *et al.*, 1999; Bouvy *et al.*, 2000; Burger *et al.*, 2000). The PHARMO data are available for research purposes, after approval of the protocol by the Scientific Board. Research projects can be conducted only through the PHARMO Institute. Inspection of discharge letters is possible after approval by the Administrative Boards of the individual hospitals.

DENMARK

COMPUTERISATION OF DANISH PHARMACIES

Similar to The Netherlands, GPs in Denmark act as gatekeepers to second-line healthcare and provide most of the medical care. The majority (97%) of citizens are assigned a GP and these GPs generate 90% of the prescriptions. Although initiatives have been taken to create GP databases, the most important source for pharmacoepidemiological studies in Denmark to date constitutes data from the Danish pharmacies that have become increasingly computerised over the last decade and have allowed for the establishment of regional and national prescription registries (Gaist *et al.*, 1997). As part of its tax-funded healthcare for all inhabitants, the Danish National Health Service (NHS) provides medical attendance free of charge and reimburses 50% of all expenditure on a wide range of prescribed medicines independently of the presenter's income and employment status. Measured in defined daily doses, 73% of all medication sold in Denmark in 1996 was on prescription (Gaist *et al.*, 1997).

The NHS is divided into 16 sections. Each community pharmacy collects data on all prescription drugs and forwards data on reimbursable medicines to their local NHS section on a monthly basis. These data form the basis for the two prescription registries, the Odense University Pharmacoepidemiological Database (OPED) and the Pharmacoepidemiological Prescription Database of North Jutland (PDNJ) (Sorensen and Larsen, 1994; Gaist *et al.*, 1997).

A third prescription register was established in 1994, the Register of Drug Statistics (RDS) at the Medicines Division of the National Board of Health, that collects information on all pharmacy transactions of prescribed drugs independent of reimbursement status and covers the entire population of 5 million inhabitants. Although drug-utilisation studies have been performed with this database, there are no official guidelines on access to RDS (Hallas *et al.*, 1995; Sorensen *et al.*, 1996; Gaist *et al.*, 1997; Gaist, 1999; Juul *et al.*, 1999).

THE OPED AND THE PDNJ

The OPED database covers the county of Funen (population approximately 470 000) persons and PDNJ covers the county of Jutland (approximately 490 000 persons). Together they have covered a representative sample of 18% of the Danish population (Gaist *et al.*, 1997; Nielsen *et al.*, 1997) since 1992. Dispensing claims data that are collected in the systems comprise a unique patient identifier, the civil registration number (CRN), which allows longitudinal tracking of the patient through different layers of the healthcare system: the date of dispensing, the product code (unique for brand, quantity and formulation) and the ATC code. The computerised drug-dispensing histories contain data concerning the dispensed drug, type of prescriber, dispensing date, dispensed amount, prescribed dose regimens, and the legend duration (prescription length). The prescribed dosing regimen (and therefore legend duration) is not recorded in the systems. Over-the-counter medication and non-reimbursed drugs (such as sedatives, hypnotics, oral contraceptives, laxatives), or in-hospital drugs use are not registered. Population data are obtained from the Central Registration System every six months to track migration or date of death. Completeness of reimbursed dispensed drugs has proven to be good (Gaist *et al.*, 1997).

Prescription data have been linked to local, regional and national hospitalisation discharge data, cancer registries, death and birth registries for specific projects through the CRN number in the PDNJ database (Dalton *et al.*, 2000; Fonager *et al.*, 2000; Larsen *et al.*, 2000; Nielsen *et al.*, 1996, 1999; Olesen *et al.*, 1999, 2001; Sorensen *et al.*, 1996, 1999, 2000a, 2000b; Steffensen *et al.*, 1997;

Thrane and Sorensen, 1999). The Danish hospital discharge registry comprises data on 99.4% of all discharges from Danish hospitals and includes the CRN code, dates of admission and discharge, the surgical procedures performed, and up to 20 diagnoses classified according to the ICD-10 classification of diseases (Andersen et al., 1999). Almost all of the OPED studies are based on prescription data only and the authors have used prescription symmetry analyses to associate drug use with specific outcomes (Bjerrum and Bergman, 2000; Bjerrum et al., 1997, 1998, 1999, 2000; Gaist, 1999; Larsen et al., 1998; Rosholm et al., 1993, 1994, 1997, 1998; Hallas and Bytzer, 1998; Hallas, 1996; Gaist et al., 1996; Hansen et al., 1996; Hallas and Hansen, 1993a, 1993b). The OPED and the PDNJ are public institution research registries. Data can be accessed upon approval of a protocol by the Steering Committees.

ITALY

HEALTHCARE

Similar to The Netherlands and the United Kingdom, GPs in Italy act as gatekeepers to second line healthcare and provide most of the medical care. Contrary to The Netherlands, however, direct feedback from specialists or hospitals to GPs is less organised. Although several initiatives have been taken to create centralised GP databases or networks (e.g. the Healthsearch project), none of the projects has produced pharmacoepidemiological papers in Medline-listed journals so far.

Italy is rather unique in having a specific paediatric primary care system for children between 0 and 14 years of age. A minority of children are cared for by family physicians (mostly those 10 years and older), whereas there are almost 7000 paediatricians throughout the country associated with the NHS that gives a flat fee for service per registered child to the paediatrician. Inscription in the National Health system is compulsory for residents; thus, every child at birth is referred to a paediatrician associated with the NHS. All consultations, prescriptions and exams that are prescribed by the paediatrician are free of charge to

the patient, thus there are no economic constraints to attend medical care (Fornaro et al., 1999). This unique feature of Italian healthcare resulted in the initiation of the Pedianet database in 1999.

As part of its tax-funded healthcare for residents, the Italian NHS provides medical attendance and prescribed medicines. Typically, new and more expensive drugs are preferred in Italy even when effective, safe and less expensive alternatives are available. Prescribers had to face a highly dynamic pharmaceutical market in which 30% of substances (among the 300 most sold) changed every five years prior to the Drug Reform Act in 1994. (Maggini et al., 1996). After the Drug Reform Act, the reimbursement status of drugs was categorised in three groups: class A drugs are reimbursed completely; class B drugs require a small patient fee dependent on age and exemption status. Class C drugs are not reimbursed at all (Rolle et al., 1995). An example of a class C drug is sedatives.

Healthcare is organised by regional and local health agencies that use the local and regional health care information systems (SISR) for the planning of resource utilisation. Historically, the most important source for pharmacoepidemiological studies in Italy has been the SISR, which accumulates data on all births, deaths, claims of dispensed drugs, hospitalisations, procedures, and vaccinations that are reimbursed by the NHS through their local health units (Menniti-Ippolito et al., 1998; Maggini et al., 1991; Arpino et al., 1995; Traversa et al., 1994, 1995, 1998; Tebano et al., 1996; Raschetti et al., 1993; Caffari and Raschetti, 1991; Degli Esposti et al., 1999). The SISR of the Friuli–Venezia–Giulia (FVG) Region in the North-east of Italy has been used most frequently for the conduct of pharmacoepidemiological research (Castellsague et al., 1999; Cattaruzzi et al., 1999; Garcia-Rodriguez et al., 1995, 1998; Ruigomez et al., 1999; Maggini et al., 1999; Mannino et al., 1998; Rossi et al., 1991; Simon et al., 1994).

THE FVG

The FVG regional health database contains accurate data on demographics (unique patient identifier, gender, date of birth, registration and end of registration date) outpatient prescriptions (drug name, strength, formulation, price, date of dispensing and number of dispensed packages, since 1992), hospitalisations (including date of admission and discharge, all discharge diagnoses, since 1985), outpatient procedures (since January, 1998) and deaths relating to the 1.2 million residents registered with the NHS.

The prescription data concern NHS reimbursed drugs sold by all private and public pharmacies; the hospitalisation data refer to all public and private hospitals in the FVG, whereas outpatient procedures are registered if reimbursed by the NHS (private non-reimbursed procedures are excluded). Data access has been complicated since the changes in the privacy legislation in Italy in 1999. Linkage of data that are collected for administrative purposes is not possible for other purposes. Access is limited to the National Institute of Health (Istituto Superiore di Sanità).

PEDIANET

Since 1999 the Società Servizi Telematici (So.-Se.Te.) based in Padova has developed a national database, called PEDIANET, which currently collects the clinical, demographic and prescription data for approximately 60 000 children that have provided informed consent and who are under the care of any of the 84 primary care paediatricians (FP) that currently provide data to the database. Recruitment of paediatricians and the informed consent of patients is ongoing and the purpose is to include a total of 250 paediatricians (covering 250 000 children) by the end of 2001.

Data are generated during routine patient care with the software JB 95® and are stored in different files, which can be linked through a unique (anonymous) numerical identifier. The identification file contains information on the demographic data of the child and the eligibility status (registration status, date of registration, date of death). The prescription file contains information on all drugs (date of prescription, ATC code, product, quantity, dosing regimen, legend duration, indication, reimbursement status) and vaccinations that are prescribed by the

paediatricians. Reasons for contact and diagnoses (free text or coded by the ICD-9 system) are collected in the medical file. In addition, the database contains information on referrals to specialists, procedures, hospitalisations, medical exams, health status (according to the Guidelines of Health Supervision of the American Academy of Paediatrics) and centile diagrams.

The database is suitable for both retrospective inspection of routinely collected data and for prospective data collection (outcomes, indirect costs of disease) (Menniti-Ippolito et al., 2000; Cantarutti et al., 2001). Data access is possible after approval of the protocol by the Scientific Board.

GENERAL CONSIDERATIONS

The use of automated data for the conduct of observational epidemiological research has been heavily discussed in the past and will continue to be discussed even more if researchers are using the same or similar data. A good example is the conflicting results of two studies on the risk of venous thromboembolism in women using third-generation oral contraceptives that were both conducted in the GPRD (Farmer et al., 2000; Kaye et al., 2000). Despite the controversies that may arise between persons with conflicting interest (researchers, producers, prescribers, patients), there is no doubt that the use of automated linkage or GP data has proven its value in pharmacoepidemiology. The recent acquisition of the GPRD database by the Medicines Control Agency (MCA), the sublicensing of the GPRD to different research groups and companies and the interest of various regulatory agencies in the use of automated databases clearly demonstrates the need for longitudinal medical databases to anticipate, evaluate and assess the use, cost and positive and adverse effects of drugs.

Large automated databases have given us the opportunity to study the rare and common effects of (in)frequently used drugs. Good examples are the studies conducted with the PDNJ database on the teratogenic effects of specific drugs (Fonager et al., 2000; Larsen et al., 2000; Nielsen et al., 1999, 2001; Sorensen et al., 1999, 2000a; Thulstrup et al.,

1999). Owing to the tax-funded healthcare structures in many European countries, it is possible to conduct population-based studies that do not suffer from potential socio-economic selection biases that may occur with the health maintenance organisation databases in the United States. In addition, the longitudinal prospective collection of routine care data eliminates recall errors that have plagued so many *ad hoc* case–control studies in the past.

Challenges remain the validation of outcomes, misclassification of exposure and the adequate control of confounding by indication, severity and contra-indication. The extent of these potential problems depends on the type of database. Record linkage databases such as PHARMO, FVG, OPED, PDNJ and also MEMO usually contain only data on hospitalisations and (reimbursed) drug use. Important confounding factors such as the indication for drug use, body mass index, smoking, family history and minor medical problems cannot easily be assessed and adjusted for. Validation of outcomes with original charts has become more difficult owing to the current privacy regulations.

The GP's databases like IPCI and Pedianet have fewer disadvantages than record linkage systems owing both to the nature of the data (90% of the patient care is conducted by the practitioners) and the fact that data are collected directly from the individual healthcare provider. The latter not only simplifies access to original data but also the insertion of project-specific modules in the software. It is possible to conduct prospective studies with additional data collection such as days of school or work lost in Pedianet (Cantarutti *et al.*, 2001). In the IPCI database we are currently exploring the conduct of large naturalistic trials that should effectively deal with confounding.

The unification of Europe and the increased computerisation of health care are promising future perspectives. Initiatives have been taken further to link hospitalisation and pharmacy claims data to GP records, and we may soon expect databases also in other countries (Sweden, Spain). Now that we transfer from data scarcity to an era of data abundance, it will be possible to choose a database that is tailored for the research question at hand. Table 32.2 may offer aid in comparing the available databases. As researchers we may want to unite forces. Effort should be put into the organisation of multinational database studies that have advantages in size but also in variability of drug use, allowing for the full evaluation of drug-and dose specific risks and comparisons between countries.

REFERENCES

Andersen T, Madsen M, Jorgensen J, Mellenmkjaer L, Olsen, J (1999) *Dan Med Bull* **46**: 263–8.

Arpino C, Da Cas R, Donini G, Pasquini P, Raschetti, R, Traversa G (1995) *Acta Psychiatr Scand* **92**: 7–9.

Bjerrum L, Bergman U (2000) *Scan J Prim Health Care* **18**: 94–8.

Bjerrum L, Rosholm JU, Hallas J, Kragstrup J (1997) *Eur J Clin Pharmacol* **53**: 7–11.

Bjerrum L, Sogaard J, Hallas J, Kragstrup J (1998) *Eur J Clin Pharmacol* **54**: 197–202.

Bjerrum L, Sogaard J, Hallas J, Kragstrup J (1999) *Br J Gen Pract* **49**: 195–8.

Bjerrum L, Sogaard J, Hallas J, Kragstrup J (2000) *Ugeskr Laeger* **162**: 2037–40.

Bouvy ML, Heerdink ER, De Bruin ML, Herings RM, Leufkens HG, Hoes AW (2000) *Arch Intern Med* **160**: 2477–80.

Burger H, Herings RM, Egberts AC, Neef C, Leufkens HG (2000) *Eur J Clin Pharmacol* **56**: 319–22.

Caffari B, Raschetti R (1991) *Ann Ist Super Sanita* **27**: 195–200.

Cantarutti L, Sturkenboom M, Bordin A, Bussi R, Cozzani S, Del Torso S, *et al.* (2001) *Medico e Bambino*, 1–9.

Castellsague J, Garcia-Rodriguez LA, Perez-Gutthann S, Agostinis L, Cattaruzi C, Troncon MG (1999) *Respir Med* **93**: 709–14.

Cattaruzzi C, Troncon MG, Agostinis L, Garcia-Rodriguez LA (1999) *J Clin Epidemiol* **52**: 499–502.

Chapple CR (2001) *Eur Urol*, **39** (Suppl 3): 31–6.

Dalton SO, Johansen C, Mellemkjaer L, Sorensen HT, McLaughlin JK, Olsen J, Olsen JH (2000) *Epidemiology* **11**: 171–6.

de Smet P (1988) *J Soc Adm Pharmacy* **5**: 49–58.

Degli Esposti E, Berto P, Buda S, Di Nardo AM, Sturani A (1999) *Am J Hypertens* **12**: 790–6.

Farmer R, Williams T, Nightingale A (2000) *Br Med J* **321**: 1352.

Fonager K, Larsen H, Pedersen L, Sorensen HT (2000) *Acta Neurol Scand* **101**: 289–94.

Fornaro P, Gandini F, Marin M, Pedrazzi C, Piccoli P, Tognetti D, Assael BM, Lucioni C, Mazzi S (1999) *Pediatr Infect Dis J* **18**: 414–9.

Gaist D (1999) *Cephalalgia* **19**: 735–61.

Gaist D, Hallas J, Hansen N, Gram L (1996) *Br J Clin Pharmacol* **41**: 285–9.

Gaist D, Sorensen HT, Hallas J (1997) *Dan Med Bull* **44**: 445–8.

Garcia-Rodriguez LA, Cattaruzzi C, Troncon MG, Agostinis L (1998) *Arch Intern Med* **158**: 33–9.

Garcia-Rodriguez LA, Cattaruzzi C, Grazia Troncon M, Agostinis, L, Simon, G (1995) *Br J Clin Pharmacol* **40**: 104–5.

Gerrits CM, Herings RM, Leufkens HG, Lammers JW (1999) *Pharm World Sci* **21**: 116–9.

Hallas J (1996) *Epidemiology* **7**: 478–84.

Hallas J, Bytzer P (1998) *Eur J Gastroenterol Hepatol* **10**: 27–32.

Hallas J, Hansen N (1993a) *J Intern Med* **234**: 65–70.

Hallas J, Hansen NC (1993b) *J Intern Med* **234**: 65–70.

Hallas J, Lauritsen J, Dalsgard Villadsen H, Gram L (1995) *Scand J Gastroenterol* **30**: 438–44.

Hansen N, Hallas J, Lauritsen J, Bytzer P (1996) *Scand J Gastroenterol* **31**: 126–30.

Heerdink ER, Leufkens HG, Herings RM, Ottervanger JP, Stricker BH, Bakker A (1998) *Arch Intern Med* **158**: 1108–2.

Herings RM (1993) *Pharmo: a record linkage system for postmarketing surveillance of prescriptions in The Netherlands. Thesis.* Utrecht: University of Utrecht.

Herings RM, Bakker A, Stricker BH, Nap G (1992) *J Epidemiol Community Health* **46**: 136–40.

Herings RM, de Boer A, Stricker BH, Bakker A, Sturmans F (1995a) *Pharm World Sci* **17**: 17–9.

Herings RM, de Boer A, Stricker BH, Leufkens HG, Porsius A (1995b) *Lancet* **345**: 1195–8.

Herings RM, Leufkens HG, Vandenbroucke JP (2000) *J Am Med Assoc* **284**: 2998–9.

Herings RM, Stricker BH (1995) *Pharm World Sci* **17**: 133–7.

Herings RM, Stricker BH, Bakker A (1990) *Ned Tijdschr Geneeskd* **134**: 1903–7.

Herings RM, Stricker BH, de Boer A, Bakker A, Sturmans F (1995c) *Arch Intern Med* **155**: 1801–7.

Herings RM, Stricker BH, de Boer A, Bakker A, Sturmans F, Stergachis A (1996) *J Clin Epidemiol* **49**: 115–9.

Herings RM, Stricker BH, Leufkens HG, Bakker A, Sturmans F, Urquhart J (1993) *Pharm World Sci* **15**: 212–8.

Herings RM, Urquhart J, Leufkens HG (1999) *Lancet* **354**: 127–8.

Juul KV, Thomsen OO, Nissen A, Hallas J, Kolmos HJ, Funch-Jensen PM, Lauritsen K (1999) *Ugeskr Laeger* **161**: 6635–8.

Kaye J, Vasilakis-Scaramozza C, Jick S, Jick H (2000) *Br Med J* **321**: 1528.

Lamberts H, Wood M (1987) *International Classification of Primary Care.* Oxford: Oxford Univeristy Press.

Larsen H, Nielsen GL, Sorensen HT, Moller M, Olsen J, Schonheyder HC (2000) *Acta Obstet Gynecol Scand* **79**: 379–83.

Larsen J, Bjerrum L, Hallas J, Kragstrup J (1998) *Ugeskr Laeger* **160**: 3544–7.

Leufkens H, Urquhart J (1994) In: Strom B, ed., *Pharmacoepidemiology.* New York: Wiley, pp. 231–44.

Logie JW, Clifford GM, Farmer RD, Meesen BP (2001) *Eur Urol*, **39** (Suppl 3): 42–7.

Maggini M, Menniti Ippolito F, Spila Alegiani S, Traversa G, Fortini M (1991) *Ann Ist Super Sanita* **27**: 201–6.

Maggini M, Raschetti R, Agostinis L, Cattaruzzi C, Troncon MG, Simon G (1999) *Ann Ist Super Sanita* **35**: 429–33.

Maggini M, Raschetti R, Traversa G (1996) *Eur J Clin Pharmacol* **49**: 429–30.

Mannino S, Troncon MG, Cattaruzzi C, Agostinis L, Wallander M, Romano F, Marighi P, Walker A (1998) *PDS* **7**.

Menniti-Ippolito F, Maggini M, Raschetti R, Da Cas R, Traversa G, Walker AM (1998) *Eur J Clin Pharmacol* **54**: 393–7.

Menniti-Ippolito F, Raschetti R, Da Cas R, Giaquinto G, Cantarutti L (2000) *Lancet* **355**: 1613–4.

Nielsen G, Sorensen H, Zhou W, Steffensen F, Olsen J (1997) *Intern J Risk Safety Med* **10**: 203–5.

Nielsen GL, Sorensen HT, Larsen H, Pedersen L (2001) *Br Med J* **322**: 266–70.

Nielsen GL, Sorensen HT, Pedersen AB, Sabroe S (1996) *J Med Syst* **20**: 1–10.

Nielsen GL, Sorensen HT, Thulstrup AM, Tage-Jensen U, Olesen C, Ekbom A (1999) *Aliment Pharmacol Ther* **13**: 1085–9.

Olesen C, De Vries CS, Thrane N, MacDonald TM, Larsen H, Sorensen HT, Group TE (2001) *Br J Clin Pharmacol* **51**: 153–7.

Olesen C, Steffensen FH, Nielsen GL, de Jong-van den Berg L, Olsen J, Sorensen HT (1999) *Eur J Clin Pharmacol* **55**: 139–44.

Raschetti R, Spila Alegiani S, Diana G, Da Cas R, Traversa G, Pasquini P (1993) *Acta Psychiatr Scand* **87**: 317–21.

Rolle C, Ferraro L, Marrazzo E, Ostino G (1995) *Pharm World Sci* **17**: 158–62.

Rosholm J, Bjerrum L, Hallas J, Worm J, Gram L (1998) *Dan Med Bull* **45**: 210–13.

Rosholm J, Gram L, Isacsson G, Hallas J, Bergman U (1997) *Eur J Clin Pharmacol* **52**: 205–9.

Rosholm J, Hallas J, Gram L (1993) *J Affect Disord* **27**: 21–8.

Rosholm J, Hallas J, Gram L (1994) *Br J Clin Pharmacol* **37**: 533–8.

Rossi P, Perraro F, Tosato F, Aulenti G, Marasco MG, Del Frate B, Scocchi A, Valentinis U (1991) *Qual Assur Health Care* **3**: 179–82.

Ruigomez A, Garcia Rodriguez LA, Cattaruzzi C, Troncon MG, Agostinis L, Wallander MA, Johansson S (1999) *Am J Epidemiol* **150**: 476–81.

Simon G, Francescutti C, Brusin S, Rosa F (1994) *Epidemiol Prev* **18**: 224–9.

Sorensen HT, Hansen I, Ejlersen E, Sabroe S, Hamburger H (1996) *J Med Syst* **20**: 57–65.

Sorensen HT, Johnsen SP, Larsen H, Pedersen L, Nielsen GL, Moller M (2000a) *Acta Obstet Gynecol Scand* **79**: 655–9.

Sorensen HT, Larsen BO (1994) *J Med Syst* **18**: 33–8.

Sorensen HT, Mellemkjaer L, Blot WJ, Nielsen GL, Steffensen FH, McLaughlin JK, Olsen JH (2000b) *Am J Gastroenterol* **95**: 2218–4.

Sorensen HT, Nielsen GL, Olesen C, Larsen H, Steffensen FH, Schonheyder HC, Olsen J, Czeizel AE (1999) *Br J Clin Pharmacol* **48**: 234–8.

Steffensen FH, Kristensen K, Ejlersen E, Dahlerup JF, Sorensen HT (1997) *J Intern Med* **242**: 497–503.

Stricker BH, Barendregt M, Herings RM, de Jong-van den Berg LT, Cornel MC, de Smet PA (1992) *Eur J Clin Pharmacol* **42**: 555–7.

Tebano MT, Traversa G, Da Cas R, Loizzo A (1996) *Aliment Pharmacol Ther* **10**: 659–3.

Thrane N, Sorensen HT (1999) *Acta Paediatr* **88**: 1131–6.

Thulstrup AM, Sorensen HT, Nielsen GL, Andersen L, Barrett D, Vilstrup H, Olsen J (1999) *Am J Perinatol* **16**: 321–6.

Traversa G, Pasquini P, Bottoni A, Da Cas R, Di Giovambattista G, Martino P, Raschetti R (1994) *Ann Ist Super Sanita* **30**: 229–35.

Traversa G, Spila-Alegiani S, Arpino C, Ferrara M (1998) *J Child Adolesc Psychopharmacol* **8**: 175–80.

Traversa G, Walker AM, Ippolito FM, Caffari B, Capurso L, Dezi A, Koch M, Maggini M, Alegiani SS, Raschetti R (1995) *Epidemiology* **6**: 49–54.

van der Klauw MM, Goudsmit R, Halie MR, van't Veer MB, Herings RM, Wilson JH, Stricker BH (1999) *Arch Intern Med* **159**: 369–74.

van der Klauw MM, Stricker BH, Herings RM, Cost WS, Valkenburg HA, Wilson JH (1993) *Br J Clin Pharmacol* **35**: 400–8.

van der Lei J, Duisterhout J, Westerhof H, van der Does E, Cromme P, Boon W, van Bemmel J (1993) *Ann Intern Med* **119**: 1036–41.

van der Linden PD, van de Lei J, Nab HW, Knol A, Stricker BH (1999) *Br J Clin Pharmacol* **48**: 433–7.

van der Linden PD, van der Lei J, Vlug AE, Stricker BH (1998) *J Clin Epidemiol* **51**: 703–8.

Visser LE, Vlug AE, van der Lei J, Stricker BH (1996) *Eur J Clin Pharmacol* **49**: 439–4.

Vlug AE, van der Lei J, Mosseveld BM, van Wijk MA, van der Linden PD, Sturkenboom MC, van Bemmel JH (1999) *Methods Inf Med* **38**: 339–44.

33

Surveillance for Medical Devices—USA

THOMAS P. GROSS

Division of Postmarket Surveillance, Office of Surveillance and Biometrics, Center for Devices and Radiological Health, US Food and Drug Administration, Rockville, MD, USA

LARRY G. KESSLER

Office of Surveillance and Biometrics, Center for Devices and Radiological Health, US Food and Drug Administration, Rockville, MD, USA

INTRODUCTION

The world of medical devices encompasses a wide variety of products from single use disposable to short- or long-term implantable to multiple use durable capital equipment, from products that are used to monitor to those used to diagnose or treat, and from products that deliver their effect through electronic means to those who do so via mechanical or chemical means. In addition, all these products involve both the user and patient (at times the same) and are used in a variety of settings (e.g. from hospital to home care).

The Center for Devices and Radiological Health (CDRH) is that part of the US Food and Drug Administration (FDA) that helps ensure that the world of medical devices (see addendum for definition) intended for human use is safe and effective and helps reduce unnecessary exposure to radiation from medical, occupational, and consumer products. The industry that the FDA regulates accounted for $129.5 billion in global business in 1996 and consisted of 3000 product lines and 84 000 individual products (Wilkerson Group, 1995; Gallivan, 1997). Furthermore, the US industry in 1997 was comprised of approximately 6000 medical and diagnostics companies, about 80% of whom employed 50 or fewer people. These small entrepreneurial entities accounted for only 10% of sales, whereas the largest 2% accounted for 45% of sales (Lewin Group, Inc., 2000).

The agency's mandate is carried out through both premarket product evaluation and postmarket oversight that continues over the lifetime of the

* The opinions or assertions presented herein are the private views of the authors and are not to be construed as conveying either an official endorsement or criticism by the US Department of Health and Human Services, the Public Health Service, or the US Food and Drug Administration.

This material fits the description in the US Copyright Act of a "United States Government Work", i.e. all authors are bona fide officers or employees of the US Government, and that the work was prepared as a part of these authors' official duties as a government employee, and therefore is not subject to US copyright. The chapter is now freely available for publication, without a copyright notice, and there are no restrictions on its use, now or subsequently, for non-commercial government purposes.

Pharmacovigilance. Edited by R.D. Mann and E.B. Andrews
© 2002 John Wiley & Sons, Ltd

product, from early design to widespread use, and
ultimately, to obsolescence. At major junctures of
a product's life cycle, the FDA must weigh the
product's benefits and risks. Central to this risk
management function is the FDA's decision for
marketing, one that must ensure that beneficial
medical products are available (and labeled with
adequate information on their benefits and risks)
while protecting the public from unsafe products
or false claims (Food and Drug Administration,
1999a). Once marketed, a product's continued
safety and effectiveness must be ensured not only
by oversight on the part of industry and the FDA,
but most importantly by healthcare providers' and
patients' appropriate product selection and use
based on the product's labeling.

PREMARKET OVERVIEW

The FDA provides reasonable assurance that the
product will be useful while not posing unacceptable risks to patients once device marketing begins.
Operationally, this goal is accomplished through
the FDA's use of regulatory controls and the
classification process. General controls include
device labeling, registration and listing, premarket
notification, good manufacturing practices, and
records and reports. Premarket notification requires any manufacturer intending to market a
medical device to submit an application at least 90
days before beginning commercial distribution. The
agency then determines if the device is substantially
equivalent to a predicate device (meaning as safe
and effective and for the same intended use). [New
intended uses or significant changes in technology
are potential reasons that a device may not be
found substantially equivalent. In these cases, a
Premarket Approval (PMA) submission may be
required (see below).] Class I devices (such as
heating pads or dentures) are those for which these
controls alone are sufficient to assure the FDA of a
product's safety and effectiveness.

Special controls are used *in addition to* general
controls for higher risk Class II devices (such as
hospital beds or surgical staplers). These controls
include patient registries, guidances, and standards. Guidance documents are non-binding and

assist industry in preparing regulatory submissions
and FDA staff in the review process. They may
interpret regulatory requirements, provide information on application content requirements for
a specific device type, or convey guidance to
sponsors on the development of preclinical and
clinical data. Standards (both national and international), on the other hand, are developed
through accredited standards development organizations with full participation of the government, industry, and academia. Most pertain to test
methods for device evaluation or material specifications for type and quality of materials used in
manufacturing. Manufacturers may declare con-
formity to FDA-recognized standards in a new
device application.

When there is insufficient information to
determine that general and special controls alone
will reasonably assure safety and effectiveness, a
product may be placed into Class III pending one
other condition. The product must either be life-
sustaining, life-supporting, or for use of a substantial importance in preventing impairment of
human health, or presents a potential unreasonable risk of illness or injury [Section 513 (a)(1)(C),
of the Federal Food, Drug, and Cosmetic Act (the
Act)]. *In addition to* general and special controls,
all Class III products (such as deep brain
stimulators and cochlear implants) require the
submission of clinical data in support of premarket submissions, known as PMA applications (in
contrast to premarket notifications noted above).

POSTMARKET SURVEILLANCE

CONTEXT

For the majority of marketed products, no, or very
limited clinical data are required. Of 783 Class I
device regulations (each of which typically pertains
to more than one device), 720 (92%) are exempt
from premarket notification. Similarly, of the 898
Class II device regulations, 75 (8%) are exempt.
For the Class I and II products requiring premarket notification, many applications do not
include clinical data. Even when clinical trial
information is provided (for Class III devices),

these data have some of the same inherent limitations noted in drug trials [i.e. limited size, duration, and select patient population (e.g. restrictions in age, gender, disease complexity)]. In addition, investigators in premarket device clinical trials tend to be those physicians at the "cutting edge" of product development and who are most familiar with the device's characteristics and application. Thus, limited information may be generated on human factor concerns such as optimal design for ease of use, optimal use environment (e.g. free of electromagnetic interference), labeling that anticipates less sophisticated use or that minimizes maintenance error, or the consequences of re-use on device performance and safety. Once in the marketplace, devices are likely be used by a wide array of physicians and other clinicians of varying skill levels, training, and experience. In addition, less stringent diagnostic and other criteria may be applied reflecting either non-optimal product choice or off-label use, the latter a hallmark of the evolving practice of medicine.

Since no device is free from adverse events and product problems, and since premarket clinical data are limited, postmarket oversight is needed as a "safety net" to ensure the continued safety and effectiveness of marketed products. Postmarket oversight refers to both postmarket surveillance (and risk assessment) as well as postmarket enforcement. The former refers to the systematic process of adverse event/product problem reporting, monitoring, and evaluation as well as the subsequent, more formal, assessments of identified potential patient risks. The latter refers to investigations of a device firm's compliance with statutory and regulatory requirements. Both processes are integral to product development and evolution. This chapter will focus on the FDA programs constituting postmarket surveillance.

GOALS

As with drugs, the goals of device postmarket surveillance and risk assessment are: (1) identification of previously unknown or not well-characterized adverse events/product problems ("signals"); (2) identification and characterization of sub-

groups at risk; (3) collection and evaluation of information on issues not directly addressed in premarket submissions (e.g. long-term effectiveness or changes in use environment, from professional to home use); and (4) development of a public health context to interpret these data. This process ultimately aims to disseminate information regarding newly emerging device problems to appropriate stakeholders (particularly health professionals and the public), incorporate the information into the device approval process, and provide findings to the device industry to aid in product corrections and improvements. The principal postmarket "tools" utilized by the agency to achieve these goals are: (1) adverse event/product problem reporting [through the Medical Device Reporting (MDR) system and MEDWatch, premarket application (PMA) conditions of approval, the pilot Medical Product Surveillance Network (MedSuN), and international vigilance]; (2) mandated postmarket studies (including conditions of approval and Section 522 studies); and (3) applied epidemiology.

ADVERSE EVENT/PRODUCT PROBLEM REPORTING

MDR and MEDWatch

The FDA monitors postmarket device-related adverse events/product problems (AEs), through both voluntary and mandatory reporting, to detect "signals" of potential public health safety issues. Voluntary reporting to the FDA began in 1973 and presently continues under MEDWatch (Kessler, 1993), a program created in 1993 to encourage voluntary reporting by all interested parties (but principally among healthcare professionals) as a critical professional and public health responsibility.

It was not until 1984 that the FDA implemented mandatory reporting as per the MDR regulation. This regulation required device manufacturers and importers to report device-related deaths, serious injuries, and malfunctions to the FDA. Additional legislative initiatives in the 1990s resulted in significant changes to mandatory reporting. Under the Safe Medical Devices Act of 1990, universal reporting of adverse events by user facilities (hospitals, nursing homes, ambulatory surgical facilities, outpatient diagnostic and treatment facilities, ambulance services, and health care entities) and distributors was enacted. Under the FDA Modernization Act (FDAMA, Section 213 of the Act), and in response to experience with distributor and user facility reporting, the US Congress mandated that distributor reporting be repealed and that universal user facility reporting be limited to a "... subset of user facilities that constitutes a representative profile of user reports ...". The conceptual framework for these "sentinel sites", collectively referred to as the Medical Product Surveillance Network (Med-SuN), is discussed below.

To better understand reporting of AEs under the current MDR regulations governing mandatory reporting [Title 21 Code of Federal Regulations (CFR) Part 803], requirements should be noted and terms defined. Manufacturers and importers are currently required to submit reports of device-related deaths, serious injuries, and malfunctions. User facilities are required to report deaths to the FDA and deaths and serious injuries to the manufacturer. Serious injuries are defined as life-threatening events, events that result in permanent impairment of a body function or permanent damage to a body structure, and events that require medical or surgical intervention to preclude permanent impairment or damage. Malfunctions are defined as the failure of a device to meet its performance specifications or otherwise perform as intended. The term "device-related" means that the event was or may have been attributable to a medical device, or that a device was or may have been a factor in an event, including those occurring as a result of device failure, malfunction, improper or inadequate design, poor manufacture, inadequate labeling, or use error. Guidance is issued to reporting entities as needed to more clearly define the reporting of specific events, for example implant failures.

Since its inception in 1973, the FDA's database of voluntary and mandatory reports of device AEs has received slightly more than 1 million reports and currently averages approximately 90 000 per year, with mandatory reports accounting for about 97% of the total. The reports are submitted on the same standardized voluntary and mandatory forms used to submit drug-related events and capture information on device specifics (e.g. brand name, model number), event description, pertinent dates (e.g. event date), and patient characteristics. The reports are also coded (either by reporters or internally) using a coding thesaurus of patient and device problem codes. Manufacturers also supply methods, results, and conclusion codes relevant to their report investigation. To enhance report handling and signal detection, the FDA has established methods of triage:

- emergency reports (e.g. a cluster of deaths or serious injuries in a dialysis facility) are handled under agency-wide standard operating procedures;
- pre-designated high priority reports are reviewed within 2 hours of receipt and include, among others, reports of pediatric death, exsanguination, explosion/fire, or anaphylaxis;
- other individual reports (account for about 38% of all reports) are reviewed within 5 days of receipt;
- autoscreen reports (account for about 11%) are those that are computer-screened (by pre-designated device and event) where events are considered to be familiar, but text may be particularly valuable in assessing event or events are coded inconsistently; 10% of screened reports are later individually reviewed; and
- summary reports (account for about 50%) capture well-characterized and well-known device events and amount to a quarterly submission by manufacturers of line-listed data. The data elements per event include the manufacturer, model-specific device, event and receipt dates, and patient and device problem codes. A system is being developed to perform automated numerator-only trend analyses looking for month-to-month variation, monthly moving averages, and 12-month trends.

When potential hazards are detected (either based on internal individual or aggregate review) or upon notification by the manufacturer (under voluntary recalls), denominator data can be obtained from manufacturers upon request. The denominator data most appropriate to the analysis tend not be generic higher-order data (such as number manufactured of that brand during the past year) but typically are model-specific, many times lot-specific (and thus time-specific), and may be sub-group-specific (e.g. pediatric use). Complicating the selection of appropriate denominator data are the myriad types of devices (e.g. single-use disposables to multi-component durable medical equipment) and the inherent difficulties in assessing potential population exposure (e.g. factoring in multiple uses, average shelf-life, component replacement).

A staff, predominantly of nurses, review the individual reports from a variety of perspectives including the potential for device failure (e.g. poor design, manufacturing defect), use error (e.g. device misassembly, incorrect clinical use, misreading instructions), packaging error, support system failure, adverse environmental factors, underlying patient disease or co-morbid conditions, idiosyncratic patient reactions (e.g. allergy), maintenance error, and adverse device interaction (e.g. electromagnetic interference) (ECRI, 1998). Since many devices involve complex human interaction, great emphasis is placed on human factor considerations. Simply put, these considerations ask: (1) To what extent did sub-optimal device design, packaging, or labeling induce human error? (2) To what extent was anticipated use (and abuse) of the product factored into device design, packaging, or labeling?

Several immediate actions, aside from routine requests for follow-up information, may be taken by the staff and include:

- Directed inspections of manufacturers. These may lead to: (a) label changes, including those affecting device instructions or training materials, (b) product modification/recall, and (c) rarely, product seizure or injunction.
- Internal *ad hoc* safety meetings. These may lead to public notifications such as safety alerts and public health advisories, recommendations for additional postmarket study, or meetings with the company to explore issues further.
- Alerting regulatory authorities outside the United States through the international vigilance program (see below).

Other internal uses of the AE data are widespread and include: input into recall classifications (involving a hazard evaluation based on AE data); monitoring of recalls (and assessing reports in similar products); input into product re-classifications and exemptions from premarket notifications (based, in part, on a product's safety profile); use in, and initiating of, standards efforts that establish device performance; input into premarket review (by providing human factor insights and information on product experience in the general population); educating the clinical community through newsletters, literature articles (peer-reviewed and professional and trade journals), and teleconferences; and as a general information resource for healthcare providers and the general public.

A recent example of reports of AEs typifies the system in action. The agency received reports alerting it to events (including deaths) related to the malfunction of crystal resonating components of a model of automatic implantable cardioverter defibrillators (AICDs). In follow-up with the firm for failure analyses, it was learned they planned a voluntary recall. To elucidate the failure mechanism, agency engineers (in concert with the company) discovered that vacuum loss in the crystal housing, secondary to sub-standard hermeticity, led to crystal oscillation malfunction resulting in degradation of timing functions and electrical signal synchronization, a failure mode that could be catastrophic (*Cardiology*, 1997; *Dickinson's FDA Review*, 1997). Subsequent to this discovery, and because this failure mode could pertain to other implantable medical devices, a public notification ("Dear Manufacturer" letter) was issued by the agency (Food and Drug Administration, 1997).

As is typical of passive surveillance systems (including those for drugs), the FDA's system has notable weaknesses as well as strengths. Among the former are:

- data may be incomplete or inaccurate and are typically not independently verified;
- events are under-reported; causes include lack of detection and/or attribution of device to event, lack of knowledge about reporting

system, liability concerns, perceived lack of utility in reporting, and limited feedback;

- data reflect reporting biases driven by factors such as event severity or uniqueness, familiarity with reporting, or publicity and litigation;
- determination of incidence and prevalence is not possible due to under-reporting and lack of denominator data; and
- causality cannot be inferred from any individual report. [In addition, devices are often not returned to manufacturers for assessment (for a variety of reasons) and therefore failure analyses of data are often inadequate or lacking.]

The system strengths are:

- it provides nationwide safety surveillance from a variety of sources, thus providing insight into AEs related to "real world" use;
- it is relatively inexpensive considering the scope of surveillance;
- data collected are uniform in terms of a standardized form with pre-specified data elements;
- it is one of only a few means to detect rare AEs; and
- it is accessible and the information is open to the public.

Supplementing this reporting system are PMA conditions of approval (applies to Class III devices). All products with approved PMAs have conditions of approval, one of those being the submission of information on AEs outside the MDR regulatory requirements [Title 21 CFR Part 814.82 (a)(9)]. Examples of this include labeled AEs occurring with unexpected severity or frequency. This requirement helps the agency cast a wider "safety net" in its surveillance of AEs.

Medical Product Surveillance Network (MedSun)

Although user facility reporting was mandated in 1990, it accounted for only 3% of all reports in 1999. Furthermore, only about 2000 reports came from hospitals in 1999, representing about 800

hospitals out of a universe of about 7000. Likewise, only 90 reports came from nursing homes, representing 50 nursing homes out of a universe of about 12 000. This lack of mandatory institutional reporting has many root causes (some alluded to above under weaknesses of AE reporting), but basically reflects a lack of educational outreach coupled with a lack of enforcement (with both tied to inadequate resources). Recognizing the need for user facility reporting but also the difficulties behind universal reporting, the US Congress mandated under FDAMA 1997 that reporting be limited to a "... subset of user facilities that constitutes a representative profile of user reports ...". This network of user facilities is currently in its developmental phase (Food and Drug Administration, 1999b). Its principal objective is to increase the utility of user facility reporting by recruiting a cadre of well-trained and motivated facilities and establish a collaborative effort to better understand device use in its natural clinical environment. It is envisioned that, in addition to enhancing the detection of emerging device problems, the network would act as a two-way communication channel between the FDA and the clinical community and serve as a setting for applied clinical research on device issues. To succeed, the effort must: train staff in the recognition and reporting of AEs, assure confidentiality to reporters, minimize burden of participation, and provide timely feedback. By 2005, it is anticipated that at least 250 hospitals and approximately 50 nursing homes will comprise the network. Aiming for a statistically representative sample, the network may allow for national estimates.

International Vigilance Reporting

The reach of AE surveillance was augmented and truly became global under the auspices of the Global Harmonization Task Force (GHTF) established in 1992. The GHTF was established to respond to the increasing need for international harmonization in the regulation of medical devices (Internet site: www.ghtf.org). The GHTF is a voluntary international consortium of public health officials, responsible for administering national medical device regulatory systems, and representatives from regulated industry. The task force acts as a vehicle for convergence in regulatory practices related to ensuring the safety, effectiveness and quality of medical devices and promoting technological innovation as well as facilitating international trade. This is principally accomplished through publication and dissemination of harmonized guidance documents on basic regulatory practices.

One of the four GHTF study groups is charged with reviewing current adverse event reporting, postmarket surveillance and other forms of vigilance for medical devices, and performing an analysis of different requirements with a view to harmonizing data collection and reporting systems. A process for the global exchange of vigilance reports between National Competent Authorities (NCAs) has been established. Standardized reports on potentially high-risk issues for which action is to be taken (even if investigations are incomplete) are submitted electronically to a shared listserver. General and specific criteria for categorizing issues as high risk have been established and include: the equivalent of US Class I and high level Class II recalls, all public health notifications, and special public health concerns (e.g. high index of preventability or particularly vulnerable populations). During its first year, the program exchanged 70 such reports.

Global Medical Device Nomenclature

Part of the information requirements for the vigilance exchange program includes the official name of the device that is the subject of the vigilance report. Only since 2001 has the medical device community had an official international source for such names, the Global Medical Device Nomenclature (GMDN). The GMDN, developed through a major international standards effort, was created largely via the merging and evaluation of six extant naming systems (including the one used by the FDA). The resultant 14 000 terms abide by specified naming rules and conventions as well as definition structure and content (e.g. incorporating intended use). The GMDN is based on the level of specificity of the "device group",

which is best described by way of example, i.e. pacemaker, cardiac, implantable or gastroduodenoscope, flexible, fibreoptic. It is meant for use by regulatory agencies, but has the potential for wider applications (e.g. inventory control or marketing) and may eventually be incorporated into administrative and other databases that could be used for public health purposes. When compared with the National Drug Classification coding system, however, the GMDN is more limited in that it does not at present include model-specific information, or other potentially useful data such as material composition, component parts, or size.

MANDATED POSTMARKET STUDIES

Another "tool" that the FDA uses to achieve its surveillance and risk assessment goals are mandated postmarket studies, conducted under either PMA conditions of approval (for Class III products) or FDAMA (Section 522) authorities. A sponsor may be required to perform a post-approval study as a condition of approval for a PMA [Title 21 CFR Part 814(a)(2)]. The study questions may relate to longer-term performance of an implant, or focus on specific safety issues that may have been identified during review of the product for which additional information is felt to be needed, postmarket. Results from these studies may be included as revisions to the product's labeling (including patient- and clinician-related material).

In addition to the PMA authority for Class III products, the agency may, under Section 522, impose postmarket study requirements on certain devices. The latter provision, originally mandated in 1990 under SMDA, allows the agency, under its discretion and for good reason, to order a manufacturer of a class II or class III device to conduct a postmarket study if the device: (1) is intended to be implanted in the human body for more than one year; (2) is life-sustaining or life-supporting (and used outside a device user facility); or (3) failure would reasonably be likely to have serious adverse health consequences. Although this discretionary authority overlaps the PMA postapproval authority for some products (e.g. PMA Class III implants), it effectively extends FDA authority to cover non-PMA products as well (i.e. those subject to premarket notification). Unless there are unusual circumstances, the Section 522 authority is typically reserved for the latter.

Prior to issuing an order, the FDA will discuss the public health concern with the firm. The concern may arise from questions about a product's long-term safety, about performance of a device in general use or involving a change in user setting (e.g. professional to home use), or notable AEs. Upon receiving an order, the firm has up to 30 days in which to submit their study plan and, by statute, studies are limited to 3-year patient follow-up (or longer if agreed to by the firm). (The FDA soon plans to issue a regulation clearly specifying the requirements for a study plan, conduct, and follow-up.)

The FDA has issued guidance on criteria used in considering order issuance as well as possible study approaches (October, 1998; http://www.fda.gov/cdrh/postsurv/index.html). Briefly, the criteria include: the public health issue must be important; other postmarket mechanisms cannot effectively address the issue; the study must be practicable (i.e. feasible, timely, not cost-prohibitive); and the issue is of high priority. The possible study approaches vary widely (designed to capture the most practical, least burdensome approach to produce a scientifically sound answer) and include: a detailed review of complaint history and the literature; non-clinical testing of the device; telephone or mail follow-up of a patient sample; use of registries; observational studies; and, rarely, randomized controlled trials.

Generally speaking, these mandated postmarket studies (both via PMA conditions of approval and Section 522) require the participation of both firms and the clinical community. Problems, however, may arise in the conduct of these studies if, for instance, it is difficult to recruit physician investigators or accrue patients or if industry lacks incentive. These issues particularly resonate with rapidly evolving technologies, where rapid device evolution may make studies of prior models obsolete by the time they are completed.

Although there may be difficulties in study conduct, an example of a Section 522 study reveals the authority's public health importance and its risk assessment role. In 1991, FDA scientists demonstrated that it was possible for polyurethane to break down under laboratory conditions to form 2,4-toluenediamine (TDA). TDA had been shown to be an animal carcinogen. Prior to this it was thought that breakdown could only occur at very high temperatures and pH extremes. The firm that manufactured polyurethane foam-coated breast implants ceased sales in 1991 and agreed to a clinical study under Section 522. The study involved comparing TDA levels in urine and serum samples from women with and without the implants. Although minute amounts of TDA were found in the majority of women with the implants, the increase in cancer risk was determined to be vanishingly small (1 in 1 million) (Hester et al., 1997; DoLuu et al., 1998). The FDA issued a public health correspondence (FDA Talk Paper) on the results and their reassuring implications (Food and Drug Administration, 1995).

APPLIED EPIDEMIOLOGY

Postmarket surveillance and risk assessment would not be complete without epidemiology, a discipline that provides the means and methods to further elucidate a device's postmarket safety and effectiveness in a population context. Through employing methods of observational (as opposed to experimental) study, epidemiologists help refine AE signals, characterize sub-groups at risk, test hypotheses, and evaluate device performance and use. The epidemiology program serves a vital postmarket function at the agency and works to inform Center and agency device policy, address relevant scientific questions, provide guidance for the development of postmarket studies, assess the effectiveness of regulatory approaches, provide risk assessments, develop new postmarket surveillance and other data resources, and provide important public health information (e.g. through peer-reviewed publications).

To accomplish its mission, the epidemiology program makes use of a variety of databases (e.g. US Medicare claims data to evaluate outpatient oxygen therapy) and develops device-specific supplements to nation-wide surveys (e.g. US National Home and Hospice Care Survey to assess home use of devices) (Bright, 2000). In addition, the program explores enhanced surveillance (e.g. through a nation-wide surveillance network of emergency departments operated by the US Consumer Products Safety Commission), develops and expands existing device registries (e.g. exploring the use of transmyocardial revascularization using the Society of Thoracic Surgeons National Adult Cardiac Surgery database), helps design and analyze mandated postmarket studies, reviews and assesses observational literature (e.g. studies of cellular phones and their relation to brain cancer), and conducts applied research (e.g. breast implants and rupture rates) (Brown et al., 2000).

The ability of drug or device epidemiologists within the agency to address issues, however, is at times limited for both practical and regulatory reasons. There may be practical resource limitations (e.g. limited staff or limited funding) or time constraints (i.e. issues requiring immediate resolution may not lend themselves to observational study). Limits imposed by the regulatory environment are most apparent when mandating postmarket studies. The agency levies these studies on specific manufacturers of specific products. In doing so, there is no intent for comparative analyses, or pooled analyses, amongst manufacturers of similar products. Nor is there any intent on assessing cost effectiveness, or conducting other economic analyses, since this is not within the agency's mandate.

Other practical limitations, with regard to medical devices, have to do with the type of information available from extant data sources. Many of the data sources used by pharmacoepidemiologists (e.g. hospital based, public health based as in Saskatchewan, or health maintenance organization based) may not have device-specific information, whether at the "device group" level such as an ultrasonic rigid laparoscope or carbon dioxide surgical laser or certainly not at the model- or brand-specific level. Other data sources, such as medical care claims records, often collect procedure-specific, but not device-specific information, leaving one to infer device use. Compounding this

situation is the relative lack of data sources for assessing device exposure and difficulties in deriving the most appropriate denominator data (as noted previously with regard to AEs) (Bright et al., 2000).

These limitations not withstanding, epidemiology continues to play a vital role in addressing agency device concerns. The role of epidemiology is exemplified by the following two cases. On the basis of both AEs and reports in the literature of possible gender-related effects, the program undertook a collaborative effort, with principal investigators of the NIH-funded New Approaches to Coronary Intervention Registry, to expand the registry to include a much larger proportion of women and to analyze data on short- and long-term outcomes related to use of the Palmaz–Schatz stent (Marinac-Dabic et al., 1998). The results of the study were reassuring for women showing that the stent was effective, revealing a low overall rate of major cardiac events during hospitalization. The results were equally encouraging in long-term follow-up. The epidemiology program was also very much involved in assessing the overall risk of connective tissue and auto-immune disease related to silicone-gel-filled breast implants (Silverman et al., 1996; Brown et al., 1998). This important public health issue had been addressed through multiple published observational studies, many of which suffered from some of the weaknesses mentioned above. The Center epidemiologists performed a systematic review of that literature to date, and determined that, if there were a risk, the risk was small.

THE FUTURE

There is no one optimal system for detecting and analyzing all medical device related AEs for at least two very significant reasons. First, as we have pointed out, the range of medical devices is vast, including latex gloves, catheters, infusion pumps, heart valves, deep brain stimulators, and magnetic resonance imaging machines. As might be expected, the kinds of problems that befall these devices span an equally large variety and this leads to difficulty in detecting these problems with one surveillance approach. The CDRH has begun crafting an interlocking system of approaches to postmarket surveillance that we believe will manage risks of medical products in as effective a way as possible given limited resources.

Each of the component parts of the future postmarket surveillance system will be part of a total product life cycle approach to medical devices (i.e. keeping in mind the life cycle of the product from initial design/testing to marketing and to obsolescence while integrating pre- and postmarket activities). In addition, each of the pieces of the system will be better suited to picking up certain kinds of problems more than the other parts of the system.

One of the key elements of the system will remain the MDR program. While the MDR system will continue to be driven by manufacturer reporting, the future will have several important features that will change in this system. First, increased use of summary reports will be made (thereby decreasing individual review of well-known events). Second, additional analytic techniques will be used with this system including the new area of data mining that has been more extensively explored with drug–adverse event reports. Third, the MDR system will become even more international as nomenclature is standardized and the exchange of vigilance reports, representing important public health signals, will grow among various countries.

Working in conjunction with the MDR is the agency's quality system requirements, designed for a wide variety of features but principally to maintain high quality control over manufacturer products. This system of quality control also includes a vigilance aspect to product complaints and product performance. We expect that as the quality system requirements become more standard throughout the device industry, more known problems with devices, previously considered as MDR reportable events, will be kept by the manufacturing firm and monitored over time. Reports of unusual trends, under the MDR program (and also agreed to internationally), will then be a signal both to the industry and to the agency suggesting possible action.

In addition to MDR and related quality systems, the second feature of the future system will be an improved program of formal postmarket studies as part of the realization of CDRH's total product life cycle concept. We will identify potentially important postmarket concerns with new devices at the time of consideration of approval. The notion of bringing products to market with a least burdensome regulatory approach will begin to more systematically include consideration of postmarket surveillance to achieve an appropriate balance between necessary pre- and postmarket information. In addition, data from these postmarket studies will be more systematically brought back to the premarket side of the agency for consideration in speeding the release of new technology to the market.

One of the most challenging aspects of device performance is long-term safety and effectiveness. More and more device products are expecting to have extremely long lifetimes, but both the manufacturer and the agency must be mindful of complications that may not be seen for many years after the use of a particular product. However, long-term monitoring of products can be among the most difficult and expensive aspects of postmarket surveillance. The agency hopes to expand its use of two separate data collection methodologies that may provide considerable assistance in discovering long-term problems. First, the agency already uses advanced epidemiologic methodology and resources with available data where possible (as noted previously). More recently, the agency has begun to examine the potential of product registries as a means for addressing critical postmarket surveillance questions. One such example is the Society of Thoracic Surgeons National Adult Cardiac Surgery database (a collaborative project on transmyocardial revascularization was mentioned previously). Since 1990, the database has captured over 1.4 million procedures from over 500 institutions. Encouraging industry to fully participate in the registries with the clinical community can be a challenge for a variety of reasons. For example, registries generally include products from all companies and there is a natural competitiveness among companies that presents a problem with issues of AE reports or information sharing.

Finally, the centerpiece of the future for the FDA is MedSun. Almost all reports of significant AEs begin with the patient and the clinician. Recognizing and understanding when a device has not performed as intended or when a device has either caused or contributed to a patient injury can be clinically complex. The MedSun system, in addition to providing "routine" reports, will also provide a laboratory for just such examination or study when appropriate, with a special focus on human factors. In addition, MedSun will provide a critical feature to almost any surveillance activity: an appropriate population of reference. The MedSun system, given certain devices, may have a sufficiently closed system to be able to estimate both numerators and denominators that approximately come from the same population of interest. This represents a significant contribution, given problems previously noted with reliable numerator and denominator data.

We believe that the efficient use of each of these components of the postmarket system will provide the most effective strategy available for the agency to mitigate risk in the postmarket period and to achieve an improved risk management perspective throughout the total product life cycle.

ADDENDUM

The definition of a medical device is: an instrument, apparatus, implement, machine, contrivance, implant, *in vitro* reagent, or other similar or related article, including any component, part, or accessory, which is: (1) recognized in the official National Formulary, or the US Pharmacopoeia, or any supplement to them; (2) intended for use in the diagnosis of disease or other conditions, or in the cure, mitigation, treatment, or prevention of disease in man or other animals; or (3) intended to affect the structure or any function of the body of man or other animals, and which does not achieve its primary intended purposes through chemical action within or on the body of man or other animals and which is not dependent upon being metabolized for the achievement of any of its primary intended purposes (Section 201 of the Act, Title 21 U.S. Code §321).

ACKNOWLEDGEMENT

The authors wish to acknowledge the contributions of Dr Celia Witten to the information conveyed regarding premarket review.

REFERENCES

Bright RA (2000) Special methodological issues in the pharmacoepidemiology studies of devices. In: Strom, BL, ed., *Pharmacoepidemiology*, 3rd edn. New York: Wiley, pp. 733–47.

Brown SL, Langone JJ, Brinton LA (1998) Silicone breast implants and autoimmune disease. *J Am Med Women Assoc* **53**: 21–4.

Brown SL, Middleton MS, Berg WA, Soo MS, Pennello G (2000) Prevalence of rupture of silicone gel breast implants revealed on magnetic resonance imaging in a population of women in Birmingham, Alabama. *Am J Radiol* **175**: 1057–64.

Cardiology (1997) FDA alerts device manufacturers. *Cardiology* **26**(10): 7.

Dickinson's FDA Review (1997) FDA detective work on implants gets grip on vacuum hazard. *Dickinson's FDA Review* **September**: 22.

DoLuu HM, Hutter JC, Bushar HF (1998) A physiologically based pharmacokinetic model 2,4-toluene-diamine leached from polyurethane foam-covered breast implants. *Environ Health Perspect* **106**(7): 393–400.

ECRI (1998) Medical device problem reporting for the betterment of healthcare. *Health Devices* **27**(8): 277–92.

Food and Drug Administration (1995) TDA and polyurethane breast implants. *Food and Drug Administration Talk Paper*. Rockville, MD: US Food and Drug Administration.

Food and Drug Administration (1997). Vacuum loss in resonating components. *FDA Dear Manufacturer Letter*. Rockville, MD: US Food and Drug Administration.

Food and Drug Administration (1999a) Designing a medical device surveillance network. *FDA Report to Congress*. Rockville, MD: US Food and Drug Administration.

Food and Drug Administration (1999b) Managing the risks from medical product use: creating a risk management framework. *Report to the FDA Commissioner from the Task Force on Risk Management*. Rockville, MD: US Food and Drug Administration.

Gallivan M (1997) *The 1997 Global Medical Technology Update: The Challenges Facing U.S. Industry and Policy Makers*. Washington, DC: Health Industry Manufacturers Association, pp. 37–51.

Hester TR Jr, Ford NF, Gale PJ, Hammett JL, Raymond R, Turnbull D, Frankos VH, Cohen MB (1997) Measurement of 2,4-toluenediamine in urine and serum samples from women with Meme or Replicon breast implants. *Plast Reconstr Surg* **100**(5): 1291–8.

Kessler DA (1993) Introducing MEDWatch: a new approach to reporting medication and device adverse effects and product problems. *J Am Med Assoc* **269**: 2765–8.

Lewin Group, Inc. (2000) *State of the Industry, Year 2000*. Report 1 for AdvaMed, pp. 3–6.

Marinac-Dabic D, Kennard ED, Torrence ME (1998) Palmaz-Schatz stenting in women: acute and long-term outcomes. *APHA 126th Annual Meeting*, Washington, DC [Abstract].

Silverman BG, Brown SL, Bright RA, Kaczmarek RG, Arrowsmith-Lowe JB, Kessler DA (1996) Reported complications of silicone gel breast implants: an epidemiologic review. *Ann Intern Med* **124**: 744–56.

Wilkerson Group (1995) *Forces Reshaping the Performance and Contribution of the U.S. Medical Device Industry*. New York, pp. 3–31.

Part III

PHARMACOVIGILANCE AND
SELECTED SYSTEM ORGAN CLASSES

34

Dermatological ADRs

LAURENCE VALEYRIE AND JEAN-CLAUDE ROUJEAU

Service de Dermatologie, Hôpital Henri Mondor, Université Paris XII, Créteil, France

INTRODUCTION

Skin is one of the most common targets of adverse drug reactions (ADRs) (Arndt and Hershel, 1976). Eruptions are observed in 0.1%–1% of treated patients in premarketing trials of most drugs, and also in the placebo groups. A number of drugs of current utilization are associated with higher rates of skin eruptions: 5%–7% for aminopenicillins, 3%–4% for antibacterial sulphonamides, and 5%–10% for many antiepileptics. In a reported series, 90% of these drug eruptions are benign. Because under-reporting is expected to be more frequent for benign reactions, one may assume that severe cutaneous ADRs account for about 2% of all skin reactions.

The Council for International Organization of Medical Sciences (CIOMS) considers as serious ADRs that "are fatal or life-threatening, or require prolonged hospitalization, or result in persistent or significant disability or incapacity" (CIOMS, 1997) Because hospitalization may depend on the socioeconomic status of the patient and on access to health care, we prefer to consider as severe those drug eruptions that are associated with a definite risk of increased mortality, even if the risk is low, and whether the risk is related to "acute skin failure", to associated visceral lesions

or to both factors. Not all severe skin ADRs develop rapidly. Many well-defined clinical entities like eosinophilia-myalgia syndrome, drug-induced pemphigus or lupus usually occur after prolonged exposure.

It is our opinion that the different clinical patterns of severe drug eruptions should be distinguished, while others prefer mixing all of them under the denomination of "hypersensitivity reactions" (Knowles *et al.*, 2000). Both conceptions are based on mechanistic considerations. The "mergers" emphasize the key role of "reactive metabolites" of drugs as common initiators of all types of reactions. The "splitters" underline the differences in clinical presentation, pathology of skin and visceral lesions, and biologic markers that suggest that the effector mechanisms are probably different (Roujeau and Stern, 1994).

PATTERNS OF CUTANEOUS ADRS

EXANTHEMATOUS DRUG ERUPTION

Exanthematous or maculo-papular eruptions, often reported as "drug rashes" or "drug eruptions" are the most common ADRs affecting the skin. The main mechanism is probably immunologic,

Pharmacovigilance. Edited by R.D. Mann and E.B. Andrews

and may correspond to type IV delayed cell-mediated hypersensitivity reaction.

The eruption usually occurs between 4 and 14 days after beginning a new therapy, and even a few days after it has ceased ("eruption of the ninth day"). However, it can develop sooner, especially in the case of rechallenge. The eruption consists of erythematous macules, papules, often symmetric. They begin on the trunk, upper extremities, and progressively become confluent (Figure 34.1, between pp. 426 and 427). The eruption is typically polymorphous: morbilliform or sometimes urticarial on the limbs, confluent on the thorax, purpuric on the feet. Mucous membranes are usually not involved. Prurit and low-grade fever are often associated with the eruption, which frequently lasts one to two weeks.

Cutaneous pathological slides exhibit a mild lymphocytic infiltrate around vessels of the dermis, and a few necrotic keratinocytes within the epidermis. This pattern is not specific and cannot help to distinguish a drug eruption from an eruption of another cause.

The differential diagnosis of exanthematous drug reactions includes viral eruptions (EBV, CMV, HHV6, Parvovirus B19, etc.), toxinic eruptions, acute Graft-vs-Host reaction, Kawasaki syndrome, Still's disease, etc. Dermatologists usually consider that viral infections are the cause of most drug eruptions in children, while drugs are more frequently responsible in adults.

Treatment is largely supportive, usually after the removal of the offending agent, associated with topical corticosteroid and systemic antipruritic agents. When the suspected drug is of paramount importance for the patient (e.g. antibacterial sulphonamides in AIDS patients) treating "through the eruption" can be considered as an option. In most instances, the eruption will disappear in about the same time as if the drug had been withdrawn. Because a few patients may experience a progressive worsening of the eruption leading to one of the severe reactions described below, the benefit–risk ratio of this attitude should be carefully weighted and the evolution of the rash strictly monitored.

Most drugs can induce an erythematous eruption in about 1% of users. The following drugs have higher risks (more than 3% of users): allopurinol, aminopenicillins, cephalosporins, antiepileptic agents and antibacterial sulphonamides.

URTICARIA AND ANGIO-OEDEMA

Urticaria is a common, transient eruption of erythematous and oedematous papules and plaques, usually associated with pruritis. When dermal and subcutaneous tissues are involved, this reaction is known as angio-oedema. Urticaria and angio-oedema are associated in 50% of cases. They can be complicated by a life-threatening anaphylactic reaction. Urticaria, angio-oedema and anaphylaxis are generally a type I hypersensitivity reaction mediated by IgE antibodies. But other "anaphylactoid" mechanisms, leading to direct and non-specific liberation of histamine or other mediators of inflammation, are also common for drug reactions.

Clinically, itchy erythematous, oedematous papules and plaques develop in variable numbers and size (Figure 34.2, between pp. 426 and 427). They are localized anywhere on the body, including the palm, soles and scalp. They frequently last a few hours and disappear within 24 hours, leaving the skin with a normal appearance. Angio-oedema is often associated with urticaria, consisting of pale or pink swellings which affect the face (eyelids, lips, ears, etc.) but also buccal mucosa, the tongue, larynx, pharynx, etc. More severe reaction, such as anaphylaxis, can involve other systems and lead to respiratory collapse, shock and death.

Urticaria is histologically non-specific with a superficial and deep scarce infiltrate of mononuclear cells accompanied by eosinophils and neutrophils, oedematous reticular dermis, vascular and lymphatic dilatation. The epidermis is uninvolved.

Urticaria has been classified into acute, when the eruption lasts less than six weeks, or chronic when it persists much longer. It usually occurs within 36 hours of drug administration, but may also occur within a few minutes.

Withdrawal of the causative agent is the main treatment. It can sometimes be associated with histamine H1 receptor blockers. Systemic steroids and an intramuscular injection of epinephrine are necessary in an emergency if severe angio-oedema and anaphylaxis occur.

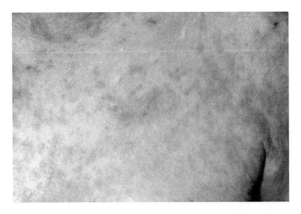

Figure 34.1. Exanthematous morbilliform eruption consisting of erythematous macules and papules of the trunk.

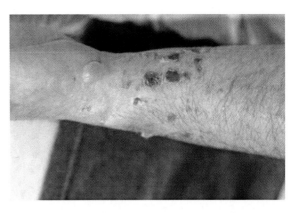

Figure 34.3. Bullous eruption of the arm corresponding to a phototoxic eruption on a sun-exposed area.

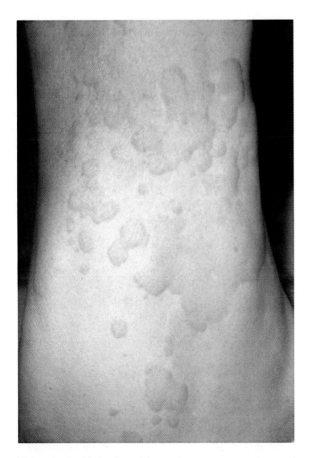

Figure 34.2. Urticaria with oedematous papules and plaques, which generally last a few hours.

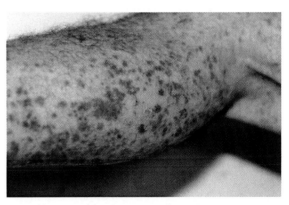

Figure 34.4. Cutaneous necrotizing vasculitis, consisting of purpuric papules, which predominate on the lower extremities.

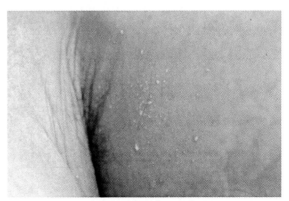

Figure 34.5. Acute generalized exanthematous pustulosis.

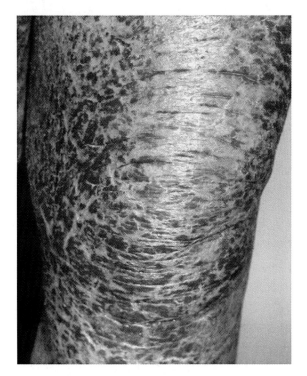

Figure 34.6. DRESS syndrome presenting as exfoliative dermatitis.

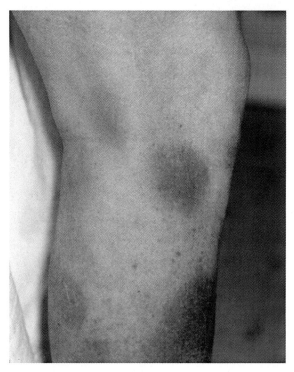

Figure 34.7. Fixed drug eruption, characterized by round, sharply demarcated erythematous plaques.

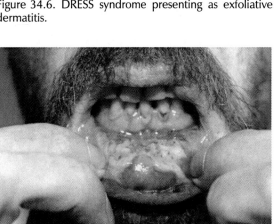

Figure 34.8. Drug-induced pemphigus with erosions of mucous membrane.

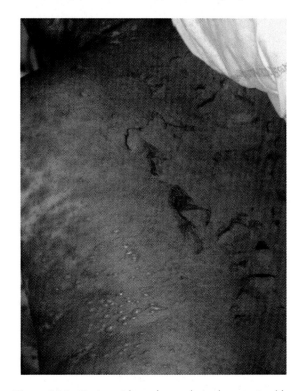

Figure 34.9. Toxic epidermal necrolysis characterized by skin necrosis, with flaccid blisters and epidermal detachment on the trunk.

Many drugs can induce urticaria (most often of the acute type). Antibiotics, especially penicillin, and general anaesthetics are classic causes of IgE-mediated hypersensitivity reaction. A radioallergosorbent test (RAST) or ELISA and skin tests (prick-tests) can be useful to confirm the diagnosis. Because they may rarely induce an anaphylactic reaction, prick-tests must be performed only by experienced physicians. The two most frequent causes of drug-induced non-IgE-mediated urticaria and angio-oedema are NSAIDs and angiotensin-converting enzyme (ACE) inhibitors. Angio-oedema occurs in 2 to 10 per 10 000 new users of ACE inhibitors (Hedner *et al.*, 1992), a rate that is probably higher than the risk associated with penicillins (about 1 per 10 000 courses).

PHOTOSENSITIVITY

Cutaneous photosensitivity diseases may be idiopathic, produced by endogenous photosensitizers (e.g. porphyrins) or associated with exogenous photosensitizers like drugs. The association of light and a drug can be responsible for acute inflammation of the skin. The photosensitivity reactions are divided into two types: phototoxicity and photoallergy (Gould *et al.*, 1995).

Phototoxicity

Phototoxic disorders are not rare and always predictable. It can occur in any person who receives sufficient quantities of a phototoxic drug, together with the proper light exposure. The reaction results directly from photochemistry involving the skin. The association of light with a photosensitizing chemical in the skin creates an unstable singlet or triplet state within the electrons. This leads to the generation of reactive oxygen, which is responsible for cell damage.

Clinical manifestations usually present as an exaggerated sunburn occurring in sun-exposed areas only (Figure 34.3, between pp. 426 and 427). This is followed by hyperpigmentation. Photo-onycholysis and pseudoporphyria (blisters on sun-exposed parts of the limbs) are less common clinical forms.

Phototoxicity is histologically characterized by epidermal cell degeneration with necrotic keratinocytes, oedema, sparse dermal lymphocytic infiltrate and vasodilatation. Phototoxicity is easily documented *in vitro* or *in vivo*. A photopatch test will be positive in all individuals and will therefore not be discriminant for a causality assessment. The minimal dose of UV (UVA more often than UVB) inducing an erythema will be decreased in all subjects during treatment.

Photoallergy

A photoallergic reaction is considered as a result of cell-mediated hypersensitivity. Ultraviolet radiation is required to convert a drug into an immunopathologically active compound (photoantigen) that induces the immune response.

Photoallergic eruption is more chronic than phototoxicity and is mainly eczematous and pruritic. A lichen planus-like reaction has also been reported. It is usually more marked in exposed sites, but may often progress outside these areas. In the chronic phase, erythema, scaling and lichenification predominate. Photoallergic reactions are usually transient and resolve after a variable length of time when the offending agent has been removed. Rarely, an extreme sensitivity to sun may persist for months or years ("persistent light reactors"). Photopatch testing is valuable when photoallergy is suspected. A multitude of drugs induce photoallergic reactions, including antibiotics (sulphonamides, pyrimethamine, fluoroquinolones), fragrances, NSAIDs, phenothiazine, thiazide diuretics, etc.

In phototoxic reactions, the treatment requires removal of the offending agent and/or avoidance of sun exposure. For a drug with a short elimination half-life, administration in the evening may be enough to decrease the risk below the clinical threshold. In photoallergy, drug withdrawal is recommended, because of the risk of worse reactions even with low UV doses. Topical corticosteroid, systemic antipruritic agents may be useful.

VASCULITIS

Vasculitis corresponds to inflammation and damage to a blood vessel's wall. It may be caused by a variety of agents, especially infections and collagen vascular diseases. Many cases remain idiopathic. Drug-induced vasculitis is believed to result from antibodies directed against drug-related haptens (Roujeau and Stern, 1994). Direct drug toxicity against a vessel's wall, autoantibodies reacting with endothelial cells and cell-mediated cytotoxic reactions against vessels were also proposed as explanations. The precise mechanism is still unknown.

This drug-induced eruption corresponds to a cutaneous necrotizing vasculitis consisting of palpable purpuric papules, which predominate on the lower extremities (Figure 34.4, between pp. 426 and 427). Urticaria-like lesions, ulcers, nodules, hemorrhagic blisters, Raynaud's disease and digital necrosis also occur. The vasculitis may involve other organs, with fever, arthralgias, myalgias, headache, dyspnea, neurological involvement and renal abnormalities, sometimes life-threatening. The histology of small blood vessels exhibits necrotizing and/or leukocytoclasic vasculitis. The direct immunofluorescence is often positive, with IgM and C3 deposits on capillary walls.

Vasculitis occurs 7 to 21 days after drug administration, and less than 3 days after rechallenge. Withdrawing the drug usually leads to a rapid resolution. A systemic corticosteroid may benefit some patients.

Drug-induced cases are a minority of cases of vasculitis (no more than 10% in a large series) and have to be differentiated from other causes of cutaneous vasculitis: infection, autoimmune diseases (polyarteritis nodosa, Wegener's granulomatosis, etc.) Schönlein-Henoch purpura, and cancer.

The main drugs implicated are: allopurinol, NSAIDs, cimetidine, penicillin, hydantoin, sulphonamides and propylthiouracil.

ACUTE GENERALIZED EXANTHEMATOUS PUSTULOSIS

In 1980, Beylot et al. described an acute pustular dermatosis named "Acute generalized exanthematous pustulosis" (AGEP) (Beylot and Bioulac, 1980). Of these eruptions, 60%–80% could be drug-induced. Hypersensitivity to mercury and infection with enteroviruses may also be responsible. The incidence of AGEP has been underestimated and many cases have been confused with pustular psoriasis. Synonyms are pustular drug rash, pustular eruption, pustuloderma (Staughton et al., 1984). Proposed diagnosis criteria (Roujeau et al., 1991) include:

1. an acute pustular eruption
2. fever above 38 °C
3. neutrophilia with or without a mild eosinophilia
4. subcorneal or intraepidermal pustules on skin biopsy
5. spontaneous resolution in less than 15 days.

AGEP is characterized by fever, which generally begins the same day as the pustular rash. Numerous, small, mostly non-follicular pustules arise on a widespread oedematous erythema, burning pruritic or both (Figure 34.5, between pp. 426 and 427). Oedema of the face and the hands, purpura, vesicles, blisters, erythema multiforme-like lesions and mucous membrane involvement have also been associated. These pustules are mainly localized on the mainfolds (neck, axillae, groins, etc.) trunk and upper extremities.

The histopathology shows spongiform pustules located under the stratum corneum, the most superficial layer of the epidermis. Papillary dermal oedema and perivascular polymorphous infiltrate are usually present. Leukocytoclasic vasculitis and focal necrotic keranocytes have also been reported.

Hyperleukocytosis with elevated neutrophils count, transient renal failure and hypocalcemia are frequently seen.

The time between the drug administration and the skin eruption is relatively short, less than two days. The eruption lasts 1 to 2 weeks, and is followed by a superficial desquamation. The withdrawal of the responsible drug is the main treatment, associated with a topical corticosteroid and sometimes a systemic antipruritic agent.

AGEP must be differentiated from acute pustular psoriasis of the von Zumbusch type. The pustules in both diseases are clinically indistinguishable; the histopathology can be helpful.

Antibiotics (β lactam, macrolides, etc.) are the main drugs implicated in AGEP.

DRESS/HYPERSENSITIVITY

"Hypersensitivity syndrome" refers to a specific severe skin reaction. The acronym of DRESS for Drug Reaction with Eosinophilia and Systemic Symptoms has been proposed as more specific than "hypersensitivity", which would be appropriate for most types of drug reaction. It has been estimated to occur in between one in 1000 and one in 10 000 exposures with drugs such as antiepileptics and sulphonamides. This syndrome is typically characterized in its complete form by a severe eruption, lymphadenopathy, fever, hepatitis, arthralgias, pulmonary infiltrates, interstitial nephritis and haematological abnormalities (Shear and Spielberg, 1988; Roujeau and Stern, 1994; Callot et al., 1996). Multivisceral involvement differentiates hypersensitivity syndrome from common exanthematous eruption. Some authors consider that Stevens–Johnson Syndrome (SJS) and toxic epidermal necrolysis (TEN) may occur as part of a "hypersensitivity syndrome". The skin lesions and visceral complications are actually different. Eosinophilia and atypical lymphocytosis are not observed in SJS and TEN.

These reactions are more frequent among black persons. They begin 2 to 6 weeks after the first drug use, later than most other skin reactions. Fever and skin rash are the most common symptoms. Cutaneous manifestations begin as a morbilliform rash, which later becomes infiltrated with an oedematous follicular accentuation (Figure 34.6, between pp. 426 and 427). Erythroderma, vesicles, tight blisters induced by dermal oedema, follicular as well as non-follicular pustules can also occur. Face, upper trunk and extremities are initially involved. Oedema of the face is frequently associated and evocative of diagnosis.

Prominent eosinophilia is common and the more characteristic biological feature of this reaction. It is often associated with atypical lymphocytosis. Liver abnormalities with raised aminotransferase concentration, alkaline phosphatase concentration, prothrombin time and bilirubin concentration are present in about 50% of patients.

Histopathology exhibits a rather dense lymphocytic infiltrate in the superficial dermis and/or perivascular, associated with eosinophils and dermal oedema.

Rash and hepatitis may persist for several weeks after drug withdrawal, and some of the manifestations may be life threatening.

The differential diagnosis includes other cutaneous drug reactions, acute viral infection, idiopathic hypereosinophilic syndrome, lymphoma and pseudolymphoma. Special attention should be paid to HHV6, since several publications suggest a possible interaction between DRESS and reactivation of HHV6.

Topical high-potency corticosteroids can be helpful in skin manifestations. Systemic corticosteroids are often proposed when internal organ involvement exists.

The aromatic antiepileptic agents (phenobarbital, carbamazepine, phenytoïn) and sulphonamides are the most frequent causes of hypersensitivity syndrome. Minocycline, allopurinol, gold salts and dapsone may also induce this syndrome.

FIXED DRUG ERUPTION

A fixed drug eruption is an exclusively drug-induced cutaneous reaction. The lesions develop usually less than two days after the drug intake. Clinically, they are characterized by a solitary or few, round, sharply demarcated erythematous and oedematous plaques, sometimes with a central blister (Figure 34.7, between pp. 426 and 427). The eruption can be located on every site of the body and may involve mucous membranes, principally the lips and genitalia. The eruption progressively fades in a few days, to leave a post-inflammatory brown pigmentation. With rechallenge with the causative drug, the lesions recur at exactly the same sites. After several relapses the eruption may involve large areas of the body. This Generalized Fixed Drug Eruption may be difficult to distinguish from TEN.

Histopathology reveals a superficial and deep dermal and perivascular infiltrate (composed of lymphocytes, eosinophils, and sometimes neutrophils) associated with necrotic keratinocytes. Dermal macrophages pigmented by melanin (melanophages) when present are considered an important clue to the diagnosis.

The drugs most frequently associated with fixed drug eruption are phenazone derivates, barbiturates, tetracycline, sulphonamides, and carbamazepine (Kauppinen and Stubb, 1984).

DRUG-INDUCED PEMPHIGUS

Pemphigus is a chronic autoimmune blistering disease provoked by autoantibodies reacting with normal constituants of desmosomes, the structures that provide attachment between epidermal cells. It presents clinically with flaccid intraepidermal blisters and erosions of the skin and mucous membranes (Figure 34.8, between pp. 426 and 427). Nikolsky's sign is found.

The histology exhibits detachment of epidermal cells (acantholysis), responsible for intraepidermal blisters located subcorneally (pemphigus foliaceus) or in the lower epidermis (pemphigus vulgaris).

Direct immunofluorescence performed to a perilesional skin biopsy specimen reveals immunoglobulin deposits around keratinocytes in the epidermis in all "spontaneous" cases but in only 50% of drug-induced cases. The presence in the serum of autoantibodies reacting against the epidermis is detected by indirect immunofluorescence, western-blot or ELISA tests.

In western countries about 10% of cases of pemphigus could be drug-induced. It begins several weeks or months after drug therapy is initiated. It presents as pemphigus foliaceus or as pemphigus vulgaris with mucosal involvement. The main drugs incriminated are d-penicillamine and other drugs containing a thiol radical, like captopril and piroxicam. The remission after drug withdrawal is not always spontaneous, particularly in cases of pemphigus attributed to drugs that do not have a thiol part.

SJS AND TEN

SJS and TEN are rare, life-threatening, drug-induced skin reactions. The incidence of TEN is evaluated to 0.4 to 1.2 cases per million person-years and of SJS from 1 to 6 cases per million person-years (Roujeau and Stern, 1994). The

immunopathologic pattern of early lesions suggests a cell-mediated cytotoxic reaction against epidermal cells. Widespread apoptosis of epidermal cells is provoked by the activation of several pathways: the interaction of Fas antigen (cell surface death receptor) and Fas ligand but also perforin plus granzyme and TNFalpha.

With others we proposed to consider SJS and TEN as severity variants of the same drug-induced disease, and to distinguish SJS from erythema multiforme major (Bastuji-Garin et al., 1993), the latter being mostly related to infections, especially with herpes (Wolkenstein et al., 1998).

According to this proposal, erythema multiforme (major when mucous membranes are involved) is characterized by typical concentric "target" lesions acrally distributed, with limited blisters (detachment rarely involves more than 2%–3% of the body surface area). The pathology shows an interface dermatitis with moderate to marked lymphocyte infiltrate in the dermis, exocytosis and mild necrosis of epidermal cells. In our experience, erythema multiforme is rarely drug-induced. Most of the cases that are reported or published as drug-induced erythema multiforme are either cases that we would label as SJS or cases of erythematous drug eruptions, because of confusion between "multiforme" and the polymorphous patterns of many erythematous eruptions.

SJS is characterized by atypical targets and more often by small blisters arising on purple macules. Lesions are widespread and usually predominate on the trunk. Confluence of blisters on limited areas leads to detachment below 10% of the body surface area. The pathology can be separated from that of erythema multiforme by less lymphocyte infiltrate and more epidermal necrosis (Wolkenstein et al., 1998).

Toxic epidermal necrolysis is characterized by the same lesions as SJS but with a confluence of blisters leading to a positive Nikolski sign and to the detachment of large epidermal sheets on more than 30% of the body surface area (cases with detachment of between 10% and 30% are labelled overlap SJS–TEN) (Figure 34.9, between pp. 426 and 427). Skin pathology shows necrosis of full-thickness epidermis and negative immunofluorescence. This is important for distinguishing TEN from exfoliative dermatitis, staphylococcal scalded skin syndrome, acute exanthematous pustulosis and paraneoplastic pemphigus, which may be misdiagnosed as SJS or TEN.

Patients with SJS or TEN have high fever. Severe erosions of mucous membranes are nearly constant. Systemic manifestations include mild elevation of hepatic enzymes (overt hepatitis in 10% of cases), intestinal and pulmonary manifestations (with sloughing of epithelia similar to what happens to the skin). Leucopenia is frequent and eosinophilia unusual. Death occurs in 5% of patients with SJS and 30% of patients with TEN, principally from sepsis or pulmonary involvement (Roujeau and Stern, 1994).

The treatment is mainly symptomatic, consisting of nursing care, maintenance of fluid and electrolyte balance and nutritional support. Early withdrawal of all potentially responsible drugs is essential. Short courses of corticosteroids early in the disease have been advocated, but their effectiveness has never been demonstrated in controlled trials. Thalidomide has been shown to be detrimental in TEN, possibly because of a paradoxical enhancement of TNFalpha production. High-dose intravenous immunoglobulins were disappointing in our experience.

Drug reactions are responsible for at least 70% of cases of both SJS and TEN (Knowles et al., 2000). Antibacterial sulphonamides, anticonvulsants, oxicam and pyrazolone NSAIDs, allopurinol and chlormezanone are the drugs associated with the higher risks. An international case–control study of SJS and TEN found relative risks of between 50 and 172 for new users (treatment duration of less than two months) of the above-mentioned drugs and also for corticosteroids (Roujeau et al., 1995). In that study, excess risks for associated drugs were in the range of 1 to 4.5 cases for 1 million users per week (Roujeau et al., 1995).

SJS and TEN typically begin within four weeks of initiating therapy, usually 7 to 21 days after the first drug exposure and sometimes a few days after the drug has been withdrawn. It occurs more rapidly with rechallenge.

OTHER DRUG-INDUCED CUTANEOUS REACTIONS

Serum Sickness-like Eruption

This syndrome is principally reported in children and typically includes fever, arthralgias and rash (morbilliform, urticaria) and lymphadenopathy (Roujeau and Stern, 1994; Knowles et al., 2000). It occurs 1 to 3 weeks after drug exposure. Unlike "true" serum sickness reaction, hypocomplementemia, immune complexes, vasculitis and renal lesions are absent. This reaction occurs in about 1 in 2000 children given cefaclor, which, with minocycline, penicillins, and propranolol are the main drugs responsible for this eruption.

Anticoagulant-induced Skin Necrosis

This reaction is a rare, sometimes life-threatening, effect of warfarin, which typically begins 3 to 5 days after therapy is initiated. Clinically, red, painful plaques evolve to necrosis, hemorrhagic blisters, ulcers, etc. as a consequence of occlusive thrombi in vessels of the skin and subcutaneous tissue (Roujeau and Stern, 1994). Of the individuals who receive warfarin, 1 in 10 000 will develop skin necrosis. People with an hereditary deficiency of protein C are at the highest risk. Therapy includes discontinuing warfarin, administering vitamin K, giving heparin as an anticoagulant, and monoclonal antibody-purified protein C concentrate.

Heparin also induces thrombosis and necrosis in the skin and other organs. In this case, the discontinuation of the drug, treatment with warfarin, or an antiplatelet drug is useful.

Pseudolymphoma

Drug-induced pseudolymphoma corresponds to an insidious disease, which simulates lymphoma clinically and histologically. It develops months or years after the beginning of the incriminated drug. Cutaneous lesions may be solitary or numerous, localized or widespread red papules, plaques or nodules. Lymphadenopathy is often associated, but can also be isolated (Callot et al., 1996).

Histologically, dense lymphocytic infiltrate mimics T-cell lymphoma and B-cell lymphoma, but the lymphocytes are polyclonal. Complete recovery occurs a few weeks after withdrawal of the responsible drug. The majority of drug-induced pseudolymphoma have been reported with hydantoin, butobarbital, carbamazepine, ACE, amiloride, D penicillamine, etc.

Erythema nodosum, acneiform eruptions, lupus erythematosus, psoriasis, oral erosions, alopecia, lipodystrophy and many other skin manifestations may also be induced by drugs. These are usually well-defined clinical entities, which we will not discuss here.

ASSESSMENT AND REPORTING OF CUTANEOUS ADRS

Case assessment should begin with an accurate description of the skin lesions. If a specific diagnosis is proposed, then it is important to know if it has been made or confirmed by a dermatologist. The use of lay words is often more informative than the use of "specific" terms when the accuracy of these terms is not certain.

Relevant clinical information includes:

1. Distribution of lesions
   - Face
   - Hands, feet
   - Photoexposed vs. covered areas
2. Number of lesions
3. Pattern of individual lesions (macules, purpura, blisters, pustules, etc.)
4. Mucous membrane involvement.

It is important to distinguish whether the cutaneous part of an orifice of the body is involved or if there are lesions of mucous membranes (e.g. lips vs. mouth, scrotum vs. glans on genitalia, etc.). Only mucous membrane lesions indicate a severe reaction.

5. Duration of the eruption
6. Associated symptoms/signs
   - Fever
   - Pruritis
   - Lymph node enlargement.

The documentation of cases should be completed by *photographic pictures*. Cheap disposable cameras can provide both easy and adequate documentation. This will be of major help for the retrospective assessment of cases by experts.

A skin biopsy is not useful in mild eruptions, but is mandatory for all severe reactions. It will allow a retrospective validation of the diagnosis and in some cases may help to exclude non-drug causes of a reaction pattern.

Information should be obtained on the presence of factors that increase the risk of drug eruptions: HIV infection, acute EBV infection, collagen-vascular disease.

The attribution to a newly released drug of a few cases of severe cutaneous reactions may lead to restrictions in the use of this drug, with important medical and economic impacts. This underlines the importance of a good assessment of cases, which should be proportional to the seriousness of the reaction.

REFERENCES

Arndt KA, Hershel J (1976) Rates of cutaneous reactions to drug. *J Am Med Assoc* **235**: 918–23.

Bastuji-Garin S, Rzany B, Stern RS, *et al.* (1993) A clinical classification of cases of toxic epidermal necrolysis, Stevens–Johnson syndrome and erythema multiforme. *Arch Dermatol* **129**: 92–6.

Beylot C, Bioulac P, Doutre MS (1980) Pustuloses exanthématiques aiguës généralisées, à propos de 4 cas. *Ann Dermatol Venereol* **107**: 37–48.

Callot V, Roujeau J-C, Bagot M, *et al.* (1996) Drug-induced pseudolymphoma and hypersensitivity syndrome: two different clinical entities. *Arch Dermatol* **138**: 1315–21.

Council for International Organization of Medical Sciences (CIOMS) (1997) Harmonizing the use of adverse drug reaction terms, definition of terms and minimum requirements for their use: respiratory disorders and skin disorders. *Pharmacoepidemiology and Drug Safety* **6**: 115–27.

Gould JW, Mercurio MG, Elmets CA (1995) Cutaneous photosensitivity diseases induced by exogenous agents. *JAAD* **33**: 551–73.

Hedner T, Samuelsson O, Lunde H, *et al.* (1992) Angio-oedema in relation to treament with angiotensin converting enzyme inhibitors. *Br Med J* **304**: 941–5.

Kauppinen K, Stubb S (1984) Drug eruptions: causative agents and clinical types. *Acta Derm Venereol (Stockh)* **64**: 320–4.

Knowles SR, Uetrecht J, Shear NH (2000) Idiosyncratic drug reactions: the reactive metabolite syndromes. *Lancet* **356**: 1587–91.

Roujeau J-C, Bioulac-Sage P, Bourseau C, *et al.* (1991) Acute generalized exanthematous pustulosis, analysis of 63 cases. *Arch Dermatol* **127**: 1333–8.

Roujeau J-C, Kelly JP, Naldi L, *et al.* (1995) Medication use and the risk of Stevens–Johnson syndrome or toxic epidermal necrolysis. *New Engl J Med* **333**: 1600–7.

Roujeau J-C, Stern RS (1994) Severe cutaneous adverse reactions to drugs. *New Engl J Med* **331**: 1272–85.

Shear NH, Spielberg SP (1988) Anticonvulsant hypersensitivity syndrome. *J Clin Invest* **82**: 1826–32.

Staughton RCD, Rowland-Payne CME, Harper JI, *et al.* (1984) Toxic pustuloderma: a new entity. *J R Soc Med* **77** (Suppl 4): 6–8.

Wolkenstein P, Latarget J, Roujeau JC, *et al.* (1998) Randomised comparison of thalidomide versus placebo in toxic epidermal necrolysis. *Lancet* **352**: 1586–89.

35

Gastrointestinal ADRs

JOHN R. WOOD
Wood and Mills Limited, Fulmer, Buckinghamshire, UK
GRAHAM A. PIPKIN
GlaxoSmithKline Research and Development, Stockley Park, Middlesex, UK

INTRODUCTION

Disturbances of gastrointestinal function are common events that can be attributed to ingestion of a wide range of drug classes. Over 30 years ago it was reported that some 20%–40% of adverse drug reactions (ADRs) in hospital monitoring were gastrointestinal in origin (Hurwitz and Wade, 1969). More recent estimates of the incidence of ADRs in hospitalised patients (Bates et al., 1993; 1995a, 1995b; Bowman et al., 1994; Lazarou et al., 1998) or of subjects admitted to hospital due to an ADR (Col et al., 1990; Einarson, 1993; Nelson and Talbert, 1996; Lazerou et al., 1998; Roughead et al., 1998; Pouyanne et al., 2000) provide only limited information specifically about gastrointestinal events.

A study in over 4000 hospitalised patients in the United States found 247 ADRs among 207 admissions (Bates et al., 1997). Examination of each by organ system affected showed that 18% of events were of gastrointestinal origin, predominantly nausea, vomiting and antibiotic-associated diarrhoea. An almost identical rate was reported in an observational study of 1024 patients in an internal medicine ward in the United States

(Bowman et al., 1994). The gastrointestinal system was the organ system affected in 17.8% of drug-related adverse events.

The findings from a prospective study in France showed that gastrointestinal events were the most frequent cause for admission to hospital for an ADR (Pouyanne et al., 2000). Of one hundred admissions, 27 were gastrointestinal, including 13 cases of gastrointestinal haemorrhage caused by anticoagulant drugs and nine caused by ingestion of non-steroidal anti-inflammatory drugs (NSAIDs).

The extent of drug-related hospital admissions in Australia was reviewed from Australian studies published between 1988 and 1996 (Roughead et al., 1998). Fourteen studies were included in the analysis although the diagnosis associated with the drug-related admissions was available from only five reports. Among the conditions commonly identified was gastrointestinal bleeding, which usually was associated with either warfarin or NSAID therapy.

Many drugs causing gastrointestinal disorders have been recognised (Bateman and Aziz, 1998). Well-established unwanted effects of drugs include changes in gastrointestinal motility, altered gastric emptying, disturbances of nutrient absorption,

Pharmacovigilance. Edited by R.D. Mann and E.B. Andrews

antimicrobial-associated colitis and pseudomem-branous colitis. Furthermore, drug-induced lesions are documented for all sections of the gastro-intestinal tract. These encompass a wide range of pathophysiological processes including inflamma-tion, formation of strictures, haemorrhage, ulcera-tion and perforation. Others consist of symptoms such as nausea and vomiting (Quigley *et al.*, 2001), diarrhoea (Fine and Schiller, 1999) or constipation (Locke *et al.*, 2000) in the absence of underlying pathology.

The medical literature on gastrointestinal ADRs is dominated by reports concerning the NSAIDs. Effects have been documented over many years but it has been during the past decade that the risk factors for upper gastrointestinal problems have been systematically examined. Over the same period, the small and large bowel toxicities of the NSAIDs have also become clearly identified.

In this chapter we summarise some of the important literature and reviews from the past 10 years concerning the adverse effects of NSAIDs on the gastrointestinal tract. We also review the medical literature for the last decade to identify adverse gastrointestinal effects with other medica-tions detected using a variety of pharmacovigi-lance techniques.

The oesophagus, despite its physiological de-fence mechanisms, is prone to injury induced by a wide variety of agents. Medication-induced oeso-phageal injury or "pill oesophagitis" was first described over 30 years go (Pemberton, 1970). In most cases direct oesophageal toxicity is the cause and the condition is generally fully reversible on withdrawal of treatment (Doman and Ginsberg, 1981; Kikendall, 1999a). Pill oesophagitis is often underdiagnosed, in many instances it is incorrectly believed to be gastro-oesophageal reflux disease (Donan and Ginsberg, 1981; Bonavina *et al.*, 1987). Almost 1000 reports in the medical litera-ture of pill oesophagitis attributable to about 100 different medications have been extensively re-viewed (Kikendall, 1999a, 1999b). Drugs most frequently implicated in pill oesophagitis (reports of ⩾ 10 cases) include antibiotics (doxycycline, tetracycline hydrochloride and other unspecified tetracyclines, oxytetracycline, pivmecillinam), po-tassium chloride, alendronate, ferrous sulphate

and ferrous succinate, quinidine, naproxen, as-pirin, emepronium bromide, pinaverium bro-mide, and alprenalol (Bott *et al.*, 1987; Baehr and McDonald, 1998; Kikendall, 1999a, 1999b; Graham, 2000).

In the upper gastrointestinal tract, NSAIDs are causally associated with peptic ulceration along with associated complications such as bleeding and perforation. NSAIDs also cause upper gastroin-testinal haemorrhage as may the selective seroto-nin re-uptake inhibitors. Studies in volunteers have shown that alendronate, one of the bisphospho-nate class of drugs, may cause acute gastric mucosal damage and gastric ulceration.

NSAIDs can also cause a low grade enteropathy in the small intestine. Additionally, in both small and large intestine, they have been associated with the formation of strictures, bleeding and perfora-tion.

Recently, an association between a rotavirus vaccine and intussusception in children has been reported and fibrosing colonopathy has been linked with the use of pancreatin supplements in children and adults with cystic fibrosis. The possibility that measles–mumps–rubella (MMR) vaccination may be a causal factor in the devel-opment of inflammatory bowel disease is currently a matter of some controversy.

Numerous drugs have been reported to have caused obstruction of the gastrointestinal tract (Iredale, 1993). Acute colonic pseudo-obstruction is characterised by massive colonic dilation with a clinical and radiological appearance of mechanical obstruction, but in the absence of primary colonic pathology. Although the underlying pathogenetic mechanisms are unknown, it is commonly asso-ciated with surgery, trauma, metabolic imbalance, neurological disease and serious systemic illness. Anecdotal case reports over the past decade have associated various drugs with colonic pseudo-obstruction including clonidine (Maganini and Pollitt, 1983; Steiger *et al.*, 1997), imipramine (Sood and Kumar, 1996), amitryptiline (McMa-hon, 1989), amitryptyline with concomitant lithium (Fava and Galizia, 1995), nimodipine (Fahy, 1996), tocolytic therapy comprising intravenous magnesium and nifedipine (Pecha and Danilewitz, 1996), interleukin-2 (Post *et al.*,

1991), diltiazem (Mantzoros *et al.*, 1994; Fauville *et al.*, 1995), morphine (Murthy *et al.*, 1998), fludarabine (Campbell *et al.*, 2000), and enteral activated charcoal alone (Brubacher *et al.*, 1996) and together with sorbitol and papaveretum (Longdon and Henderson 1992) when given for management of theophylline overdose.

NSAIDS

When grouped by category, NSAIDs are the most commonly prescribed of all drugs. More than 20 million prescriptions per year are written in the United Kingdom alone (Langman, 1988). In the United States, 2–3 million patients take daily NSAIDs and world-wide, it has been estimated that over 30 million people take NSAIDs each day (Gibson, 1988). The use of NSAIDs has been rising steadily since the 1970s, particularly amongst the elderly (Walt *et al.*, 1986). Approximately 50% of all NSAID prescriptions are for persons over 60 years old (Langman, 1988; Fries *et al.*, 1990).

Although NSAIDs reduce pain and inflammation and improve quality of life for patients with inflammatory disorders, it is widely recognised that such benefit is achieved at the risk of gastrointestinal injury. In the upper gastrointestinal tract this may range from clinically insignificant blood loss and minor erosive changes to deep ulceration with the associated risk of haemorrhage or perforation. Adverse effects of NSAIDs are also recognised in the small and large intestine and range from asymptomatic enteropathy to severe complications such as ulceration, bleeding, perforation, and stricture (Bjarnason *et al.*, 1993; Aabakken, 1999; Faucheron, 1999).

UPPER GASTROINTESTINAL LESIONS

The annual incidence of upper gastrointestinal bleeding associated with the use of NSAIDs has been reported to be from 50 to 150 cases per 100 000 (Gilbert, 1990; Laporte *et al.*, 1991) with chronic NSAID users experiencing a 1%–4% annual incidence of gastroduodenal perforation, ulcer or bleeding (Singh, 1998). In the United States gastrointestinal injury induced by NSAIDs is responsible for an estimated 107 000 hospitalised patients and 16 500 deaths annually (Singh, 1998; Wolfe *et al.*, 1999). Estimates for the United Kingdom suggest that some 12 000 emergency upper gastrointestinal admissions (including over 2200 deaths) per annum are due to NSAID use (Blower *et al.*, 1997).

Studies of the prevalence of peptic ulceration in arthritic patients receiving NSAIDs have been reviewed (McCarthy, 1989). Crude prevalence rates of gastric and duodenal ulcer were 13% and 11%, respectively. Similar findings were reported from an endoscopic screening study of over 1800 rheumatoid or osteoarthritic patients (Geis *et al.*, 1991). Gastric ulcers were present in 14.8% of patients and duodenal ulcers in 10.2%.

A number of investigators have addressed the question of the relative gastrointestinal toxicities of NSAIDs. Most assessments of relative toxicity have been derived from case–control studies. Despite the difficulties in interpretation of these data, such as NSAIDs being used in different populations for diverse indications and at a range of doses, some clear differences have been found. In general, studies have shown that the risk of adverse upper gastrointestinal effects is lowest with ibuprofen and diclofenac. Piroxicam and azapropazone have consistently been associated with a high risk of upper gastrointestinal toxicity (Committee on Safety of Medicines, 1986; Somerville *et al.*, 1986; Carson *et al.*, 1987a; Rossi *et al.*, 1987; Gabriel *et al.*, 1991; Garcia-Rodriguez and Jick, 1994; Griffin *et al.*, 1991; Laporte *et al.*, 1991; Henry *et al.*, 1993; Kaufman *et al.*, 1993; Savage *et al.*, 1993; Langman *et al.*, 1994).

These studies and others have been included in a meta-analysis to examine the relative risks of serious gastrointestinal complications reported with NSAIDs (Henry *et al.*, 1996). This showed that there are wide differences between individual NSAIDs in the risk of inducing gastrointestinal bleeding and ulcer perforation. Overall, ibuprofen was associated with the lowest relative risk, followed by diclofenac. Ranked highest for risk was tolmetin, piroxicam and ketoprofen, with the greatest risk being with azapropazone.

A meta-analysis of studies has also shown that long-term therapy with aspirin is associated with a significant increase in the incidence of gastro-intestinal haemorrhage (Derry and Loke, 2000). This occurred in 2.4% of patients taking aspirin compared with 1.42% taking placebo. Furthermore, it was shown that neither reducing the dose nor using modified release preparations reduced the incidence of gastrointestinal haemorrhage.

The risk of developing peptic ulcer disease and complications exists for the duration of NSAID treatment. However, the risk may be greatest in the first month of taking NSAIDs (Gabriel et al., 1991; Griffin et al., 1991; Henry et al., 1993). Griffin et al. reported that persons with a shorter duration of exposure to NSAIDs had an increased risk for the development of peptic ulcer disease (Griffin et al., 1991). The relative risk was 7.2 for those with a total duration of use of no more than 30 days, significantly greater than the relative risks of 3.7 and 3.9 for persons with 31–90 days, and more than 90 days of use, respectively.

Meta-analysis of studies resulted in similar findings (Gabriel et al., 1991). The highest measures of risk for adverse gastrointestinal events related to NSAID use were obtained from studies in which the duration of NSAID consumption was less than one month.

Higher doses of NSAIDs increase the risk of gastroduodenal ulceration and upper gastrointestinal complications (Carson et al., 1987b; Gabriel et al., 1991; Griffin et al., 1991; Henry et al., 1993; Garcia-Rodriguez and Jick, 1994; Langman et al., 1994). The relative risk of developing peptic ulcer disease as a function of the dose of NSAID was investigated in a nested case–control study of 1400 patients over 65 years old enrolled in a Medicaid programme in the United States (Griffin et al., 1991). Patients had been hospitalised for confirmed peptic ulcer and relative risks were compared with over 7000 controls. For users of NSAIDs, the risk increased with increasing dose, from a relative risk of 2.8 for the lowest, to a relative risk of 8.0 for the highest dose category.

Similar findings were reported from a study in the United Kingdom (Langman et al., 1994). The previous use of NSAIDs in 1144 patients aged 60 years or older and admitted to hospital with peptic ulcer bleeding was compared with matched hospital and community controls. Among subjects who took a non-aspirin NSAID during the previous month, the risk of ulcer complications increased with dose.

NSAID users with a prior history of gastro-intestinal disease are more likely to experience adverse gastrointestinal events when taking NSAIDs (Gabriel et al., 1991; Garcia-Rodriguez and Jick, 1994; Weil et al., 2000). Patients with a past history of peptic ulcer disease who are receiving NSAIDs are at a three- to four-fold higher risk of another episode of upper gastro-intestinal bleeding than are NSAID users with no past history of ulcer (Garcia-Rodriguez and Jick, 1991; Weil et al., 2000).

Elderly women are often believed to be at particular risk of NSAID-associated peptic ulcer complications. Whilst elderly patients are at greater risk than younger patients (Garcia-Rodriguez and Jick, 1994), the effect of gender is less clear. Findings from studies have been inconsistent and whilst some investigators report that the risk for a serious gastrointestinal event appears approximately equal amongst men and women, others suggest that women may be at a somewhat greater risk (e.g. Griffin et al., 1991; Henry et al., 1993; Neutel et al., 2000).

The combined use of NSAIDs and corticosteroids is associated with approximately two to three-times the risk of gastrointestinal toxicity than is the use of NSAIDs alone (Carson et al., 1987a; Gabriel et al., 1991; Piper et al., 1991; Garcia-Rodriguez and Jick, 1994; Weil et al., 2000).

Concomitant treatment with NSAIDs and corticosteroids increased the risk of hospitalisation due to gastroduodenal events in elderly patients (Piper et al., 1991). Relative risk of hospitalisation was 1.1 with corticosteroids alone, 4.1 with NSAIDs alone, but was increased 15-fold when both were combined. It should be noted that peptic ulcer is a rare complication of corticosteroid therapy alone (Conn and Poynard, 1994). The concurrent use of selective serotonin re-uptake inhibitors with NSAIDs has also been shown to potentiate the risk of upper gastrointestinal bleeding (de Abajo et al., 1999) as has the concomitant use of NSAIDs and anticoagulants (Shorr et al., 1993; Weil et al., 2000).

NSAIDs are effective in the management of inflammatory disease because they inhibit cyclo-oxygenase (COX) and hence inhibit the production of prostaglandins (Vane, 1971). Two COX isoforms exist, namely COX-1 and COX-2. Prostaglandins protect the upper gastrointestinal mucosa from damage and are a product of the activity of COX-1, a constitutive isoform. COX-2, however, is an enzyme that is induced to generate other prostaglandins that mediate pain and inflammation. The beneficial therapeutic effects of the non-selective NSAIDs are hence attributable to inhibition of the COX-2 enzyme, whereas the toxic effects on the upper gastrointestinal tract are a result of COX-1 inhibition (Vane and Botting, 1998).

The development of cyclooxygenase-2 (COX-2) selective NSAIDs (Jackson and Hawkey, 2000), such as celecoxib (Clemett and Goa, 2000) and rofecoxib (Hawkey et al., 2001), promises to reduce the gastrointestinal problems of patients needing anti-inflammatory drug therapy. Studies suggest that in osteoarthritis and in rheumatoid arthritis, COX-2 inhibitors have similar efficacy to conventional NSAIDs in relieving pain and improving functional status, but are associated with a lower incidence of upper gastrointestinal perforations, ulcers and bleeding (Clemett and Goa, 2000; Hawkey et al., 2001).

INTESTINAL LESIONS

In the small intestine NSAIDs may cause a low grade enteropathy (increased intestinal permeability, low grade inflammation with blood and protein loss), strictures, bleeding, lesions and perforation (Bjarnason et al., 1993; Aabakken, 1999).

An estimate of the prevalence of NSAID-induced lesions in the small intestine is available from a prospective autopsy study involving over 700 subjects (Allison et al., 1992). Non-specific small intestinal ulceration was found in 8.4% of 249 users of NSAIDs compared with 0.6% of 464 non-users. The prevalence of non-specific ulceration was higher in long-term users of NSAIDs (13.5%) compared with short-term users (6.3%). Three

patients (4.1%) in the long-term NSAID group died as a direct consequence of peritonitis from perforated, non-specific small intestinal ulcers.

Ingestion of NSAIDs has also been associated with colonic ulcers, large intestinal perforation and bleeding, complications of diverticular disease (perforation, fistulae and bleeding) and with relapse of inflammatory bowel disease (Bjarnason et al., 1993; Faucheron, 1999). In addition, over the past 10 years or so there have been an increasing number of anecdotal reports of NSAID-associated colonic strictures or NSAID-induced colonic diaphragm disease in patients receiving diclofenac, indomethacin, sulindac, phenylbutazone, ibuprofen, and etodolac (Eis et al., 1997; Ribeiro et al., 1998; Faucheron, 1999; Weinstock et al., 1999; Smith and Pineau, 2000).

In the large intestine NSAIDs, in particular the fenemates (mefenamic and flufenamic acid) may cause colitis. This may range from proctitis to pancolitis, although most histological reports are of mild non-specific colitis. NSAIDs have also been implicated in causing eosinophilic, pseudo-membranous and collagenous colitis.

BISPHOSPHONATES

The bisphosphonate group of drugs is used for the management of disorders typified by enhanced bone resorption such as Paget's disease and osteoporosis. Alendronate, a drug that is indicated for the treatment of osteoporosis, has been associated with adverse oesophageal and gastric events. Case reports of oesophagitis, oesophageal ulcer and of oesophageal stricture have been reported (Maconi and Bianchi Porro, 1995; Abdelmalek and Douglas, 1996; Colina et al., 1997, de Groen et al., 1996; Liberman and Hirsch, 1996; Naylor and Davies, 1996; Rimmer and Rawls, 1996; Kelly and Taggart, 1997; Levine and Nelson, 1997). Pamidronate also has been associated with oesophagitis (Lufkin et al., 1994).

In addition to causing oesophageal injury, it has been shown in endoscopic studies in volunteers that alendronate, and likely risedronate, can cause acute gastric mucosal damage and gastric ulceration (Graham, 2000). The incidence of adverse gastrointestinal events in users of alendronate was assessed from computerised pharmacy claims of the United Health Group–affiliated health plans in the United States (Park *et al.*, 2000). Over 1400 persons who received alendronate prescriptions were identified. Amongst those who had no prior oesophageal or gastric diagnoses, the cumulative incidence of upper gastrointestinal events was 3.3% in females, 2% in males and 3% overall. This included 22 patients with oesophagitis, 2 with oesophageal ulcer, 1 with gastric ulcer and 15 with gastritis/duodenitis.

SELECTIVE SEROTONIN RE-UPTAKE INHIBITORS

It has recently been suggested that the ingestion of selective serotonin re-uptake inhibitors is associated with upper gastrointestinal bleeding (de Abajo *et al.*, 1999). From a general practice research database, 1651 cases of gastrointestinal bleeding were identified along with 10 000 controls matched for age, gender and year of identification. Current use of selective serotonin re-uptake inhibitors or other antidepressants within 30 days before gastrointestinal bleeding was assessed. Use of selective serotonin re-uptake inhibitors was identified in 3.1% of patients with upper gastrointestinal bleeding compared with 1% of controls. The relative risk was unaffected by gender, age, dose or duration of treatment. The absolute risk of upper gastrointestinal bleeding was estimated as one case per 8000 prescriptions or one case per 1300 users. The authors also reported that the risk of upper gastrointestinal bleeding was greatly potentiated by the concomitant use of NSAIDs and, to a lesser extent, low-dose aspirin (de Abajo *et al.*, 1999). Further studies using alternative methods to confirm these observations have been recommended (Po, 1999).

PANCREATIC ENZYME SUPPLEMENTS

Some 90% of patients with cystic fibrosis receive pancreatic enzyme supplements for management of the symptoms of exocrine pancreatic insuffi-

ciency (FitzSimmons, 1993). By reducing steatorrhea and faecal fat excretion, the supplements improve the nutritional status of the patient. Pancreatic extracts have been used for many years, but in 1994 five cases of stricture of the ascending colon in children with cystic fibrosis who were receiving extracts were published (Smyth *et al.*, 1994). Additional cases (Campbell *et al.*, 1994; McHugh *et al.*, 1994; Oades *et al.*, 1994; Freiman and FitzSimmons, 1996; FitzSmmons *et al.*, 1997) suggested that the strictures appeared to be temporally related to the recent introduction of high-dose pancreatic supplements.

These reports, and a further 35 cases of colonic stricture reported to the US Cystic Fibrosis Foundation, prompted the Foundation to organise a Consensus Conference to examine the use of pancreatic enzymes in patients with cystic fibrosis (Borowitz *et al.*, 1995). The Conference used the term fibrosing colonopathy to describe "a condition associated with ingestion of large quantities of pancreatic enzyme supplements" and which leads to colonic strictures. It was considered that patients at highest risk were those who were less than 12 years of age, have taken more than 6000 lipase units per kg per meal for more than six months, have a history of meconium ileus or distal intestinal obstruction, have had intestinal surgery, or have a diagnosis of inflammatory bowel disease.

Although it was initially suspected that it was high-dose pancreatic supplements only that were causing fibrosing colonopathy, subsequently there were reports of the condition in children with cystic fibrosis who were receiving low-dose preparations (Jones *et al.*, 1995; Taylor and Steiner, 1995; Freiman and FitzSimmons, 1996; O'Keefe, 1996). However, a dose-related risk for the development of fibrosing colonopathy has been suggested (Smythe *et al.*, 1995; Bakowski and Prescott, 1997; FitzSimmons *et al.*, 1997).

A detailed review of early cases of fibrosing colonopathy and the chronology of events following the introduction in the United Kingdom and the United States of new forms of pancreatic supplements has been published (Bakowski and Prescott, 1997). The authors suggest that the patterns of use of the pancreatic supplements and the development of fibrosing colonopathy is highly suggestive of a dose-related causal role for preparations of which methacrylic acid co-polymer is a constituent of the enteric coating. This confirmed an earlier observation that methacrylic acid could be a key factor in the development of fibrosing colonopathy (van Velzen, 1995).

More recently there have been anecdotal case reports of fibrosing colonopathy in two adult patients receiving pancreatic enzyme supplements (Hausler et al., 1998; Bansi et al., 2000). The first was of a 25-year-old woman who developed symptomatic fibrosing colonopathy several months after beginning high-dose (17 000 units lipase per kg per day) pancreatic enzyme therapy (Hausler et al., 1998). The second involved a woman in her late 20s who had undergone cholecystectomy for gallstone disease followed thereafter by endoscopic management of common bile duct stones (Bansi et al., 2000). She later underwent a pylorus-preserving pancreaticoduodenectomy and in the subsequent seven years received large amounts of pancreatic enzyme supplements. After developing a large bowel obstruction, a right hemicolectomy was undertaken and fibrosing colonopathy of the ascending colon and caecum was confirmed by histology.

ROTAVIRUS VACCINE

Rotaviruses are the main cause of severe dehydrating diarrhoea in young children world-wide, accounting for 125 million cases of diarrhoeal disease with more than 800 000 associated deaths (Greenberg et al., 1999). Estimates vary, but in the United States, rotavirus is a common cause of severe gastroenteritis in children where it accounts for 50 000–65 000 hospitalisations and for 20–70 deaths per annum (Greenberg et al., 1999; US Department of Health and Human Services, 1999a).

In 1998, a tetravalent rhesus-based rotavirus vaccine was licensed in the United States for vaccination of infants. During the following 11 months, 15 cases of radiographically confirmed intussusception in vaccinated infants were reported to the United States Vaccine Adverse Events Reporting System (US Department of

Health and Human Services, 1999a). Of the 15, most (87%) developed intussusception following the first dose of the three-dose vaccination schedule. Eight of the children required surgical reduction and one, resection of part of the distal ileum and proximal colon. Following review of the data it was concluded that intussusception occurred with a significantly increased frequency after rotavirus vaccination (US Department of Health and Human Services, 1999b). Recommendations to vaccinate infants in the United States were subsequently withdrawn.

The above reports of intussusception prompted an investigation to further evaluate the potential association with the vaccine (Murphy et al., 2001). Infants aged at least 1 month, but less than 12 months, and who were hospitalised in 19 states of the United States between 1 November, 1998 and 30 June, 1999 were identified. Of 446 infants with intussusception, 429 were eligible to be included in a case–control analysis with 1763 matched controls. Four hundred and thirty-two of the 446 infants were also included in a case–series analysis. Among the infants with intussusception, 17.2% had received the rotavirus vaccine compared with 12.8% of the controls ($p = 0.02$). There was an increased risk of intussusception for the period of 3–14 days after the first dose of the vaccine. Case–series analysis showed the risk was also increased following the second dose of the vaccine, although this was smaller than the risk after the first dose. The authors concluded that the strong association between the rotavirus vaccine and intussusception supports the existence of a causal relationship.

MEASLES–MUMPS–RUBELLA VACCINE

A study published in 1995 suggested that there may be a link between measles vaccination and the subsequent development of Crohn's disease and ulcerative colitis (Thompson et al., 1995). The study was reported by the Inflammatory Bowel Disease Study Group at the Royal Free Hospital School of Medicine in London.

The prevalence of Crohn's disease and ulcerative colitis were determined in three cohorts: (a) a vaccinated group of 3545 people who had received measles vaccine in 1964 as part of a measles vaccine trial, (b) a control group of 11 407 people born in 1958 who were unlikely to have been vaccinated due to their age and of whom 89% had reported measles by age 11, and (c) a second control group of 2541 partners of individuals in the vaccinated group whose vaccination history was not known.

Disease prevalence data were collected by means of a postal questionnaire. The vaccinated group and their partners were asked whether they had, or had ever been told, by a doctor, that they had Crohn's disease, ulcerative colitis, coeliac disease or peptic ulcer disease. The unvaccinated group were asked about any condition that required regular medical supervision, the presence of any long-standing illness, disability, or infirmity, and details of all out-patient appointments and hospital admissions. Reports of Crohn's disease and ulcerative colitis were confirmed with the subject's physicians in the vaccinated and unvaccinated groups only.

Respondents were assumed to have inflammatory bowel disease if they reported it and the diagnosis was not refuted by their physician. Reports of inflammatory bowel disease where no confirmation could be made were included.

Crohn's disease and ulcerative colitis were reported more often among the measles vaccine group than among the control groups. The difference in the prevalence of inflammatory bowel disease was significantly higher in the vaccinated group when compared with the unvaccinated group. It was reported that, compared with the birth cohort, there was a relative risk of 3.01 (95% confidence interval: 1.45–6.23) of developing Crohn's disease in the vaccinated group. The relative risk of developing ulcerative colitis was 2.53 (95% confidence interval: 1.15—5.58). There was no difference in the rates for coeliac disease.

In contrast, a case–control study in the United Kingdom, which included 140 patients with inflammatory bowel disease (83 with Crohn's disease), was unable to show an association with measles vaccination (Feeney et al., 1997).

The Inflammatory Bowel Disease Study Group reported another study in 1998 that suggested an association between the combined measles, mumps and rubella (MMR) vaccine and gastrointestinal disease resulting in malabsorption, neurological damage and autism (Wakefield et al., 1998).

Twelve children between the ages of 3 years and 10 years were studied. All had been referred to a paediatric gastroenterology unit with a history of normal development followed by loss of acquired skills, together with diarrhoea and abdominal pain. Gastroenterological, neurological and developmental assessments, and a review of developmental records were performed.

All 12 children had intestinal abnormalities, including lymphoid nodular hyperplasia in 10. Histology showed patchy chronic inflammation in the colon in 11 children and reactive ileal lymphoid hyperplasia in 7, but no granulomas. Behavioural disorders included autism in 9 children, disintegrative psychosis in 1 and possible postviral or postvaccinal encephalitis in 2.

The onset of behavioural symptoms was associated, by the parents or the child's physician, with MMR vaccination in 8 of the 12 children, with measles infection in 1 child and otitis media in another. The average interval from MMR vaccination to the onset of behavioural symptoms was 6.3 days (range 1–14). Parents were less sure about the timing of onset of abdominal symptoms because children were not toilet trained at the time or because behavioural features made children unable to communicate symptoms.

Conflicting findings have been reported by long-term follow-up data for children receiving MMR vaccination in Finland (Peltola et al., 1998; Patja et al., 2000). A national surveillance system to detect serious adverse events was established in Finland when their MMR vaccination programme was launched in 1982. A potentially serious adverse event was defined as an event in any temporal association (no time limit was imposed) with MMR vaccination that fulfilled one or more of three characteristics: a potentially life-threatening disorder; the possibility that a chronic disease had been triggered by the vaccination; or the patient had been hospitalised for reasons possibly attributable to MMR vaccine. Reports were collected from all hospitals and health centres from 1982 to 1996. During this period about 3 million vaccine doses had been administered to 1.8 million individuals.

The health of children who had developed gastrointestinal symptoms, lasting 24 hours or more following vaccination, was reviewed (Peltola *et al.*, 1998). The time between the reported event and the health review ranged from 1 year and 4 months to 15 years (mean 9 years 3 months). Thirty-one children had gastrointestinal symptoms, of whom 20 were admitted to hospital. The most common symptom was diarrhoea (55%). The time from MMR vaccination to the onset of symptoms ranged from 20 hours to 15 days. Symptoms generally resolved within a week. No evidence of an association between MMR and inflammatory bowel disease or developmental disorder was found.

All serious adverse event reports collected in the Finnish 14-year surveillance programme were analysed with the finding that serious events causally related to MMR vaccine were rare (Patja *et al.*, 2000). No cases of inflammatory bowel disease were detected.

The proposal continues (Wakefield and Montgomery, 2000) although it is apparent that other studies have failed to confirm associations between either Crohn's disease or autism and MMR vaccination (Elliman and Bedford, 2001). Independent prospective studies are urgently needed to resolve this important issue as parents in the United Kingdom vote with their feet and abstain from vaccinating their children.

REFERENCES

Aabakken L (1999) Small bowel side effects of non-steroidal anti-inflammatory drugs. *Eur J Gastroenterol and Hepatol* **11**: 383–8.

Abdelmalek MF, Douglas DD (1996) Alendronate-induced ulcerative esophagitis. *Am J Gastroenterol* **91**: 1282–3.

Allison MC, Howatson AC, Torrance CJ, Lee FD, Russell RI (1992) Gastrointestinal damage associated with the use of nonsteroidal anti-inflammatory drugs. *New Engl J Med* **327**: 749–54.

Baehr PH, McDonald GB (1998) Esophageal disorders caused by infection, systemic illness, medications, radiation, and trauma. In: Feldman M, Scharschmidt BF, Sleisenger MH, eds, *Sleisenger & Fordtran's Gastrointestinal and Liver Disease*. Philadephia: WB Saunders, pp. 519–39.

Bakowski MT, Prescott P (1997) Patterns of use of pancreatic enzyme supplements in fibrosing colonopathy: Implications for pathogenesis. *Pharmacoepidemiology and Drug Safety* **6**: 347–58.

Bansi DS, Price A, Russell C, Sarner M (2000) Fibrosing colonopathy in an adult owing to overuse of pancreatic enzyme supplements. *Gut* **46**: 283–5.

Bates DW, Boyle DL, Vander Vliek MB, Scheider J, Leape LL (1995a) Relationship between medication errors and adverse drug reactions. *J Gen Intern Med* **10**: 199–205.

Bates DW, Cullen DJ, Laird N, Petersen LA, Small SD, Servi D, Laffel G, Sweitzer BJ, Shea BF, Hallisey R, Vander Vliet M, Nemeskal R, Leape LL (1995b) Incidence of adverse drug events and potential adverse drug events: implications for prevention. *J Am Med Assoc* **274**: 29–34.

Bates DB, Leape LL, Petrycki S (1993) Incidence and preventability of adverse drug events in hospitalized adults. *J Gen Intern Med* **8**: 289–94.

Bates DW, Spell N, Cullen DJ, Burdick E, Laird N, Petersen LA, Small SD, Sweitzer BJ, Leape LL (1997) The costs of adverse drug events in hospitalized patients. *J Am Med Assoc* **277**: 307–11.

Bateman DN, Aziz EE (1998) Gastrointestinal disorders. In: Davies DM, Ferner RE, deGlanville H, eds, *Davies's Textbook of Adverse Drug Reactions*, 5th edn. London: Chapman & Hall Medical, pp. 259–74.

Bjarnason I, Hallyar J, Macpherson AJ, Russell AS (1993) Side effects of nonsteroidal anti-inflammatory drugs on the small and large intestine in humans. *Gastroenterology* **104**: 1832–47.

Blower AL, Brooks A, Fenn GC, Hills A, Pearce MY, Morant S, Bardhan KD (1997) Emergency admissions for upper gastrointestinal disease and their relation to NSAID use. *Alimentary Pharmacol Ther* **11**: 283–91.

Bonavina L, DeMeester TR, McChesney LM, Schwizer W, Albertucci M, Bailey RT (1987) Drug-induced oesophageal strictures. *Ann Surg* **206**: 173–83.

Borowitz DS, Grand RJ, Drurie PR and the Consensus Committee (1995) Use of pancreatic enzyme supplements for patients with cystic fibrosis in the context of fibrosing colonopathy. *J Pediatr* **127**, 681–4.

Bott S, Prakash C, McCallum RW (1987) Medication-induced esophageal injury: survey of the literature. *Am J Gastroenterol* **82**: 758–63.

Bowman L, Carlstedt BC, Black CD (1994) Incidence of adverse drug reactions in adult medical inpatients. *Can J Hosp Phar* **47**: 209–16.

Brubacher JR, Levine B, Hoffman RS (1996) Intestinal pseudo-obstruction (Ogilvie's syndrome) in theophylline overdose. *Vet Human Toxicol* **38**: 368–70.

Campbell CA, Forrest J, Musgrove C (1994) High-strength pancreatic enzyme supplements and large-bowel stricture in cystic fibrosis. *Lancet* **343**: 109–10.

Campbell S, Thomas R, Parker A, Ghosh S (2000) Fludarabine induced intestinal pseudo-obstruction: case report and literature review. *Eur J Gastroenterol Hepatol* **12**: 711–3.

Carson JL, Strom BL, Morse ML, West SL, Soper KA, Stolley PD, Jones JK (1987a) The relative gastrointestinal toxicity of the non-steroidal anti-inflammatory drugs. *Arch Intern Med* **147**: 1054–9.

Carson JL, Strom BL, Soper KA, West SL, Morse ML (1987b) The association of non-steroidal anti-inflammatory drugs with upper gastrointestinal tract bleeding. *Arch Intern Med* **147**: 85–8.

Clemett D, Goa KL (2000) Celecoxib. A review of its use in osteoarthritis, rheumatoid arthritis and acute pain. *Drugs* **59**: 957–80.

Col N, Fanale JE, Kronholm P (1990) The role of medication noncompliance and adverse drug reactions in hospitalizations of the elderly. *Arch Intern Med* **150**: 841–5.

Colina RE, Smith M, Kikendall JW, Wong RK (1997) A new probable increasing cause of esophageal ulceration: alendronate. *Am J Gastroenterol* **92**: 704–6.

Committee on Safety of Medicines (1986) Non-steroidal anti-inflammatory drugs and serious gastrointestinal adverse reactions. *Br Med J* **292**: 1190–1.

Conn HO, Poynard T (1994) Corticosteroids and peptic ulcer: meta-analysis of adverse events during steroid therapy. *J Intern Med* **236**: 619–32.

de Abajo FJ, Garcia-Rodriguez LA, Montero D (1999) Association between selective serotonin reuptake inhibitors and upper gastrointestinal bleeding: population based case–control study. *Br Med J* **319**: 1106–9.

de Groen PC, Lubbe DF, Hirsch LJ, Daifotis A, Stephenson W, Freedholm D, Pryor-Tillotson S, Seleznick MJ, Pinkas H, Wang KK (1996) Esophagitis associated with the use of alendronate. *New Engl J Med* **335**: 1016–21.

Derry S, Loke YK (2000) Risk of gastrointestinal haemorrhage with long-term use of aspirin: meta analysis. *Br Med J* **321**: 1183–7.

Doman DB, Ginsberg AL (1981) The hazard of drug-induced esophagitis. *Hosp Practice* **June**: 17–25.

Einarson TR (1993) Drug-related hospital admissions. *Ann Pharmacother* **27**: 832–40.

Eis MJ, Watkins BM, Philip A, Welling RE (1997) Nonsteroidal-induced benign strictures of the colon: a case report and review of the literature. *Am J Gastroenterol* **93**: 120–1.

Elliman D, Bedford H (2001) MMR vaccine: the continuing saga. *Br Med J* **322**: 183–4.

Fahy BG (1996) Pseudoobstruction of the colon: early recognition and therapy. *J Neurosurg Anaesthesiol* **8**: 133–5.

Faucheron J-L (1999) Toxicity of non-steroidal anti-inflammatory drugs in the large bowel. *Eur J Gastroenterol Hepatol* **11**: 389–92.

Fauville JP, Hantson P, Honore P, Belpaire F, Rosseel MT, Mahieu P (1995) Severe diltiazem poisoning with intestinal pseudo-obstruction: case report and toxicological data. *J Toxicol Clin Toxicol* **33**: 273–7.

Fava S, Galizia AC (1995) Neuroleptic malignant syndrome and lithium carbonate. *J Psychiatry Neurosci* **20**: 305–6.

Feeney M, Clegg A, Winwood P, Snook J (1997) A case control study of measles vaccination and inflammatory bowel disease. *Lancet* **350**: 764–6.

Fine KD, Schiller LR (1999) AGA technical review on the evaluation and management of chronic diarrhea. *Gastroenterology* **116**: 1464–86.

FitzSimmons SC (1993) The changing epidemiology of cystic fibrosis. *J Pediatr* **122**: 1–9.

FitzSimmons SC, Burkhart GA, Borowitz D, Grand RJ, Hammerstrom T, Durie PR, Lloyd-Still JD, Lowenfels AB (1997) High dose pancreatic enzyme supplements and fibrosing colonopathy in children with cystic fibrosis. *New Engl J Med* **336**: 1283–9.

Freiman JP, FitzSimmons SC (1996) Colonic strictures in patients with cystic fibrosis. Results of a survey of 114 cystic fibrosis care centres in the United States. *J Pediatr Gastroenterol Nutrition* **22**: 153–6.

Fries JF, Miller SR, Spitz PW, Williams CA, Hubert HB, Bloch DA (1990) Identification of patients at risk for gastropathy associated with NSAID use. *J Rheumatol* **17** (Suppl 20): 12–9.

Gabriel SE, Jaakkimainen L, Bombardier C (1991) Risk for serious gastrointestinal complications related to the use of non-steroidal anti-inflammatory drugs. A meta-analysis. *Ann Intern Med* **115**: 787–96.

Garcia-Rodriguez LA, Jick H (1994) Risk of upper gastrointestinal bleeding and perforation associated with individual non-steroidal anti-inflammatory drugs. *Lancet* **343**: 769–72.

Geis GS, Stead H, Wallemark CB, Nicholson PA (1991) Prevalence of mucosal lesions in the stomach and duodenum due to chronic use of NSAIDs in patients with rheumatoid arthritis or osteoarthritis, and an interim report on prevention by misoprostil of diclofenac-associated lesions. *J Rheumatol* **18** (Suppl 28): 11–4.

Gibson T (1988) Non-steroidal anti-inflammatory drugs—another look. *Br Rheumatol* **27**: 87–90.

Gilbert DA (1990) Epidemiology of upper gastrointestinal bleeding. *Gastrointestinal Endoscopy* **36**: S8-S13.

Graham DY (2000) Bisphosphonate gastrointestinal damage: perspective and research needs. *Pharmacoepidemiology and Drug Safety* **9**: 377–81.

Greenberg HB, Matsui SM, Loutit JS (1999) Small intestine: infections with common bacterial and viral pathogens. In: Yamada T, Alpers DH, Laine L, Owyang C, Powell DN, eds, *Textbook of Gastroenterology*. Philadelphia: Lippincott, Williams & Wilkins, pp 1611–40.

Griffin MR, Piper JM, Daughert JR, Snowden M, Ray WA (1991) Non-steroidal anti-inflammatory drug use and increased risk for peptic ulcer disease in elderly persons. *Ann Intern Med* **114**: 257–63.

Hausler M, Meilicke R, Biesterfeld S, Heinann G (1998) First adult patient with fibrosing colonopathy. *Am J Gastroenterol* **93**: 1171–2.

Hawkey CJ, Jackson L, Harper SE, Semon TJ, Mortensen E, Lines CR (2001) Review article: the gastrointestinal safety profile of rofecoxib, a highly selective inhibitor of cyclooxygenase-2, in humans. *Alimentary Pharmacol Ther* **15**: 1–9.

Henry D, Dobson A, Turner C (1993) Variability in the risk of major gastrointestinal complications from non-aspirin non-steroidal anti-inflammatory drugs. *Gastroenterology* **105**: 1078–88.

Henry D, Lim LL-Y, Garcia-Rodriguez LA, Gutthan SP, Carlon JL, Griffin M, Savage R, Logan R, Moride Y, Hawkey C, Hill S, Fries JT (1996) Variability in risk of gastrointestinal complications with individual non-steroidal anti-inflammatory drugs: results of a collaborative meta-analysis. *Br Med J* **312**: 1563–6.

Hurwitz N, Wade OL (1969) Intensive hospital monitoring of adverse reactions to drugs. *Br Med J* **i**: 531.

Iredale JP (1993) Drugs causing gastrointestinal obstruction. *Adv Drug Reactions Toxicol Rev* **12**: 163–75.

Jackson LM, Hawkey CJ (2000) COX-2 selective nonsteroidal anti-inflammatory drugs. Do they really offer any advantages? *Drugs* **59**: 1207–16.

Jones R, Franklin K, Spicer R, Berry J (1995) Colonic strictures in children with cystic fibrosis on low-strength pancreatic enzymes. *Lancet* **346**: 499.

Kaufman DW, Kelly JP, Sheehan JE, Laslo A, Wilholm BE, Alfredsson L, Koff RS, Shapiro S (1993) Non-steroidal anti-inflammatory drug use in relation to major upper gastrointestinal bleeding. *Clin Pharmacol Ther* **53**: 485–94.

Kelly R, Taggart H (1997) Incidence of gastrointestinal side effects due to alendronate is high in clinical practice. *Br Med J* **315**: 1235.

Kikendall JW (1999a) Pill esophagitis. *J Clin Gastroenterol* **28**: 298–305.

Kikendall JW (1999b) Pill-induced esophageal injury. In: Castell DO, Richter JE, eds, *The Esophagus*. Philadelphia: Lippincott Williams & Wilkins, pp. 527–37.

Langman MJS (1988) Ulcer complications and non-steroidal anti-inflammatory drugs. *Am J Med* **84** (Suppl 2A): 15–9.

Langman MJS, Weil J, Wainwright P, Lawson DH, Rawlins MD, Logan RFA, Murphy M, Vessey MP, Colin-Jones DG (1994) Risks of bleeding peptic ulcer associated with individual non-steroidal anti-inflammatory drugs. *Lancet* **343**: 1075–8.

Laporte JR, Carne X, Vidal X, Moreno V, Juan J (1991) Upper gastrointestinal bleeding in relation to previous use of analgesics and non-steroidal anti-inflammatory drugs. *Lancet* **337**: 85–9.

Lazarou J, Pomeranz BH, Corey PN (1998) Incidence of adverse drug reactions in hospitalized patients. A meta-analysis of prospective studies. *J Am Med Assoc* **279**: 1200–5.

Levine J, Nelson D (1997) Esophageal stricture associated with alendronate therapy. *Am J Med* **102**: 489–91.

Liberman UI, Hirsch LJ (1996) Esophagitis and alendronate. *New Engl J Med* **355**: 1069–70.

Locke GR, Pemberton JH, Phillips SF (2000) AGA technical review on constipation. *Gastroenterology* **119**: 1766–78.

Longdon P, Henderson A (1992) Intestinal pseudo-obstruction following the use of enteral charcoal and sorbitol and mechanical ventilation with papaveretum sedation for theophylline poisoning. *Drug Safety* **7**: 74–7.

Lufkin EG, Argueta R, Whitaker MD, Cameron AL, Wong VH, Egan KS, O'Fallon WM, Riggs BC (1994) Pamidronate: an unrecognized problem in gastrointestinal tolerability. *Osteoporosis Intnl* **4**: 320–2.

Maganini RJ, Pollitt JB (1983) Pseudo-obstruction of the colon (Ogilvie's syndrome) associated with clonidine administration. *J Abdom Surg* **27**: 27–9.

Manconi G, Bianchi Porro G (1995) Multiple ulcerative esophagitis caused by alendronate. *Am J Gastroenterol* **90**: 1889–90.

Mantzoros CS, Prabhu AS, Sowers JR (1994) Paralytic ileus as a result of diltiazem treatment. *J Intern Med* **235**: 613–4.

McCarthy DM (1989) Non-steroidal anti-inflammatory drug-induced ulcers: management by traditional therapies. *Gastroenterology* **96**: 662–74.

McHugh K, Thomson A, Tam P (1994) Case report: colonic stricture and fibrosis associated with high-strength pancreatic enzymes in a child with cystic fibrosis. *Br J Radiol* **67**: 900–1.

McMahon AJ (1989) Amitryptiline overdose complicated by intestinal pseudo-obstruction and caecal perforation. *Postgrad Med J* **65**: 948–9.

Murphy TV, Gargiullo PM, Massoudi MS, Nelson DB, Jumaan AO, Okoro CA, Zanardi LR, Setia S, Fair E, LeBaron CW, Wharton M, Livingwood JR (2001) Intussusception among infants given an oral rotavirus vaccine. *New Engl J Med* **344**: 564–72.

Murthy BV, Ion F, Winstanley JR (1998) Intestinal pseudo-obstruction associated with oral morphine. *Eur J Anaesthesiol* **15**: 370–1.

Naylor G, Davies MH (1996) Oesophageal stricture associated with alendronic acid. *Lancet* **348**: 1030–1.

Nelson KM, Talbert RL (1996) Drug-related hospital admissions. *Pharmacotherapy* **16**: 701–7.

Neutel CI, Maxwell CJ, Appel WC (2000) Differences between males and females in risk of NSAID-related severe gastrointestinal events. *Pharmacoepidemiology and Drug Safety* **8**: 501–7.

Oades PJ, Bush A, Ong PS, Brereton RJ (1994) High-strength pancreatic enzyme supplements and large-bowel stricture in cystic fibrosis. *Lancet* **343**: 109.

O'Keefe P (1996) Case report. *Postgrad Med J* **72**: S23–S25.

Park B-J, Clouse J, Shatin D, Stergachis A (2000) Incidence of adverse oesophageal and gastric events in alendronate users. *Pharmacoepidemiology and Drug Safety* **9**: 371–6.

Patja A, Davidkin I, Kurki T, Kallio MJT, Valle M, Peltola H (2000) Serious adverse events after measles–mumps–rubella vaccination during a fourteen-year prospective follow-up. *Pediatr Inf Dis J* **19**: 1127–34.

Pecha RE, Danilewitz MD (1996) Acute pseudo-obstruction of the colon (Ogilvie's syndrome) resulting from combination tocolytic therapy. *Am J Gastroenterol* **91**: 1265–6.

Peltola H, Patja A, Leinikki P, Valle M, Davidkin I, Paunio M (1998) No evidence for measles, mumps and rubella vaccine-associated inflammatory bowel disease or autism in a 14-year prospective study. *Lancet* **351**: 1327–8.

Pemberton J (1970) Oesophageal obstruction and ulceration caused by oral potassium therapy. *Br Heart J* **32**: 267.

Piper JM, Ray WA, Daugherty JR, Griffin MR (1991) Corticosteroid use and peptic ulcer disease: rise of non-steroidal anti-inflammatory drugs. *Ann Intern Med* **114**: 735–40.

Po ALW (1999) Antidepressants and upper gastrointestinal bleeding. New results suggest a link. *Br Med J* **319**: 1081–2.

Post AB, Falk GW, Bukowski RM (1991) Acute colonic pseudo-obstruction associated with interleukin-2 therapy. *Am J Gastroenterol* **86**: 1539–41.

Pouyanne P, Haramburu F, Imbs JL, Bégaud B (2000) Admissions to hospital caused by adverse drug reactions: cross sectional incidence study. *Br Med J* **320**: 316.

Quigley EMM, Hasler WL, Parkman HP (2001) AGA technical review on nausea and vomiting. *Gastroenterology* **120**: 263–86.

Ribeiro A, Wolfsen HC, Wolfe JT, Loeb DS (1998) Colonic strictures induced by nonsteroidal anti-inflammatory drugs. *South Med J* **91**: 568–72.

Rimmer DE, Rawls DE (1996) Improper alendronate administration and a case of pill esophagitis. *Am J Med* **91**: 2648–9.

Rossi AC, Hsu JP, Faich GA (1987) Ulcerogenicity of piroxicam: an analysis of spontaneously reported data. *Br Med J* **294**, 147–9.

Roughead EE, Gilbert AL, Primrose JG, Sansom LN (1998) Drug-related hospital admissions: a review of Australian studies published 1988–96. *Med J Austr* **168**: 405–8.

Savage RL, Moller PW, Ballantyne CL, Wells JE (1993) Variation in the risk of peptic ulcer complications

with non-steroidal anti-inflammatory drug therapy. *Arthritis and Rheumatism* **36**: 84–90.

Shorr RI, Ray WA, Daugherty JR, Griffin MR (1993) Concurrent use of nonsteroidal anti-inflammatory drugs and oral anticoagulants places elderly persons at high risk for haemorrhagic peptic ulcer disease. *Arch Intern Med* **153**: 1665–70.

Singh G (1998) Recent considerations in nonsteroidal anti-inflammatory drug gastropathy. *Am J Med* **105** (Suppl II): S31–S8.

Smith JA, Pineau BC (2000) Endoscopic therapy of NSAID-induced colonic diaphragm disease: two cases and a review of published reports. *Gastrointest Endosc* **52**: 120–5.

Smythe RL, Ashby D, O'Hea U, Burrows E, Lewis P, van Velzen D, Dodge JA (1995) Fibrosing colonopathy in cystic fibrosis: results of a case–controlled study. *Lancet* **346**: 1247–51.

Smyth RL, van Velzen D, Smyth AR, Lloyd DA, Heaf DP (1994) Strictures of ascending colon in cystic fibrosis and high-strength pancreatic enzymes. *Lancet* **343**: 85–6.

Somerville K, Faulkener G, Langman M (1986) Non-steroidal anti-inflammatory drugs and bleeding peptic ulcer. *Lancet* **i**: 462–4.

Sood A, Kumar R (1996) Imipramine induced acute colonic pseudo-obstruction (Ogilvie's syndrome): a report of two cases. *Ind J Gastroenterol* **15**: 70–1.

Stieger DS, Cantieni R, Frutiger A (1997) Acute colonic pseudoobstruction (Ogilvie's syndrome) in two patients receiving high dose clonidine for delirium tremens. *Intens Care Med* **23**: 780–2.

Taylor CJ, Steiner GM (1995) Fibrosing colonopathy in a child on low-dose pancreatin. *Lancet* **346**: 1106–7.

Thompson NP, Montgomery SM, Pounder RE, Wakefield AJ (1995) Is measles vaccine a risk factor for inflammatory bowel disease? *Lancet* **345**: 1071–4.

US Department of Health and Human Services (1999a) Intussusception among recipients of rotavirus vaccine—United States, 1998–9. *Morbidity and Mortality Weekly Rep* **48**: 577–81.

US Department of Health and Human Services (1999b) Withdrawal of rotavirus vaccine recommendations. *Morbidity Mortality Weekly Rep* **48**: 1007.

van Velzen D (1995) Colonic strictures in children with cystic fibrosis on low-strength pancreatic enzymes. *Lancet* **346**: 499–500.

Vane JR (1971) Inhibition of prostaglandin synthesis as a mechanism of action for aspirin-like drugs. *Nature* **231**: 232–5.

Vane JR, Botting RM (1998) Mechanism of action of nonsteroidal anti-inflammatory drugs. *Am J Med* **104** (Suppl 1): S2–S8.

Wakefield AJ, Montgomery SM (2000) Mumps measles rubella vaccine: through a glass darkly. *Adv Drug Reactions Toxicol Rev* **19**: 265–83.

Wakefield AJ, Murch SH, Anthony A, Linnell J, Casson DM, Malik M, Berelowitz M, Dhillon AP, Thompson MA, Harvey P, Valentine A, Davies SE, Walker-Smith JA (1998) Ileal-lymphoid-nodular hyperplasia, non-specific colitis, and pervasive developmental disorder in children. *Lancet* **351**: 637–41.

Walt R, Katschinski B, Logan R, Ashley J, Langman M (1986) Ulcer complications and non-steroidal anti-inflammatory drugs. *Lancet* **i**: 489–92.

Weil J, Langman MJS, Wainwright P, Lawson DH, Rawlins M, Logan RFA, Brown TP, Vessey MP, Murphy M, Colin-Jones DG (2000) Peptic ulcer bleeding: accessory risk factors and interactions with non-steroidal anti-inflammatory drugs. *Gut* **46**: 27–31.

Weinstock LB, Hammond Z, Brandwin L (1999) Nonsteroidal anti-inflammatory drug-induced colonic stricture and ulceration treated with balloon dilation and prednisone. *Gastrointest Endosc* **50**: 564–6.

Wolfe MM, Lichtenstein DR, Singh G (1999) Gastrointestinal toxicity of nonsteroidal antiinflammatory drugs. *New Engl J Med* **340**: 1888–99.

36

Haematological ADRs

SARAH DAVIS
Post-Licensing Division, Medicines Control Agency, London, UK

RONALD D. MANN
Waterlooville, Hampshire, UK

INTRODUCTION

This chapter has the specific objective of looking at what one national adverse drug reaction reporting scheme can provide, by way of data, regarding suspected drug toxicity affecting the haematological system in man. The reporting system chosen has been the UK "Yellow Card" Scheme begun in 1964 by the Committee on Safety of Drugs (the forerunner of today's Committee on Safety of Medicines) under the chairmanship of Sir Derrick Dunlop. The written assurances given to prescribing doctors by Sir Derrick at the beginning of this scheme (see Mann, 1998) have been honoured over the intervening years and have allowed the accumulation of a database that can be used to explore many aspects of the clinical toxicity of drugs. These various aspects have been summarized elsewhere (Rawlins, 1986).

There are three other chapters in this volume that relate to the subject of haematological adverse drug reactions (ADRs). First, the Introduction (Mann and Andrews) provides a table listing drugs withdrawn during or since 1975 in the United Kingdom by the Marketing Authorization holder or suspended or revoked by the Licensing Author-

ity for safety reasons. This list of 31 drugs includes two—nomifensine (major safety concern, haemolytic anaemia) and remoxipride (major safety concern, aplastic anaemia)—which were withdrawn due to reports of haematological reactions. Remoxipride was an unpleasant reminder of oxyphenbutazone and phenylbutazone—also strongly associated with reports of aplastic anaemia—which will be discussed further in this chapter.

The second chapter directly concerned with haematological ADRs is that by Stonier and Edwards (Chapter 12) on nomifensine and haemolytic anaemia. The remarkable story of the long period that elapsed after nomifensine was marketed and before its toxic effects were recognized—and the way in which these effects led to the withdrawal of the drug world-wide—was first told in Peter Stonier's courageous paper of nine years ago (Stonier, 1992). The literature contains few accounts of a crucial drug disaster as experienced by a physician with keynote responsibilities within the company concerned and the relevant account is, therefore, informative.

The third chapter, which has special relevance, is that by Curel and Stather (Chapter 40). This

Pharmacovigilance. Edited by R.D. Mann and E.B. Andrews
© 2002 John Wiley & Sons, Ltd

provides a list of "ADR headlines from 1999" and a similar list for the year 2000. The entry for ticlopidine regarding thrombotic thrombocytopenic purpura, liver failure and agranulocytosis will be noted along with that for Rho(D) immunoglobulin regarding reports of intravascular haemolysis in Rho(D)-positive patients with immune thrombocytopenic purpura. However, these useful listings show that over these two years haematological problems formed a minority of the big ADR highlights that occupied the attention of those concerned with pharmacovigilance.

HAEMOPOIETIC REPORTS VIA THE "YELLOW CARD" SCHEME

The data available relate to UK spontaneous reports of suspected ADRs committed onto the Adverse Drug Reactions On-line Information Tracking (ADROIT) database of the Medicines Division and Committee on Safety of Medicines as of 7 March 2001. An early account of this database was given by Wood and Coulson (1993), the late Susan Wood having been instrumental in establishing this facility.

DEFINITIONS

1. "Total reactions reported": the overall number of reactions reported for a given drug substance or class, regardless of the body system affected by the reaction.
2. "Haemopoietic reactions reported": the overall number of reactions in the haemopoietic system/organ class reported for a given drug substance or therapeutic class.
3. "Serious haemopoietic reactions": the number of haemopoietic reactions reported for a given drug substance/class which are defined as serious on the ADROIT Medical Dictionary; see Appendices A and B for lists of serious and non-serious reactions.
4. "Fatal haemopoietic reactions": the number of haemopoietic reactions reported for a given drug substance/class, where the outcome of the reaction was stated as being "fatal" by the reporter.

THE DATA

Table 36.1 lists those drug substances/ multiconstituent preparations for which over 75

Table 36.1. Drug substances/multiconstituent preparations for which there are >75 haemopoietic reactions on the ADROIT database.

Drug	Total reactions reported	Haemopoietic reactions reported	Haemopoietic reactions reported as % of total reactions reported	Serious haemopoietic reactions	Fatal haemopoietic reactions	Fatal haemopoietic reactions as a % of haemopoietic reactions reported	Class
Clozapine	4475	1196	26.7	1151	3	0.3	Anti-psychotics
Phenylbutazone	2483	657	26.6	652	305	46.2	NSAIDs
Co-trimoxazole	6299	623	9.9	618	62	10	Antibiotics
Methyldopa	2319	589	25.4	500	50	8.5	Anti-hypertensives
Carbamazepine	6017	521	8.7	498	14	2.7	Anti-epileptics
Warfarin	2088	512	24.5	498	36	7	Anti-coagulants
Sulphasalazine	2734	511	18.7	500	42	8.2	Aminosalicylates
Valproic acid	3016	341	11.3	324	9	2.6	Anti-epileptics
Mianserin	2910	319	11	314	23	7.2	Anti-depressants
Indomethacin	6889	284	4.1	281	41	14.4	NSAIDs
Naproxen	5270	269	5.1	259	24	8.9	NSAIDs

Table 36.1. *Continued*.

Drug	Total reactions reported	Haemopoietic reactions reported	Haemopoietic reactions reported as % of total reactions reported	Serious haemopoietic reactions	Fatal haemopoietic reactions	Fatal haemopoietic reactions as a % of haemopoietic reactions reported	Class
Diclofenac	8194	266	3.2	254	11	4.1	NSAIDs
Ibuprofen	5293	260	4.9	256	20	7.7	NSAIDs
Cimetidine	7632	258	3.4	252	15	5.8	H2 antagonists
Carbimazole	1079	242	22.4	241	29	12	Anti-thyroid
Oxyphenbutazone	779	237	30.4	237	112	47.3	NSAIDs
Fluoxetine	13396	227	1.7	203	1	0.4	Anti-depressants
Penicillamine	1371	223	16.3	220	26	11.7	Anti-rheumatic
Ranitidine	5330	213	4	204	9	4.2	H2 antagonists
Mefenamic acid	2981	206	6.9	200	14	7	NSAIDs
Methotrexate	1170	191	16.3	187	64	33.5	Cytotoxics
Piroxicam	5582	187	3.4	182	12	6.4	NSAIDs
Trimethoprim	3003	184	6.1	177	13	7.1	Antibiotics
Captopril	5259	184	3.5	177	9	4.9	ACE inhibitor
Lamotrigine	3246	180	5.5	165	7	3.9	Anti-epileptics
Azathioprine	1298	176	13.6	170	24	13.6	Immunosuppressant
Azapropazone	3130	172	5.5	161	7	4.1	NSAIDs
Phenytoin	1672	167	10	160	23	13.8	Anti-epileptics
Omeprazole	6871	141	2.1	129	11	7.8	PPI
Sodium aurothiomalate	715	138	19.3	137	30	21.7	Anti-rheumatic
Chlorpromazine	1313	135	10.3	131	35	25.9	Anti-psychotics
Nomifensine	1087	128	11.8	117	6	4.7	Anti-depressants
Ciprofloxacin	4733	127	2.7	117	6	4.7	Antibiotics
Paroxetine	17531	119	0.7	106	3	2.5	Anti-depressants
Fenbufen	9902	118	1.2	115	7	5.9	NSAIDs
Tryptophan + ascorbic acid + pyridoxine	382	114	29.8	112	0	0	Anti-depressants
Frusemide	1155	114	9.9	113	13	11.4	Diuretics
Ketoprofen	2929	113	3.9	111	4	3.5	NSAIDs
Enalapril	6295	111	1.8	103	3	2.7	ACE inhibitor
Benoxaprofen	5752	110	1.9	107	14	12.7	NSAIDs
Heparin	558	105	18.8	100	27	25.7	Anti-coagulants
Mesalazine	1281	103	8	97	8	7.8	Aminosalicylates
Lofepramine	4753	99	2.1	93	8	8.1	Anti-depressants
Amiodarone	3024	97	3.2	94	3	3.1	Anti-arrhythmic
Thioridazine	836	95	11.4	95	11	11.6	Anti-psychotics
Zidovudine	319	90	28.2	89	4	4.4	Anti-retroviral
Allopurinol	1679	89	5.3	88	6	6.7	Anti-gout
Chloramphenicol	368	83	22.6	83	41	49.4	Antibiotics
Rifampicin	793	81	10.2	80	1	1.2	Antibiotics
Latamoxef	164	78	47.6	73	4	5.1	Antibiotics
Dothiepin	1597	77	4.8	76	4	5.2	Anti-depressants
Lansoprazole	3964	77	1.9	72	1	1.3	PPI

Table 36.2. Cumulative data for NSAIDs, antibiotics, anti-psychotics, anti-depressants and anti-epileptics.

Drug class	Total reactions reported	Haemopoietic reactions reported	Haemopoietic reactions reported as % of total reactions reported	Serious haemopoietic reactions	Fatal haemopoietic reactions	Fatal haemopoietic reactions as a % of haemopoietic reactions reported
NSAIDs	55 271	3191	5.8	3090	448	14
Antibiotics	27 532	2108	7.7	2049	173	8.2
Anti-psychotics	11 423	1870	16.4	1779	77	4.1
Anti-depressants	39 316	1642	4.2	1540	80	4.9
Anti-epileptics	10 046	1283	12.8	1217	55	4.3

Table 36.3. Clozapine.

Haemopoietic reaction (preferred term)	Number of reports
Neutropenia	680
Agranulocytosis	200
Leucopenia NOS	199
Leucocytosis NOS	23
Thrombocytopenia	18
Anaemia	13
Eosinophilia (exc pulmonary)	13
Neutrophilia	11
Thrombocythaemia	9
Haemoglobin decreased	6
Lymphopenia	6
Decreased lymphocyte count	4
Decreased platelet count	3
White blood cell abnormalities	3
Atypical lymphocytes	1
Blood dyscrasia NOS	1
Bone marrow depression	1
Coagulation disorder NOS	1
Haemolytic anaemia	1
Iron deficiency anaemia	1
Splenomegaly	1
Thrombocytopenic purpura NOS	1
Total	1196

haemopoietic reactions have been reported. This number was selected for convenience and includes 52 drugs/preparations. The data presented relate to each of the above definitions.

Table 36.2 provides data for each of 5 classes of drug—non-steroidal anti-inflammatory drugs (NSAIDs), antibiotics, anti-psychotics, anti-depressants and anti-epileptics. The data include information on drugs listed in the relevant sections of the current British National Formulary (BNF) and older drugs in these therapeutic classes that are no longer marketed (e.g. oxyphenbutazone is included in the NSAIDs and nomifensine in the anti-depressants).

Table 36.3 provides for clozapine (the drug for which the highest number of haemopoietic reactions have been received) a breakdown of the haemopoietic reactions reported, and the number of reports for each of these reactions. Table 36.4 provides similar data for phenylbutazone.

Table 36.5 provides, for phenylbutazone, a breakdown showing the number of haemopoietic reactions reported each year since 1964.

INTERPRETATION OF THE DATA

It needs to be kept in mind that the data represent reports of suspected adverse reactions. In considering the possibility of causation the temporal relationship between exposure and the onset of the reaction needs to be considered along

Table 36.4. Phenylbutazone.

Haemopoietic reaction (preferred term)	Number of reports
Aplastic anaemia	289
Thrombocytopenia	96
Agranulocytosis	74
Pancytopenia	49
Neutropenia	40
Bone marrow depression	20
Anaemia	19
Hypoplastic anaemia	15
Haemorrhage NOS	10
Haemolytic anaemia	6
Coagulation time increased	5
Eosinophilia (exc pulmonary)	4
Leucopenia NOS	4
Prothrombin decreased	3
Thrombotic thrombocytopenic purpura	3
B12 deficiency anaemia	2
Capillary fragility increased	2
Coombs positive haemolytic anaemia	2
Leucocytosis NOS	2
Macrocytic anaemia NOS	2
Splenomegaly	2
Folate deficiency anaemia	1
Iron deficiency anaemia	1
Leukaemoid reaction	1
Megaloblastic anaemia NOS	1
Myelogfibrosis	1
Myeloproliferative disorder NOS	1
Polycythaemia NOS	1
Thrombocythaemia	1
Total	657

Table 36.5. Haemopoietic reactions associated with phenylbutazone, by year.

Year of receipt of report	Number of haemopoietic reactions reported in association with phenylbutazone
1964	25
1965	51
1966	48
1967	46
1968	41
1969	39
1970	33
1971	35
1972	32
1973	40
1974	34
1975	66
1976	41
1977	30
1978	38
1979	16
1980	9
1981	6
1982	13
1983	4
1984	6
1985	2
1992	2
Total	657

with the nature of the patient's underlying disease, the presence of concomitant drug therapy, carry-over effects of previous medication, data on rechallenge or dechallenge, and convincing reports from other sources involving patients given monotherapy.

The data, being devoid of a reliable numerator, cannot be used to calculate the incidence of the reaction. It is misleading to make numerical comparisons for the same reaction between different drugs or drug classes since many factors, other than the number of reports, are involved. These include the level of reporting and underreporting, the level of use of the drug in the population, variations in populations and the time the drug has been in clinical usage; the data are also frequently affected by biases due to media coverage, regulatory and professional warnings and other extraneous factors.

Many additional factors influence the number of reports received for a particular drug and reaction. These factors include the seriousness of the reaction, the ease of recognition of the reaction, and the reporting requirements and practices in the country concerned.

OVERVIEW OF THE DATA

Although it is not possible to compare the drugs listed in Table 36.1 simply on the basis of the numbers of haemopoietic reports included in the ADROIT database, it is evident that Table 36.1 contains no real surprises. The drugs in this list are generally all recognized to have haematological side-effects and this is reflected in their approved prescribing information.

The list includes a number of drugs that, in the United Kingdom, have been withdrawn from the market or had their use severely restricted due to haematological adverse reactions. These include: phenylbutazone, clozapine, oxyphenbutazone, and nomifensine.

Table 36.1 is headed by clozapine which, from two points of view, provides findings of the greatest interest to those concerned with pharmacovigilance. This drug was withdrawn and all clinical trials were suspended in 1974 when eight patients in Finland died from agranulocytosis attributed to the drug (Amsler et al., 1977). The compound was of valuable use in the treatment of severe schizophrenia and was reintroduced into clinical practice by means of the closely monitored "Clozaril Patient Monitoring Service" (Committee on Safety of Medicines, 1990). That Table 36.1 shows only three fatal haemopoietic reaction reports strongly suggests that this service (run by the relevant pharmaceutical company) has been highly effective. The findings provide an example of the effective use of a patient/disease monitoring registry in controlling a known life-threatening iatrogenic disease relating to the use of a drug active in a major indication (drug-resistant schizophrenia). The second point about clozapine in Table 36.1 is that the total number of reports of haemopoietic reactions is a splendid example of bias: doctors cannot use the drug without doing blood counts in the prescribed fashion and there are, as a result, a very large number of reports. In addition, the relevant pharmaceutical company

runs the monitoring scheme and is obliged to report suspected reactions to the Medicines Control Agency. This factor is of obvious importance since a search of the ADROIT database shows that over 90% of the reports of haemopoietic reactions are received from the pharmaceutical company rather than from a health professional. This finding contrasts with overall UK experience which shows that the majority of reports are received from health professionals (the converse of the situation in the United States).

The column of "fatal haemopoietic reactions" in Table 36.1 shows the special place of phenylbutazone (305 relevant reports, 46.2% of all haemopoietic reactions) and oxyphenbutazone (112 fatal reports comprising 47.3% of all haemopoietic reports for the drug). The contrasting adverse reaction profiles of these two drugs compared with the other NSAIDs have been considered elsewhere (Mann, 1988) but the known haematological toxicity of both drugs was tolerated for a number of years because of their efficacy and the paucity, over those years, of equally effective agents. Once reasonably useful alternatives became available they were withdrawn or their use severely restricted.

Table 36.1 shows columns of percentage values. This reflects interest in calculating Proportional Reporting Ratios (PRRs) (Evans et al., 1998). When the whole of the ADROIT database is considered, haemopoietic reactions comprise 2.7% of all UK spontaneous reports on the database; this figure can loosely be taken as an indicator of the "background" levels of reporting for these suspected reactions. If a more precise indicator were required, then the same calculation could be made excluding reports for clozapine, oxyphenbutazone and phenylbutazone, to give a more accurate measure of background levels of reporting; excluding reports for these drugs, 2.2% of UK spontaneous reactions relate to haemopoietic reactions. When haemopoietic reactions are considered as a percentage of the total number of reactions reported for each drug, it is notable that for some drugs (e.g. paroxetine, fluoxetine, omeprazole, enalapril, lanzoprazole) haemopoietic reactions are reported at a lower value than the background rate. This may reflect extremely wide usage and the volume of reports received. The finding is likely to be coincidental. High PRR values can be due to bias (the reporting requirements with clozapine) or can reflect the known pharmacology/toxicity of the drug (phenylbutazone, oxyphenbutazone, systemic chloramphenicol, the anti-coagulants). Table 36.1 contains no surprises in this context.

In respect of individual drugs, it is not possible to compare classes of drugs simply on the basis of the numbers of haemopoietic reports received. When these reactions are considered as a proportion of the total number of reactions received for each drug class, it is the anti-psychotics and anti-epileptics that stand out (Table 36.2) as having a high proportion of reactions of this type. Given the high level of reporting of these reactions for clozapine, this is not unexpected for the anti-psychotics. In addition, since these drug classes were selected for investigation based on the appearance of drugs in the "Top 52", the fact that these classes of drugs have higher then average proportions of haemopoietic reactions is not unexpected. The relatively high proportion of fatal haemopoietic reactions shown in Table 36.2 in respect of the NSAIDs is clearly a result of the experience with phenylbutazone and oxyphenbutazone.

Additional data for clozapine are given in Table 36.3. This shows the dominant place of neutropenia, agranulocytosis and leucopenia among the reactions reported with this drug. The data clearly reflect the clinically beneficial findings produced by the Clozaril Patient Monitoring Service. Table 36.4 shows the massive numbers of blood dyscrasias associated with the use of phenylbutazone and Table 36.5 shows the decline in the number of haemopoietic reactions reported for phenylbutazone. The table shows the effect of the regulatory restrictions on the use of this drug.

CONCLUSION

Pharmacovigilance has to be conducted with the realization that behind every adverse reaction report there is a patient's face and one seeks to avoid that face reflecting the effects of serious iatrogenic disease. Table 36.5 and the data given above suggest that this has been largely achieved in respect of haemopoietic ADRs associated with the use of phenylbutazone. In the United Kingdom the ADROIT database facilitates continued observation to preserve and augment this type of improvement.

ACKNOWLEDGEMENTS

We gratefully acknowledge the assistance of Victoria Newbould in the preparation of the data included in this chapter. We also express our thanks to the doctors and other healthcare professionals who have provided reports in support of the "Yellow Card" Scheme.

APPENDIX A

Haemopoietic reactions defined as serious on the ADROIT Medical Dictionary

Acquired abnormal karyotype	Afibrinogenaemia neonatal
Acquired afibrinogenaemia	Agranulocytosis
Acquired anti-VIII inhibitor	Aleukaemic blood picture
Acquired anti-VIII inhibitor increased	Anaemia
Acquired anti-XIII inhibitor	Anaemia aggravated
Acquired Factor IX deficiency haemorrhage	Angioimmunoblastic lymphadenopathy
Acquired Factor VIII deficiency	Aplastic anaemia
Acquired haemophilia NOS	Autoimmune haemolytic disease NOS
Acquired sideroblastic anaemia	B12 deficiency anaemia
Activated partial thromboplastin time decreased	Bence Jones proteinuria
Activated partial thromboplastin time increased	Benign monoclonal gammopathy
Addisonian pernicious anaemia	Blast cell proliferation

Bleeding tendency
Bleeding tendency aggravated
Bleeding time increased
Blood dyscrasia NOS
Bone marrow depression
Bone marrow failure
Bone marrow hypocellular
Bone marrow necrosis
Burst capillaries
Carboxyhaemoglobinaemia
Chemotherapy-induced anaemia
Childhood haemolytic anaemia
Coagulation disorder NOS
Coagulation factor deficiency NOS
Coagulation time increased
Congenital anaemia
Coombs negative haemolytic anaemia
Coombs positive haemolytic anaemia
Cryoglobulinaemia
Cryoglobulinaemia aggravated
Decreased lymphocyte count
Decreased white cell count aggravated
Disseminated intravascular coagulation
Disseminated intravascular coagulation aggravated
Eosinophilia (exc pulmonary)
Eosinophilia myalgia syndrome
Erythropoieis depression
Essential thrombocythaemia
Evan's syndrome
Extravascular haemolysis
Factor V decreased
Factor X deficiency
Factor XII deficiency
Foetal anaemia
Folate deficiency anaemia
Fragmented red cells
Glucose-6-phosphate dehydrogenase deficiency
Granulomatous marrow reaction
Haemoglobinopathy NOS
Haemolysis NOS
Haemolysis NOS aggravated
Haemolytic anaemia aggravated
Haemophilia A (Factor VIII)
Haemophilia A haemorrhage
Haemophilia B (Factor IX)
Haemophilia B haemorrhage
Haemophilia C (Factor XI)
Haemophilia NOS
Haemophiliac pseudotumour
Haemophiliac pseudotumour exacerbated
Haemorrhage NOS
Haemorrhage NOS aggravated
Haemorrhagic disease of newborn
Heinz bodies
Hereditary haemolytic anaemia NOS
Hereditary sideroblastic anaemia
Hereditary spherocytosis

Hyperchromic anaemia
Hypereosinophilic syndrome
Hypersplenism
Hyperviscosity syndrome
Hypoplastic anaemia
Idiopathic thrombocytopenic purpura
Idiopathic thrombocytopenic purpura aggravated
Increased frequency of bleeding
International normalized ratio decreased
International normalized ratio increased
Intravascular coagulation NOS
Intravascular haemolysis
Iron deficiency anaemia
Isoimmune haemolytic disease
Leucoerythroblastic anaemia
Leucopenia aggravated
Leucopenia NOS
Lymphohistiocytosis
Lymphohistiocytosis aggravated
Lymphopenia
Macrocytic anaemia NOS
Macrocytosis
Macrophage haemophagocytosis
Malin's syndrome
Marrow hyperplasia
Mastocytosis
Megablastic anaemia NOS
Microangiopathic haemolytic anaemia
Microcytic anaemia
Microcytosis
Monoclonal gammopathy NOS
Myeloblastic syndrome
Myelodysplastic syndrome
Myelofibrosis
Myeliod dysplasia
Myeloproliferative disorder NOS
Myelosuppression
Neutropenia
Neutropenia aggravated
Normochromic normocytic anaemia
Nucleated red cells
Pancytopenia
Pancytopenia aggravated
Paroxysmal nocturnal haemoglobinuria
Platelet abnormalities
Platelet storage defect
Polycythaemia aggravated
Polycythaemia NOS
Polycythaemia rubra vera
Prothrombin decreased
Punctate basophilia
Recurrence of haemolytic anaemia NOS
Recurrence of idiopathic thrombocytopenic purpura
Red blood cell abnormalities NOS
Red cell hypoplasia
Refractory anaemia
Reticulocytosis

Reticulofibrosis
Rouleaux formation
Secondary anaemia
Secondary polycythaemia
Secondary thrombocytopenic purpura
Sickle cell crisis
Sickle cell disorders
Spherocytosis acquired
Splenic haemorrhage
Splenic infarct
Splenic rupture
Splenomegaly
Thalassaemia
Thrombin decreased
Thrombin increased

Thrombocythaemia
Thrombocythaemia aggravated
Thrombocytopenia
Thrombocytopenia aggravated
Thrombocytopenia purpura NOS
Thromboplastin decreased
Thromboplastin increased
Thrombotic tendency
Thrombotic thrombocytopenic purpura
Thrombotic thrombocytopenic purpura aggravated
Von Willebrand's disease (exc congenital)
Waldenstrom's macroglobulinaemia
White blood cell abnormalities
White clot syndrome

APPENDIX B

Haemopoietic reactions defined as non-serious on the ADROIT Medical Dictionary

Atypical lymphocytes
Basophilia
Capillary fragility increased
Capillary permeability increased
Capillary resistance decreased
Clot retraction accelerated
Clot retraction retarded
Coagulation time decreased
Coombs direct test negative
Coombs direct test positive
Coombs test NOS positive
Decreased platelet count
Extramedullary haemopoeisis
Factor V deficiency
Factor VII deficiency
Familial polycythaemia
Fibrin decreased
Fibrin increased
Fibrinogen plasma decreased
Fibrinogen plasma increased
Fibrinolysis decreased
Fibrinolysis increased
Haemoglobin decreased
Haemoglobin electrophoresis abnormal
Haeoglobinaemia

Idiopathic purpura
Inhibitory antibodies to Factor IX
Inhibitory antibodies to Factor VIII
Inhibitory antibodies to Factor VIII C
Leucocytosis NOS
Leukaemoid reaction
Lymph node tenderness
Lymphocytosis
March haemoglobinuria
Monocytosis
Neutrophilia
Plasma viscosity decreased
Plasma viscosity increased
Polychromatophilia
Prothrombin time decreased
Reticuloendothelial system stimulated
Schilling test abnormal
Schumm's test positive
Serum iron abnormal
Spherocytic anaemia (exc congenital)
Spleen disorder NOS
Stress polycythaemia
Thrombasthenia
Total iron binding capacity abnormal

REFERENCES

Amsler HA, Teerenhovi L, Bartha E, Harjuia K, Vuopic P (1977) Agranulocytosis in patients treated with clozapine: a study of the Finnish epidemic. *Acta Psychiatr Scand* **56**: 214–48.

Committee on Safety of Medicines (1990) Clozaril induced neutropenia and the Clozaril Patient Monitoring Service. *Current Problems* **No. 30** (December): 1.

Evans SJW, Waller P, Davis S (1998) Proportional Reporting Ratios: the uses of epidemiological methods for signal generation. *Pharmacoepidemiology and Drug Safety* **7** (Suppl 2): S102.

Mann RD (1988) The history of the non-steroidal anti-inflammatory agents. In: Mann RD, ed., *The History of the Management of Pain*. Carnforth, UK: Parthenon, pp. 77–126.

Mann RD (1998) A memorable letter. *Br Med J* **316**: 837.

Rawlins MD (1986) Spontaneous reporting of adverse drug reactions. *Q J Med (New Series 59)* **230**: 531–4.

Stonier PD (1992) Nomifensine and haemolytic anaemia—Experience of a post-marketing alert. *Pharmacoepidemiology and Drug Safety* **1**(4): 177–85.

Wood SM, Coulson R (1993) Adverse drug reactions on-line information tracking (ADROIT). *Pharmaceut Med* **7**: 203–13.

37

Hepatic Adverse Drug Reactions

GURUPRASAD P. AITHAL

Queen's Medical Centre, University Hospital, Nottingham, UK

CHRISTOPHER P. DAY

Centre for Liver Research, The Medical School, Newcastle upon Tyne, UK

INTRODUCTION

Since the liver is central to the biotransformation of virtually all drugs and foreign substances, drug-induced liver injury is a potential complication of nearly every medication that is prescribed. The liver is the most common target organ for toxicity encountered during the course of drug development (Ballet, 1997). Despite considerable progress in toxicological studies, the correlation between liver toxicity in animals and man remains poor (Lumley, 1990). This was highlighted by the tragic fialuridine trial, wherein potential mitochondrial injury leading to hepatic failure (resulting in 5 deaths and 2 liver transplantations among 15 treated patients) was not detected during preclinical testing in rats, dogs, monkeys and woodchucks (infected with the woodchuck hepatitis virus) treated with the drug for a month (McKenzie et al., 1995; Josephson, 1996). Hepatotoxicity remains the principal cause of termination in clinical trials of new chemical entities, accounting for one-third of such terminations. Adverse hepatic reactions accounted for 18% of postmarketing withdrawals in France, Germany, the United Kingdom and the United States between 1961 and 1992 (Spriet-Pourra and Auriche, 1994) and have continued to be the leading cause of such withdrawals in the last few years. Furthermore, the number of prescription drugs, including the new molecular entities, on the market has increased dramatically over the last two decades (Friedman et al., 1999). Hence, a larger number of agents now appear to contribute to the total burden of drug-induced liver disease. Physician awareness of this constantly changing pattern of drug-induced hepatotoxicity is essential for early recognition.

DEFINITIONS

An adverse drug reaction (ADR) is defined as any response to a drug that is noxious, unintended, and which occurs at doses normally used in man for the prophylaxis, diagnosis, or therapy of disease (Anon., 1969). These idiosyncratic or "unexpected" reactions, which are the focus of this chapter, are to be distinguished from predictable reactions due to overdoses. The problems of case definition and causality assessment of drug-induced liver injury have been

Pharmacovigilance. Edited by R.D. Mann and E.B. Andrews

addressed by an international group of experts and their recommendations have provided a standardised framework for evaluation of drug-induced hepatotoxicity (Benichou, 1990). When liver biopsy or autopsy has been performed, hepatotoxicity should be classified according to the histology. In the absence of histological data, the term "liver injury" has been used to signify abnormalities of the biochemical tests. Liver injury is designated "hepatocellular" when there is a twofold (or more) increase in alanine aminotransferase (ALT) alone, or when the ratio of serum activity (activity is expressed as a multiple of upper limit of normal) of ALT to alkaline phosphatase (ALP) is 5 or more. Liver injury is designated "cholestatic" when there is a twofold (or more) increase in ALP alone, or when the ratio of serum activity of ALT to ALP is 2 or less. Liver injury is termed "mixed" when the ratio of the serum activity of ALT to ALP is between 2 and 5. When increases in the liver tests have been of less than 3 months' duration, the liver injury is considered "acute", and when the increase lasted more than 3 months, "chronic liver injury" is considered to be present.

EPIDEMIOLOGY

METHODS OF ESTIMATING THE FREQUENCY OF HEPATIC ADVERSE REACTIONS

The epidemiology of adverse hepatic reaction remains poorly documented. Controlled clinical trials have the advantages of close and prospective surveillance as well as a control group. However, the median number of subjects exposed to a new drug at the time of marketing is usually around 1500, with rarely more than 100 patients receiving the product for more than a year (Rawlins, 1995). This is clearly inadequate since around 30 000 treated subjects need to be observed to identify, with a power 0.95, at least one with drug hepatotoxicity when the incidence is 1 in 10 000 patient years (Stricher, 1992). The debate surrounding the initial approval and the recent withdrawal from the market of troglitazone high-lights the realities of drug development and the need for postmarketing surveillance. In the clinical trials of troglitazone (representing a novel class of oral antihyperglycaemic agents), 1.9% of 2510 patients receiving the drug had elevated liver enzymes, two of which developed reversible jaundice (Watkins and Whitcomb, 1998). It took more than 3 years and 90 deaths or liver transplantations (in over a million patients treated), before the drug was withdrawn from the market (Lumpkin, 2000). Furthermore, clinical trials usually include selected patients and the findings may therefore not be generalisable to a wider population. Hence, in the United Kingdom and many other countries, postmarketing surveillance relies largely on spontaneous reporting (Rawlins, 1995), and data on adverse hepatic reactions have come most often from this source. Spontaneous reporting allows surveillance to continue throughout the life of a marketed drug when a large number of individuals have been exposed to the drug, and hence relatively rare adverse reactions have been recognised. However, only 10% of the serious and 2%–4% of non-serious reactions are usually reported (Rawlins, 1995). A relatively high rate of reporting may result from a high frequency of adverse reactions or may simply be due to the publicity or novelty of a new agent. One such "apparent epidemic" of flucloxacillin-induced jaundice in Australia (reporting 357 ADRs and 17 deaths) has been considered to be a reporting artefact (Devereaux et al., 1995; Roughead et al., 1999). In addition to the variability in reporting, identification of cases in a non-systematic way introduces significant inaccuracy to the data. In a recent survey in the United Kingdom, about half of the reported adverse hepatic reactions were classified as "unrelated" to the drugs under systematic evaluation (Aithal et al., 1999). A further difficulty with spontaneous reporting is that the denominator is usually unknown, although drug sales figures could be used to estimate the frequency of adverse reactions.

Record linkage studies connect information on drug exposure from prescription data with outcome, and have the advantages of prospective design and comprehensive identification of cases.

Established linkages such as the General Practice Research Database in the United Kingdom and Group Health Cooperative of Puget Sound in the United States have contributed valuable epidemiological information regarding drug-induced liver disease (Beard et al., 1986; Derby et al., 1993; Jick et al., 1999). However, most often the outcomes such as deaths, hospital admissions and discharge diagnoses, used in linkage studies are those that pertain only to the more serious reactions or those that occur while the patient is in the hospital. The latter underestimates the frequency of adverse hepatic reactions since acute hospital inpatient stays are usually shorter than the latent period (5 days to 3 months) of most types of drug-induced liver disease.

Case–control studies are particularly useful when the outcome is rare. In the field of drug-induced liver disease, they have been applied to hepatic tumors, industrial hepatotoxicity and the role of aspirin in Reye's syndrome (Farrell, 1994).

FREQUENCY OF HEPATIC ADVERSE REACTIONS

Despite increasing awareness of hepatotoxicity and the availability of less toxic alternatives, the absolute frequency of hepatic drug reactions has not decreased in the last decade, in keeping with the increasing number of prescriptions and pharmacological agents available (Larrey, 2000). Hepatic injury accounts for 3.5%–9.5% of all ADR reports and up to 14.7% of fatal adverse reactions (Friis and Andreasen, 1992). Using data from the computerised Danish National Hospital Registry, the incidence of drug-induced liver disease was calculated as 19 and 22 per million person-years for men and women, respectively (Almdal and Sorensen, 1991). Another study from the United States estimated the overall incidence of drug-induced liver disease requiring hospitalisation to be 1 per 100 000 person-years (Beard et al., 1986). Drug-induced liver disease accounts for between 1 in 666 and 1 in 3000 hospital admissions in Denmark and United States (Jick et al., 1981; Hallas et al., 1992).

THE CONTRIBUTION OF DRUG-INDUCED HEPATOTOXICITY TO THE OVERALL BURDEN OF LIVER DISEASE

Drugs are responsible for between 2% and 6% of jaundice and about 10% of cases of "acute hepatitis" (Lewis and Zimmerman, 1989; Whitehead et al., 2001). In industrialised nations such as the United States, France and Denmark ADRs account for up to 20% of cases of acute hepatic failure, while it is less common (5%) in tropical countries such as India (Acharya et al., 1996; Ostapowicz et al., 1999). Drug-induced chronic hepatitis has been considered rare, even though it accounts for up to 6% of all chronic hepatitis (Aithal and Day, 1999). Drug hepatotoxicity almost certainly remains an important and often neglected cause of cholestasis, although its relative frequency among other cholestatic syndromes has not been reported. Drugs probably contribute to the aetiology of less than 1% of all liver tumors (Farrell, 1994).

RELATIVE FREQUENCIES OF DRUGS IMPLICATED

Advances in drug development have allowed the replacement of many potentially toxic drugs with "safer" alternatives. For example, oxyphenisatin has been withdrawn as a laxative in most countries, alpha-methyldopa is now rarely used as an antihypertensive agent, and perhexilene has been replaced by alternative, safer agents. As might be expected, this has led to a change in the pattern of implicated drugs causing hepatotoxicity over the last few decades. In the 1960s chlorpromazine was most commonly associated with hepatotoxicity (Cook and Sherlock, 1965) and in the 1970s halothane was responsible for 25% of hepatotoxic drug reactions reported (Dossing and Andreasen, 1982). Even though this has led to a significant reduction in use in the United Kingdom, halothane continues to account for significant numbers of hepatotoxic adverse reactions in Europe and New Zealand (Friis and Andreasen, 1992; Pillans, 1996). Similarly, liver injury secondary to antitubercular drugs such as isoniazid continues to be reported worldwide (Acharya et

Table 37.1. Drugs causing adverse hepatic reactions.

Acute hepatocellular and mixed pattern of liver injury (or acute hepatitis)
NSAIDs: diclofenac, ibuprofen, naproxen, nimesulide, piroxicam, sulindac

Anaesthetics: enflurane, halothane, isoflurane

Antimicrobials: ketoconozole, ofloxacin, sulphamides, sulphones, terbinafine, tetracyclines; antimycobacterials such as isoniazid, pyrazinamide, rifampicin; anti-HIV agents such as didanosine, indinavir, zidovudine

Neuropsychotropics: tricyclics (most), fluoxetine, paroxitine, pemoline, sertraline, tacrine, riluzole; illegal compounds such as cocaine and Ecstasy

Antiepileptics: carbamazapine, phenytoin, valproate

Cardiovascular drugs: bezafibrate, captopril, diltiazem, enalapril, lisinopril, lovastatin, simvastatin, ticlopidine

Antineoplastic and immunomodulatory agents: cyclophosphamide, cis-platinum, doxorubcine, granulocyte colony stimulating factor, interleukin (IL)-2, IL-12, tamoxifen

Others: etretinate, glipizide, herbal remedies, ranitidine

Acute cholestatic pattern of liver injury and cholestatic hepatitis
Hormonal preparations: androgens, oral contraceptives, tamoxifen

Antimicrobials: clindamycin, co-amoxiclav, co-trimoxazole, erythromycin, flucloxacillin, troleandomycin

Analgesic/anti-inflammatory drugs: gold salts, propoxyphene, sulindac

Neuropsychiatric drugs: carbamazapine, chlorpromazine, tricyclic antidepressants

Antineoplastic and immunomodulatory agents: asparaginase, azathioprine, cyclosporin

Cardiovascular drugs: ajmaline, captopril, propafenone, ticlopidine

Others: allopurinol, chlorpropamide

Chronic hepatitis and/or cirrhosis
Aspirin, diclofenac, halothane, herbal medicine (germander), isoniazide, methotrexate, methyldopa, nitrofurantoin, papaverine, vitamin A

Chronic cholestasis and ductopenia
Ajmaline, carbamazepine, chlorpromazine, co-amoxiclav, co-trimoxazole, erythromycin, flucloxacillin, methyltestosterone, phenytoin

Granulomatous hepatitis
Allopurinol, carbamazepine, cephalexin, dapsone, diltiazem, gold salts, hydralazine, isoniazid, methyldopa, nitrofurantoin, penicillin, penicillamine, phenytoin, procainamide, quinidine, sulphonamides, sulphfonylureas

Macro and microvesicular steatosis
Amiodarone, asparaginase, buprenorphine, corticosteroids, flutamide, female sex hormone, methotrexate, perhexiline, salicylate, tacrine, tetracycline, valproate, zidovudine

Hepatic vascular lesions
Hepatic vein thrombosis/veno-occlusve disease: azathioprine, dacarbazine, combination chemotherapy (carmustine, cytarabine, mitomycin, thioguanine, urethane), oral contraceptives

Sinusoidal dilation/peliosis: anabolic steroids, azathioprine, hydroxyurea, oral contraceptives

Perisinusidal fibrosis: azathioprine, methotrexate, vitamin A

Tumors
Androgens, oral contraceptives

For more comprehensive lists see Farrell (1994), Pillans (1996), Desmet (1997), Erlinger (1997), Larrey (2000), Krahenbuhl (2001), and Lucena *et al.* (2001).

al., 1996; Ostapowicz et al., 1999; Lucena et al., 2001). As the relatively "high-risk" agents have been replaced, relatively rare reactions to commonly prescribed "low-risk" agents have become the most important cause of hepatotoxicity. In the last few years, non-steroidal anti-inflammatory drugs (NSAIDs) such as diclofenac and sulindac, antimicrobials such as co-amoxiclav, flucloxacillin and erythromycin, and H2 antagonists have become important causes of hepatotoxicity (Pillans, 1996; Lucena et al., 2001). In addition, hepatotoxicity due to substances that were previously thought to have little toxicity, such as "Ecstasy" (recreational amphetamine) and herbal remedies, are being increasingly recognised (Larrey, 1997; Andreu et al., 1998). A brief list of the drugs which are important causes of hepatotoxicity and the pattern of the liver injury are shown in Table 37.1.

DIAGNOSIS OF ADVERSE HEPATIC REACTION

The importance of drugs as a cause of liver injury lies not in the overall number of cases, but in the severity of some reactions and their potential reversibility, provided the drug aetiology is promptly recognised. Adverse hepatic reactions can mimic a wide spectrum of hepatobiliary diseases. Early recognition and prompt withdrawal of the drug is essential in preventing serious hepatic failure and is the critical step in the management of adverse reactions (Nolan et al., 1999). Failure to detect hepatotoxicity at an early stage has led to mortality in many reported cases of hepatotoxicity (Moulding, 1999). The long-term prognosis of drug-induced hepatotoxicity may be worse if the responsible agent is continued (Aithal and Day, 1999).

CAUSALITY ASSESSMENT METHODS

The lack of specific tests for diagnosing drug hepatotoxicity poses particular problems for definitively attributing a liver reaction to an implicated drug. The approach to the diagnosis of a drug-induced liver disease involves physician awareness,

exclusion of other causes of the reaction and an objective weighing of the circumstantial evidence. These considerations have been termed "causality assessment" and form the cornerstone to the diagnosis of drug-induced hepatotoxicity.

Decision Tree Model

An algorithm-based model developed by Stricker considers three factors:

1. the specificity of the clinico-pathological pattern and its course;
2. the temporal relationship between intake/discontinuation of the suspected drug and onset/disappearance of hepatic injury; and
3. exclusion of other possible causes for the observed pattern (Stricher, 1992).

The model assesses the degree of certainty of a causal relationship between hepatic injury and drug intake; however, it has several major disadvantages. First, all the factors are given equal weight; second, the quantitative data are reduced to qualitative "yes" or "no" answers. Finally, categories such as "probable" and "possible" lead to a semantic cause of inter-observer variation.

Bayesian Model

A logical approach to the problem of causality assessment is based on Bayes' theorem. This model uses the background incidence of an event, the individual clinical features of a particular case and the probability of other potential causes. The model estimates the probability of a specific reaction in a particular individual in a given situation being related to the drug therapy. However, the Bayesian model is time consuming and, hence, impracticable to use in the evaluation of a large number of adverse hepatotoxic reactions. In addition, the background incidence of a given reaction may not be known, thus further limiting its use. In a large survey, the Bayesian model had an accuracy of only 45% in the diagnosis of drug-induced liver disease when compared with the final diagnosis after investigations (Lavelle and Kavanagh, 1995).

International Consensus Criteria

In 1990, under the auspices of the Council for International Organizations of Medical Sciences (CIOMS), an international group of "experts" proposed definitions of adverse hepatotoxic reactions and criteria for assessing causality of drug-induced liver diseases in order to standardise the evaluation of drug hepatotoxicity by physicians, health authorities of different countries and pharmaceutical manufacturers (Benichou, 1990). For causality assessment the French method of ADR assessment was adapted to suit the evaluation of drug-induced liver disease (Danan, 1988). "International consensus criteria" combined the basic principles of "chronological criteria" (establishing a temporal relationship between the drug treatment and the reaction) and "clinical criteria" (exclusion of alternative causes for the particular pattern of liver injury) to determine the probability of the reaction being related to the drug. A detailed scoring system was developed (CIOMS scale) and validated using cases of drug-induced liver injury with known positive rechallenge (Danan and Benichou, 1993). The CIOMS scale performed well when these cases were assessed using the data prior to rechallenge. In a recent study (Aithal *et al.*, 1999) 86% of the suspected hepatic ADRs could be classified as "drug-related" or "unrelated" using a simplified form of consensus classification (see Table 37.2).

Even though the "International consensus criteria" are considered to be "state of the art", they cannot be used rigidly in all circumstances, especially to exclude a drug as a cause of a given reaction. For example, the classification of a causal relationship between a drug and cholestatic injury as "incompatible" if the onset occurs more than one month after the last drug intake would unduly refute such cases attributable to co-amoxiclav intake (Larrey *et al.*, 1992a). Similarly, flucloxacillin-induced cholestasis which, in one-third of patients may take up to 18 months after the drug withdrawal to resolve (Turner *et al.*, 1989), may be classified as "inconclusive" according to the consensus criteria. The CIOMS scale also defines alcohol, pregnancy and age over 55 years as risk factors which would reduce the

Table 37.2. Classification of suspected adverse reactions using International Consensus Criteria (simplified version).

Drug-related
1. The time from drug intake and withdrawal to the apparent onset of the reaction was "suggestive" of drug hepatotoxicity (5–90 days from initial drug intake) or "compatible" with drug hepatotoxicity (<5 or >90 days from initial drug intake and ≤15 days from drug withdrawal for "hepatocellular" reactions or ≤30 days from drug withdrawal for "cholestatic" reactions).
2. The course of the reaction after cessation of the drug was "very suggestive" (decrease in the liver enzymes by ≥50% of the excess over the upper limit of normal within 8 days) or "suggestive" (decrease in the liver enzymes by ≥50% within 30 days for "hepatocellular" reactions and 180 days for "cholestatic" reactions) of drug hepatotoxicity.
3. Alternative cause of the reaction had been excluded by relevant investigations.
4. There was a positive response to rechallenge (at least a doubling of liver enzymes) when such information was available.

Reactions were classified as "drug-related" if all of the first three criteria were met or if two out of the first three criteria were met in the presence of a positive rechallenge response.

Drug-unrelated
1. The time from drug intake and withdrawal to the apparent onset of the reaction was "incompatible" with drug hepatotoxicity (drug taken after the onset of the reaction or reaction >15 days from cessation of the drug except for slowly metabolised drugs).
2. Time course of the reaction after drug withdrawal "not suggestive" of drug hepatotoxicity (decrease in liver enzymes <50% decrease in liver enzymes within 30 days for hepatocellular reactions and 180 days for cholestatic reactions). Both "indeterminate" and "inconclusive" cholestatic reactions were included in this group.
3. The presence of an alternative cause for the reaction.

A reaction was classified as drug-unrelated if one or both of the first two criteria were met in the presence of an alternative cause for the reaction.

Indeterminate
1. A temporal relationship between drug intake and the reaction in the presence of a likely alternative cause for the reaction.

    Or

2. A temporal relationship between drug intake and the reaction not suggestive of drug-induced hepatotoxicity but no alternative cause for the reaction.

flexibility to weigh other risk factors relevant to the clinical setting.

Clinical Diagnostic Scale

More recently, a simplified scoring system called the "Clinical Diagnostic Scale" (CDS) (otherwise called the Maria & Victorino scale) has been developed (Maria and Victorino, 1997). Scores are attributed in seven different components of a given reaction (Table 37.3) and the reactions are graded according to the final score. The original validation of the CDS used real and fictitious cases and

the opinion of a panel of experts as the gold standard. A detailed comparison of the CIOMS scale and the CDS concluded that the latter performed poorly while evaluating reactions with long latency periods and evolution to chronicity after withdrawal (e.g. cholestasis due to amoxiclav) (Lucena *et al.*, 2001).

The CDS generally underscores the reactions. Even in the initial study, only four (all of which had positive rechallenge) were classified as definite adverse hepatic reaction (score >17) (Maria and Victorino, 1997). The reason for low scoring is due to the emphasis given to positive rechallenge as

Table 37.3. Description of Clinical Diagnostic Scale (Maria & Victorino scale) (Maria and Victorino, 1997).

Component elements	Scores attributed
I. Temporal Relationship between drug intake and the reaction	
A. *Time from Drug intake until the onset of first clinical or laboratory manifestations*	
4 days to 8 weeks (or less than 4 days in cases of re-exposure	3
Less than 4 days or more than 8 weeks	1
B. *Time from withdrawal of the drug until the onset of manifestations*	
0 to 7 days	3
8 to 15 days	0
More than 15 days (except in cases of prolonged persistence of the drug in the body after withdrawal; e.g. Amiodarone)	−3
C. *Time from withdrawal of the drug until normalisation of laboratory values*	
(Decrease to values 2× the upper limit of normal values)	
Less than 6 months (cholestatic or mixed pattern) or 2 months (hepatocellular)	3
More than 6 months (cholestatic or mixed pattern) or 2 months (hepatocellular)	0
II. Exclusion of alternative causes (viral hepatitis, alcoholic liver disease, biliary obstruction, pre-existing liver disease, ischaemic hepatitis)	
Complete exclusion	3
Partial exclusion	0
Possible alternative cause detected	−1
Probable alternative cause detected	−3
III. Extrahepatic manifestations (rash, fever, arthralgia, eosinophilia, cytopenia)	
4 or more	3
2 or 3	2
1	1
None	0
IV. Intentional or accidental re-exposure to the drug	
Positive rechallenge	3
Negative or absent rechallenge	0
V. Previous report in the literature of cases of hepatotoxicity associated with the drug	
Yes	2
No (drugs marketed for up to 5 years)	0
No (drugs marketed for more than 5 years)	−3

Final classification of the reaction as definite (score >17), probable (14–17), possible (10–13), unlikely (6–9), and excluded (<6).

well as extrahepatic manifestations (maximum of 3 scores each). Deliberate rechallenge of an incriminated drug is ethically unjustifiable and inadvertent re-exposure is reported in a minority (8.8%) of hepatic ADRs (unpublished data). Extrahepatic manifestations, considered to represent immunoallergic reaction, are infrequent with hepatotoxicity due to many of the currently used drugs (Banks *et al.*, 1995; Hautekeete *et al.*, 1999). None of the 180 patients in a large series of diclofenac hepatotoxicity would have scored maximum points for this component on the CDS (Banks *et al.*, 1995). Even though underscoring by the CDS attributes a lower level of probability to an individual drug-related hepatotoxic reaction, a cut-off CDS score of >9 still remains useful in grouping the reactions that require further investigations and those wherein withdrawal of the drug is justified (Aithal *et al.*, 2000). Moreover, a numerical "cut-off" is far easier to apply in routine clinical practice.

Systematic evaluation using causality assessment methods such as international consensus criteria or a clinical diagnostic scale provides objectivity and consistency to the assessment of suspected adverse hepatic drug reactions. Their more widespread adoption should enhance the accuracy of case definition for epidemiological studies.

RECHALLENGE

The recurrence of liver injury after re-administration (often inadvertent) of a suspected drug is the most definitive evidence for drug-induced liver disease and may outweigh other considerations in causality assessment. The biochemical criteria for a positive rechallenge have been outlined by the consensus group (Benichou, 1990). But, rechallenge of an incriminated drug can be dangerous and may even be fatal (Ransohoff and Jacobs, 1981; Lo *et al.*, 1998). Deliberate rechallenge may only be justified when continued treatment with the implicated agent is highly desirable.

ROLE OF LIVER BIOPSY

Drug-induced liver injury can cause any known pattern of liver pathology, although certain histological features are particularly suggestive of a drug-induced aetiology (Anon., 1974). Liver biopsy is also an important way to exclude alternative causes of a given pattern of liver injury. However, liver biopsy is an invasive procedure with significant morbidity in 0.24% and mortality in 0.11% of subjects (Cohen *et al.*, 1992). Hence, benefits should be weighed against the risk and liver biopsy should be considered only in circumstances where discontinuation of the suspected medication is undesirable or when a patient appears to have an as yet unrecognised form of drug-induced liver injury.

SPECIFIC TESTS

The exceptions to the lack of "specific" markers of drug hepatotoxicity are the detection of liver–kidney microsomal type 2 (anti-P450 2C9) antibodies in tienilic acid-induced hepatitis, antimitochondrial type 6 antibody in iproniazid-induced hepatitis (Homberg *et al.*, 1985), and liver microsomal antibody (anti-P450 1A2) in dihydralazine-related liver injury (Bourdi *et al.*, 1990). Both tienilic acid and iproniazid were withdrawn because of the high incidence of hepatotoxicity, and dihydralazine is rarely used now in clinical practice.

IN VITRO TESTS

The difficulties encountered in the diagnosis of drug-induced liver injury have led to attempts to develop *in vitro* diagnostic tests. Assays have been devised to study the cytotoxic effect of metabolites generated by a hepatic microsomal drug-metabolising system on the peripheral blood mononuclear cells from patients suffering hepatotoxicity due to phenytoin and sulphonamides (Rieder *et al.*, 1989; Gennis *et al.*, 1991). The lymphocyte transformation test aims to demonstrate *in vitro* proliferation of a patient's lymphocytes in response to the drug in question. Considering the complexity of the immunological events necessary for the *in vivo* induction of specifically sensitised T-cells, it is not surprising that the test is positive only in 30% of all patients with suspected drug-induced liver injuries (Berg and Becker, 1995). The use of sera collected from healthy volunteers after drug intake (containing *ex vivo* drug antigens) and the addition of prostaglandin inhibitors to the cultures (to prevent inhibition of lymphocyte response by prostaglandin-producing suppresser cells) can increase the sensitivity of the test up to 56% (Maria and Victorino, 1998). However, the fact that these *in vitro* tests are extremely tedious and operator-dependent has limited their widespread use.

MECHANISMS OF DRUG-INDUCED LIVER INJURY

The general mechanism by which most drugs induce liver injury is based on the unusual susceptibility of individual patients. For some drugs, the idiosyncratic reaction is immunologically mediated and for others metabolic idiosyncrasy may be responsible. Even though the molecular basis of the idiosyncratic drug-induced liver injury is poorly understood, some key events have emerged as being particularly important.

METABOLIC IDIOSYNCRASY

The suggestion of dose dependence in some cases of drug-induced liver injury indicates that a host-dependent idiosyncrasy in the metabolism or excretion of these drugs may be responsible for hepatotoxicity. Although several xenobiotics are transformed by the cytochrome P450 system (CYPs) into stable metabolites, many others are oxidised into unstable, chemically reactive intermediates. These reactive intermediates attack hepatic constituents such as unsaturated lipids, proteins or DNA and can lead to liver cell death (Pessayre, 1995). The abundance of CYPs in the liver explains the major role of these metabolites in drug-induced hepatotoxicity. Furthermore, the centrilobular location of most CYPs accounts for the pericentral location of these lesions. When small amounts of reactive metabolites are formed, glutathione serves as a decoy target, sparing critical hepatic macromolecules. However, when large amounts of the reactive metabolite are formed, the formation of glutathione conjugates exceeds the capacity of the liver to synthesise

glutathione. The resulting depletion of glutathione together with direct covalent binding of the metabolite to protein thiols has serious consequences. The oxidation of protein thiol groups results in the formation of disulphur bonds between different molecules of actin, resulting in destruction of the microfilamentous network beneath the plasma membrane (Mirabelli *et al.*, 1988). Depletion of protein thiol groups also decreases the activity of calcium translocases resulting in increases in intracellular Ca^{2+} which further damages the cytoskeleton (Bellomo and Orrenius, 1985). These and other effects of oxidative stress lead to the swelling and disruption of intracellular organelles ultimately resulting in hepatocyte necrosis.

Although it was initially thought that the toxicity of reactive metabolites only caused cell necrosis, this idea has been challenged in recent years (Pessayre *et al.*, 1999). It is now clear that the extensive formation of reactive metabolites can cause apoptosis, necrosis or both (Fau *et al.*, 1997; Shi *et al.*, 1998). Several compounds, such as acetaminophen and cocaine, transformed into reactive metabolites have been shown to cause DNA fragmentation of hepatocytes indicative of apoptosis (Shen *et al.*, 1992; Cascales *et al.*, 1994). The cellular mechanisms causing metabolite-induced apoptosis have been studied with germander, a medicinal plant used in weight control diets, the widespread use of which led to an epidemic of hepatitis in France (Larrey *et al.*, 1992b). Germander contains furano diterpenoids, which are activated by CYP 3A into electrophilic metabolites (Lekehal *et al.*, 1996). Extensive formation of glutathione conjugates results in glutathione depletion which, in combination with covalent binding of the metabolites, results in protein thiol oxidation (Lekehal *et al.*, 1996). Oxidation of protein thiols inactivates plasma membrane calcium translocases and increases the permeability of the mitochondrial inner membrane (the mitochondrial membrane permeability transit or MMPT) which, through the release of cytochrome C, leads to the activation of caspases (Fagian *et al.*, 1990). Caspases are cysteine proteases that cut proteins after an aspartate residue and are the major executioners of apoptosis (Thornberry and Lazebnik, 1998). Caspase activation in conjunction with increased intra-cellular calcium activates calcium-dependent endonucleases, which cut the DNA between nucleosomes, eventually resulting in apoptosis (Fau et al., 1997). Germander-induced apoptotic hepatocyte death is prevented by troleandomycin, which inhibits its metabolic activation by CYP 3A4 or by preventing depletion of glutathione with cysteine (Fau et al., 1997)

Factors Influencing Direct Toxicity Due to Reactive Metabolites

Hepatotoxicity from the reactive metabolites of drugs is a significant problem with drugs where the formation of reactive metabolites is low enough to ensure the absence of hepatotoxicity in most recipients (and therefore allowing the marketing of the drug), but is high enough to lead to "idiosyncratic" toxicity in some "susceptible" subjects. The reason for susceptibility could be either genetically determined or acquired.

Genetic Factors

The amount of reactive metabolite formed depends on a particular isoenzyme the hepatic level of which may vary between individuals. Genetic polymorphisms of drug metabolising enzymes may contribute to an individual's risk to an ADR. Polymorphism in debrisoquine oxidation (CYP 2D6) leads to accumulation of perhexiline resulting in liver injury in poor metabolisers (Morgan et al., 1984) and increases the formation of reactive metabolites leading to chlorpromazine hepatotoxicity in extensive metabolisers (Watson et al., 1988). Polymorphism in mephenytoin hydroxylation (CYP 2C19) may predispose poor metabolisers to atrium (phenobarbital, febarbamate and difebarbamate) induced hepatotoxicity (Horsmans et al., 1994).

Acquired Factors

Individual susceptibility to hepatotoxicity due to reactive metabolites may also be related to physiological, nutritional or therapeutic modifications in drug metabolism. For example, fasting leads to glycogen depletion and decreased glucuronidation, depletion of glutathione and induction of CYP2E1 leading to an increased risk of paracetamol-induced liver injury (Price et al., 1987; Whitcomb and Block, 1994). Acquired factors enhancing the rate of biotransformation of a drug to its reactive metabolites through the induction of cytochrome P450 isoenzymes play an important role in increasing the direct toxicity. Alcohol is a potent inducer of CYP2E1 and to a lesser extent CYP3A4. Subjects who consume alcohol regularly may therefore have increased bioactivation of paracetamol (which is metabolised by CYP2E1 and 3A4), resulting in hepatotoxicity at conventional "therapeutic" doses (Zimmerman and Maddrey, 1995). In individuals with heavy alcohol intake this is compounded by reduced glutathione synthesis and low glutathione stores due to inhibition of glutathione synthatase and ethanol-related oxidative stress, respectively. Isoniazid also increases the toxicity of paracetamol by inducing CYP2E1, while rifampicin, another microsomal enzyme inducer, increases the risk of hepatotoxicity due to isoniazid (Pessayre et al., 1977; Moulding et al., 1991). Anticonvulsants (phenytoin, carbamazepine, and phenobarbital) induce CYP3A4 and can also enhance the toxic effects of paracetamol (Bray et al., 1992). As an alternative mechanism of drug interaction leading to an increased risk of paracetamol-induced liver injury, zidovudine competes for glucuronidation of the toxic metabolite, thus reducing its excretion (Shriner and Goetz, 1992). Drug accumulation can result from metabolic inhibition caused by another drug. For instance, troleandomycin increases the risk of cholestasis with oral contraceptives by inhibiting the CYP3A responsible for estrogen oxidation (Miguet et al., 1980).

The presence of underlying liver disease may predispose to dose-dependent drug toxicity, especially if the margin between therapeutic and toxic concentrations is small (Schenker et al., 1999). It is generally believed that pre-existing liver disease would neither induce nor worsen idiosyncratic hepatotoxicity, although this issue has not been studied adequately. However, a recent study demonstrated a higher incidence of hepatotoxicity as well as more severe liver injury secondary to antituberculosis agents in hepatitis B virus (HBV) carriers when compared with non-carriers and with HBV carriers who did not receive antituberculosis therapy (Wong *et al.*, 2000).

IMMUNOLOGIC IDIOSYNCRASY

The clinico-pathologic features of some idiosyncratic drug reactions suggest that immunological mechanisms could play an important role in the pathogenesis of drug hepatotoxicity. These include (a) fever, rash, lymphadenopathy, eosinophilia and involvement of other organs; (b) hepatic inflammatory infiltrates; (c) low frequency (<1/1000 users); (d) delay in appearance of the disease (2 weeks to several months); and (e) accelerated onset after rechallenge (Beaune and Lecoeur, 1997; Robin *et al.*, 1997). In hepatitis secondary to sulphonamides, phenytoin and nitrofurantoin, the liver is implicated as part of a systemic hypersensitivity reaction, and evidence for immunological responsiveness to these drugs can be obtained by *in vitro* rechallenge with the drug or its metabolite (Spielberg *et al.*, 1981; Shear and Spielberg, 1988; Rieder *et al.*, 1989). Interestingly, the immune response may not be directed at the drug *per se*, but at compounds arising as a result of its metabolism. Drug hepatotoxicity may therefore be the result of both metabolic and immunological idiosyncrasy. In this respect the superimposition of cytochrome P-450 and the immune system in the liver has potential disadvantages. The covalent binding of the reactive metabolites to "self" proteins results in the formation of neoantigens that "mislead" the immune system into mounting an immune response against hepatocytes.

The initial and crucial event underlying so-called immuno-allergic hepatitis is the oxidative metabolism of a drug by a cytochrome P-450 enzyme resulting in the formation of reactive metabolites. Electrophilic metabolites react with and covalently bind to nucleophilic groups of proteins to form protein adducts. The best-studied example is that of halothane which is oxidised into a reactive acyl chloride (CF_3COCl) by cytochrome P450 2E1. The metabolite reacts with the $\varepsilon-NH_2$ group of the lysine residues of proteins to form trifluoroacety-

lated proteins (CF_3CO–lysine proteins) (Gut *et al.*, 1993). The reactive metabolite may also bind covalently to the CYP 2E1 protein itself (Eliasson and Kenna, 1996). Alkylation of cytochrome P450 proteins may lead both to anti-P450 autoantibodies and to antibodies against the modified part of the protein. Therefore a single drug such as halothane may concomitantly give rise to both "immuno-allergic" as well as "autoimmune" hepatitis.

Factors Influencing Immunologically Mediated Drug Hepatotoxicity

Genetic factors influencing the development of immune-mediated drug hepatotoxicity can be grouped into factors affecting the amount of the reactive metabolite and therefore protein adduct formed and factors affecting the immune response to the adducts. Dihydralazine hepatitis is a good example of how a "metabolic" genetic factor can contribute to susceptibility to immune-mediated hepatotoxicity. Dihydralazine is predominantly acetylated by the polymorphic N-acetyl transferase 2. In slow acetylators, the majority of the drug is available for metabolic activation by CYP 1A2 into a free radical. The alkylation of hepatic proteins is more extensive and the incidence of immune-mediated hepatitis is higher (Bourdi *et al.*, 1994).

The second group of genetic factors influencing susceptibility to immune-mediated hepatic drug reactions is the genes whose products are involved in immune regulation. Genetic polymorphism in major histocompatibility complex (MHC) molecules is the most obvious example. The presence or absence of a given human leukocyte antigen (HLA) molecule may determine the efficient presentation of an alkylated immunogenic peptide. Associations have been reported between HLA A11 and hepatotoxicity due to halothane, tricyclic antidepressants and diclofenac, HLA DR6 and liver injury secondary to chlorpromazine and nitrofurantoin, HLA B8 and clometacine hepatitis (Berson *et al.*, 1994). More recently, the often serious co-amoxiclav-induced jaundice has been strongly associated with HLA DRB1*1501–DQA1*0102–DQB1*0602 haplotype in the northern European population (Hautekeete *et al.*, 1999).

SPECIFIC HISTOLOGICAL TYPES OF DRUG-INDUCED LIVER INJURY

Cholestasis

From experimental models, several mechanisms have been postulated for impaired bile secretion. They are inhibition of Na+, K+ ATPase resulting in reduced uptake of bile acids, increased pericellular permeability and regurgitation into plasma of bile constituents, impaired intracellular transport due to cytoskeletal dysfunction, altered intracellular calcium homeostasis or altered canalicular carriers (Erlinger, 1997). A recent study demonstrated that oestrogen metabolites trans-inhibit the bile salt export pump in rat liver providing a molecular basis for drug-induced cholestasis (Stieger et al., 2000).

Steatosis

Microvesicular steatosis occurs in conditions characterised by severe impairment of the mitochondrial β-oxidation process. Drugs can sequester coenzyme A (aspirin, valproic acid), inhibit mitochondrial β-oxidation enzymes (tetracycline), and, in addition, inhibit oxidative phosphorylation (amiodarone, perhexiline). When β-oxidation is severely impaired, fatty acids, which are poorly oxidized by mitochondria, are mainly esterified into triglycerides and accumulate as small vesicles (Fromenty et al., 1997).

MANAGEMENT OF IDIOSYNCRATIC HEPATOTOXICITY

Early detection and withdrawal of the causative drug is the single most important step in the management of adverse hepatic reaction. Cases of serious and often fatal hepatotoxicity due to isoniazid, halothane, valproate, notrofurantoin and perhexiline are often linked to continuation or resumption of the drug following symptoms that could have been attributable to drug-induced liver reaction (Farrell, 1994; Lo et al., 1998; Moulding, 1999). The Seattle–King County Public Health Department used a protocol to monitor isoniazid therapy, which included advising the patient at each visit to stop the medication and call the clinic if symptoms of hepatotoxicity occurred. With such careful monitoring, the rate of hepatotoxicity in 11 141 patients was much lower (0.1%–0.15%) than previously reported (1%) and there were no deaths (Nolan et al., 1999). Prompt withdrawal of the drug is also important because the long-term prognosis may be worse if the responsible agent is continued. In a retrospective study, one-third of patients with drug-induced liver disease had persistently abnormal liver tests (liver enzymes and/or imaging) at median follow-up of 5 years, and detection of fibrosis in the liver biopsy and continued drug intake after the initial liver injury predicted adverse outcome (Aithal and Day, 1999).

Management of acute hepatic failure secondary to idiosyncratic hepatic reaction is similar to that of viral hepatitis. The overall mortality of drug-induced hepatic failure (excluding paracetamol overdose) appears to be higher than that for viral hepatitis. Despite the availability of liver transplantation, the mortality from severe hepatotoxicity ranges from 2% to 7% with drugs such as pemoline, ketoconazole and diclofenac, up to 50% in the case of halothane (Lewis et al., 1984; Nehra et al., 1990; Banks et al., 1995; Lo et al., 1998). Corticosteroid treatment has not been shown to be beneficial in the management of drug-induced hepatitis. There is no clear evidence that ursodeoxycholic acid therapy changes outcome in chronic cholestasis.

PREVENTION

Experience gained by wide clinical usage of a drug following marketing may assist in recognising individual risk factors and better definition of safe dosage. Strategies of avoiding the prescription in "at-risk situations" and safer dosage regimes have reduced adverse hepatic reactions due to several drugs. Some such examples include, avoidance of reuse of halothane within 3 months, parenteral administration of large doses of tetracycline as well as its use in pregnancy and renal disease, aspirin in children, and valproic acid in combination therapy in children under 3 years of age

(Farrell, 1994; Neuberger, 1998). The incidence of hepatic fibrosis with weekly low-dose methotrexate regimes is much lower than that reported with daily dose regimes (Boffa *et al.*, 1995; Aithal *et al.*, 2001).

Of even greater importance in the determination of individual risk are the inherited factors that affect the kinetics and dynamics of numerous drugs. Susceptibility to hepatic drug reaction depends principally on genetic factors that determine the metabolism, as well as the biochemical and immunological responses, to the metabolites. A major difference between genetic and environmental variation is that an inherited trait has to be tested for only once in a lifetime, whereas environmental effects change continuously. In the future, the discovery of pharmacogenetic traits will change with new technologies based on genomics. Rapid sequencing and single-nucleotide polymorphisms (SNPs) will play a major role in the linking of sequence variations with heritable phenotypes of drug response (Meyer, 2000). In fact, pharmacogenetics technology may enable a significantly better postmarketing surveillance system. In this proposed concept (Roses, 2000) hundreds of thousands of patients who receive the drug would have blood taken and stored in an approved location. As rare, serious adverse events are documented, DNA from patients who experienced the ADR could be compared with that from controls, who did not have adverse reaction while on the drug. This would enable "genetic fingerprints" (SNP profiles) of the subjects susceptible to the adverse event to be determined. These adverse event profiles would be combined with efficacy profiles to produce a comprehensive medicine response profile. This would allow selection of patients for both efficacy and lower complications of drug therapy.

REFERENCES

Acharya SK, Dasarathy S, Kumer TL, Sushma S, Prasanna KS, Tandon A, Sreenivas V, Nijhawan S, Panda SK, Nanda SK, Irshad M, Joshi YK, Duttagupta S, Tandon RK, Tandon BN (1996) Fulminant hepatitis in a tropical population: clinical course, cause, and early predictors of outcome. *Hepatology* **23**: 1448–55.

Aithal GP, Day CP (1999) The natural history of histologically proved drug induced liver disease. *Gut* **44**: 731–5.

Aithal GP, Haugk B, Gumustop B, Burt AD, Record CO (2001) Monitoring methotrexate induced hepatic fibrosis in patients with psoriasis: are serial biopsies justified? *Hepatology* **34**: 342A.

Aithal GP, Rawlins MD, Day CP (1999) Accuracy of hepatic adverse drug reaction reporting in one English health region. *Br Med J* **319**: 1541.

Aithal GP, Rawlins MD, Day CP (2000) Clinical diagnostic scale: a useful tool in the evaluation of suspected hepatotoxic adverse drug reactions. *J Hepatol* **33**: 949–52.

Almdal TP, Sorensen TI (1991) Incidence of parenchymal liver diseases in Denmark, 1981 to 1985: analysis of hospitalization registry data. The Danish Association for the Study of the Liver. *Hepatology* **13**: 650–5.

Andreu V, Mas A, Bruguera M, Salmeron JM, Moreno V, Nogue S, Rodes J (1998) Ecstasy: a common cause of severe acute hepatotoxicity. *J Hepatol* **29**: 394–7.

Anon. (1969) International drug monitoring. The role of the hospital. *World Health Organization Technical Report Series* **425**: 5–24.

Anon. (1974) Guidelines for diagnosis of therapeutic drug-induced liver injury in liver biopsies. *Lancet* **1**: 854–7.

Ballet F (1997) Hepatotoxicity in drug development: detection, significance and solutions. *J Hepatol* **26** (Suppl 2): 26–36.

Banks AT, Zimmerman HJ, Ishak KG, Harter JG (1995) Diclofenac-associated hepatotoxicity: analysis of 180 cases reported to the Food and Drug Administration as adverse reactions. *Hepatology* **22**: 820–7.

Beard K, Belic L, Aselton P, Perera DR, Jick H (1986) Outpatient drug-induced parenchymal liver disease requiring hospitalization. *Clin Pharmacol* **26**: 633–7.

Beaune PH, Lecoeur S (1997) Immunotoxicology of the liver: adverse reactions to drugs. *J Hepatol* **26** (Suppl 2): 37–42.

Bellomo G, Orrenius S (1985) Altered thiol and calcium homeostasis in oxidative hepatocellular injury. *Hepatology* **5**: 876–82.

Benichou C (1990) Criteria of drug-induced liver disorders. Report of an international consensus meeting. *J Hepatol* **11**: 272–6.

Berg PA, Becker EW (1995) The lymphocyte transformation test—a debated method for the evaluation of drug allergic hepatic injury. *J Hepatol* **22**: 115–8.

Berson A, Freneaux E, Larrey D, Lepage V, Douay C, Mallet C, Fromenty, Benhamou JP, Pessayre D (1994) Possible role of HLA in hepatotoxicity. An exploratory study in 71 patients with drug-induced idiosyncratic hepatitis. *J Hepatol* **20**: 336–42.

Boffa MJ, Chalmers RJ, Haboubi NY, Shomaf M, Mitchell DM (1995) Sequential liver biopsies during long-term methotrexate treatment for psoriasis: a reappraisal. *Br J Dermatol* **133**: 774–8.

Bourdi M, Larrey D, Nataf J, Bernuau J, Pessayre D, Iwasaki M, Guengerich FP, Beaune PH (1990) Anti-liver endoplasmic reticulum autoantibodies are directed against human cytochrome P-450IA2. A specific marker of dihydralazine-induced hepatitis. *J Clin Invest* **85**: 1967–73.

Bourdi M, Tinel M, Beaune PH, Pessayre D (1994) Interactions of dihydralazine with cytochromes P4501A: a possible explanation for the appearance of anti-cytochrome P4501A2 autoantibodies. *Molec Pharmacol* **45**: 1287–95.

Bray GP, Harrison PM, O'Grady JG, Tredger JM, Williams R (1992) Long-term anticonvulsant therapy worsens outcome in paracetamol-induced fulminant hepatic failure. *Human Exp Toxicol* **11**: 265–70.

Cascales M, Alvarez A, Gasco P, Fernandez-Simon L, Sanz N, Bosca L (1994) Cocaine-induced liver injury in mice elicits specific changes in DNA ploidy and induces programmed death of hepatocytes. *Hepatology* **20**: 992–1001.

Cohen MB, Kader HH, Lambers D, Heubi JE (1992) Complications of percutaneous liver biopsy in children. *Gastroenterology* **102**: 629–32.

Cook GC, Sherlock S (1965) Jaundice and its relation to therapeutic agents. *Lancet* **1**: 175–9.

Danan G (1988) Consensus meeting on causality assessment of drug-induced liver injury. *J Hepatol* **7**: 132–6.

Danan G, Benichou C (1993) Causality assessment of adverse reactions to drugs—I. A novel method based on the conclusions of international consensus meetings: application to drug-induced liver injuries. *J Clin Epidemiol* **46**: 1323–30.

Derby LE, Jick H, Henry DA, Dean AD (1993) Cholestatic hepatitis associated with flucloxacillin. *Med J Austr* **158**: 596–600.

Desmet VJ (1997) Vanishing bile duct syndrome in drug-induced liver disease. *J Hepatol* **26** (Suppl 1): 31–5.

Devereaux BM, Crawford DH, Purcell P, Powell LW, Roeser HP (1995) Flucloxacillin associated cholestatic hepatitis. An Australian and Swedish epidemic? *Eur J Clin Pharmacol* **49**: 81–5.

Dossing M, Andreasen PB (1982) Drug-induced liver disease in Denmark. An analysis of 572 cases of hepatotoxicity reported to the Danish Board of Adverse Reactions to Drugs. *Scand J Gastroenterol* **17**: 205–11.

Eliasson E, Kenna JG (1996) Cytochrome P450 2E1 is a cell surface autoantigen in halothane hepatitis. *Molec Pharmacol* **50**: 573–82.

Erlinger S (1997) Drug-induced cholestasis. *J Hepatol* **26** (Suppl 1): 1–4.

Fagian MM, Pereira-da-Silva L, Martins IS, Vercesi AE (1990) Membrane protein thiol cross-linking associated with the permeabilization of the inner mitochondrial membrane by Ca^{2+} plus prooxidants. *J Biol Chem* **265**: 19955–60.

Farrell GC (1994) *Drug-Induced Liver Disease*. London: Churchill Livingstone.

Fau D, Lekehal M, Farrell G, Moreau A, Moulis C, Feldmann G, Haouzi D, Pessayre D (1997) Diterpenoids from germander, an herbal medicine, induce apoptosis in isolated rat hepatocytes. *Gastroenterology* **113**: 1334–46.

Friedman MA, Woodcock J, Lumpkin MM, Shuren JE, Hass AE, Thompson LJ (1999) The safety of newly approved medicines: do recent market removals mean there is a problem? *J Am Med Assoc* **281**: 1728–34.

Friis H, Andreasen PB (1992) Drug-induced hepatic injury: an analysis of 1100 cases reported to the Danish Committee on Adverse Drug Reactions between 1978 and 1987. *J Intern Med* **232**: 133–8.

Fromenty B, Berson A, Pessayre D (1997) Microvesicular steatosis and steatohepatitis: role of mitochondrial dysfunction and lipid peroxidation. *J Hepatol* **26** (Suppl 1): 13–22.

Gennis MA, Vemuri R, Burns EA, Hill JV, Miller MA, Spielberg SP (1991) Familial occurrence of hypersensitivity to phenytoin. *Am J Med* **91**: 631–4.

Gut J, Christen U, Huwyler J (1993) Mechanisms of halothane toxicity: novel insights. *Pharmacol Ther* **58**: 133–55.

Hallas J, Gram LF, Grodum E, Damsbo N, Brosen K, Haghfelt T, Harvald B, Beck-Nielsen J, Worm J, Jensen KB (1992) Drug related admissions to medical wards: a population based survey. *Br J Clin Pharmacol* **33**: 61–8.

Hautekeete ML, Horsmans Y, Van Waeyenberge C, Demanet C, Henrion J, Verbist L, Brenard R, Sempoux C, Michielsen PP, Yap PS, Rahier J, Geubel AP (1999) HLA association of amoxicillin-clavulanate-induced hepatitis. *Gastroenterology* **117**: 1181–6.

Homberg JC, Abuaf N, Helmy-Khalil S, Biour M, Poupon R, Islam S, Darnis F, Levy VG, Opolon P, Beaugrand M (1985) Drug-induced hepatitis associated with anticytoplasmic organelle autoantibodies. *Hepatology* **5**: 722–7.

Horsmans Y, Lannes D, Pessayre D, Larrey D (1994) Possible association between poor metabolism of mephenytoin and hepatotoxicity caused by Atrium, a fixed combination preparation containing phenobarbital, febarbamate and difebarbamate. *J Hepatol* **21**: 1075–9.

Jick SS, Stender M, Myers MW (1999) Frequency of liver disease in type 2 diabetic patients treated with oral antidiabetic agents. *Diabetes Care* **22**: 2067–71.

Jick H, Walker AM, Porter J (1981) Drug-induced liver disease. *J Clin Pharmacol* **21**: 359–64.

Josephson L (1996) Severe toxicity of fialuridine (FIAU). *New Engl J Med* **334**: 1135–6.

Krahenbuhl S (2001) Mitochondria: important target for drug toxicity? *J Hepatol* **34**: 334–6.

Larrey D (1997) Hepatotoxicity of herbal remedies. *J Hepatol* **26** (Suppl 1): 47–51.

Larrey D (2000) Drug-induced liver diseases. *J Hepatol* **32**: 77–88.

Larrey D, Vial T, Micaleff A, Babany G, Morichau-Beauchant M, Michel H, Benhamou JP (1992a) Hepatitis associated with amoxycillin-clavulanic acid combination report of 15 cases. *Gut* **33**: 368–71.

Larrey D, Vial T, Pauwels A, Castot A, Biour M, David M, Michel H (1992b) Hepatitis after germander (Teucrium chamaedrys) administration: another instance of herbal medicine hepatotoxicity. *Ann Intern Med* **117**: 129–32.

Lavelle SM, Kavanagh JM (1995) *Clinical Presentation of Jaundice in Europe: Occurrence and Diagnostic Value of Clinical Findings.* Galway, Ireland: Project Management Group—Ericterus Project.

Lekehal M, Pessayre D, Lereau JM, Moulis C, Fouraste I, Fau D (1996) Hepatotoxicity of the herbal medicine germander: metabolic activation of its furano diterpenoids by cytochrome P450 3A Depletes cytoskeleton-associated protein thiols and forms plasma membrane blebs in rat hepatocytes. *Hepatology* **24**: 212–8.

Lewis JH, Zimmerman HJ (1989) Drug-induced liver disease. *Med Clin N Am* **73**: 775–92.

Lewis JH, Zimmerman HJ, Benson GD, Ishak KG (1984) Hepatic injury associated with ketoconazole therapy. Analysis of 33 cases. *Gastroenterology* **86**: 503–13.

Lo SK, Wendon J, Mieli-Vergani G, Williams R (1998) Halothane-induced acute liver failure: continuing occurrence and use of liver transplantation. *Eur J Gastroenterol Hepatol* **10**: 635–9.

Lucena MI, Camargo R, Andrade RJ, Perez-Sanchez CJ, Cuesta FSDL (2001) Comparison of two clinical scales for causality assessment in hepatotoxicity. *Hepatology* **33**: 123–30.

Lumley C (1990) Clinical toxicity: could it have been predicted? Pre-marketing experience. In: Lumley CE, Walker SR, eds., *Animal Toxicity Studies. Their Relevance to Man.* Lancaster: Quay Publishing, pp. 49–57.

Lumpkin MM (2000) Troglitazone: Presentation to advisory committee, FDA.

Maria VA, Victorino RM (1997) Development and validation of a clinical scale for the diagnosis of drug-induced hepatitis. *Hepatology* **26**: 664–9.

Maria VA, Victorino RM (1998) Immunological investigation in hepatic drug reactions. *Clin Exp Allergy* **28** (Suppl 4): 71–7.

McKenzie R, Fried MW, Sallie R, Conjeevaram H, Di Bisceglie AM, Park Y, Savarese B, Kleiner D, Tsokos M, Luciano C, *et al.* (1995) Hepatic failure and lactic acidosis due to fialuridine (FIAU), an investigational nucleoside analogue for chronic hepatitis B. *New Engl J Med* **333**: 1099–1105.

Meyer UA (2000) Pharmacogenetics and adverse drug reactions. *Lancet* **356**: 1667–71.

Miguet JP, Vuitton D, Pessayre D, Allemand H, Metreau, JM, Poupon R, Capron JP, Blanc F (1980) Jaundice from troleandomycin and oral contraceptives. *Ann Intern Med* **92**: 434

Mirabelli F, Salis A, Marinoni V, Finardi G, Bellomo G, Thor H, Orrenius S (1988) Menadione-induced bleb formation in hepatocytes is associated with the oxidation of thiol groups in actin. *Arch Biochem Biophys* **264**: 261–9.

Morgan MY, Reshef R, Shah RR, Oates NS, Smith RL, Sherlock S (1984) Impaired oxidation of debrisoquine in patients with perhexiline liver injury. *Gut* **25**: 1057–64.

Moulding T (1999) Toxicity associated with isoniazid preventive therapy. *J Am Med Assoc* **282**: 2207–8.

Moulding TS, Redeker AG, Kanel GC (1991) Acetaminophen, isoniazid, and hepatic toxicity. *Ann Intern Med* **114**: 431

Nehra A, Mullick F, Ishak KG, Zimmerman HJ (1990) Pemoline-associated hepatic injury. *Gastroenterology* **99**: 1517–9.

Neuberger J (1998) Halothane hepatitis. *Eur J Gastroenterol Hepatol* **10**: 631–3.

Nolan CM, Goldberg SV, Buskin SE (1999) Hepatotoxicity associated with isoniazid preventive therapy: a 7-year survey from a public health tuberculosis clinic. *J Am Med Assoc* **281**: 1014–8.

Ostapowicz G, Fontana RJ, Larson AM, Davern T, Lee WM and the Acute Liver Failure Study Group (1999) Etiology and outcome of acute liver failure in the USA: preliminary results of a prospective multi-center study. *Hepatology* **30**: 221A.

Pessayre D (1995) Role of reactive metabolites in drug-induced hepatitis. *J Hepatol* **23** (Suppl 1): 16–24.

Pessayre D, Bentata M, Degott C, Nouel O, Miguet JP, Rueff B, Benhamou JP (1977) Isoniazid-rifampin fulminant hepatitis. A possible consequence of the enhancement of isoniazid hepatotoxicity by enzyme induction. *Gastroenterology* **72**: 284–9.

Pessayre D, Haouzi D, Fau D, Robin MA, Mansouri A, Berson A (1999) Withdrawal of life support, altruistic suicide, fratricidal killing and euthanasia by lymphocytes: different forms of drug-induced hepatic apoptosis. *J Hepatol* **31**: 760–70.

Pillans PI (1996) Drug associated hepatic reactions in New Zealand: 21 years experience. *N Z Med J* **109**: 315–9.

Price VF, Miller MG, Jollow DJ (1987) Mechanisms of

fasting-induced potentiation of acetaminophen hepatotoxicity in the rat. *Biochem Pharmacol* **36**: 427–33.

Ransohoff DF, Jacobs G (1981) Terminal hepatic failure following a small dose of sulfamethoxazole-trimethoprim. *Gastroenterology* **80**: 816–9.

Rawlins MD (1995) Pharmacovigilance: paradise lost, regained or postponed? The William Withering Lecture 1994. *J R Coll Phys London* **29**: 41–9.

Rieder MJ, Uetrecht J, Shear NH, Cannon M, Miller M, Spielberg SP (1989) Diagnosis of sulfonamide hypersensitivity reactions by in-vitro "rechallenge" with hydroxylamine metabolites. *Ann Intern Med* **110**: 286–9.

Robin MA, Le Roy M, Descatoire V, Pessayre D (1997) Plasma membrane cytochromes P450 as neoantigens and autoimmune targets in drug-induced hepatitis. *J Hepatol* **26** (Suppl 1): 23–30.

Roses AD (2000) Pharmacogenetics and the practice of medicine. *Nature* **405**: 857–65.

Roughead EE, Gilbert AL, Primrose JG (1999) Improving drug use: a case study of events which led to changes in use of flucloxacillin in Australia. *Soc Sci Med* **48**: 845–53.

Schenker S, Martin RR, Hoyumpa AM (1999) Antecedent liver disease and drug toxicity. *J Hepatol* **31**: 1098–1105.

Shear NH, Spielberg SP (1988) Anticonvulsant hypersensitivity syndrome. In vitro assessment of risk. *J Clin Invest* **82**: 1826–32.

Shen W, Kamendulis LM, Ray SD, Corcoran GB (1992) Acetaminophen-induced cytotoxicity in cultured mouse hepatocytes: effects of Ca(2+)-endonuclease, DNA repair, and glutathione depletion inhibitors on DNA fragmentation and cell death. *Toxicol App Pharmacol* **112**: 32–40.

Shi J, Aisaki K, Ikawa Y, Wake K (1998) Evidence of hepatocyte apoptosis in rat liver after the administration of carbon tetrachloride. *Am J Pathol* **153**: 515–25.

Shriner K, Goetz MB (1992) Severe hepatotoxicity in a patient receiving both acetaminophen and zidovudine. *Am J Med* **93**: 94–6.

Spielberg SP, Gordon GB, Blake DA, Goldstein DA, Herlong HF (1981) Predisposition to phenytoin hepatotoxicity assessed in vitro. *New Engl J Med* **305**: 722–7.

Spriet-Pourra C, Auriche M (1994) *Drug Withdrawal from Sales*, 2nd edn. Richmond: PJB Publications.

Stieger B, Fattinger K, Madon J, Kullak-Ublick GA, Meier PJ (2000) Drug- and estrogen-induced cholestasis through inhibition of the hepatocellular bile salt export pump (Bsep) of rat liver. *Gastroenterology* **118**: 422–30.

Stricher BHCh (1992) *Drug-Induced Hepatic Injury*, 2nd edn. Amsterdam: Elsevier Science.

Thornberry NA, Lazebnik Y (1998) Caspases: enemies within. *Science* **281**: 1312–6.

Turner IB, Eckstein RP, Riley JW, Lunzer MR (1989) Prolonged hepatic cholestasis after flucloxacillin therapy. *Med J Austr* **151**: 701–5.

Watkins PB, Whitcomb RW (1998) Hepatic dysfunction associated with troglitazone. *New Engl J Med* **338**: 916–7.

Watson RG, Olomu A, Clements D, Waring RH, Mitchell S, Elias E (1988) A proposed mechanism for chlorpromazine jaundice—defective hepatic sulphoxidation combined with rapid hydroxylation. *J Hepatol* **7**: 72–8.

Whitcomb DC, Block GD (1994) Association of acetaminophen hepatotoxicity with fasting and ethanol use. *J Am Med Assoc* **272**: 1845–50.

Whitehead MW, Hainsworth I, Kingham JGC (2001) The causes of obvious jaundice in South West Wales: perception versus reality. *Gut* **48**: 409–13.

Wong WM, Wu PC, Yuen MF, Cheng CC, Yew WW, Wong PC, Tam CM, Leung CC, Lai CL (2000) Antituberculosis drug-related liver dysfunction in chronic hepatitis B infection. *Hepatology* **31**: 201–6.

Zimmerman HJ, Maddrey WC (1995) Acetaminophen (paracetamol) hepatotoxicity with regular intake of alcohol: analysis of instances of therapeutic misadventure. *Hepatology* **22**: 767–73.

38

Ocular ADRs

F.W. FRAUNFELDER AND F.T. FRAUNFELDER
Casey Eye Institute, Portland, OR, USA

INTRODUCTION

The eye is one of the more common organs of the body which prevents a drug from reaching the market place. While the liver and kidney are the most common areas that develop drug toxicity, a majority of the organs may have to be damaged before an abnormal laboratory finding becomes evident. However, with the eye, if the macula is involved, even a small fraction of 1% may show a significant abnormality on testing. In addition, the eye has so many different tissues, i.e. pigment, connective tissue, blood vessels, muscles, the lens, central and peripheral nervous tissue, mucous membranes, multiple glands, etc. that many different classes of drugs may affect the eye. Adverse drug-induced ocular effects occur from topical medication, including their preservatives, or from systemic medications. Drugs (especially antimetabolites) may concentrate in the tears, causing marked irritation to the mucous membrane overlying the eye, including scarring. Acute glaucoma can occur by dilation of the pupil (atropine-like agents), or open angle glaucoma by the deposition of mucopolysaccarides in the ocular outflow channels (oral or topical steroids). Opacification of the lens (steroids, allopurinol), or

disruption of the pigmented tissue of the macula (chloroquine or hydroxychloroquine) are not uncommon.

The key to suspecting an adverse ocular effect is a high degree of clinical suspicion—being aware that the signs and symptoms of a disease process do not fit the expected clinical picture. The busy clinician can easily miss a drug-related ocular event, especially if patients are on multiple topical or systemic medications. It is estimated that the incidence of adverse drug events from topical ocular medications alone is 13% (Wilson, 1983). How best to determine whether an adverse drug event has occurred is shown in Table 38.1. The World Health Organization (WHO) has defined these events, as shown in Table 38.2 (WHO, 1972; Edwards and Biriell, 1995).

With over 30 000 prescription drugs in the United States alone, and obviously many more world-wide, plus a multitude of over-the-counter and herbal products available, it is impossible to cover this subject entirely in this short chapter. Probably the two most encompassing textbooks are Grant and Schuman's *Toxicology of the Eye* (Grant and Schuman, 1993) and *Drug-Induced Ocular Side Effects*, 5th edition (Fraunfelder and Fraunfelder, 2001).

Pharmacovigilance. Edited by R.D. Mann and E.B. Andrews

Table 38.1. How to possibly tell if a drug causes an adverse effect.

- Temporal association—time of onset, pattern, etc.
- Dose response
- Positive dechallenge
- Positive rechallenge
- Scientific explanation as to the mechanism of action
- Similar effects from others in this "class" of drugs
- No alternative explanation

The National Registry of Drug-Induced Ocular Side Effects is also a source of help to the busy clinician (Fraunfelder, 1985). The objectives of the Registry are:

1. to establish a national center where possible drug-induced ocular side effects can be accumulated,
2. to add to this data base the spontaneous reporting data of possible drug-induced ocular side effects collected from the Food and Drug Administration (FDA) (Rockville, MD) and the World Health Organization (WHO) (Uppsala, Sweden),
3. to compile the data in the world literature on reports of possible drug-induced ocular side effects in humans,
4. to publish some of this data every 4 to 5 years in book form, and
5. to make available this data to physicians who feel they have a possible drug-induced ocular side effect.

You can contact us to help you with: a suspected drug reaction, access to data in the Registry, or to report a case. When sending data, it would be ideal to include: name of drug, dosage, length of time on drug, suspected reaction, what happened if the drug was stopped, if rechallenged, concomitant drugs, and the name and address of person reporting the case (optional, but encouraged).

Reports can be mailed to:

National Registry of Drug-Induced Ocular Side Effects
Casey Eye Institute
3375 SW Terwilliger Blvd.
Portland, OR 97201-4197, USA

or faxed: (503) 494-4286
or e-mailed: www.eyedrugregistry.com

DRUGS WITH OCULAR SIDE-EFFECTS OF RECENT CLINICAL IMPORTANCE

HYDROXYCHLOROQUINE (PLAQUENIL®)

Primary Use

Hydroxychloroquine is used primarily for the treatment of rheumatoid arthritis and lupus erythematosis, dermatologic conditions, and various inflammatory disorders.

Table 38.2. World Health Organization (WHO) definitions—causality assessment of suspected adverse reactions.

- Certain: A clinical event, including laboratory test abnormality, occurring in a plausible time relationship to drug administration, and which cannot be explained by concurrent disease or other drugs or chemicals. The response to withdrawal of the drug (dechallenge) should be clinically plausible. The event must be definitive pharmacologically or phenomenologically, using a satisfactory rechallenge procedure if necessary.
- Probable/Likely: A clinical event, including laboratory test abnormality, with a reasonable time sequence to administration of the drug, unlikely to be attributed to concurrent disease or other drugs or chemicals, and which follows a clinically reasonable response on withdrawal (dechallenge). Rechallenge information is not required to fulfill this definition.
- Possible: A clinical event, including laboratory test abnormality, with a reasonable time sequence to administration of the drug, but which could also be explained by concurrent disease or other drugs or chemicals. Information on drug withdrawal may be lacking or unclear.
- Unlikely: A clinical event, including laboratory test abnormality, with a temporal relationship to drug administration which makes a causal relationship improbable, and in which other drugs, chemicals or underlying disease provide plausible explanations.
- Conditional/Unclassified: A clinical event, including laboratory test abnormality, reported as an adverse reaction, about which more data are essential for a proper assessment or the additional data are under examination.
- Unassessable/Unclassifiable: A report suggesting an adverse reaction which cannot be judged because information is insufficient or contradictory, and which cannot be supplemented or verified.

Definition of Hydroxychloroquine Maculopathy

Maculopathy must be bilateral and reproducible by Amsler grid and visual field testing. Transient or unilateral defects are not sufficient reasons to implicate the drug, and are not an indication to stop therapy.

The Goal

The goal is to find early changes, i.e. relative scotomas. Later findings include retinal changes, color vision loss, absolute scotoma or decreased vision, since even if the drug is stopped, two-thirds of these patients may continue to lose some vision and/or peripheral fields. Patients with early paracentral relative scotomas seldom advance when the drug is discontinued.

Guidelines for Following Patients (modified after Easterbook, 1999)

- *Baseline examination.* Within the first 1 to 2 years after starting this drug, a complete— dilated—ophthalmic examination should be done, including some type of informed consent of possible permanent visual problems in rare instances. This baseline examination should include visual acuity, Amsler grids (with instructions for monthly home use), and color vision (preferably including the blue–yellow axis, such as the pseudo-isochromatic plates for color by American Optical Corporation). If any abnormality of the macular area is seen, it would be ideal to obtain fundus photographs. If you have any suspicion of an ocular abnormality of a progressive type, consider a baseline Humphrey 10–2 or other automated perimetry.
- *Follow-up examinations.* If the patient is not obese, frail, elderly or extremely thin, or does not have significant renal or hepaatic disease or macular disease of any type, and is below age 40, he or she does not need another complete examination for 2–4 years. They need to see you sooner if:

  — they experience any persistent visual symptoms, or
  — their dosage exceeds 6.5 mg/kg

If between 40 and 64 years:

— same as above.

If age 64 and above:

— same as above, however need to see you every 1–2 years.

- *Annual examinations should be done if:*

  — over 5 years of therapy,
  — obese, or lean and small—especially elderly,
  — progressive macular disease of any type,
  — significant renal or liver disease,
  — dosage exceeds 6.5 mg/kg.

- Follow-up examinations:

  — Repeat baseline examination.
  — Fundus photography if any macular abnormality noted.
  — Consider fluorescein angiography only if suspect pigmentary changes of any cause.
  — Automated central visual fields
  — If available, but not essential, in selected cases, multifocal electroretinogram (ERG).

Chloroquine

Perform same tests as above. See at least annually if dosage is less than 3.0 mg/kg of ideal body weight. See every 6 months if dosage greater than 3.0 mg/kg body weight, if short/obese or if renal and/or liver impairment.

ISOTRETINOIN (ACCUTANE®)

Primary Use

Cystic acne, psoriasis and various skin disorders.

Clinical Importance

The drug competes with binding sites with retinoic acid and retinol in the retina. Isotretinoin can cause decreased dark adaptation. However, only recent data suggests the probability of rare cases of *permanent night blindness* (Fraunfelder et al., 2001). Therefore, the Physicians' Desk Reference (PDR) in the year 2001 will list a warning about this in the package insert. This drug can cause meibomitis, blepharitis, atrophy of the meibomian gland (in animals—complete destruction) (Mathers *et al.*, 1991), often with increased staphylococcus disease. Any or all of these may decrease tear film break-up time and increase tear osmolality. Therefore, isotretinoin probably can cause a permanent "evaporative" form of sicca.

Isotretinoin is secreted in the tears, causing an irritative conjunctivitis, superficial punctate keratitis, drug deposits in the superficial cornea, and decreased tolerance for contact lens wear. Some sicca patients are made worse, or latent sicca becomes manifest. This photosensitizer can cause or significantly aggravate existing lid disease, especially blepharitis. Other known side-effects include: acute myopia, papilledema secondary to pseudotumor cerebri and optic neuritis. Recently, isotretinoin has also been shown probably to cause reversible color vision defects.

Guidelines for following patients

It is not practical to have all patients receive an eye examination prior to starting these agents. However, if the patient is below age 40 and has not had an eye examination in the past few years, or if above age 40 and has not had one in 1–2 years, it may be prudent to do so. This is especially true if the patient has any other ocular problems prior to starting the drug, to prevent aggravation of above conditions or have the drug unfairly blamed for latent ocular disease.

Explain risk–benefit ratio in patients with:

- Retinitis pigmentosa
- Dystrophic or degenerative retinal disease
- Severe or chronic blepharoconjunctivitis
- Significant tear film abnormalities
- Pre-existing night blindness

In select patients with anterior segment or retinal pathology, consider UV blocking lenses since the drug is a photosensitizer. Consider discontinuing or delaying fitting of contact lenses while on these drugs. Patients on chronic long-term isotretinoin should have an annual eye examination. Suggest that patients see you sooner

if any significant ocular signs or symptoms occur. Quiz on night blindness; if progressive or persistent, consider stopping the drug. Since many cases are transitory, this is not an indication for stopping the drug. However, if this persists for a number of weeks, consider closer monitoring and possibly further testing, i.e. electroretinography, visual field testing, and dark adaptometry testing.

Stop the drug if any of the following occur:

- pseudotumor cerebri
- optic neuritis
- persistent night blindness

Permanent night blindness, permanent sicca, and transitory loss of color vision only occur in patients on long-term, chronic therapy, and are indeed rare events.

SILDENAFIL (VIAGRA®) (LATIES AND FRAUNFELDER, 2000)

Primary Use

For the management of erectile dysfunction.

Clinical Importance—minimal

Ocular side-effects are uncommon, dosage dependent and thus far all have been fully reversible.

Reported Side-Effects

- *Changes in color perception*
  - Objects have colored tinges—usually blue or blue/green, maybe pink or yellow
  - Diminished color vision
  - Dark colors appear darker

- *Blurred vision*
  - Central haze
  - Transitory decreased vision

- *Changes in light perception*
  - Increased perception of brightness
  - Flashing lights—especially when blinking

- *Conjunctiva*
  - Hyperemia

— Subconjunctival hemorrhages—not proven to be drug-related
— Ocular pain
— Photophobia

The above ocular side-effects are dose dependent and occur at the following incidence:

50 mg	3%
100 mg	10%
200 mg	40%–50%

Ocular side-effects are directly proportional to blood drug levels.

The side-effects based on dosage start at 15–30 minutes, and usually peak 1 hour after ingestion of drug.

50 mg	gone 1 hour
100 mg	gone 2 hours
200 mg	gone 4–6 hours

● *Contraindicated* or use extreme caution in patients with:
  — retinitis pigmentosa
  — congenital stationary night blindness
  — deficiency or mutation of photoreceptor cGMP PDF
  — informed consent advised; no data to prove it is harmful, but it theoretically could be.

VIGABATRIN (SABRIL®) (RUETHER *ET AL.*, 1998)

Primary Use

Used in over 50 countries for the treatment of refractory epilepsy, generalized tonic-clonic seizures and infantile spasm.

Reports include:

● Symptomatic or asymptomatic field loss, mainly bilateral concentric peripheral constriction with variable degree of visual field defects. Cases of severe tunnel vision have occurred.
● Can occur anytime within 1 month to 6+ years of therapy.

● Incidence unknown—from 0.5% up to 10%–20% on long-term therapy. May be dose-related.
● Cause may be increased levels of gamma-aminobutyric acid (GABA) in the retina.
● Visual field changes not progressive with discontinuation of the drug; however, the visual defect may persist and may be irreversible in up to 80% of cases.
● Some visual changes are dramatic, with over 50% of visual field loss.
● Some groups have asked for the drug to be recalled because of visual side-effects; however, in some patients this is the only drug that controls their seizures.

Recommendations (as per Drug Company—Hoechst Marion Roussel):

● Visual field testing every 6 months.
● Question patients regularly for visual symptoms.
● If visual symptoms reported, might be drug-related—repeat fields.
● If field reproducible, access risk–benefit ratio for stopping the drug.
● If the drug is discontinued, it must be tapered over a 2–4 week period.

CAPECITABINE (XELODA®) (WAIKHOM *ET AL.*, 2000)

Capecitabine is a new, widely used anticancer agent (metastatic breast, colon and many solid tumors). It is metabolized in a three-step process to the active agent, 5-fluorouracil, a known ocular irritant which is secreted in tears.

Ocular findings in patients on capecitabine:

● 10% have ocular irritation, probably secondary to the drug or its byproducts being present in tears.
● Superficial punctate keratitis may be present, especially inferonasally.
● In patients on high dosages, and probably if sicca is present, can cause white granular deep epithelial or subepithelial deposits.

- Deposits may be associated with significant ocular pain and decreased vision to 20/60.
- Complete clearing of superficial punctate keratitis (SPK) and corneal deposits occurs within 3 to 6+ weeks after the drug is discontinued.

CORTICOSTEROIDS—INHALED (BECLOMETHASONE—BECLOVENT®, BECONASE®, VANCENASE®, VANCERIL®); (BUDESONIDE—RHINOCORT®)

Primary Use

For use in asthmatic, allergic and chronic lung diseases.

Clinical Significance

A report in the *Journal of the American Medical Association* (Garbe *et al.*, 1998) states that inhaled corticosteroids at high doses for over 3 years had a three-fold increased risk of cataract extraction compared to a control group.

Comments

- Inhaled induced steroid-induced glaucoma is well documented.
- Statistical analysis based on 416 patients using inhaled steroids who had not used systemic steroids for at least 5 years shows increased incidence of cataract surgery.
- This is first report to investigate risk according to daily dose of inhaled steroids and duration of use (> 1 mg of beclomethasone or budesonide per day).
- Systemic steroid use after only one year duration causes a statistically significant increase in the incidence of cataract surgery in the elderly in this same study.
- As study points out, while there are many variables in this research, this indirect evidence suggests that we may have markedly underestimated the potential of steroids as a cataractogenic co-factor in the elderly.

TAMOXIFEN (NOLVADEX®)

Primary Use

For metastatic breast cancer, pancreatic cancer and malignant melanoma. Beginning to be used for long-term therapy as a prophylaxis in patients with a strong family history of breast cancer. Expect to see more patients on long-term tamoxifen for follow-up ocular examinations.

Clinical Concern

There is minimal data on long-term exposure (4–5+ years) with a drug with documented significant ocular side-effects, so the data are preliminary.

Known Side-Effects

- Posterior subcapsular cataracts
- Decreased color perception
- Decreased vision
- Retina or macula—refractile bodies, edema, degeneration, pigmentary changes and hemorrhages
- Visual fields—constriction, scotomas
- Papilledema
- Optic neuritis
- Corneal deposits
- ERG changes

Guidelines for Following Patients (Modified after Gorin *et al.*, 1998)

1. Baseline ophthalmic examination within the first year of starting tamoxifen. This should include slit lamp biomicroscopy of the anterior and posterior segments in combination with an indirect ophthalmoscope or contact lens. Baseline color vision testing is important.
2. In keeping with the American Academy of Ophthalmology's current recommendations, in normal adults, do a complete eye examination at least every 2 years.
3. More frequent examinations are required if ocular symptoms occur.

4. The discovery of a limited number of intraretinal crystals in the absence of macular edema or visual impairment does not seem to warrant discontinuation of the drug.
5. Consultation with the oncologist is essential if significant ocular findings occur.
6. Presence of age-related maculopathy is not a contraindication to the use of tamoxifen. However, informed consent may be advisable in our litigious society.
7. Presence of posterior subcapsular cataracts is not an indication to stop the drug since the condition usually progresses even if the drug is discontinued.
8. Significant color loss may be a valid reason to consider discontinuing the drug. Gorin *et al.* recommend considering stopping the drug for 3 months (in patients on prophylactic therapy), and retest. If the color vision returns to normal, restart the drug and retest in 3 months. If, at any time, there is no recovery after stopping the drug, or continued progression, then one may need to consult the oncologist and re-evaluate the risk–benefit.

Comments

- The incidence of ocular toxicity reported in the literature is from 1.5% to 12%; however, incidence requiring stopping the drug due to an ocular complication is less than 1%.
- Indications for stopping the drug require consultation with the oncologist since there are many variables. Decreasing the dosage may be an option if frequent ophthalmic observations are performed. Indications to stop the drug include:
  — macular edema,
  — decreased vision (with or without refractile bodies or pigmentary change),
  — optic neuritis, or
  — decreased color vision.
- Retinal crystals, *per se*, are not an indication to stop the drug.
- Retinal changes can occur even at 20 mg dosage levels.
- Optic neuritis has been reported at a total dosage of only 2–3 grams.

AMIODARONE (CORDONE®) (MACALUSO ET AL., 1999)

Primary Use

Primarily used in the treatment of various cardiac arrhythmias.

Known Ocular Side-Effects

- Corneal deposits (100%)—may interfere with vision, especially with night driving
- Color vision defects
- Photosensitizing drug—eyelids and conjunctiva (yellow–brown, gray–blue) discoloration
- Cataracts—anterior subcapsular, seldom interfere with vision

Guidelines for Following Patients

- Baseline ophthalmic examination
- See every 6 months (controversial)
- Any visual disturbance, patient to see ophthalmologist promptly

An important recent finding is that of amiodarone-induced optic neuropathy. Since it may be impossible to distinguish non-arteritic anterior ischemic optic neuropathy (NAION) from amiodarone optic neuropathy in many cases, a neuro-ophthalmologist consult may be necessary. Many of these patients may already have a compromised optic nerve due to vascular disease, and the amiodarone deposition in the axons further impedes neural function, causing vision loss.

- The cause of amiodarone neuropathy is unknown, but may be due to selective accumulation of intracytoplasmic or its by-product inclusions (primary lipidosis) in optic nerve axons which may mechanically or biochemically decrease axoplasmic flow.
- Resultant optic nerve head edema may persist as long as transport is inhibited, i.e. as long as several months following discontinuation of amiodarone, which has up to a 100-day half-life, while with NAION, edema resolves much more rapidly.

- No reported cases of amiodarone neuropathy causing no light perception (NLP).
- The degree of amiodarone neuropathy may not be equal in each eye for a few months, but usually will be if the drug is continued.
- Stopping the drug, in consultation with the cardiologist, at the first signs of optic nerve involvement must be considered unless very confident of the diagnosis of NAION.

REFERENCES

Easterbrook M (1999) Detection and prevention of maculopathy associated with antimalarial agents. *Intl Ophthalmol Clin* **39**: 49–57.

Edwards IR, Biriell C (1995) Harmonisation in pharmacovigilance. *Drug Safety* **10**: 93–102.

Fraunfelder FT (1985) National Registry of Drug-Induced Ocular Side Effects. In: Inman WH, ed., *Monitoring for Drug Safety*. London: MTP Press, pp. 363–9.

Fraunfelder FT, Fraunfelder FW (2001) *Drug-Induced Ocular Side Effects*, 5th edn. Woburn, MA: Butterworth Heinemann.

Fraunfelder FT, Fraunfelder FW, Edwards R (2001) Ocular side effects possibly associated with isotretinoin usage. *Am J Ophthalmol* **132**: 299–305.

Garbe E, Suissa S, Lelorier J (1998) Association of inhaled corticosteroid use with cataract extraction in elderly patients. *J Am Med Assoc* **280**: 539–44.

Gorin MB, Day R, Costantino JP, Fisher B, Redmond CK, Wickerham L, Gomolin JE, Margolese RG, Mathen MK, Bowman DM, Kaufmann, D, Dimitrov NV, Singerman LJ, Bornstein R, Wolmark N (1998) Long-term tamoxifen citrate use and potential ocular toxicity. *Am J Ophthalmol* **125**: 493–501.

Grant WM, Schuman JS (1993) *Toxicology of the Eye*, 4th edn. Springfield: Charles C. Thomas.

Laties A, Fraunfelder FT (2000) Visual side effects possibly associated with sildenafil (Viagra®). *J Toxicol: Cutaneous and Ocular Toxicol* **19**: 21–5.

Macaluso DC, Shults WT, Fraunfelder FT (1999) Features of amiodarone-induced optic neuropathy. *Am J Ophthalmol* **127**: 610–12.

Mathers WD, Shields WJ, Schdev MS, Petroll WM, Jester JV (1991) Meibomian gland morphology and tear osmolarity: changes with Accutane therapy. *Cornea* **10**: 286–90.

Ruether K, Pung T, Kellner U, Schmitz B, Hartmann C (1998) Electrophysiologic evaluation of a patient with peripheral visual field constriction associated with vigabatrin. *Arch Ophthalmol*, **116**: 817–19.

Waikhom B, Fraunfelder FT, Henner WD (2000) Severe ocular irritation and corneal deposits associated with capecitabine use. *New Engl J Med* **343**: 740–1.

Wilson FM (1983) Adverse ocular effects of topical ophthalmic therapy: an epidemiological, laboratory, and clinical study. *Trans Am Ophthalmol* **81**: 854.

World Health Organization (WHO) (1972) International drug monitoring: the role of national centres. *The WHO Technical Report Series No. 498*. Geneva: World Health Organization.

39

Drug Safety in Pregnancy

CHRISTINA D. CHAMBERS
Department of Pediatrics, University of California at San Diego, CA, USA
ELIZABETH B. ANDREWS
RTI Health Solutions, Research Triangle Institute, Research Triangle Park, NC, USA, and School of Public Health and School of Pharmacy, University of North Carolina at Chapel Hill, NC, USA

INTRODUCTION

Following the recognition that thalidomide, when used by pregnant women, induced a characteristic pattern of severe congenital anomalies in many of the offspring, pharmaceutical manufacturers, regulatory agencies and a variety of public health entities have faced the challenge and responsibility of assessing the safety of medication with respect to the developing fetus (Lenz, 1961; McBride, 1961). This is a daunting task for a variety of reasons, not the least of which is the number and variety of medications to which a pregnant woman is likely to be exposed. Although pharmacovigilance for a variety of adverse reproductive outcomes, ranging from spontaneous abortion to long-term postnatal functional deficits or learning disabilities, is appropriate in assessing pharmaceutical safety during pregnancy, the focus of this chapter will be limited to major congenital anomalies. As congenital anomalies are the leading cause of infant mortality in the United States, prevention of even the small proportion that are likely to be attributable to maternal medication use is a worthy goal of any pharmacovigilance effort (Rosenberg et al., 1996).

FREQUENCY AND VARIETY OF MEDICATION USE AMONG PREGNANT WOMEN

In the United States alone, 639 new drug applications were approved by the Food and Drug Administration (FDA) between 1993 and 1999, and of these, 232 were new molecular entities (CDER, 1999). New drugs do not come to market with clinical trial safety data specifically designed to address questions related to human pregnancy. Once a new drug is available for clinical use, the frequency with which it is prescribed and the specific medical conditions that it is used to treat influence the likelihood that women of reproductive age will use the drug. However, numerous studies have demonstrated that pregnant women are commonly using several medications over the course of gestation. For example, in a review of drug utilization studies, Bonati et al. (1990) identified 13 publications originating from sites

Pharmacovigilance. Edited by R.D. Mann and E.B. Andrews
© 2002 John Wiley & Sons, Ltd

in the United States and Europe in which pregnant women used an average of 4.7 drugs per person with the mean number ranging from 3 to 11. A 1996 survey of records of the French Health Insurance Service demonstrated that in a sample of 1000 women living in southwest France, 99% of women received a prescription for at least one drug during pregnancy with a mean of 13.6 medications prescribed per woman (Lacroix *et al.*, 2000).

Given that a significant proportion of pregnancies occur without prior planning—in the United States estimates are as high as 56%—women may be inadvertently exposed to medications before pregnancy is recognized, and this vulnerable period may extend into the first 4 to 6 weeks or longer following conception (Forrest, 1994). Thus, unintentional fetal exposures can occur during part or all of the most critical period in embryonic development for drug-induced malformations.

In addition to medication exposures that take place prior to pregnancy recognition, many maternal conditions, both acute and chronic, may require treatment after pregnancy is verified. A variety of relatively common diseases that occur in women of reproductive age may necessitate treatment throughout the course of pregnancy. For example, the prevalence of clinical depression is estimated to be as high as 8.0%–20.0% (Kessler *et al.*, 1993), asthma 0.4%–1.3% (Wen *et al.*, 2001), epilepsy 0.4%–1.0% (Holmes *et al.*, 1994; Yerby, 2000), and rheumatoid arthritis 1.0%–2.0% (Belios and Carsons 1998) among women in their reproductive years. For some of these maternal conditions a decision not to treat could lead to events, such as uncontrolled seizure activity or psychiatric episodes, which could be detrimental to the pregnancy and/or the fetus itself (Goldberg and Nissim, 1994).

PRE-MARKETING SOURCES OF DATA REGARDING REPRODUCTIVE SAFETY

The traditional methods for evaluating drug safety in the pre-marketing phases of drug development, i.e. animal reproductive toxicity studies and randomized clinical trials, have limited application with respect to human pregnancy. Owing to species specificity and sensitivity to reproductive toxins, it is difficult to extrapolate with confidence from pre-marketing animal studies to human pregnancy. The species, dose of medication, route of drug administration and maternal toxic effects are some of the experimental variables that can influence findings and limit the interpretability and predictive value of these studies (Brent, 1986).

Clinical trials are the second traditional method of evaluating drug safety. For obvious ethical reasons, pregnant women typically are not recruited for trials during any phase of drug development. If and when unintended pregnancies occur during the course of a trial, pregnancy outcomes can provide preliminary information regarding the risks of exposure. However, these data usually involve very few subjects. There is a trend to include larger numbers of women of childbearing age in clinical trials, and this will undoubtedly result in a larger number of exposed pregnancies in such trials. Nevertheless, these numbers will still be too small to provide meaningful information.

POST-MARKETING SOURCES OF DATA REGARDING REPRODUCTIVE SAFETY

Once a medication is marketed, there are a number of resources that can provide observational data regarding drug safety in pregnancy.

1. *Clinician case reports* published in the medical literature can delineate a phenotype in an affected infant born to a mother with a specific prenatal medication exposure. However, these reports must be initiated spontaneously, and therefore may involve investigator as well as publication bias. Furthermore, without a known denominator of exposed pregnancies that do not result in infants with the specific malformation, it is difficult to determine if the reported defects represent an increase over baseline. If the phenotype is sufficiently unique, e.g. the isotretinoin embryopathy (Lammer *et al.*, 1985), then a series of case reports can strongly suggest a hypothesis that can be confirmed using other methods.

2. *Centralized adverse event reporting systems* can provide a systematic method for accumulation of case reports from a variety of resources. For example, under the US FDA's Adverse Event Reporting System (AERS), manufacturers, and distributors of FDA approved pharmaceuticals are mandated to report events such as congenital anomalies as they are reported to them, or are published in the scientific literature and have been associated with their drugs. The FDA receives additional reports through the MedWatch program, an educational and promotional effort which facilitates spontaneous reporting from healthcare providers (Kessler, 1993; Goldman and Kennedy, 1998). And finally, consumers may provide information to the manufacturer or directly to the FDA.

The advantages of such a system are that reports can be accumulated from a variety of resources in a timely fashion and can be reviewed and investigated further with respect to any potential concerns. For example, the angiotensin II converting enzyme inhibitor (ACE inhibitor) fetopathy, which includes a unique pattern of renal tubular dysplasia and hypocalvaria occurring in association with second or third trimester use of one of the drugs in the ACE inhibitor group, was first reported by a clinician (Pryde *et al.*, 1993). However, the frequency of similar or related abnormalities in relation to gestational timing and dose of the drug was identifiable through review of a series of 110 ACE inhibitor adverse event reports submitted to the FDA through 1999 (Tabacova *et al.*, 2000).

The primary limitations of such systems are similar to those of case reports appearing in the medical literature, i.e. that reports must be initiated spontaneously, and this may involve bias, and that there is no known denominator of exposed, unaffected pregnancies that could be used to develop a birth prevalence rate for purposes of comparison. In addition this system relies on the "prepared mind" to make a link between medication exposure and pregnancy outcome, a link more likely for outcomes normally rare and extremely severe, and less likely for outcomes considered common or with subtle presentation.

3. *Drug registries* have been one method of evaluating drug safety in pregnancy dating back to the Swedish lithium registry established in 1962 (Schou *et al.*, 1973). Similar manufacturer-sponsored registries have been successfully completed for fluoxetine (Goldstein *et al.*, 1997) and acyclovir (Andrews *et al.*, 1992; Preboth, 2000) while several others are presently ongoing (White and Andrews, 1999). All involve spontaneous reporting of exposed pregnancies. The collection of outcome data is usually accomplished through the healthcare provider who initiates contact with the registry, but in some registry designs outcome data are collected from the pregnant woman herself. Although pregnancy outcome reports can be collected retrospectively, most current drug registries identify exposed women prospectively, i.e. during gestation, and collect exposure and other information prior to the known outcome of that pregnancy. In these cases, the registry may be considered a targeted follow-up study.

The registry approach has a number of advantages including timely and centralized ascertainment of exposed pregnancies which can parallel prescribing practices for newly-marketed medications. Particularly if the exposure is rare, this may be the most efficient method for collecting pregnancy outcome data. In addition, the registry approach provides a defined denominator of exposed women which facilitates comparisons of congenital anomaly rates with those of a reference group. These studies generally have the ability to detect a meaningful increase in the overall frequency of major birth defects that are evident at birth.

Limitations of such registries typically include the following. As these studies depend on spontaneous reporting of exposed pregnancies, it is difficult to project sample sizes, and therefore there may be insufficient power to adequately evaluate increased risks for specific congenital anomalies. In addition, some current registries rely on externally derived reference rates while others use as controls other drugs monitored in the same study. Depending on the characteristics of women in the exposed group, the use of external reference statistics may not represent the most appropriate comparison. And finally, as most registries rely on a wide variety of individual healthcare providers to report outcome, there is potential misclassification bias with respect to the accurate diagnosis of some congenital anomalies.

4. *Birth defects monitoring or surveillance systems* are designed to provide population- or hospital-based identification of congenital anomalies in order to measure trends and to respond to unusual clusters of events. At this level of information gathering, if an upward trend in the birth prevalence of a certain defect or a time-related cluster of an unusual pattern of defects coincides with widespread use of a new medication, then surveillance programs can function as an early warning system (Khoury *et al.*, 1993). Because an unusual pattern of congenital anomalies may occur with extreme rarity within any one surveillance system, these efforts are enhanced by collaborations such as the International Clearinghouse of Birth Defects Monitoring Systems (ICBDMS) which has been in existence since 1974 (Erickson, 1991; Khoury *et al.*, 1994a).

5. *Birth defects case–control studies* can be classified into one of two general approaches. The first group might be termed classical hypothesis-testing case–control designs while the second involves on-going case–control surveillance for drug-induced congenital malformations.

Using the first design, cases and controls are identified with the specific intent to measure the association between a risk factor and a specified birth defect or group of defects. This approach requires that a priori decisions be made regarding the research questions, selection of the appropriate control group, and adequate power and sample size. For example, based on concerns raised in the literature, this design was successfully used to document an association between congenital facial nerve paralysis, or Möebius' Syndrome, and first-trimester use of misoprostol (Pastuszak *et al.*, 1998).

The second approach, case–control surveillance, has been incorporated into several birth defects monitoring programs in the United States. This design is also used on an on-going basis programs such as the Slone Epidemiology Unit's hospital-based surveillance program based at Boston University (Mitchell *et al.*, 1981; Hernández-Díaz *et al.*, 2000), the Latin American Collaborative Study of Congenital Malformations (ECLAMC) which involves over 70 hospitals in several South American countries (Castilla and Peters, 1992), and the population-based Hungarian Congenital Malformation Registry (Czeizel *et al.*, 2000). These programs usually involve ascertainment of malformed cases as well as systematic sample selection of non-malformed infants who can be used as controls. Exposure and other risk factor information is generally gathered by post-natal maternal interview and review of medical records. However, rather than being hypothesis-driven from the outset, case–control surveillance is designed to collect information on a wide variety of congenital anomalies as well as a broad spectrum of exposures, facilitating multiple hypothesis testing at any future date. In addition, some designs have incorporated DNA sampling and banking from case and control children and their parents so that future hypotheses regarding genetic susceptibility can be tested.

The primary of advantage of any case–control approach in studies of rare events such as congenital anomalies is the enhanced power to detect an association for a given sample size. Additional advantages of case–control surveillance include, to a varying degree, relatively complete ascertainment of the congenital anomalies of interest within a defined population, concurrent selection of controls from the same population, and the ability to validate the classification of diagnoses. In addition, this approach provides flexibility in the ultimate use of the data, i.e. based on the needs of a given analysis, subsets of cases and controls can be selected from the entire data set to test or confirm specific hypotheses. For example, this method was useful in confirming the protective effect of antenatal folic acid supplementation in reducing the incidence of neural tube defects (Werler *et al.*, 1993). Furthermore, case–control surveillance data are amenable to hypothesis generation. For example, these data were used to first raise the question of an association between pseudoephedrine and gastroschisis (Werler *et al.*, 1992).

The limitations of case–control studies of any type generally relate to the use of retrospective data collection and the selection of controls. For example, maternal interviews may be conducted in some cases many months after completion of the pregnancy, which raises the possibility, although controversial, of limited recall of early pregnancy medication use (Tomeo *et al.*, 1999). In addition, the potential for serious differential recall bias among mothers of malformed infants relative to mothers of non-malformed controls has been cited by some (Khoury *et al.*, 1994b), while the bias associated with the use of malformed controls has been suggested by others (Prieto and Martínez-Frias, 2000). With respect to the use of appropriate controls, case–control surveillance studies have the advantage of flexibility in selection of one or multiple control groups, malformed or not, from the larger data set as judged necessary for any specific analysis.

Because case–control surveillance programs are on-going, they have the potential to recognize an association with a newly-marketed medication; however, they may have limited sensitivity in this regard. These studies may miss an association if the medication of interest is related to a relatively unusual congenital anomaly and/or that specific defect is not included in the range of selected anomalies for which maternal interviews are conducted. In addition, if new medications are infrequently used among pregnant women, then weak or moderate associations may be difficult to detect. However, given the rarity of congenital anomalies in general, these approaches provide a relatively powerful method of hypothesis testing and hypothesis generating and can be effectively used alone and in conjunction with other methods.

6. *Large cohort studies* can involve open cohorts that are population-based and ongoing, or can be hospital-based and of limited duration. For example, the Swedish Registry of Congenital Malformations in combination with the Swedish Medical Birth Registry encompasses all births in Sweden and utilizes exposure interviews conducted by midwives during the first trimester of pregnancy as well as data recorded prospectively in medical records (Ericson *et al.*, 1999). The Collaborative Perinatal Project conducted in the 1960s was a study involving over 50 000 mother–child pairs identified at multiple sites throughout the United States (Chung and Myrianthopoulos,

1975). These studies have the advantage of prospective ascertainment of exposure information as well as data regarding a variety of potential confounders. In addition, women with and without the exposure of interest are concurrently enrolled as members of the cohort, facilitating the identification of an appropriate reference group. Like on-going case–control designs, studies of this type can address multiple hypotheses that need not be formulated a priori. However, even in large cohort studies, issues of sample size can be a limitation. For example, the Collaborative Perinatal Project had inadequate power to detect weak to moderate associations with any but the most common major congenital malformations. In contrast, the Swedish Registry with approximately 120 000 annual births, accumulated over more than a 25-year span of time, has enhanced power to identify these associations. Of course, the caveat with any large cohort study is the substantial cost involved in such efforts.

7. *Small cohort studies* focused on specific medications have been conducted by Teratology Information Services (TIS) both in North America and Europe. These studies draw on a base of callers who contact a TIS seeking counseling regarding the safety of a medication used in pregnancy. Follow-up of pregnancy outcome is obtained for selected exposures. These studies have strengths similar to the registries described above with respect to the potential for rapid identification of exposed women as well as prospective collection of exposure and other risk factor information. Also, similar to other registries, TIS studies rely on spontaneous callers for recruitment of subjects which may result in a biased sample. TIS studies usually employ a concurrently enrolled unexposed control group which may provide the most appropriate reference in this context. The primary limitation of TIS studies relates to sample size. TIS sites either independently or in collaboration have published studies typically involving between 100 and 200 exposed subjects (Pastuszak *et al.*, 1993; McElhatton *et al.*, 1999). Collaborative projects among networks of TIS sites in North America are conducted through the Organization of Teratology Information Services (OTIS) (Scialli, 1999) and in Europe through the European

Network of Teratology Information Services (ENTIS) (Schaefer *et al.*, 1996).

These formal collaborations can shorten recruitment time, add to the variability and possibly the representativeness of subjects in the sample, and increase the obtainable sample size. However, these studies usually are not capable of adequately evaluating any but the most dramatic increased risks for single major malformations. The primary strength of TIS studies is the focus on a spectrum of pregnancy outcomes and, in some designs, the evaluation of exposed children for a pattern of major and minor malformations (Jones *et al.*, 1989). This unique advantage can generate hypotheses that might not be conceived using any other method.

8. *Database linkage studies*, as technological advances permit, can offer many of the advantages of large cohort studies at potentially far less cost. Early efforts along these lines utilized the Michigan Medicaid database, a government health insurance program within which maternal prescription records could be linked to pediatric billing records to identify children born with and without congenital anomalies (Rosa, 1999). Similar approaches have been used successfully elsewhere in North America and Europe. For example, investigators in Denmark have linked prescription database records to hospital discharge and medical birth register records for children with and without congenital anomalies to investigate the safety of a widely used antibiotic (Larsen *et al.*, 2000). In countries where there is universal and standardized healthcare delivery and record-keeping, or in countries where healthcare maintenance or other large membership-based providers serve a significant proportion of the population, linked prescription and birth records provide an attractive alternative method for testing hypotheses regarding drug safety in pregnancy. This approach has been used successfully to evaluate pregnancy exposure to clarithromycin using longitudinal claims data for members from 12 geographically diverse United Health Group-affiliated health plans (Drinkard *et al.*, 2000). Similarly, information from the Group Health Cooperative of Puget Sound in the United States has been used to examine the association between topical tretinoin (Retin-A) and major birth defects (Jick *et al.*, 1993). The General Practice Research Database in the United Kingdom is another potentially fruitful resource (Jick and Terris, 1997; Jick, 1999). The primary advantages are the availability of large numbers of subjects and ease of access to data. This approach also avoids some of the biases involved in studies that rely entirely on maternal report to classify exposure. These strengths must be weighed against the limitations inherent in a study design that does not involve subject contact. For example, these studies usually cannot ensure that the medication prescribed was actually taken by the mother, or taken during the period of time critical for development of any specific birth defect. There are also issues related to misclassification of outcome depending on the quality of records used to determine or exclude the diagnosis of a congenital anomaly. However, as a relatively efficient method for surfacing and testing hypotheses related to prescription medications, these studies hold significant promise. Moreover, in some settings the use of automated records can be supplemented with chart abstraction and/or patient interviews to optimally match methods and purpose.

CHALLENGES FOR THE FUTURE

Existing methods of pharmacovigilance for medication-induced birth defects, taken as a whole, are limited in capacity to recognize a problem with a new pharmaceutical agent. These limitations are amplified if the drug is infrequently used by women of reproductive age, if the relative risk for congenital anomalies is not high, or if the associated birth defect(s) pattern is not unique, is difficult to diagnose, or is not likely to be diagnosed at birth. Existing methods also suffer from the need for large enough sample sizes, and the costs associated with supporting studies that are adequately powered.

One area of opportunity is improvement in the designs of pre-marketing reproductive toxicity studies. If the cross-species predictive value of these experiments can be increased, then it may be possible to avoid human exposure to new teratogens (Moore *et al.*, 1995; Lau *et al.*, 2000; Selevan *et al.*, 2000). Another possibility for the future is to take advantage of the large existing databases to "screen" for possible signals of major teratogenic effects of new and older medications. When strong signals are identified, other methods, such as case–control studies or small follow-up studies, might be appropriate for confirmation or refutation.

It is important to recognize that no single study design or methodology is sufficient to provide reassurance that new teratogens will be identified in a timely fashion. Therefore, a coordinated and systematic approach to evaluating new medications, both on a national and international basis, could contribute to more effective pharmacovigilance for birth defects, and provide information that is critically needed by clinicians and pregnant women.

REFERENCES

Andrews EB, Yankaskas BC, Cordero JF, Schoeffler K, Hampp S (1992) Acyclovir in pregnancy registry. *Obstet Gynecol* **79**: 7–13.

Belios E, Carsons S (1998) Rheumatologic disorders in women. *Med Clin N Am* **82**: 77–101.

Bonati M, Bortolus R, Marchetti F, Romero M, Tognoni G (1990) Drug use in pregnancy: an overview of epidemiological (drug utilization) studies. *Eur J Clin Pharmacol* **38**: 325–28.

Brent RL (1986) The complexities of solving the problem of human malformations. *Clinics in Perinatol* **13**: 491–503.

Castilla E, Peters PWJ (1992) Impact of monitoring systems: national and international efforts. In: Kuliev A, *et al.*, eds *Genetic Services Provision: An International Perspective. Birth Defects: Original Article Series*, Vol. 28. White Plains, NY: March of Dimes Birth Defects Foundation.

CDER (1999) *Report to the Nation: Improving Public Health Through Human Drugs*. US Department of Health and Human Services, Food and Drug Administration, Center for Drug Evaluation and Research.

Chung CS, Myrianthopoulos NC (1975) Factors affecting risks of congenital malformations. I. Analysis of epidemiologic factors in congenital malformations. Report from the Collaborative Perinatal Project. *Birth Defects* **11**: 1–22.

Czeizel AE, Rockenbauer M, Sørensen HT, Olsen J (2000) A population-based case–control teratologic study of oral chloramphenicol treatment during pregnancy. *Eur J Epidemiol* **16**: 323–7.

Derby LE, Myers MW, Jick H (1999) Use of dexfenfluramine, fenfluramine and phentermine and the risk of stroke *Br J Clin Pharmacol* **47**: 565–9.

Drinkard CR, Shatin D, Clouse J (2000) Postmarketing surveillance of medications and pregnancy outcomes: clarithromycin and birth malformations. *Pharmacoepidemiology and Drug Safety* **9**: 549–56.

Erickson JD (1991) The International Clearinghouse for Birth Defects Monitoring Systems: past, present, and future. *Intnl J Risk Safety Med* **2**: 255–70.

Ericson, A, Källén B, Wiholm B (1999) Delivery outcome after the use of antidepressants in early pregnancy. *Eur J Clin Pharmacol* **55**: 503–8.

Forrest JD (1994) Epidemiology of unintended pregnancy and contraceptive use. *Am J Obstet Gynecol* **170**: 1485–89.

Goldberg HL, Nissim R (1994) Psychotropic drugs in pregnancy and lactation. *Intnl J Psych Med* **24**: 129–49.

Goldman SA, Kennedy DL (1998) MedWatch FDA's medical products reporting program. *Postgrad Med* **103**: 13–6.

Goldstein DJ, Corbin LA, Sundell KL (1997) Effects of first-trimester fluoxetine exposure on the newborn. *Obstet Gynecol* **89**: 713–18.

Hernández-Díaz S, Werler MM, Walker AM, Mitchell AA (2000) Folic acid antagonists during pregnancy and the risk of birth defects. *New Engl J Med* **343**: 1608–14.

Holmes LB, Harvey EA, Brown KS, Hayes AM, Khoshbin S (1994) Anticonvulsant teratogenesis: I. A study design for newborn infants. *Teratology* **49**: 202–7.

Jick SS (1999) Pregnancy outcomes after maternal exposure to fluconazole. *Pharmacotherapy* **19**: 221–2.

Jick SS, Terris BZ (1997) Anticonvulsants and congenital malformations. *Pharmacotherapy* **17**: 561–4.

Jick SS, Terris BZ, Jick H (1993) First trimester topical tretinoin and congenital disorders. *Lancet* **341**: 1181–2.

Jones KL, Lacro RV, Johnson KA, Adams J (1989) Pattern of malformations in the children of women treated with carbamazepine during pregnancy. *New Engl J Med* **320**: 1661–6.

Kessler DA (1993) Introducing MedWatch: a new approach to reporting medication and device adverse effects and product problems. *J Am Med Assoc* **269**: 2765–8.

Kessler RC, McGonagie KA, Swartz M, Blazer DG, Nelson CB (1993) Sex and depression in the National Cormorbidity Survey. I: lifetime prevalence, chronicity and recurrence. *J Affective Disorders* **29**: 85–96.

Khoury MJ, Botto L, Mastriacovo P, Skjaerven R, Castilla E, Erickson JD (1994a) Monitoring for multiple congenital anomalies: an international perspective. *Epidemiol Rev* **16**: 35–50.

Khoury MJ, Botto L, Waters GD, Mastroiacovo P, Castilla E, Erickson JD (1993) Monitoring for new multiple congenital anomalies in the search for human teratogens. *Am J Med Gen* **46**: 460–66.

Khoury MJ, James LM, Erickson JD (1994b) On the use of affected controls to address recall bias in case–control studies of birth defects. *Teratology* **49**: 273–81.

Lacroix I, Damase-Michele C, Lapeyre-Mestre M, Montastruc JL (2000) Prescription of drugs during pregnancy in France. *Lancet* **356**: 1735–6.

Lammer EJ, Chen DT, Hoar RM, *et al.* (1985) Retinoic acid embryopathy. *New Engl J Med* **313**: 837–41.

Larsen H, Nielsen GL, Sorensen HT, Moller M, Olsen J, Schonheyder HC (2000) A follow-up study of birth outcome in users of pivampicillin during pregnancy. *Acta Obstet Gynecol Scand* **79**: 379–83.

Lau C, Andersen ME, Crawford-Brown DJ, Kavlock RJ, Kimmel CA, Knudsen TB, Muneoka K, Rogers JM, Setzer RW, Smith G, Tyl R (2000) Evaluation of biologically based dose-response modeling for developmental toxicity: a workshop report. *Regulat Toxicol Pharmacol* **31**: 190–9.

Lenz W (1961) Diskussionsbemerkung zu dem Vortrag von R.A. Pfeiffer und K. Kosenow: zur Frage der exogenen Entstehung schwere Extremitatenmissbildungen. *Tagung Rheinischwestfal Kinderarztevere Dusseldorf* **19**: 11.

McBride WG (1961) Thalidomide and congenital abnormalities. *Lancet* **2**: 1358.

McElhatton PR, Bateman DN, Evans C, Pughe KR, Thomas SH (1999) Congenital anomalies after prenatal ecstasy exposure. *Lancet* **354**: 1441–2.

Mitchell AA, Rosenberg L, Shapiro S, Slone D (1981) Birth defects related to Bendectin use in pregnancy: 1. oral clefts and cardiac defects. *J Am Med Assoc* **245**: 2311–4.

Moore JA, Daston GP, Faustman E, Golub MS, Hart WL, Huges C Jr, Kimmel CA, Lamb JC IV, Schwetz BA, Scialli AR (1995) An evaluative process of assessing human reproductive and developmental toxicity of agents. *Reproduc Toxicol* **9**: 61–95.

Pastuszak A, Schick-Boschetto, B, Zuber, C, Feldkamp M, Pinelli M, Sihn S, Donnenfeld A, McCormack M, Leen-Mitchell M, Woodland C, *et al.* (1993) Pregnancy outcome following first-trimester exposure to fluoxetine (Prozac). *J Am Med Assoc* **269**: 2246–8.

Pastuszak, AL, Schüler L, Speck-Martins, CE, Coelho KE, Cordello SM, *et al.* (1998) Use of misoprostol during pregnancy and Möbius' syndrome in infants. *New Engl J Med* **338**: 1881–5.

Preboth, M. (2000) The antiretroviral pregnancy registry interim report. *Am Fam Physician* **61**: 2265.

Prieto L, Martínez-Frias ML (2000) Response to "What kind of controls to use in case control studies of

malformed infants: recall bias versus 'teratogen nonspecificity' bias". *Teratology* **62**: 372–3.

Pryde PG, Sedman AB, Nugent CE, Barr M, Jr (1993) Angiotensin-convering enzyme inhibitor fetopathy. *J Am Soc Nephrol* **3**: 1575–82.

Rosa F. (1999) Databases in the assessment of the effects of drugs during pregnancy. *J Allergy Clin Immunol* **103**: S360–1.

Rosenberg HM, Bentura SG, Maurer JD, *et al.* (1996) *Births and Deaths, United States, 1994.* Hyattsville, MD: US Department of Health and Human Services, Public Health Service, CDC, National Center for Health Statistics. (Monthly vital statistics report; vol. 45, no 3, suppl.)

Schaefer C, Amoura-Elefant E, Vial T, Ornoy A, Garbis H, Robert E, Rodriguez-Pinilla E, Pexieder T, Prapas N, Merlob P (1996) Pregnancy outcome after prenatal quinolone exposure. Evaluation of a case registry of the European Network of Teratology Information Services (ENTIS) *Eur J Obstet, Gynecol, Reproduc Biol* **69**: 83–9.

Schou M; Goldfield MD, Weinstein MR (1973) A Villeneuve, lithium and pregnancy. I. Report from the Register of Lithium Babies. *Br Med J* **2**: 135–6.

Scialli, AR. (1999) The Organization of Teratology Information Services (OTIS) Registry Study. *J Allergy Clin Immunol* **103**: S373–6.

Selevan SG, Kimmel CA, Mendola P (2000) Identifying critical windows of exposure for children's health. *Teratology* **61**: 448.

Tabacova S, Vega A, McCloskey C, Kimmel CA (2000) Enalapril exposure during pregnancy: adverse developmental outcomes reported to FDA. *Teratology* **61**: 520.

Tomeo CA, Rich-Edwards JW, Michels KB, Berkey CS, Hunter DJ, *et al.* (1999) Reproducibility and validity of maternal recall of pregnancy-related events. *Epidemiology* **10**: 774–7.

Wen SW, Demissie K, Liu S (2001) Adverse outcomes in pregnancies of asthmatic women: results from a Canadian population. *Ann Epidemiol* **11**: 7–12.

Werler MM, Mitchell AA, Shapiro S (1992) First trimester maternal medication use in relation to gastroschisis. *Teratology* **45**: 361–7.

Werler MM, Shapiro S, Mitchell AA (1993) Periconceptional folic acid exposure and risk of occurrent neural tube defects. *J Am Med Assoc* **269**: 1257–61.

White AD, Andrews EB (1999) The pregnancy registry program at Glaxo Wellcome Company. *J Allergy Clin Immunol* **103**: S362–3.

Yerby MS (2000) Quality of life, epilepsy advances, and the evolving role of anticonvulsants in women with epilepsy. *Neurology* **55** (Suppl 1): S21–S31.

40

ADRs and Drug Safety 1999–2000

PAULINE CUREL AND ROSIE STATHER

Adis International Ltd, Aukland, New Zealand

INTRODUCTION

At the invitation of the editors of this textbook on *Pharmacovigilance* in this chapter we provide listings of adverse drug reaction (ADR) highlights for the years 1999 and 2000. These listings were first published in the Adis publication *Reactions Weekly*. They are reproduced in this volume with the consent of Adis International Ltd, a Wolters Kluwer Company, and because the editors believe them to be informative and of special relevance. Particular attention is drawn to those sections of this material concerned with market withdrawals/ suspensions and additional labelling changes and regulatory actions.

These listings allow the reader to consider which drugs and drug classes attracted attention and regulatory action in the relevant years. They also allow consideration of which bodily systems and system-organ classes were affected by the adverse events that precipitated regulatory action or were the cause of concern.

The small superscript numbers in the text indicate the issue and page number of *Reactions Weekly* in which the relevant information originally appeared and from where that information can be retrieved.

ADR HEADLINES FROM 1999

In 1999, confidence in vaccinations received another blow following the withdrawal of rota-virus vaccine ("RotaShield") because of reports of intussusception, and there was misleading press coverage regarding the safety of the measles, mumps and rubella (MMR) vaccine. Investigations continued into the link between anorectic agents and valvular heart disease, the safety of sildenafil, and metabolic disorders associated with protease inhibitors. Fluoroquino-lones came into the spotlight when marketing of trovafloxacin and its IV formulation alatro-floxacin was suspended in Europe because of hepatotoxicity, and grepafloxacin was withdrawn worldwide later in the year following reports of fatal cardiovascular events.

"ROTASHIELD" WITHDRAWN IN THE UNITED STATES

In July 1999, the US Centers for Disease Control and Prevention (CDC) and the American Academy of Pediatrics (AAP) recommended tempora-rily suspending the use of rotavirus vaccine

Pharmacovigilance. Edited by R.D. Mann and E.B. Andrews
© 2002 John Wiley & Sons, Ltd

("RotaShield") in infants, pending results of a case–control study to investigate a possible link between the vaccine and intussusception.[761:3] At this time, there had been 20 cases of intussusception in infants vaccinated with "RotaShield". Manufacturers of "RotaShield", Wyeth Lederle, suspended shipments of the vaccine at this time and sent out a letter to US physicians. The CDC subsequently began a review to determine whether intussusception is associated with rotavirus vaccine and other vaccines, in particular orally delivered vaccines.[772:2]

As of 9 September 1999, 99 cases of intussusception in children vaccinated with "RotaShield" had been reported to the US Vaccine Adverse Events Reporting System (VAERS).[772:2] In October, Wyeth Lederle withdrew "RotaShield" from distribution in the United States, stating that the data continued to suggest a temporal association between administration of the vaccine and intussusception.[774:2]

THIOMERSAL TO BE REMOVED FROM VACCINES

Because of the potential risks associated with thiomersal-containing vaccines, the US Public Health Service (PHS) and the AAP, along with vaccine manufacturers, the US Food and Drug Administration (FDA) and European regulatory agencies, have agreed that thiomersal should be removed from vaccines as soon as possible.[760:2] The PHS and the AAP worked together to ensure that the replacement of vaccines containing thiomersal is managed as quickly as possible while maintaining high vaccination coverage levels in children.

In September, the AAP published interim guidelines to clinicians on infant immunisation practices in light of concerns over thiomersal.[777:2] The AAP believes that physicians should minimise children's exposure to thiomersal. However, they emphasised that the use of vaccines containing thiomersal is preferable to withholding vaccinations. In their opinion, "the larger risks of not vaccinating children far outweigh any known risk of exposure to thiomersal-containing vaccines".

MORE BAD PRESS FOR MMR VACCINE

The safety of the MMR vaccination was brought into question in 1998 following a report by UK researchers suggesting a link with inflammatory bowel disease (IBD) and autism.[691:2] Concerns over the MMR vaccine were raised again in 1999 following the publication of another study by the same researchers in April linking atypical viral infections in childhood with IBD in later life.[757:2] However, one of the study researchers, Dr Scott Montgomery, later emphasised that this study did not show any link between IBD and MMR vaccine, because they did not study the vaccine. The media coverage of the study findings was criticised by the UK Department of Health. Furthermore, a panel investigating the study concluded that there was no evidence indicating a link between the MMR vaccine and IBD (or autism) so there is no reason to change the MMR vaccination policy. Results of another study conducted by Professor Brent Taylor and colleagues from the United Kingdom also indicated that there is no causal association between the MMR vaccine and autism.[756:5]

OTHER VACCINE ADRS REFUTED

In January, the safety of hepatitis B vaccine was questioned again by a US patient advocacy group who were concerned about the number of reports of serious adverse events and deaths in American children linked with hepatitis B vaccination.[736:3] The hepatitis B school vaccination campaign was suspended in France in 1998 amidst concerns over a possible link with the onset or reactivation of multiple sclerosis and other demyelinating diseases. However, the available evidence does not demonstrate a causal association between hepatitis B vaccination and such diseases, according to the Viral Hepatitis Prevention Board, a WHO Collaborating Centre for the prevention and control of viral hepatitis.[741:3] The Board concluded that there is no need to change current hepatitis B immunisation public health policies. Results of a large population-based study published in September also showed no evidence that recombinant hepatitis B vaccination is linked with demyelinating diseases.[773:5]

The possible association between vaccination and type I diabetes mellitus that was previously found in animal studies has also been refuted by several researchers. After reviewing the available information, the Institute for Vaccine Safety at the Johns Hopkins School of Public Health concluded that there is no evidence that any childhood vaccines increase the risk of type I diabetes mellitus in humans.[746:2]

ANORECTICS AND HEART VALVE DISORDERS

In 1999, investigation into the link between anorectic agents and valvular heart disease continued following the worldwide market withdrawal of fenfluramine and dexfenfluramine in September 1997. US research suggested that the risk of valvular heart disease may be related to the dosage and duration of therapy, and that the risk may decrease after discontinuation of therapy.

Dr Neil Weissman and colleagues reported that their previous finding of a slight increase in heart valve regurgitation with short-term (2–3 months') dexfenfluramine,[719:3] is no longer present 4–5 months after discontinuation of the agent.[757:3]

Dr D.H. Ryan and colleagues reported that 16.5% of patients treated with fenfluramine or dexfenfluramine in combination with mazindol or phentermine developed new valvular regurgitation.[767:5] They found that duration of anorectic therapy >6 months was the only factor significantly associated with the development of valvular regurgitation in the study patients.

Dr R. Li and colleagues reported that the severity of valvulopathy may increase with increasing fenfluramine dosage in patients receiving a combination of fenfluramine and phentermine.[781:4]

OVERALL RISK IS LOW

Dr Andrew Burger and colleagues reported that combination treatment with fenfluramine and phentermine for up to 30 months for obesity is associated with a low prevalence of significant valvular heart disease.[779:5] Overall, 8% of their patients developed significant valvular regurgita-

tion as defined by US FDA criteria. This incidence is similar to that previously reported in a population-based cohort from the Framingham Heart Study. Thus, the researchers suggested that the valvular abnormalities seen in their study may be associated with age-related degenerative changes.

Dr Christina Wee and colleagues also reported that the risk of new or progressive valvular heart disease associated with the use of fenfluramine and dexfenfluramine (for ≥ 14 days) may be lower than previously reported.[735:6] Results of their study showed an incidence of only 4.3%, as compared with previously reported incidences ranging up to more than 30%.

Dr B.K. Shively and colleagues reported a significantly lower prevalence of aortic regurgitation in dexfenfluramine recipients who had undergone echocardiogram ≥ 8 months after discontinuing the agent, compared with those who underwent echocardiogram earlier.[780:6]

UNRESOLVED ISSUES WITH "VIAGRA"

Following its launch in 1998, sildenafil ("Viagra") continued to attract a lot of interest in 1999. In August 1998, the American College of Cardiology (ACC) and the American Heart Association (AHA) issued interim recommendations for sildenafil prescribing in patients with cardiovascular disease.[717:2] Subsequently, in January 1999, an expert consensus document was released by the ACC and AHA reiterating their previously released recommendations.[738:2]

The ACC and AHA also stated that more research is needed into the effects of sildenafil in certain high-risk patients with significant cardiovascular disease. Other unresolved issues identified by the ACC and AHA included interactions with non-aspirin antiplatelet agents, interactions with other phosphodiesterase inhibitors, central nervous system (CNS) effects, hypotensive effects in high-risk cardiac patients (e.g. those with severe heart failure), and musculoskeletal effects (myalgia and chest pains) that may be mistaken for angina.

In January, findings reported by German researchers suggested that sildenafil is associated with reversible retinal dysfunction in healthy volunteers.[737:4] They suggested that retinal function should be monitored in patients taking sildenafil. Other researchers from Germany stated that such monitoring was unnecessary, but they suggested that people with retinal impairment related to genetic phosphodiesterase effects should be advised not to take sildenafil.

INTERACTION WITH PROTEASE INHIBITORS

Concerns were also raised in 1999 of a probable interaction between sildenafil and protease inhibitors leading to a potentiation of the effects of sildenafil and an increased likelihood of adverse effects.[742:3] In Europe, Pfizer and European Union regulators agreed to a sildenafil labelling change that concomitant treatment with ritonavir is not advised, and planned to expand the drug interaction precaution to include other protease inhibitors.[751:2] Similarly, in the United States, the FDA and Pfizer discussed updating the labelling of sildenafil to include a warning about possible interactions with protease inhibitors.[751:2]

In September, the Japanese Ministry of Health and Welfare issued another warning against unregulated use of sildenafil without proper consultation with a physician.[769:2] At the time, a total of 33 adverse reactions associated with sildenafil had been reported in Japan, including 2 deaths; sildenafil had been prescribed by a doctor in only 8 of the 33 cases. Also, in September, the UK Medicines Control Agency (MCA) had received 31 reports of death possibly associated with sildenafil[770:2] and the French Health Products Safety Agency had received 33 such reports.[775:5]

METABOLIC DISORDERS COMMON WITH PROTEASE INHIBITORS

The association between protease inhibitors and metabolic disorders such as hyperglycaemia, insulin resistance, hyperlipidaemia and lipodystrophy is becoming increasingly recognised and study findings reported in 1999 indicate that such disorders are common with these antiretrovirals. In June, Dr Andrew Carr and colleagues from

Australia reported an 83% incidence of lipodystrophy syndrome in HIV-positive patients after a mean of 21 months' therapy with protease inhibitors.[757:5] Thus, they recommended that patients receiving protease inhibitors should have glucose tolerance and fasting lipid levels assessed early in therapy and regularly (perhaps annually) thereafter. The following month, Dr G. Behrens and colleagues from Germany reported that 46% of patients taking protease inhibitors had impaired oral glucose tolerance, 13% had diabetes mellitus and 71% had hyperlipidaemia.[768:4] Furthermore, in September, researchers from Germany suggested that protease inhibitors may increase the risk of myocardial infarction 5-fold[773:6] and researchers from the United States reported that indinavir is associated with a significantly increased risk of hypertension.[776:6]

PROTEASE INHIBITORS MAY NOT BE THE CULPRIT

Other research reported in 1999 raised the possibility that protease inhibitors may not be the cause of metabolic disorders in patients with HIV infection. Researchers from Roche, US, suggested that the lipodystrophy syndrome may be related to HIV infection itself, and may be unmasked by prolonged survival during treatment with protease inhibitors.[734:2]

UK researchers reported that lipodystrophy occurred in 16% of patients receiving nevirapine-containing highly active antiretroviral therapy; none of these patients received protease inhibitors.[767:4] Researchers from France reported a significant association between lipodystrophy and lamivudine and stavudine therapy.[768:5] However, they stated that this finding may be biased and that intensification of therapy with a protease inhibitor does seem to increase the risk of lipodystrophy. Other researchers from France reported that lipodystrophy is associated with long-term treatment with nucleoside reverse transcriptase inhibitors, providing further evidence of the occurrence of lipodystrophy in HIV-positive patients treated with non protease inhibitor-containing regimens.[774:5]

Table 40.1. Additional labelling changes and regulatory actions in 1999.

Drug/drug class	Labelling changes/regulatory action
Cefoselis ("Wincef")	"Dear Doctor" letter issued in Japan and labelling strengthened regarding CNS disorders.[735:2]
Butyrolactone and related agents	US FDA requested manufacturers to recall butyrolactone-containing products following reports of serious adverse effects[736:2] and later issued a warning to consumers regarding other related agents such as 1,4 butanediol.[752:3]
Urokinase ("Abbokinase")	US FDA issues warning about potential risk of transmission of infectious agents because of serious manufacturing deficiencies.[737:2] Product labelling updated by Abbott.
Fluvastatin ("Lescol")	Labelling amended to reduce liver function monitoring requirements.[745:3]
Troglitazone ("Romozin"; "Rezulin")	Glaxo Wellcome's application to reintroduce troglitazone in the UK is rejected.[745:2] "Dear Healthcare Professional" letter issued and prescribing information updated in the US.[757:3]
Pramipexole ("Mirapex"/ "Mirapexin"/"Sifrol")	Labelling updated in the European Union warning about the possibility of sudden onset of sleep.[763:3] "Dear Healthcare Professional" letter issued and labelling changes in the US.[771:2]
Ropinirole ("ReQuip")	"Dear Healthcare Professional" letter issued and labelling updated in the EU about sudden onset of sleep.[781:2]
Etanercept ("Enbrel")	"Dear Doctor" letter issued and labelling updated in the US about serious infections.[752:2]
Cisapride ("Propulsid")	"Dear Doctor" letter issued and labelling updated in the US regarding new contraindications and drug interactions.[756:2]
Pemoline ("Cylert")	"Dear Healthcare Professional" letter issued and labelling updated about an association with life-threatening liver failure.[757:4]
Ticlopidine	"Dear Doctor" letter issued and labelling updated regarding thrombotic thrombocytopenic purpura liver failure and agranulocytosis.[761:2]
Aristolochia	Products containing *Aristolochia* banned in the UK.[763:2]
Ophthalmic diclofenac	Additional labelled warnings regarding serious corneal adverse events.[768:3]
Pimozide ("Orap")	"Dear Healthcare Provider" letter issued and labelling updated in the US regarding unexpected deaths with high doses.[771:3] Revised labelling also states that drugs that are inhibitors of CYP3A are contraindicated with pimozide.
IV human immunoglobulins	Canadian Bureau of Drug Surveillance issues warning about precautions that should be taken to decrease the risk of acute renal failure.[748:2] Similar action taken by the US FDA.[772:2]
Flutamide ("Eulexin")	"Dear Health Professional" letter issued and labelling revised in the US regarding liver toxicity.[771:3]
Leflunomide ("Arava")	European Medicines Evaluation Agency issues urgent safety information regarding the possibility of rare serious adverse effects including pancytopenia and skin reactions.[777:2] Launch of the drug delayed in the EU.
Didanosine ("Videx")	"Dear Healthcare Provider" letter issued and labelling revised about pancreatitis.[779:3]

VISUAL FIELD DEFECTS COMMON WITH VIGABATRIN

The reporting in 1997 of visual field defects, almost always asymptomatic, in several patients receiving long-term vigabatrin has led to extensive re-evaluation of its use. Preliminary data suggest that this defect occurs in approximately one-third of vigabatrin recipients, although two studies presented at the 23rd International Epilepsy Congress in the Czech Republic in September 1999 reported a slightly higher rate (52% and 45%).[773:3] Also in September, researchers from Finland reported a 40% incidence of visual field defects in patients receiving vigabatrin.[779:6] Furthermore, interim results of a large prescription event monitoring study have shown objective evidence of visual field defects in 0.8% of patients treated with vigabatrin.[776:6] In view of the risk of irreversible visual field defects with vigabatrin, the UK Committee on Safety of Medicines (CSM) and the MCA advised of new prescribing restrictions for the agent in November.[779:2] In effect, the agent can only be prescribed when all other appropriate anticonvulsant drug combinations are ineffective or poorly tolerated. However, vigabatrin remains first-line therapy for infantile spasms. The European Union (EU) product information for vigabatrin was updated to include the new prescribing restrictions.

MARKET WITHDRAWALS/SUSPENSIONS

In January 1999, Servier announced plans to withdraw amineptine ("Survector") from the market in France because of the risk of addiction associated with the agent.[737:2] Amineptine was subsequently withdrawn in Spain,[739:4] Portugal[741:3] and Italy.[743:3]

Paediatric formulations of nimesulide were suspended in Portugal in April by Infarmed, the Portugese Pharmacy and Medicines institute.[750:2] The move followed reports of serious adverse reactions, including hepatotoxicity, in children receiving nimesulide that were received by Portugal's National Pharmacovigilance centre.

In May, prescribing information for trovafloxacin ("Trovan") and its IV formulation, alatrofloxacin, were strengthened in Europe following reports of severe hepatotoxicity.[755:2] In the United States, the FDA issued a public health advisory to physicians regarding the risk of hepatotoxicity and recommended restricted use of these agents. In June, marketing of trovafloxacin and alatrofloxacin was suspended in Europe.[758:2]

Janssen announced the voluntary withdrawal of astemizole from all markets in June.[757:2] The decision was supported by the US FDA in light of the choice of other antihistamines now available and the overall risk/benefit profile of astemizole.

In 1999, the European Commission's Committee on Proprietary Medicinal Products (CPMP) recommended that various anorectics should be withdrawn from the market because of their questionable efficacy and risk of dependency. The anorectic agents concerned were amfepramone, phentermine, clobenzorex, fenproporex, mefenorex, norpseudoephedrine and phendimetrazine. The relevant products were subsequently suspended in Spain,[772:3] France and Portugal.[773:2]

Glaxo Wellcome voluntarily withdrew grepafloxacin ("Raxar") in October from > 30 countries worldwide due to cardiovascular safety concerns.[776:2] The company had received 7 reports of cardiovascular event-related fatalities associated with the drug. Glaxo Wellcome stated that, while these cardiovascular events are infrequent, it was no longer convinced that the benefits of grepafloxacin therapy outweighed the potential risk to patients, considering the availability of alternative antibacterials.

In October, Wyeth Lederle's live oral rotavirus vaccine ("RotaShield") was withdrawn in the United States because of concerns about a possible association with intussusception (*see above*).

Additional labelling changes and regulatory actions that occurred in 1999 are given in Table 40.1.

ADR HIGHLIGHTS FROM 2000

The 2000 drug safety arena was notable for the large number of labelling changes and regulatory actions that resulted from safety concerns. Investigations into the association between antiretroviral drugs and metabolic disorders continued. After receiving a lot of bad press in previous years, the news on vaccines in 2000 was more positive.

In 2000, two drugs that have been on the market for many years, cisapride and phenylpropanolamine, were withdrawn in some markets due to concern over adverse reactions. Action was taken with cisapride because of continued reports of heart disorders and deaths associated with this agent, and with phenylpropanolamine after this drug was linked to stroke in a US study.

CISAPRIDE WITHDRAWN/SUSPENDED IN MANY MARKETS

Since cisapride ("Propulsid") was approved in the United States in 1993, labelling has been strengthened several times because of reports of heart rhythm disorders and deaths. In January 2000, the US FDA again strengthened the labelled warnings for cisapride because of continued reports of heart disorders and deaths, particularly in patients taking certain concomitant drugs or in patients with underlying risk factors.[786:2] Up to 31 December 1999, cisapride had been associated with 341 reports of heart rhythm abnormalities, including 80 deaths. In March, Janssen announced that it would stop marketing cisapride in the United States in July.[795:2] However, cisapride will remain available for certain US patients through a limited access programme.

In June, Health Canada requested that Janssen–Ortho withdraw cisapride ("Prepulsid") in Canada after receiving 44 reports of potential heart rhythm abnormalities, including 10 deaths in patients receiving the agent; pharmacy sales of the product were stopped in Canada in August.[807:2] However, cisapride remains available through Health Canada's Special Access Programme for patients who do not respond to alternative therapies for gastro-oesophageal reflux. Also in June, the German regulatory authority announced that it intended to suspend the marketing of two cisapride products, "Propulsin" and "Alimix" in Germany.[810:2]

SIMILAR ACTION TAKEN IN THE UNITED KINGDOM

The following month, the UK CSM issued a "Dear Health Professional" letter advising that the marketing of cisapride ("Prepulsid") would be suspended in the United Kingdom.[812:2] At this time, there had been 60 reports of serious cardiovascular events, 5 of which were fatal, reported via the "yellow card" scheme since the authorisation of cisapride in the United Kingdom in 1988. The CSM had previously issued warnings about cisapride, but serious cardiovascular events and fatalities continued to be reported. Also in July, the French health products safety agency announced that cisapride would remain on the market in France, but its use would be restricted.[813:3]

Later in the year, manufacturers of cisapride in Japan temporarily halted the production and sale of cisapride products ("Acenalin", "Risamol").[826:5] Since cisapride was launched in Japan in 1989, 41 cardiovascular adverse events have been reported; 19 of these were relatively serious.

PHENYLPROPANOLAMINE LINKED WITH STROKE

In November, the US FDA issued a public health advisory concerning the potential risk of stroke with phenylpropanolamine and took steps to remove the agent from all drug products, including nasal decongestants and bodyweight control products.[827:2] These steps came following the findings of a US study that showed an increased risk of haemorrhagic stroke associated with phenylpropanolamine use.[827:5] The findings of this study were due to be published in the 21 December issue of *New England Journal of Medicine*, but were released in early November because of the potential public health implications.

FURTHER MARKET WITHDRAWALS

Within a week of the release of these study findings, phenylpropanolamine products were voluntarily withdrawn by several companies in the United States.[828:2] Novartis Consumer Health voluntarily withdrew its phenylpropanolamine-containing cold and allergy products and announced that they had started to reformulate the products using pseudoephedrine as the decongestant ingredient. Over-the-counter phenylpropanolamine-containing products were also voluntarily withdrawn in the United States by the Eckerd Corporation, one of the largest retail drug chains in the United States, and by Longs Drugs. Furthermore, a leading online wholesaler of nutritional supplements, vitacost.com, now refuses to sell products containing phenylpropanolamine and has urged other online retailers to do the same.

In Canada, SmithKline Beecham announced that it was voluntarily withdrawing phenylpropanolamine-containing products in view of the FDA public health advisory which was reinforced by Health Canada's subsequent health advisory.[828:2] Other countries, including Brazil, Singapore, Thailand and Malaysia, are also following the line of the US FDA in recommending the withdrawal of phenylpropanolamine-containing products from their markets.[831:2]

APPROACH DIFFERS IN THE UNITED KINGDOM AND EUROPE

In the United Kingdom, the CSM issued a "Dear Healthcare Professional" letter regarding the evidence of a link between phenylpropanolamine and stroke.[829:2] After conducting an initial review, the CSM concluded that the evidence for the link was weak and mainly associated with indications which are not licensed in the United Kingdom. European regulatory authorities are taking a similar approach as in the United Kingdom.[831:2] Statements have been issued by all European authorities advising that all phenylpropanolamine-containing products should remain on the market pending a review of the situation.

ALOSETRON WITHDRAWN IN THE UNITED STATES

In August, Glaxo Wellcome issued a "Dear Health Care Professional" letter in the United States advising of important new safety information regarding constipation and ischaemic colitis associated with alosetron ("Lotronex"), and the product labelling was updated accordingly.[817:2] The warnings followed post-marketing reports of serious complications of constipation associated with the use of this treatment for irritable bowel

syndrome, including obstruction, impaction, toxic megacolon, perforation, secondary ischaemia and ischaemic colitis. The US Public Citizen group demanded that the US FDA remove alosetron from the market in view of the increasing number of reports of these complications.[829:2] Subsequently, in November, Glaxo Wellcome voluntarily withdrew alosetron from the US market in response to a request by the US FDA.[830:2] However, the company stated that they believed that the benefits of using alosetron outweigh the risks and that they greatly regret withdrawing the drug from the US market. Glaxo Wellcome has abandoned plans to launch alosetron in other markets.

METABOLIC DISORDERS WITH PROTEASE INHIBITORS ...

Investigation into the association between protease inhibitors and metabolic disorders, such as hyperlipidaemia, hyperglycaemia, insulin resistance and lipodystrophy, continued in 2000. In January, Dr J.Q. Purnell and colleagues from the United States reported that ritonavir therapy in healthy volunteers results in increased triglyceride and cholesterol levels that are independent of changes in body composition or interactions with inflammatory conditions associated with HIV infection.[790:3] Dr K. Mulligan and colleagues from the United States also reported that the effects of protease inhibitors on glucose control and lipid metabolism occurred in the absence of significant increases in bodyweight or changes in body fat distribution in HIV-positive patients.[796:3] In view of their findings, they concluded that these metabolic effects may be a direct effect of protease inhibitors rather than the result of central fat accumulation.

... AND NRTIs

Also in January, Dr T. Saint-Marc and colleagues from France reported that lipodystrophy syndrome in HIV-positive patients should be subdivided into three main types: a lipoatrophy syndrome associated with increased triglyceride levels; a subcutaneous adiposity syndrome (obesity); and a mixed or fat redistribution syndrome.[790:4] In their study, they found that stavudine therapy was significantly associated with lipoatrophy, compared with zidovudine. Lamivudine and didanosine therapy were not significantly associated with fat distribution abnormalities, and neither was protease inhibitor therapy. In February, Dr A. Carr and colleagues from Australia reported that both protease inhibitors and nucleoside reverse transcriptase inhibitors (NRTIs) can contribute to the lipodystrophy syndrome, but the symptoms and metabolic features of the syndrome differ between these two drug classes.[802:4] And in July, Dr Simon Mallal and colleagues from Australia reported that NRTIs independently contribute to fat wasting in HIV infection and this effect is greatest with stavudine.[812:4] Furthermore, they found that the combination of NRTI and protease inhibitor is synergistic in terms of leading to fat wasting.

PROTEASE INHIBITORS LINKED WITH BONE DISORDERS

In March, Dr P. Tebas and colleagues from the United States reported that bone mineral loss is accelerated in HIV-infected patients receiving potent antiretroviral therapy that includes protease inhibitors.[798:3] They also found that bone mineral loss and body fat redistribution occur independently, suggesting that these adverse effects may be mediated through different mechanisms. Subsequently, at the annual meeting of the American Orthopedic Association in June, Dr Guy Paiement reported a link between protease inhibitor therapy and avascular necrosis of the femoral head.[807:4]

GOOD NEWS FOR VACCINES

After receiving a lot of bad press in 1998 and 1999, vaccines received mostly positive attention in 2000. The safety of hepatitis B virus (HBV) vaccine was questioned in 1999 because of a possible link with neonatal death in the United States. However, a review of reports received by the US national Vaccine Adverse Event Reporting System (VAERS) provided reassurance that HBV vaccine is not associated with an increased risk of unexplained neonatal death.[786:2] The HBV school vaccination programme was suspended in France in 1998 amidst concerns over a possible link with the onset or reactivation of multiple sclerosis or other demyelinating diseases. However, results of a Canadian study published in February 2000 showed no evidence of an association between HBV vaccine and multiple sclerosis or post-infectious encephalomyelitis.[789:4]

Concerns over a potential link between measles, mumps and rubella (MMR) virus vaccine and inflammatory bowel disease and autism were first raised in 1998, but were subsequently refuted by the UK Department of Health. In 2000, the potential links were refuted again by the American Academy of Pediatrics, by Britain's Medical Research Council,[798:2] and by a study conducted by the US Centers for Disease Control and Prevention.[823:3]

In June, the UK Department of Health urged parents to continue to have their children immunised with the meningococcal group C conjugate vaccine, despite reports about adverse reactions, such as blackouts, seizures and headaches, that appeared in the UK media.[808:2] The department stated that the benefits of the vaccine are "overwhelming" and that the vaccine is "very safe". Also, in August, the UK CSM and the Joint Committee on Vaccination and Immunisation issued a "Dear Doctor" letter in the United Kingdom stating that the balance of risk and benefit associated with the meningococcal group C conjugate vaccine is "overwhelmingly favourable".[818:2]

NUMEROUS REGULATORY ACTIONS

The year 2000 was notable for the number of "Dear Healthcare Professional" letters, public health advisories, labelling changes and other regulatory actions that occurred in the United States and other major markets.

Rho(D) immunoglobulin: In January, the prescribing information for Rho(D) immunoglobulin ("WinRho SDF") was revised in the United States following reports of intravascular haemolysis in Rho(D)-positive patients with immune thrombocytopenic purpura receiving the product.[785:2] The revised product insert stated that such patients should be monitored for the development of intravascular haemolysis.

Zanamivir: The US FDA issued a public health advisory in January regarding serious respiratory problems associated with zanamivir ("Relenza") and recommended caution when using in patients with underlying respiratory problems.[785:2] A similar warning was issued in Europe.[788:2] Subsequently, in July, Glaxo Wellcome advised that the safety labelling of zanamivir had been revised accordingly.[811:3]

Abacavir: In January, Glaxo Wellcome issued a "Dear Health Care Provider" letter in the United States advising of revised labelling for abacavir ("Ziagen") regarding fatal hypersensitivity reactions in patients presenting with respiratory symptoms.[787:2] In July, the company issued another warning and advised of further labelling changes regarding serious hypersensitivity reactions after rechallenge with the product.[813:2] The following month, the European Agency for the Evaluation of Medicinal Products (EMEA) also issued a public statement on abacavir.[816:2]

Hypericum: In February, the US FDA issued a Public Health Advisory regarding an interaction between hypericum (St John's Wort) and indinavir and recommended against the concomitant use of hypericum and protease inhibitors.[789:2] In the United Kingdom, the CSM warned against the use of hypericum with indinavir, warfarin, cyclosporin, oral contraceptives, digoxin, theophylline and other products;[792:2] a similar warning was also issued by the EMEA[792:2] and by Health Canada.[808:2] In May, the US Consumer Healthcare Products Association announced that it had adopted a voluntary labelled warning programme for hypericum.[804:2] In Japan, the Ministry of Health and Welfare has also told manufacturers of many drugs to add a labelled warning regarding possible interactions with hypericum.[804:2]

Halothane: In March, Wyeth–Ayerst issued a "Dear Health Care Professional" letter in the United States regarding changes to the prescribing information for halothane ("Fluothane") because of an association with ventricular arrhythmias when used in outpatient dental surgery.[794:2]

Troglitazone: In March, the US FDA asked Parke-Davis/Warner-Lambert to withdraw troglitazone ("Rezulin") from the US market because of its association with severe liver toxicity.[795:2] Labelling of troglitazone has previously been strengthened in the United States several times and close monitoring of liver function has been recommended in patients receiving this agent.[757:3] Sankyo also decided to halt sales of troglitazone ("Noscal") in Japan.

Sodium citrate: In April, the US FDA issued an urgent warning to all hospital pharmacies and haemodialysis units to stop using the 46.7% sodium citrate anticoagulant ("TriCitrasol") as a haemodialysis catheter anticoagulant following a report of cardiac arrest and reports of other incidents.[798:2]

Amprenavir: In May, Glaxo Wellcome sent out a "Dear Health Care Professional" letter in the United States about potential safety concerns regarding amprenavir oral solution ("Agenerase") due to a high content of the excipient propylene glycol.[800:2]

Trastuzumab: Genentech sent out a "Dear Health Care Provider" letter in the United States in May regarding serious adverse events associated with trastuzumab ("Herceptin"), including severe hypersensitivity reactions, infusion reactions and pulmonary events.[802:2] Labelling of the product was subsequently updated accordingly.[826:5]

Aristolochic acid: In June, the US FDA sent out a "Dear Health Care Professional" letter outlining concerns over nephrotoxicity and potential carcinogenicity with products containing aristolochic acid.[805:2] In 1999, the UK CSM issued a temporary ban on the importation, sale and supply of such products in the United Kingdom,[763:2] and following the expiry of this ban, the Medicines Control Agency (MCA) proposed a permanent ban.[788:2]

Thioridazine: In July 2000, Novartis announced that a new boxed warning would be added to thioridazine ("Mellaril") in the United States regarding potentially life-threatening QTc interval prolongation following a request by the US FDA.[811:2] A similar warning letter was sent in Canada for thioridazine ("Melleril") the following month.[818:2] Then in December, the UK CSM issued a "Dear Health Care Professional" letter advising that thioridazine use would be restricted in the United Kingdom.[833:7]

Valproate: Labelling of Abbott's tablet and capsule formulations of valproate products ("Depakote", "Depacon" and "Depakene") were updated in the US in July to include a pancreatitis warning.[813:2]

Zafirlukast: In September, AstraZeneca sent a "Dear Health Care Provider" letter in the United States advising about changes to the labelling of zafirlukast ("Accolate") to reflect additional adverse events that have been reported over the past three years.[820:3]

Table 40.2. Additional labelling changes and regulatory actions in 2000.

Drug/drug class	Labelling changes/regulatory action
Anorectics	Licences for amfepramone and phentermine withdrawn in the European Union by the European Commission because of their unfavourable benefit/risk balance. The UK MCA later lifted the ban on amfepramone and then phentermine. Anorectic warnings strengthened in Switzerland.
Sertindole ("Serdolect")	European-wide suspension of marketing authorisation. Previously withdrawn in the UK in 1998 because of reports of cardiac arrhythmias and sudden cardiac death.
Pumactant ("Alec")	Marketing suspended in the UK due to higher mortality in premature neonates treated with this synthetic lung surfactant, compared with those treated with the porcine-derived surfactant poractant alfa.
Tick-borne encephalitis vaccine ("TicoVac")	Use suspended in children < 3 years of age in Germany because of reports of high fever.
Ropinirole ("ReQuip")	Sudden onset of sleep warning issued in Canada. Similar warning previously issued in the EU.
Benzbromarone	"Dear Doctor" letter issued in Japan regarding reports of hepatitis.
Loxoprofen ("Loxonin")	Hepatic warnings strengthened in Japan.
Cefcapene pivoxil ("Flomox")	Labelling updated in Japan to warn about hepatic effects and reduced platelet count.
Interferon-α ("Sumiferon")	Labelling updated in Japan to warn about haemolytic uraemic syndrome.
Budipine ("Parkinsan")	Marketing authorisation withdrawn in Germany in view of severe cardiovascular risks.
Selective serotonin reuptake inhibitors	UK MCA recommends a warning about suicide should be included in patient information leaflets.
Pioglitazone ("Actos")	"Dear Doctor" letter issued and labelling updated in Japan regarding oedema-linked heart failure.
Ursodeoxycholic acid	Labelling updated in Japan to warn about interstitial pneumonia.
Ozagrel sodium	Labelling updated in Japan to warn about renal dysfunction.
Diclofenac	"Dear Doctor" letter issued in Japan warning against use in patients with influenza-related encephalitis or encephalopathy.

Mesoridazine: In September, Novartis sent a "Dear Doctor or Pharmacist" letter in the United States advising of changes to the labelling of mesoridazine ("Serentil") regarding prolongation of the QTc interval.[824:3]

Basiliximab: In October, Novartis, sent a "Dear Health Care Provider" letter in the United States to advise of reports of severe hypersensitivity reactions following initial use of, or re-exposure to, basiliximab ("Simulect"); labelling was revised accordingly.[824:2]

Etanercept: In October, Wyeth–Ayerst and Immunex issued a "Dear Health Care Professional" letter in the United States warning about CNS disorders and blood dyscrasias associated with etanercept ("Enbrel") and of a revision to prescribing information.[824:2] EMEA had previously issued a similar warning for etanercept.[823:2]

Nevirapine: Labelled warnings on the risk of hepatotoxicity with nevirapine ("Viramune") were strengthened in the United States by Boehringer Ingelheim/Roxane Laboratories in November in view of the continued reports of severe, and in some cases fatal, hepatotoxicity.[828:2] Labelled warnings of nevirapine were also strengthened in Europe earlier in the year because of hepatic and cutaneous reactions.[801:2]

Tiratricol: In November, the US FDA issued a warning to consumers to stop taking dietary supplements that contain tiratricol (triiodothyroacetic acid), because it is a potent thyroid hormone that may cause serious adverse effects including heart attack and stroke.[830:3]

Capecitabine: ("Xeloda") labelling was also updated by Roche in November to warn about increased rates of adverse events in patients with renal impairment.[831:4]

Additional labelling changes and regulatory actions that occurred in 2000 are given in Table 40.2.

Part IV

LESSONS AND DIRECTIONS

41

Teaching Pharmacovigilance

RONALD MEYBOOM AND STEN OLSSON
The Uppsala Monitoring Centre, Stora Torget 3, Uppsala, Sweden
MARGARET THOROGOOD
London School of Hygiene and Tropical Medicine, London, UK

INTRODUCTION

Pharmacovigilance is concerned with the study of medicines after their approval and with the use of the ensuing information for education and drug regulation. Its ultimate aim is to foster the rational and safe use of medicines. The expertise needed in pharmacovigilance includes pharmacology, epidemiology, clinical medicine and drug legislation. A further need is the skill to write drug safety information in a clear but balanced way, to ensure that healthcare practitioners and patients are given reliable information that they can understand and use. Here is a link with the drug information profession.

Pharmacovigilance is not an established academic specialism and the current curricula of the training programmes of professions such as clinical medicine, clinical pharmacy, clinical pharmacology or medical biology do not cover all the skills needed in pharmacovigilance. Therefore, there is a need for the provision of special training packages for the (further) education of professionals in pharmacovigilance, either working at health authorities, pharmaceutical companies, universities, hospitals or health maintenance organisations. Another reason is that pharmacovigilance is in a comparatively early phase of development. Its procedures frequently change and novel approaches are enriching our armamentarium. One of the tasks of a pharmacovigilance centre is the creation of a "reporting culture". Healthcare professionals need to be made aware that all medicines can cause adverse reactions and that they have a responsibility to participate in the national pharmacovigilance system and to contribute to other drug evaluation studies, recommended by the health authorities or the professional associations. Therefore, already in the curricula of undergraduate medical and pharmaceutical students attention should be paid to adverse drug reactions (ADRs) and pharmacovigilance.

Up till the present day, national and international "spontaneous reporting" schemes for suspected ADFs have been a major source of information in pharmacovigilance. As is shown in Table 41.1, spontaneous reporting has four different "layers". First, there is the organisational structure needed to ensure that the necessary data are reported, assessed, stored, processed and distributed. Second, there is the use of these data

Pharmacovigilance. Edited by R.D. Mann and E.B. Andrews

Table 41.1. Spontaneous reporting has four different "layers".

1. The collection, assessment, processing and distribution of data (organisation, routines)
2. Drug regulation (risk management, legislation)
3. Science: methodology and procedures, data interpretation
4. Communication and education (feed-back)

Table 41.2. Outline of a pharmacovigilance course.

- Needs for and aims of pharmacovigilance
- Clinical medicine, pathology, pharmacology and epidemiology of adverse drug reactions
  - Drug interactions
  - Drugs in pregnancy
  - Drugs and lactation
- Practice of spontaneous reporting
  - Organisation and maintenance of a pharmacovigilance centre
  - IT aspects of spontaneous reporting
  - Case report assessment, terminologies, coding, standardised causality assessment
  - Principles of signal detection and follow-up
  - International collaboration; the WHO-UMC International Pharmacovigilance Programme
- Drug legislation and regulation; requirements and guidelines. International harmonisation and standardisation
- Principles of pharmacoepidemiology and the practice of other methods (e.g. prescription–event monitoring, case–control surveillance, database mining, nested case–control studies, comparative follow-up studies)
- Special fields, e.g.
  - Vaccine vigilance
  - Pharmaceutical defects; counterfeit
  - Drug dependence
- Literature sources
- Benefit–risk assessment
- Communications
  - Writing a report or a publication

for the postmarketing evaluation of medicines by a country's regulatory authority, in dialogue with the pharmaceutical companies. Here the emphasis is on prompt risk management, i.e. the taking of timely and appropriate actions (ranging from a data sheet change to the suspension or withdrawal of a licence). Third is the scientific basis of spontaneous reporting: the principles underlying the method, the appropriateness of procedures and routines, and the credibility of data interpretation. Finally, there is communication and education, in particular the dissemination of information to prescribers, pharmacists and patients.

THE UMC

Experience with the organisation of pharmacovigilance training courses at the WHO Uppsala Monitoring Centre (UMC) has shown that a number of basic components of a training programme can be put forward (see Table 41.2). Training programmes can be organised by academic units in a country, specialised in clinical pharmacology, clinical pharmacy or pharmacoepidemiology. As a rule, collaboration is recommended with the pharmacovigilance agency in the country and with additional disciplines in order to provide appropriate teaching in, for example, the clinical manifestations and pathology of ADRs, the practicalities of spontaneous reporting and drug regulation. Some examples of institutes regularly organising such programmes in Europe are given in Table 41.3. In addition, several commercial educational organisations in countries around the world organise more or less comprehensive training programmes, incidentally or regularly. At the international level, the UMC organises every other

year a training course for a mixed audience, coming from governmental agencies, academia and pharmaceutical companies. In addition, the UMC is committed to provide teaching material to national or regional teaching initiatives regarding, in particular, the practice of spontaneous reporting, the organisation of a pharmacovigilance centre, information technology, terminologies, harmonisation and standardisation, signal detection methodology and communications. An example is the recently published *Guidelines for Setting Up and Running a Pharmacovigilance Centre* (also in Spanish and available on the Internet: www.who-umc.org). As the global organisation of professionals working in pharmacovigilance, the International Society of

Table 41.3. Examples of institutes offering recurrent training in pharmacovigilance.

The Uppsala Monitoring Centre (WHO Collaborating Centre for International Drug Monitoring)	Stora Torget 3 S-753 20 Uppsala Sweden	tel: +46-18-656060 fax: +46-18-656080 e-mail: `info@who-umc.org` `www.who-umc.org`
London School of Hygiene and Tropical Medicine	50 Bedford Square London WC1B 3DP UK	tel: +44-20-72994648 fax: +44-20-73230638 e-mail: `shortcourses@lshtm.ac.uk` `www.lshtm.ac.uk`
University of Hertfordshire	Hatfield Campus College Lane, Hatfield Herts, AL10 9AB UK	tel: +44-1707 284800 fax: +44-1707 284870 e-mail: `admissions@herts.ac.uk` `www.herts.ac.uk`
University of Wales	Department of Pharmacology, Therapeutics & Toxicology, UWCM, Heath Park, Cardiff CF14 4XN, UK	tel: +44-29 20 747747 fax: +44-29 20 748316 `www.uwcm.ac.uk`
Vigilex	Oudedijk 9^B 3062 AB Rotterdam The Netherlands	tel: +31 10 244 7399 fax: +31 10 244 7319 `www.vigilex.com`

Pharmacovigilance (ISOP: `http://www.who-umc.org/isoponline`) is a platform for the further development of pharmacovigilance, as a science and as a profession. ISOP is preparing programmes for the stimulation of pharmacovigilance teaching activities and for the development of quality standards and "good practices". Furthermore, related organisations, such as the International Society of Pharmacoepidemiology (ISPE) and the Drug Information Association (DIA) are increasing their contributions to teaching pharmacovigilance.

THE LSHTM

The London School of Hygiene and Tropical Medicine (LSHTM) has been running a course in pharmacoepidemiology and pharmacovigilence for the last five years. The course was first planned in response to several requests received for some specialised training from people working in pharmacoepidemiology in the United Kingdom.

LSHTM was already well established as one of the foremost teaching institutions for epidemiology, and there were several staff actively engaged on research work around drug safety. First thoughts were to set up a one-year's masters programme in the subject, but early research on likely consumer demand indicated that few people would be able to take the time for such a course because they and their employers would be unwilling for them to the such a long break from the workplace. A shorter course was therefore designed which was nevertheless rigorous, with a requirement to pass a written examination and to submit a student project on an assigned topic that required an understanding of the complexity of safety decisions. There are three teaching blocks, one of four days and two of three days. Each student is assigned an academic tutor to advise on the preparation of the 3000 word student project.

Early on in the course the wide range of people who registered was surprising. It was expected that the constituencies for the course would be people working in pharmacovigilence departments in industry, people working for regulatory authorities, and a few people working in pharmacy policy in health authorities. The first two groups registered in abundance, but each year the course has been enriched by the presence of other interests that have ranged from a medical journalist to an academic studying the safety of alternative therapies. An increasing number of participants come from outside the United Kingdom, while less than half of the people registering for the course are medically qualified.

The aim is to give a wide view of the issues surrounding drug safety, so that all students understand the wider context. In keeping with the educational philosophy of the LSHTM there is a strong emphasis on student participation at all stages, so that formal lectures are interspersed with a variety of coursework sessions and workshops. To allow teachers to give individual attention to students, course numbers each year are strictly limited. The course includes a considerable amount of epidemiological and statistical methods, together with an in-depth review of the regulatory issues and the problems that are faced in industry. Students are encouraged to develop critical skills for appraising the nature and value of the evidence they are faced with.

This course is generously supported by many other organisations whose staff give their teaching time for free. In particular, many of the teachers are drawn from the Medicines Control Agency, but heartfelt thanks are also due to the many industry personnel, independent consultants and fellow academics who give their time every year to ensure that students are exposed to the widest possible range of perspectives. It is hoped that this course makes a valuable contribution to the conduct of pharmacovigilence activity throughout Europe.

42

Medical Errors and Lessons from Drug-Related Deaths

R.E. FERNER
City Hospital, Birmingham, UK

R.M. WHITTINGTON
Formerly HM Coroner for Birmingham and Solihull Districts, Coroner's Court, Newton Street, Birmingham, UK

INTRODUCTION

Adverse drug events are harmful consequences from the therapeutic use of drugs. They include adverse consequences from reactions to drugs, adverse interactions between drugs, and the harm that comes from medication errors. They can be fatal. However, fatal adverse drug events are relatively rare, and most spontaneous reporting schemes and post-marketing studies contain few such cases. There is considerable uncertainty about both the incidence of fatal reactions and their likely causes.

The Institute of Medicine in the United States, extrapolating from information obtained in two relatively restricted hospital surveys, has suggested that as many as 98 000 deaths a year in the United States may be due to "medical error" (Kohn *et al.*, 1999). Lazarou *et al.* (1998) examined the evidence from 16 studies published between 1964 and 1995, and concluded that adverse drug reactions (ADRs) alone accounted for over 100 000 deaths in the United States in one year. This would mean that

doctors and their treatments caused about 4% of all deaths. The extrapolation was based on a total of 78 deaths, the majority observed in studies conducted prior to 1976. The US General Accounting Office (2000) subsequently reported that "the magnitude of health risk [from adverse drug events] is uncertain, because of limited incidence data".

Medication errors, that is, errors in prescribing, drawing up, and administering drugs, are a particularly important group of adverse drug events, because they are potentially preventable. The precise definition has proved difficult, but we have previously suggested the following: "a medication error is a failure in the treatment process that leads to, or has the potential to lead to, harm to the patient" (Ferner and Aronson, 1999). "Failure" in this context signifies that the process has fallen below some attainable standard.

The contribution of medication errors to the overall figure for deaths from "medical error" is not clearly established, but surveys of hospital in-patients (Bates *et al.*, 1995) and of nursing homes

Pharmacovigilance. Edited by R.D. Mann and E.B. Andrews

(Barker *et al.*, 1982) have shown that medication errors are extremely common. Anecdotal reports from several sources, including Coroners' Inquests (Whittington and Thompson, 1983; Ayers *et al.*, 1987; Whittington, 1991), and the medical defence societies (Ferner, 1995) have alerted doctors to some of the dangers.

One source of information which is potentially useful for investigating the epidemiology of adverse drug events is the records kept by Coroners in England and Wales.

INFORMATION FROM CORONERS' INQUESTS

Coroners in England and Wales have to determine how a person dies, if death is from a violent, unnatural, or unknown cause. Deaths due to errors in prescribing, dispensing, or giving drugs, and those caused by ADRs, fall within these categories. Coroners have extensive powers of investigation.

There are some caveats. The facts are not always clear, and so some deaths may be regarded as natural which in fact are due to therapy. Even if the facts are clear, the decision to report a death to the Coroner is not always straightforward, so some deaths might be reported by one doctor but not another. The extent of under-reporting is unknown. Each Coroner's Court covers deaths occurring in a defined area, so that, broadly speaking, the size of the population served by the Court is known. Local circumstances, such as the presence of a regional referral centre for some condition that is often fatal (such as liver failure), can however inflate the apparent incidence of deaths due to that cause.

We have previously described the findings in cases of death due to ADRs or to medication errors in one Coroner's district, Birmingham and Solihull, between 1986 and 1991 (Ferner and Whittington, 1994). Here we extend those data to cover the period January 1986 to June 2000.

The population in 1991 was 1.21 million people, and the number of deaths was approximately 15 000 per year, of which about a third were

reported to the Coroner. An index of cases has been kept on computer since 1995, and prior to that, a card index was kept. The database was searched for "therapeutic/accident", "therapeutic/misadventure", "medical mishap" and "medical misadventure".

PREVIOUS RESULTS

There were 10 deaths due to errors in medication and 36 due to adverse reactions in the years 1986–1991, as determined at inquest (Table 42.1). The 46 deaths represented about one in two thousand of the deaths occurring during the six years studied. Non-steroidal anti-inflammatory drugs (NSAIDs) accounted for 14/36 (39%) of the deaths due to adverse reactions—12 cases of gastrointestinal bleeding or perforation, one asthmatic attack, and one case of acute tubular necrosis. Warfarin accounted for only one fatal adverse reaction and two deaths due to error in these patients.

Errors in this earlier series of cases also contributed to the death of two patients treated with opiates, and one each with chlorpromazine, dantrolene, lithium carbonate, haloperidol (insufficient), intravenous potassium chloride, and inhaled oxygen.

RESULTS FOR 1992–2000

In the $8\frac{1}{2}$ year period 1992–June 2000, we identified a further 40 cases of death due to adverse drug events. We did not consider an adverse reaction "preventable" if its prevention would have required unusually close monitoring or care. All 40 cases were classed as due to adverse reaction alone, error alone, or both, by each of us independently. We agreed on all but three cases: these were classified after discussion between us. By these criteria, there were 24 cases of clear-cut ADRs, 3 cases where death was likely to have been due to a medication error alone, and 13 cases in which there were elements of both. In addition, one death due to an adverse reaction was compounded by a diagnostic error.

Table 42.1. Drugs associated with fatal adverse drug events in Birmingham, 1986–1991 and 1992–June 2000. The events include errors, adverse reactions, and adverse reactions as a result of errors.

First series 1986–1991	Second series 1992–June 2000
Psychotropics (5) fluoxetine lithium (2) haloperidol chlorpromazine	Psychotropics (7) amitriptyline chlorpromazine dothiepin [dosulepin] + chlorpromazine pipothiazine lithium (2) clozapine
Antibiotics (8) co-trimoxazole (3) isoniazid and others (4) oxytetracycline	Antibiotics (4) ciprofloxacin isoniazid levofloxacin penicillins
Endocrine drugs (1) cyproterone acetate	Endocrine drugs (2) dexamethasone anabolic steroids
NSAIDs (14) aspirin azapropazone + warfarin diclofenac (2) ibuprofen (3) indometacin + prednisolone ketoprofen naproxen (4) piroxicam	NSAIDs (14) aspirin diclofenac (5) flurbiprofen ibuprofen indometacin (3) mefenamic acid naproxen piroxicam
Other antirheumatic (2) methotrexate penicillamine	Other antirheumatic (1) methotrexate
Opioids (2)	Anticoagulants (9) warfarin (7) heparin (2)
Anticoagulants (3) warfarin (3)	Miscellaneous (3) theophylline + prednisolone phenytoin ethanol + various drugs
Miscellaneous (11) captopril contrast media dantrolene (2) oxygen (2) potassium chloride slow release potassium chloride solution spironolactone suxamethonium unknown	

Adverse reactions in this second series were again predominantly due to NSAIDs, which accounted for 13/37 cases (35%) in which ADRs were wholly or partly to blame for the adverse drug event. The two drugs most often implicated were diclofenac (4 cases) and indometacin (3 cases).

Warfarin was responsible for seven deaths, three due to error, and heparin for two, one of which was the result of error (Table 42.1). The 16 cases in which error played some part are as follows:

Case A: A 21-year-old man treated with dothiepin 75 milligrams twice daily became psychotic, and was admitted to a psychiatric hospital and injected with 150 milligrams of chlorpromazine intramuscularly. He suffered an asystolic cardiac arrest 11 hours later and could not be resuscitated.

Comment: The British National Formulary warns of the dangers of injecting large doses of antipsychotic agents intramuscularly, and of the potential for adverse interactions between antipsychotic agents and other drugs that can affect heart rhythm, including tricyclic antidepressants.

Case B: A 72-year-old woman with asthma was prescribed slow release theophylline tablets, 225 milligrams two tablets twice daily. Prednisolone 30 milligrams daily was added during an exacerbation, and she suffered a gastrointestinal haemorrhage. The serum theophylline concentration was over twice the upper limit of the therapeutic range.

Comment: Theophylline is difficult to use, because it has a narrow therapeutic range; gastric irritation is a recognized adverse effect of theophylline, and might have been potentiated by prednisolone.

Case C: A woman of 64 years was prescribed lithium carbonate by a psychiatrist, and her general practitioner continued to treat her with the drug for two and a half years without monitoring the serum lithium concentration. She became seriously unwell from lithium poisoning, developed renal failure and pneumonia, and died.

Comment: Lithium is another drug with a narrow therapeutic range. One adverse effect is renal impairment, which reduces elimination of lithium, causing a further increase in concentration. Since lithium concentrations can fluctuate, they should be measured every few months, even in patients apparently well established on the drug, so that the dose may be altered if necessary.

Case D: A 77-year-old woman treated with lithium carbonate for some years was admitted to a geriatric hospital with deteriorating physical and mental health. By the time lithium concentration was measured over a week after admission, she had developed renal failure, lithium toxicity, and inhalation pneumonia which proved fatal.

Case E: An elderly woman with multiple pulmonary emboli was treated with intravenous heparin by infusion. After a change of syringe, the syringe driver was set at a rate ten times higher than intended, and the woman suffered an intracranial haemorrhage and died.

Case F: An 81-year-old woman was prescribed indometacin 25 milligrams three times daily; she had previously suffered from "indigestion" and sporadically took tablets of ranitidine. Less than a month after starting indometacin treatment, she had a haematemesis and died.

Comment: The risk of gastrointestinal haemorrhage is substantially greater in patients taking NSAIDs, and especially if they are elderly. These drugs should not be used in a patient with active peptic ulceration.

Case G: An 82-year-old woman who took indometacin 75 milligrams daily for arthritis, began to vomit, and developed colicky abdominal pain. The general practitioner visited twice but did not stop indometacin treatment. She died of a massive gastrointestinal haemorrhage, and a chronic gastric ulcer was found at post mortem.

Case H: A 79-year-old woman was treated with diclofenac 150 milligrams daily for arthritis. After about a year's treatment she developed dyspepsia, which resolved when she stopped taking diclofenac. Diclofenac treatment was subsequently

resumed, and she died two weeks later in hospital from a perforated duodenal ulcer.

Case I: A man of 88 years took flurbiprofen 50 milligrams as needed for arthritis for 10 years. He also took ranitidine and omeprazole. He was admitted to hospital with anaemia and died. A giant gastric ulcer was found at post mortem.

Case J: A man of 76 years was taking warfarin regularly after aortic valve replacement. He developed diverticulitis, was treated with metronidazole, and collapsed with gastrointestinal haemorrhage, then died. The international normalised ratio (INR) was 9.

Comment: Metronidazole increases the anticoagulant action of warfarin.

Case K: A 77-year-old woman with atrial fibrillation took warfarin after suffering small strokes. An instruction to continue the dosage of 3.5 milligrams daily (one blue tablet and half a brown tablet) was misheard as one to change to 9.5 milligrams daily (three blue tablets and half a brown tablet). She sustained a subdural haemorrhage and died.

Case L: A 56-year-old woman with atrial fibrillation took warfarin after suffering a serious stroke. Anticoagulant control was erratic, and she had frequent clotting tests performed by a domiciliary phlebotomist. Ten weeks before the patient died, a phlebotomist called but could not gain entry. Later the patient was transferred to a residential home, where she was given in error a dose of warfarin 4 times higher than before, without further checks on anticoagulant control. She suddenly collapsed, and was taken to hospital where the INR was greater than 10. She died soon after from an intracranial haemorrhage.

Case M: A man aged 42 years abused alcohol and suffered from depression. He was found dead in bed, and substantial quantities of alcohol and medicines were found in post mortem samples. The pathologist considered death to be due to "acute left ventricular failure associated with high alcohol (232 milligrams per 100 millilitres) and therapeutic levels of paroxetine, carbamazepine, and thioridazine."

Comment: The patient also had prescribed to him—codeine, propranolol, zopiclone, nitrazepam, clomethiazole, and procyclidine. The dangers of polypharmacy can be considerably augmented by ethanol.

Case N: A 16-year-old schoolgirl with severe asthma had been advised by a respiratory physician never to take aspirin, but developed a headache at school, was given an aspirin tablet, and collapsed and died within two hours from acute severe asthma.

Case O: A man in his early 50s, a devoted bodybuilder and marksman, persuaded an elderly private general practitioner to furnish him with a series of prescriptions for anabolic steroids. While taking these drugs, the man had a trivial argument with his partner as to who was to buy cat food, went upstairs, and shot himself. The abuse of anabolic steroids was judged to have affected his mind and made him irrational.

Comment: The general practitioner was referred to the General Medical Council, and he voluntarily removed his own name from the Medical Register, and retired from practice.

Case P: A 59-year-old man with paranoid schizophrenia was transferred from one psychiatric hospital to another. He had been treated briefly at the first hospital with the atypical antipsychotic drug clozapine, but this had caused neutropenia. Two months after transfer, clozapine treatment was begun at the second hospital, where doctors did not realize that the man had previously suffered from neutropenia. After about six weeks of renewed treatment, he developed severe neutropenia, which eventually proved fatal.

THE GENESIS OF MEDICATION ERRORS

Errors can be classified into two broad categories, "mistakes" and "slips or lapses". The former

occur when something is wrong with the premise on which an action is based. For example, the action in Case A, when the patient was intentionally given a high dose of intramuscular chlorpromazine while taking the tricyclic antidepressant dothiepin, represents two mistakes—using the wrong dose in the circumstances, and failing to take account of the presence of a second drug in planning treatment. By contrast, Case E, in which a momentary lapse led to a syringe driver being run at a rate ten times higher than intended, illustrates a slip, which is an error of the second sort, occurring during the execution of a planned action (Reason, 1990). To some extent, training and education will help to overcome mistakes, but it is difficult to prevent slips and lapses by training, because they represent defects in tasks that are not under conscious control.

THE LESSONS FROM DEATHS RELATED TO MEDICATION

Previous studies have highlighted slips as a major cause of medication errors (Koren *et al.*, 1986). The drama of patients dying from overdoses of drugs as a result of a misplaced decimal point, or because the names of two drugs were confused, only emphasises the difficulties. However, in this series, we found that slips were much rarer than mistakes, and that medication errors were themselves a rare cause of death as determined at Coroner's Inquest. The "system" in which drugs are used needs to be improved, and that system includes both prescribers and patients. Better education, and more relevant information at the point when doctors prescribe, will help. Some drugs, notably warfarin, lithium, opioids, and potassium chloride, are difficult to use safely, and require especially careful prescribing and monitoring. Nonetheless, however safe systems for prescribing, dispensing, and administering drugs become, patients will continue to die from ADRs. That problem can only be mitigated by a more careful assessment of risks and benefits in prescribing for each patient and every drug, and by the development of safer drugs.

REFERENCES

Ayers JG, Fleming DM, Whittington RM (1987) Asthma death due to ibuprofen. *Lancet* **i**: 1082.

Barker KN, Mikeal RL, Pearson RE, Illig NA, Morse ML (1982) Medication errors in nursing homes and small hospitals. *Am J Hosp Pharm* **39**: 987–91.

Bates DW, Cullen DJ, Laird N, *et al.* (1995) Incidence of adverse drug events and potential adverse drug events. Implications for prevention. *J Am Med Assoc* **274**: 29–34.

Ferner RE (1995) More errors in prescribing and giving medicines. *J Med Defence Union* **11**: 80–2.

Ferner RE, Aronson JK (1999) Errors in prescribing, preparing, and giving medicines—definition, classification, and prevention. In: Aronson JK, ed., *Side Effects of Drugs Annual*, Vol. 22. Amsterdam: Elsevier, pp. xxiii–xxxvi.

Ferner RE, Whittington RM (1994) Coroner's cases of death due to errors in prescribing or giving medicines or to adverse drug reactions: Birmingham 1986–1991. *J R Soc Med* **87**: 145–8.

Kohn L, Corrigan J, Donaldson M (1999) *To Err is Human: Building a Safer Health System.* Washington, DC: Institute of Medicine.

Koren G, Barzilay Z, Greenwald M (1986) Tenfold errors in administration of drug doses: a neglected iatrogenic disease in pediatrics. *Pediatrics* **77**: 848–9.

Lazarou J, Pomeranz BH, Corey PN (1998) Incidence of adverse reactions in hospitalized patients. *J Am Med Assoc* **279**: 1200–5.

Reason JT (1990) *Human Error.* New York: Cambridge University Press.

US General Accounting Office (2000) *Adverse Drug Events. The Magnitude of the Health Risk is Uncertain Because of Limited Incidence Data.* GAO/HEHS-00-21.

Whittington RM (1991) Fatal hepatotoxicity of anti-tubercular chemotherapy. *Lancet* **338**: 1083–4.

Whittington RM, Thompson IMcK (1983) Possible hazard of plastic matrix from slow-release tablets. *Lancet* **i**: 184.

43

Pharmacogenetics and the Genetic Basis of ADRs

PENELOPE K. MANASCO
First Genetic Trust, Deerfield, IL, USA

PATRICIA RIESER, GAILE RENEGAR AND MICHAEL MOSTELLER
GlaxoSmithKline, Research Triangle Park, NC, USA

INTRODUCTION

Health care providers and patients have long recognized that people often respond differently to the same medicine, both in terms of efficacy and "side effects," or adverse drug reactions (ADRs). There are many factors that contribute to this inter-individual variability in response to medications, including: the pathogenesis and severity of the disease being treated; concomitant medications and drug interactions; and the patient's age, renal and liver function, concomitant illnesses, nutrition and lifestyle (smoking, alcohol use, weight, fitness) (Meyer, 2000). Genetic factors that affect the kinetics and dynamics of drugs play an even greater role in determining an individual's risk of non-response or toxicity (Evans and Relling, 1999). Although it is difficult to define the relative contribution of genetic and environmental effects in an individual, it is clear that variation in genes coding for drug-metabolizing enzymes, drug transporters, and drug receptors and targets accounts for a significant portion of the observed heterogeneity in drug response across populations.

The study of ADRs has been hampered by the use of ambiguous and inconsistent terminology and reporting. Edwards and Aronson (2000) recently proposed the following definition of an adverse drug reaction: "an appreciably harmful or unpleasant reaction, resulting from an intervention related to the use of a medicinal product, which predicts hazard from future administration and warrants prevention or specific treatment, alteration of the dosage regimen, or withdrawal of the product". ADRs may result from health care provider, pharmacy or patient error or from a variety of genetic and environmental factors. Although definitions and figures vary, it is clear that ADRs are a significant cause of morbidity, mortality and health care expense. Lazarou et al. (1998) performed a meta-analysis of 39 prospective studies from US hospitals and found that 6.7% of inpatients have a serious ADR while hospitalized, resulting in ~106 000 deaths per year. White et al. (1999) estimates that hospitalizations due to ADRs in the United States cost between $30 billion and $150 billion per year, and Destenaves and Thomas (2000) report that ADRs are a major cause of

Pharmacovigilance. Edited by R.D. Mann and E.B. Andrews

non-compliance and treatment failure, especially for patients with chronic diseases. If lack of efficacy ("unexpected failure of therapy") is included in the definition of ADRs, as suggested by Edwards and Aronson (2000), then their deleterious human and financial cost becomes even greater.

The number, severity and cost of ADRs is now recognized as a significant public health issue and has triggered interest in discovering what causes them and if and how their occurrence can be predicted and prevented. In this chapter, we will focus on the current state of knowledge regarding the genetic basis of ADRs and the important role that pharmacogenetics will play in meeting the ultimate goal of providing safer, more effective medicines.

PHARMACOGENETICS

Pharmacogenetics is the study of genetic factors related to human variability in response to medicines. Its modern root lies in the work of Archibald Garrod, whose work on alcaptonuria in 1902 comprised the first proof of Mendel's laws of genetics in humans. Garrod hypothesized that adverse reactions after drug ingestion could result from genetically determined differences in biochemical processes, and further suggested that enzymes play a role in the detoxification of foreign substances and that the lack of an enzyme in an individual might cause that mechanism to fail (Garrod, 1902).

Incidental clinical observations during the late 1940s and 1950s resulted in the discovery of several relatively common genetic variations related to ADRs. Hemolysis related to anti-malarial treatment was much more common among African–American soldiers during World War II, leading to the identification of inherited variants of glucose-6-phosphate dehydrogenase (G-6-PD). Prolonged muscle relaxation and apnea after suxamethonium was found to be caused by an inherited deficiency of a plasma cholinesterase. Peripheral neuropathy was observed in a significant number of patients treated with the anti-tuberculosis drug isoniazid, leading to the identification of genetic differences in acetylation pathways.

The genetic variations related to these observations are called *polymorphisms*—inter-individual differences in DNA sequences at a specific chromosomal location that exist at a frequency of more than 1% in the general population. The two *alleles* (alternate forms of a gene) present at a given gene locus comprise the *genotype*, which now can be characterized at the DNA level. The progress of The Human Genome Project and advances in genomic technology enhance the likelihood that high-density human whole-genome scans will become feasible and cost-efficient in the next five to ten years. The influence of genotype on *phenotype* (observable features resulting from the action of one or more genes)—in this case, the influence of genes on drug kinetics or dynamics—now can be measured using advanced analytical methods for metabolite detection and clinical investigation tools such as receptor-density studies by positron emission tomography (Meyer, 2000).

Pharmacogenetic mechanisms related to polymorphisms can result in clinically relevant sequelae in at least three ways:

● via genes associated with altered drug metabolism and transport: increased or decreased metabolism of a drug can affect the concentration of the drug and its active, inactive and toxic metabolites (e.g. metabolism of tricyclic antidepressants),
● via genes associated with unexpected drug effects (e.g. hemolysis in G-6-PD deficiency), and
● via genes associated with genetic variation in drug targets, resulting in altered clinical response and frequency of ADRs (e.g. β-adrenergic receptor variants and altered response to β-agonists in asthmatic patients) (Meyer, 2000).

Inherited variations related to drug metabolism generally are monogenic (single gene) traits, and their clinical relevance in terms of pharmacokinetics and dynamics depends on their importance for the activation or inactivation of drug substrates (Evans and Relling, 1999). The most important effects include toxicity for medicines that have a narrow therapeutic window and are inactivated by a polymorphic enzyme (e.g. thioguanine, flourouracil, mercaptopurine, azathioprine) and decreased efficacy of medicines that require activation by an enzyme that exhibits a polymorphism (e.g. codeine). These variant genes and the enzymes they code for also may be involved in some drug–drug interactions. Most of these monogenic traits have been identified on the basis of dramatic observed differences in response (efficacy and toxicity) among individuals. Although still not in common clinical use, functional enzyme analyses or genotyping to detect some of the common monogenic traits affecting drug metabolism are beginning to be used more frequently, especially in the field of cancer chemotherapy (Iyer and Ratain, 1998; Mancinelli *et al.*, 2000).

While these monogenic traits affecting drug metabolism are important, the overall pharmacologic effects of drugs are more likely to be related to the interaction of several genes (*polygenic*), all encoding proteins that are involved in multiple pathways of metabolism, transport, disposition and action (Evans and Relling, 1999). These polygenic traits, which also may play a role in drug–drug interactions, are more challenging to uncover during clinical trials, especially when the mechanisms of drug metabolism and action are unknown. In contrast with the past, when clinical observations of individual differences in drug response prompted biochemical and genetic research into the underlying causes, recent advances in molecular sequencing technology may reverse that process: laboratory identification of polymorphisms (especially those in gene regulatory or coding regions) may be the initiating observation, followed by biochemical and human studies to ascertain their phenotypic and clinical consequences (Evans and Relling, 1999).

Continued research in pharmacogenetics has the potential to result in the elucidation of the genetic basis of drug metabolism, disposition and response. In some cases, the results of research may provide clinicians with the ability to subclassify patients using pharmacogenetic-based diagnostic criteria. If research efforts are successful, then it will become possible, in many circumstances, to select medicines and determine appropriate dosing on the basis of an individual patient's inherited ability to metabolize and respond to specific drugs, thus reducing the enormous individual, societal

and economic burdens currently related to treatment failures and ADRs.

The US National Institute of General Medical Sciences (NIGMS) and other components of the National Institutes of Health (NIH) are sponsoring a major research initiative, the Pharmacogenetics Research Network, in order to reach this goal. This network, established in 2000, initially comprises nine teams of investigators across the United States, with research projects including asthma treatments, tamoxifen and other cancer drugs, ethnic differences in response to anti-depressants, drug transporters, database design, and ethical, legal and social ramifications of pharmacogenetic research (<http://www.nigms.nih.gov/news/releases/pharmacogenetics.html>).

A major component of the network will be a publicly available library (Stanford Pharmacogenetics Knowledge Base, PharmGKB) of shared information from all the projects. Initially, this library will house data regarding genetic variations of research volunteers who have had a particular response to a specific medicine. All individual data will be coded to protect individual privacy. Access to information regarding the Pharmacogenetics Research Network and PharmGKB is via the NIGMS website: <http://www.nigms.nih.gov/funding/pharmacogenetics.html>.

THE GENETIC BASIS OF ADRS

POLYMORPHISMS AFFECTING DRUG METABOLISM

Most drugs are degraded via a limited number of metabolic pathways, most of which involve microsomal hepatic enzymes. Ingelman-Sundberg *et al.* (1999) reported that about 40% of this human cytochrome (CYP) P450-dependent drug metabolism is carried out by polymorphic enzymes capable of altering these metabolic pathways. The CYP P450 monooxygenase system of enzymes detoxifies xenobiotics and activates procarcinogens and promutagens in the body via oxidative metabolic pathways. These enzymes play an important role in the elimination of endogenous substrates (such as cholesterol) and lipophilic compounds (such as central nervous system (CNS) drugs that cross the blood–brain barrier), which otherwise tend to accumulate to toxic concentrations. This very large and well-studied gene family consists of many isoforms; for example, over 70 variant alleles of the CYP2D6 locus have been described (Ingelman-Sundberg *et al.*, 1999). The distribution of variant alleles for these enzymes differs among ethnic and racial subpopulations, with significant implications for clinical practice in various areas (Table 43.1). Alleles causing altered (enhanced or diminished) rates of drug metabolism have been described for many of the P450 enzymes, and the underlying molecular mechanisms have been identified for some. Table 43.2 summarizes some clinically significant polymorphisms affecting drug metabolism and the drugs and drug effects associated with them; a comprehensive summary is available at <http://www.sciencemag.org/feature/data/1044449.shl>. Continuously updated descriptions of these alleles and accompanying references can be found at <http://www.imm.ki.se/CYPalleles/>

CYP2D6, which encodes debrisoquin hydroxylase, was the first of these enzyme-coding genes to be cloned and characterized, and it remains among the most studied. It is involved in the metabolism of many commonly used drugs, including tricyclic anti-depressants, neuroleptics, anti-arrhythmics and other cardiovascular drugs, and opioids. Variant alleles may differ from the wild-type (normal) gene by one or more point mutations, gene deletions, duplications, multiduplications or amplification. These may have no effect on enzyme activity or may code for an enzyme with reduced, absent or increased activity. The genetics and related biochemistry of these pathways are still being elucidated and are more complex than the following simplistic descriptions imply. *Extensive metabolizers*, 75%–85% of the general population, are homozygous or heterozygous for the wild-type, normal activity enzyme. *Intermediate* (10–15% of the population) and *poor* (5%–10%) *metabolizers* carry two reduced or loss-of-activity alleles. These individuals are likely to exhibit increased drug plasma concentrations when given standard doses of drugs that are metabolized by this enzyme; this

Table 43.1. Population distribution of selected polymorphic drug-metabolizing enzymes.[a]

Enzyme	Major polymorphisms	Functional consequences	Allelle frequency (%)			
			Caucasian	Asian	Black African	Ethiopian and Saudi Arabian
CYP2A6	CYP2A6*2	Inactive enzyme	1–3	0	—	—
	CYP2A6del	No enzyme	1	15	—	—
CYP2C9	CYP2C9*2	↓ Affinity for P450 oxidoreductase	8–13	0	—	—
	CYP2C9*3	Altered substrate specificity	6–9	2–3	—	—
CYP2C19	CYP2C19*2	Inactive enzyme	13	23–32	13	14–15
	CYP2C19*3	Inactive enzyme	0	6–10	—	0–2
CYP2D6	CYP2D6*2xN	↑ Enzyme activity	1–5	0–2	2	10–16
	CYP2D6*4	Inactive enzyme	12–21	1	2	1–4
	CYP2D6*5	No enzyme	2–7	6	4	1–3
	CYP2D6*10	Unstable enzyme	1–2	51	6	3–9
	CYP2D6*17	↓ Substrate affinity	0	—	34	3–9
N-acetyl-transferase 2	NAT2	↓ function	40–70	10–20	50–60	—

[a] Compiled from Ingelman-Sundberg *et al.* (1999), Meyer (2000) and references therein.

Table 43.2. Selected polymorphic enzymes associated with altered drug response.[a]

Enzyme	Variant phenotypes	Selected drugs	Altered response
CYP2D6	Ultra-rapid metabolizers Poor metabolizers Extensive metabolizers	Anti-arrhythmics (some) Anti-depressants (some) Anti-psychotics (some) Opioids ß-Adrenoreceptor antagonists (some) Debrisoquin Dextromethorphan Guanoxan Sparteine Phenformine Phenacetin	Poor: ↑ risk of toxicity Ultra-rapid: ↓ efficacy
CYP2C19	Poor and extensive hydroxylators	Mephenytoin Hexobarbital Omeprazole Proguanil Diazepam	Poor: ↑ risk of toxicity Extensive: ↓ efficacy
CYP2C9	Poor metabolizers	Warfarin Tolbutamide Glipazide Phenytoin Non-steroidal anti-inflammatories Imipramine Losartan	↑ Response and risk of toxicity
CYP2A6	Poor nicotine metabolizers	Nicotine	Possibly ↓ risk of addiction
N-acetyltransferase 2	Slow and rapid acetylators	Isoniazid Sulfamethazine Procainamide Amonifide Dapson Sufasalazine Paraminosalicylic acid Heterocyclic amines (food mutagens)	Slow: ↓ clearance and ↑ risk of toxicity, including toxic neuritis, lupus erythematosus, bladder cancer Rapid: ↓ efficacy, ↑ risk of toxicity in some cases (amonifide); colorectal cancer
Thiopurine methyltransferase	Poor TPMT methylators	6-Mercaptopurine 6-Thioguanine Azathiopurine	Bone marrow toxicity, liver damage
Dihydropyrimadine dehydrogenase	Slow inactivation	5-Fluorouracil	↑ Risk of toxicity
Plasma pseudocholinesterase	Slow ester hydrolysis	Succinylcholine	Prolonged apnea
Aldehyde dehydrogenase	Rapid and slow metabolizers	Ethanol	Slow: facial flushing Rapid: protection from liver cirrhosis
Catechol O-methyltransferase	Poor and rapid methylators	Levodopa Methyldopa	Poor: increased efficacy
Glucose-6-phosphate dehydrogenase	Poor metabolizers	Primaquine	Hemolysis
UGT-glucuronosyltransferase	Poor metabolizers	Irinotecan	Myelosuppression and diarrhea

[a]Compiled from Ingleman-Sundberg *et al.* (1999), Meyer (2000), Evans and Relling (1999), Sadee (2000) and Manicelli *et al.* (2000) and references therein.

functional overdose results in increased risk of dose-dependent ADRs associated with these drugs. These individuals also are likely to experience lack of efficacy with prodrugs that require activation by this enzyme; lack of morphine-related analgesic response to the prodrug codeine is one example. *Ultrarapid metabolizers* (1%–10%) carry duplicated or multiduplicated active genes; they will metabolize some drugs very rapidly, never achieving a therapeutic plasma drug concentration (and hence expected efficacy) at a standard dose. Alternately, an ultrarapid metabolizer given codeine may experience an ADR usually associated with morphine because of the increased conversion of prodrug to active drug; this often is true of active metabolites, as well.

Two variant alleles of CYP2C9, which result in reduced affinity for P450 oxidoreductase or altered substrate specificity, are associated with increased risk of hemorrhage with standard doses of the anticoagulant warfarin. The clearance of S-warfarin in patients who are homozygous for one of the polymorphisms is reduced by 90% compared with patients who are homozygous for the wild-type allele (Ingleman-Sundberg *et al.*, 1999). Similar reductions in drug clearance related to one of these polymorphisms have been documented with other CYP2C9 substrates such as ibuprofen and naproxen (non-steroidal anti-inflammatories), phenytoin (anti-epileptic), tolbutamide (hypoglycemic/anti-diabetic) and losartan (angiotensin II receptor antagonist) (Daly, 1995). The high frequency of these polymorphisms (up to 37% of one British population was heterozygous for one mutant CYP2C9 allele) and the severity of the potential ADR (hemorrhage with warfarin treatment) make this an important consideration in the selection and dose of warfarin and other affected drugs.

Patients who are homozygous for the null allele of CYP2C19 (poor metabolizers) are extremely sensitive to the effects of omeprazole (anti-ulcer), diazepam (anti-anxiolytic), propranolol (β-blocker), amitriptyline (tricyclic anti-depressant) and other drugs (Touw, 1997). CYP2C19 also is involved in the oxidation of the anti-malarial prodrug proguanil to cycloguanil, although it is unknown whether the polymorphism relates to its anti-malarial effects. The frequency of this polymorphism (3%–6% in Caucasians and 8%–23% in Asians) defines it as clinically significant.

Polymorphic alleles have been identified for several Phase II (conjugation) enzymes, and many of these are as important in drug metabolism as those associated with the Phase I (oxidation) enzymes discussed above. N-acetyltransferase 2, sulfotransferases, glucuronosyltransferases, catechol O-methyltransferase, dihydropyrimidine dehydrogenase (DPyDH), and thiopurine methyltransferase (TPMT) are among the Phase II enzymes known to have clinically significant effects on drug metabolism (Mancinelli *et al.*, 2000); some of these are summarized in Table 43.2. Polymorphisms of genes coding for these enzymes are particularly relevant in cancer chemotherapy (severe toxicity for homozygotes of null alleles of TPMT with thioguanine and azathioprine treatment and of DPyDH with 5-flourouracil treatment) and the treatment of Parkinson's disease with L-dopa (low methylators have an increased response to the drug).

POLYMORPHISMS AFFECTING DRUG TRANSPORT

Although cellular uptake of some drugs occurs via passive diffusion, membrane transporters also play a role in the absorption of medicines through the intestines, their excretion into bile and urine and their uptake into sites of action (such as brain, testes and cardiovascular tissue; tumor cells; synaptic cleft; and infectious microorganisms) (Evans and Relling, 1999). Increasing attention is being focused on the possible role of polymorphisms of genes encoding drug transporters, some of which are summarized in Table 43.3.

One example of a transporter with relevance to drug response is p-glycoprotein (Pgp), an ATP-dependent transmembrane efflux pump that serves to extrude numerous drugs and other substances out of cells. Pgp is coded for by the multidrug resistance locus, MDR-1. Hoffmeyer *et al.* (2000) reported that a specific polymorphism, present in homozygous form in 24% of their Caucasian sample population, correlated with expression levels and function of MDR-1. Homozygous individuals had significantly lower MDR-1 expression and exhibited a four-fold increase in plasma digoxin

Table 43.3. Selected polymorphisms of drug transporters, receptors, targets and disease genes associated with altered drug response.[a]

Drug transporter, receptor, or target	Variant phenotype	Drugs	Altered response
Multidrug resistance protein MDR-1	Overexpression in tumors	Adriamycin Paclitaxel Other anti-neoplastics	Resistance to treatment
	Low tissue expression	Digoxin Anti-neoplastics Verapamil Terfenadine Fexofenadine Protease inhibitors (most)	Possibly ↑ plasma drug concentration, risk of toxicity
$\beta 2$ adrenergic receptor	↑ Receptor downregulation	Albuterol Ventolin	↓ Response, poor control of asthma
5-HT2A serotonergic receptor	Multiple	Clozapine	Variable drug efficacy
Sulphonylurea receptor (SUR1)	Altered β-cell ATP-dependent potassium channel activity	Tolbutamide	↓ Insulin response
HER2 receptor	Overexpression in some breast and other cancers	Trastuzumab	Receptor overexpression associated with ↑ drug efficacy
Thymidylate synthase and dihydrofolate reductase	Overexpression in some tumor cells	5-Fluorouracil Methotrexate	Overexpression linked to development of resistance to drug anti-metabolites in tumor cells
Cardiac ion channels (HERG, KvLQT1, hKCNE2)	Delayed cardiac repolarization	Quinidine Cisapride Terfenadine Disopyramide Meflaquine Clarithromycin	Long Q-T syndrome, arrhythmias, torsade de pointes
Cholesteryl ester transport protein (CETP), lipoprotein lipase (LDL), β-fibrinogen		Pravastatin	Polymorphisms associated with atherosclerosis progression and response to pravastatin
Apolipoprotein E4		Tacrine Simvastatin	Presence of allele predicts poor response to tacrine, reduced cardiovascular mortality with simvastatin

[a]Compiled from Ingleman-Sundberg et al. (1999), Meyer (2000), Evans and Relling (1999), Sadee (2000) and Manicelli et al. (2000) and references therein.

concentration after a single oral dose of the drug. Other substrates of Pgp include important drugs with narrow therapeutic indices, such as chemotherapeutic agents, cyclosporin A, verapamil, terfenadine, fexofenadine and most HIV-1 protease inhibitors (Meyer, 2000). In addition, overexpression of MDR-1 in cancer tumors has been associated with resistance to adriamycin, paclitaxel and other anti-neoplastic agents, and additional similar extrusion pumps are reported to contribute to drug resistance in various tumors (Sadee, 2000).

Another potentially important gene family with a number of reported variants that may affect function is that of the biogenic amine transporters, which play a role in the regulation of neurotransmitter concentrations (including serotonin, dopamine and GABA) in synaptic transmission (Jonsson et al., 1998). These transporters are the direct target receptors for many drugs such as anti-depressants and cocaine; polymorphisms of the serotonin transporter, in particular, have been associated with the modulation of complex behavior (Heils et al., 1996) and may play a role in treatment with specific serotonin transporter inhibitors.

Mutations in other transporter-like proteins such as the sulfonylurea receptor (SUR) that regulates ATP-sensitive K + channels and insulin secretion and the Na+/H + exchanger (NHE1) that serves as one of the target receptors for amiloride (an anti-hypertensive diuretic) are being studied and may have clinical significance in modulating the activity of many medicines (Sadee, 2000).

POLYMORPHISMS AFFECTING DRUG RECEPTORS AND TARGETS

Many drugs interact with specific targets such as receptors, enzymes and other proteins involved with cell cycle control, signal transduction and other cellular events. Genes encoding these targets occur in polymorphic forms that may alter their pharmacologic response to specific medicines. For example, variants affecting β-adrenergic receptors are a major determinant of β-agonist bronchodilator (e.g. albuterol) response in asthmatic patients. A specific common polymorphism has been linked to increased β-2 receptor down-regulation in response to treatment with albuterol, which may result in

decreased drug efficacy and duration of action (Tan et al., 1997; Liggett, 2000). However, other studies have failed to show the expected correlation between the variant and clinical response (Lipworth et al., 1999). Drysdale et al. (2000) suggested that specific haplotypes (the array of alleles on a given chromosome) may have greater predictive value regarding response to β-agonist bronchodilators than the presence of individual polymorphisms. They reported marked variation in the ethnic distribution of the most frequently observed haplotypes (>20-fold differences) and in the mean β-agonist responses by haplotype pair (>2-fold differences). These authors suggested that the interactions of multiple polymorphisms within a haplotype may affect biologic and therapeutic phenotype and that haplotypes may be useful as pharmacologically relevant predictive markers.

Arranz et al. (2000) recently completed a comprehensive study of variants in multiple neurotransmitters and receptors in 200 schizophrenic patients. They reported that a set of six sequence variants involving the 5-hydroxytryptamine (serotonin) receptor, the histamine receptor (H2) and the promoter region of the serotonin transporter gene successfully predicted response to treatment with clozapine (a neuroleptic) in 76% of patients, with a sensitivity of 95% for satisfactory response. Several of these individual polymorphisms had been previously studied in this context, but with inconsistent findings. If the results of this retrospective study are prospectively validated, then they will form the basis of a simple test to optimize the usefulness of this expensive drug in a heterogeneously responsive group of patients.

The risk of drug-induced long QT syndrome, a cause of sudden cardiac death in individuals without structural heart disease, has been linked to five gene variants, each encoding structural subunits of cardiac ion channels that affect sodium or potassium transport and are affected by anti-arrhythmics and other drugs (Priori et al., 1999). Priori et al. (1999) reported that a significant number of individuals carry "silent mutations" of these genes; the resulting alterations are insufficient to prolong the QT interval at rest, but affected individuals may be especially sensitive to any drug that affects potassium currents. The combination of these silent mutations with even modest blockade induced by a variety of drugs used for many purposes can result in prolongation in action potential that is sufficient to trigger the onset of a serious ventricular arrhythmia (torsade de pointes).

Polymorphisms affecting steroid hormone nuclear receptors may affect individual response to drugs and hormones. For example, glucocorticoid resistance in asthma patients has been associated with increased expression of the glucocorticoid receptor β-isoform (Sousa et al., 2000); activating mutations of the mineralocorticoid receptor have been linked to hypertension exacerbated by pregnancy (Geller et al., 2000); and dominant negative mutations of peroxisome proliferator-activated receptor gamma (PPAR gamma) have been associated with severe insulin resistance, diabetes mellitus and hypertension (Barosso et al., 1999). Huizenga et al. (1998) identified a polymorphism affecting the glucocorticoid receptor that was present in 6% of their elderly study population. These individuals appeared healthy, but exhibited increased sensitivity (reflected in cortisol suppression and insulin response) to exogenously administered glucocorticoids. The authors postulated that this increased lifelong sensitivity to endogenous glucocorticoids might be reflected in the observed trends towards increased body mass index and decreased bone mineral density in affected individuals. This polymorphism also may be related to the development of early or serious ADRs with exogenous glucocorticoid treatment in carriers, but this has not yet been established.

Some investigators have reported a relationship between variants in the angiotensin converting enzyme (ACE) gene and individual sensitivity to ACE inhibitors such as enalapril, lisinopril and captopril, but the results reported by other teams fail to show an association, so this finding remains to be confirmed (Navis et al., 1999).

POLYMORPHISMS RELEVANT TO CANCER CHEMOTHERAPY

The basis of many forms of cancer chemotherapy involves the administration of maximum tolerated dosages with the goal of inflicting the greatest damage to malignant cells while causing the least damage to normal tissue. Genetic variations of drug-inactivating enzymes in normal tissues may increase the risk of severe toxicity or even death. As mentioned above, TMPT-deficient (homozygous; ~0.3% of the population) individuals treated for acute lymphoblastic leukemia with standard doses of mercaptopurine, thioguanine and azathioprine (immunosuppressant) may experience severe and potentially lethal bone marrow toxicity. A dose-reduction of up to 15-fold may be needed to avoid hematotoxicity in these patients (Evans et al., 1991). TPMT genotyping or phenotyping (by assessing red blood cell enzyme levels) prior to the institution of therapy with any of these agents has become accepted practice at some medical centers (Sadee, 2000).

Several similar examples have been documented (Iyer and Ratain, 1998): patients with variant DPyDH cannot inactivate 5-fluorouracil, resulting in myelosuppression and neurotoxicity, while overexpression of DPyDH in tumors is linked to resistance to that drug; N-acetyltransferase 2 rapid acetylators (30%–60% of Caucasians and 80%–90% of Asians) are at risk of greater bone marrow toxicity with amonafide treatment (topoisomerase II inhibitor); and patients who have a genetic deficiency of glucuronidation because of a variant promoter of UGT-glucuronosyltransferase UGT1A1 are at increased risk of myelosuppression and diarrhea when treated with the topoisomerase I inhibitor irinotecan. At least one example of an *activating* variant of a co-factor/enzyme has been reported: mutations of NAD(P)H(nicotinamide-adenine dinucleotide phosphate, reduced form):quinone oxidoreductase (which activates cytotoxic anti-tumor quinones such as mitomycin C) protect against cytoxic metabolites, but also may reduce anti-tumor efficacy (Gaedigk et al., 1998).

Growth factor receptors may be overexpressed in some tumors, potentially affecting the efficacy of chemotherapy. One example of this involves the humanized monoclonal antibody trastuzumab (Herceptin™), which was designed to target an oncogene (HER2/neu) that is overexpressed in some breast cancers and other cancers with poor prognoses. Trastuzumab, when given with paclitaxel and doxorubicin, enhances the cytotoxic effects of the anti-neoplastic agents in breast cancer tissues with high HER2/neu expression (Baselge *et al.*, 1998). Some researchers suggest that an optimal approach to cancer chemotherapy would involve genotyping both malignant and normal cells when feasible (Sadee, 2000).

OTHER RELEVANT POLYMORPHISMS

Some sequence polymorphisms that are involved in disease pathogenesis also may be involved in determining drug response, directly or indirectly. One example is apolipoprotein E4 (Apo-E4), a risk factor for familial late-onset and sporadic Alzheimer's Disease (AD) that has been reported to predict poor response to the cholinesterase inhibitor tacrine (Farlow *et al.*, 1996). The presence of the E4 allele also may be a factor in the success of prophylactic estrogen therapy for AD (Sadee, 2000). In addition, Apo-E4 is associated with increased risk of coronary artery disease (CAD). Gerdes *et al.* (2000) reported that presence of this allele is associated with an almost 2-fold increased risk of death in myocardial infarct survivors and that this increased mortality rate can be abolished by treatment with simvastatin (HMG-CoA/3-hydroxy-3methylglutaryl coenzyme A reductase inhibitor). Increased understanding of the underlying multigenic causes of AD, CAD and other diseases and neurodegenerative disorders may lead to the development of strategies for disease treatment and even prophylaxis for those at high risk of developing a disease.

Another example of a disease-related polymorphism that is predictive of drug response involves cholesteryl ester transfer protein (CETP) and pravastatin (HMG-CoA reductase inhibitor used to treat hypercholesterolemia). Kuivenhoven *et al.* (1998) reported a significant relationship between variation of the CETP gene and the progression of coronary atherosclerosis, independent of lipolytic plasma enzyme activity and plasma HDL cholesterol concentration. If these results are replicated, then the presence of a homozygous polymorphism at this site could be used to predict whether treatment with pravastatin would delay the progression of coronary atherosclerosis in men with CAD.

THE CHANGING PARADIGM OF DRUG DEVELOPMENT AND DELIVERY

CURRENT CHALLENGES IN THE CLINICAL APPLICATION OF PHARMACOGENETIC KNOWLEDGE

It is clear from this cursory review of the current state of knowledge regarding the genetic basis of ADRs that many clinically significant genetic polymorphisms affecting drug response in humans have been described already. The emphasis to date has been on identification of mutant alleles at a single gene locus (e.g. Phase I and II hepatic enzymes, TPMT, DPyDH), and this research has been fruitful. However, drug response depends on the drug's interaction with the many proteins involved in its absorption, distribution, excretion and target site, each of which is coded for by genes that may be associated with common variants that may affect response. For example, one individual may exhibit polymorphisms of genes coding for two drug-related proteins: one that affects the degree of drug inactivation and one that determines the sensitivity of the drug receptor. The polymorphism affecting the drug's metabolism would determine the plasma concentrations to which the individual is exposed, and the polymorphic receptor would determine the nature of the individual's response at a given drug concentration. These polygenic interactions are much more difficult to establish during the course of clinical drug trials than are the monogenic effects discussed above, but may have an even more significant impact on drug response.

The effects of environmental factors may be modified by wild-type or polymorphic genes, as well, introducing more confounding variables. The majority of these gene variants are relatively uncommon in the general population, making it difficult to establish their role in drug response and demonstrate clinical relevance, especially for heterozygous individuals who are likely to exhibit more subtle effects than homozygotes.

Clinical research in disease genetics and pharmacogenetics has, at times, produced discordant and contradictory results, creating confusion and resulting in a lack of credibility in the minds of many health care providers. Inconsistent results may be due to several factors, including the lack of strict diagnostic criteria for study entry, the heterogeneous nature of the diseases being studied, the use of different end points and scales for assessing drug efficacy and ADRs, the presence of unknown or unidentified environmental factors and the polygenic nature of many drug effects (Evans and Relling, 1999). It is crucial in clinical pharmacogenetic research that the study sample be of adequate size to demonstrate the necessary statistical power and that the results be rigorously confirmed in comparable populations by other researchers (Manasco *et al.*, 2000). In addition, once a drug has been approved, ongoing, systematic centralized collection of meaningful, evaluable data regarding drug efficacy and ADRs does not occur routinely, and pharmacogenetic data are rarely collected at all. As a result, opportunities for increasing our knowledge of dramatic and subtle genetic effects on drug response both in large numbers of diverse patients and specific diagnostic subsets of patients are lost.

Much pharmacogenetic research to date has involved identifying and categorizing drug-related polymorphisms, while relatively little has been done to determine clinical relevance in well-defined populations. Clinicians do not know which variants should be assessed; how and by whom that should be done; what drugs might be affected; what course of action would be appropriate based on the information obtained; and who will cover the cost of the test. Should the dose be altered? By how much? Should the drug be avoided entirely? What about related drugs and polymorphisms? Must each be tested separately? What effects do the variants have on drug–drug and drug–environment interactions? What issues exist around professional liability and the ethical, legal and social aspects of such testing? Carefully designed, well-controlled clinical studies in appropriate populations must be carried out to begin to answer these pressing questions, and the information then must be made available to clinicians and reflected in ethically grounded standards of clinical practice and compensation procedures.

In addition, standard pharmacotherapy references and treatment guidelines formulated by various health care organizations rarely contain relevant pharmacogenetic information even when it is known, making it difficult for clinicians to gain access to existing data. Consumers, health care providers, payers and regulatory agencies lack basic education with regard to pharmacogenetics and timely access to relevant new data as they emerge. Although the lay press occasionally spotlights a tragedy that could have been averted through the application of existing pharmacogenetic knowledge (such as "overdose" deaths of slow drug metabolizers; Stipp, 2000), the need for increased professional and public awareness and education in this arena is equal to the need for continuing research.

Until recently, genotyping an individual was a laborious, time-consuming and costly proposition that was undertaken only if there was a high index of suspicion of an identified genetic disorder. The Human Genome Project and the multitude of high technology spin-offs from it are changing this situation. Automated instrumentation, new bioinformatics systems and novel strategies derived from genomic research will enable researchers to evaluate and analyze the wealth of genetic information that will continue to emerge. High-throughput DNA sequencing, gene mapping and transcriptional analyses are becoming economically and scientifically feasible as a result of innovations such as DNA, cDNA ("edited" version of a gene, containing only the parts that will be expressed as proteins) and oligonucleotide microarrays and microfluidic analytical devices (Mancinelli *et al.*, 2000). Increasingly simple and inexpensive gene analysis systems based on these technologies eventually will result in practical, timely, cost-effective point-of-care screening of patients for relevant polymorphisms before treatment with a specific drug is initiated.

SINGLE NUCLEOTIDE POLYMORPHISMS, MEDICINE RESPONSE TESTS AND "GENETIC TESTS"

Many of the previously mentioned polymorphisms directly alter the metabolism, transport, action or excretion of medicines via identified (or identifiable) structural or functional effects; there is a causal relationship between the polymorphism and the phenotype. New genomic techniques such as those mentioned above are making it possible to detect *associations* (which may or may not be causal) between specific genetic markers and individual response to medicines. Single nucleotide polymorphisms (SNPs, pronounced "snips"), single-base differences in DNA sequence, are the most common form of human polymorphisms. They occur with an average frequency of about 1 per 1300 base pairs, serving as easily identifiable virtual mileposts along the 3 billion base pair human genome (International Human Genome Sequencing Consortium, 2001).

The SNP Consortium (a not-for-profit organization of pharmaceutical and bioinformational companies, academic centers, and a charitable trust) has produced an ordered high-density SNP map (containing 600–800 000 SNPs) of the human genome, which is publicly available at <http://snp.cshl.org>. This map will be used to find disease genes and to correlate genetic information with individual responses to medicines. Although few of these SNPs are expected to be involved directly with disease or medicine response, they will be useful as analytical tools to track small segments of the genome. Individuals who carry a particular gene variant (allele) are likely to carry variants of several SNP markers that are close to or within that allele because of the phenomenon of linkage disequilibrium (LD; when alleles are in close physical proximity, they are likely to be inherited together).

The results of whole-genome SNP scanning obtained during Phase II clinical trials of a medicine can be used to identify specific SNP markers, patterns or haplotypes that correlate to patient responses (efficacy and ADRs), forming a SNP Print[SM] (Figure 43.1), one type of medicine response test (MRT; a genetic or laboratory test used to predict an individual's response to a specific medicine or class of medicines). These medicine response-related data could form the basis for the selection of patients most likely to respond well in Phase III trials, possibly making these trials smaller, faster and more efficient (Bonnie *et al.*, 2000). MRTs also could be used to predict subtle polygenic effects on response, as well as drug–drug and drug–environment interactions that have a genetic component.

Medicine response tests may be based on SNPs of no known clinical significance, as discussed above; they also may be based on polymorphisms within genes having defined functions (e.g. identified polymorphisms such as those affecting Phase I and II metabolic enzymes, Apo-E4, new polymorphisms identified using the candidate gene approach, etc.) and on RNA or proteins. For example, a European company has developed and plans to market a gene-specific test based on polymorphisms in the renin–angiotensin–aldosterone system (through which angiotensin converting enzyme/ACE inhibitors act) to screen hypertensive patients for their responsiveness to ACE inhibitors.

Functional enzyme analysis of TPMT in red blood cells before treatment with specific cancer chemotherapy drugs is one example of an MRT in current use in the United States. Another is HercepTest®, which uses a polyclonal antibody to detect HER2 protein, reflecting HER2 expression in breast cancer cells; it is used to predict patient response to trastuzumab (Herceptin®), a humanized monoclonal antibody against the HER2 receptor. Researchers already have developed other tools for assessing HER2 expression, including a monoclonal antibody test for the HER2 protein; a test for circulating HER2 protein (in the extracellular domain); and a test using fluorescence *in situ* hybridization (FISH) directly to determine the number of copies of the HER2 gene (not its protein product). Because of the strong correlation between overexpression of HER2 protein and response to Herceptin®, the US Food and Drug Administration (FDA) required that a test kit to assess HER2 protein expression be commercially available prior to drug approval—an example of a regulatory agency

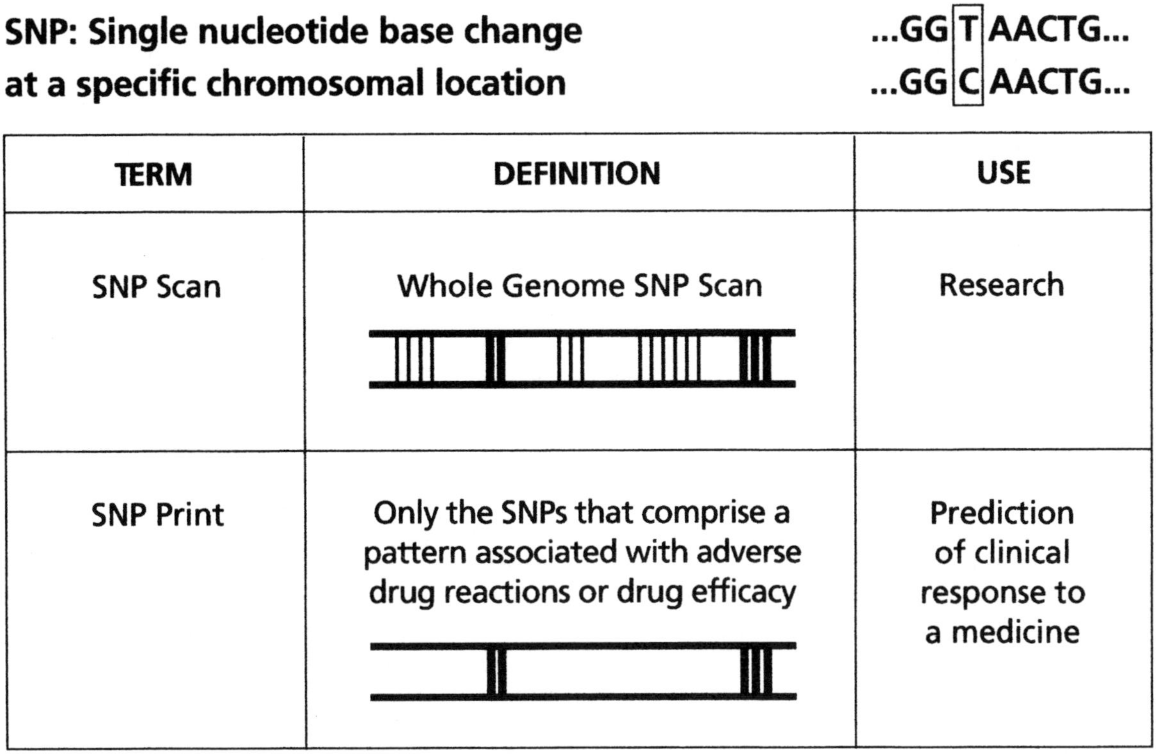

SNP: Single nucleotide base change
at a specific chromosomal location

...GG|T|AACTG...
...GG|C|AACTG...

TERM	DEFINITION	USE
SNP Scan	Whole Genome SNP Scan	Research
SNP Print	Only the SNPs that comprise a pattern associated with adverse drug reactions or drug efficacy	Prediction of clinical response to a medicine

Figure 43.1. SNPs, SNP-scans and SNP Prints[SM].

mandating the availability of an MRT linked to use of a specific drug.

Transcriptional analyses, in which the expression levels of DNA are measured, may provide another approach for MRTs (Kleyn and Vesell, 1998). RNA obtained from biopsied tissue and surgical specimens can be used for expression-based studies in some cancers, allowing detection of somatic changes associated with the development of some tumors and their response to chemotherapy. For example, the amplification of the oncogene *erb-B2* predicts a good response to treatment with a specific adjuvant therapy (cyclophosphamide-methotrexate-5-fluorouracil) for breast cancer (Muss *et al.*, 1994). Alternately, the expression of genes predicting drug response can be assayed at the protein level using antibody-based tests of serum or other tissues (Kleyn and Vesell, 2000).

Ongoing genetic and genomic research undoubtedly will result in the development of additional tools that can be incorporated into or used as the basis of MRTs. The rationale exists for conducting pharmacogenetic analyses to look for associations between drug responses (safety and efficacy) and genotype, and the technology exists for conducting these analyses (which soon will be feasible in terms of efficiency and cost). The missing piece is a pool of DNA samples with associated medical and medicine response data to facilitate the efficient conduct of pharmacogenetic research. Eventually, MRTs based on SNP Prints[SM] and other genetic tools will enable health care providers to identify patients at high risk of developing a given disease, implement preventive therapy and lifestyle adjustments when appropriate and choose the medicines that are most likely to benefit the patient and least likely to result in serious ADRs (Mancinelli *et al.*, 2000).

In the past, the term "genetic testing" often has been associated with the diagnosis of monogenic diseases such as cystic fibrosis and Huntingdon disease—conditions for which a causative, often single, genetic mutation has been identified. A newer area of genetic research and testing involves identification of genes related to the occurrence of common complex diseases such as asthma, heart disease and migraine. These diseases are likely to result from the interaction of multiple "increased risk" or susceptibility genes with each other and possibly with environmental factors. These types of genetic research and testing (related to mono-genic diseases and susceptibility genes) involve determining the likelihood of occurrence (predic-tion) or the presence (diagnosis) of disease in individuals. Although very useful and important, there are social and ethical risks related to the nature of the information revealed by these tests— what it means, who has access to it and how it can be used. There is general agreement on the need for genetic counseling to help patients and families understand and process the results of these disease- and risk-related genetic tests.

In contrast, the risks associated with tests to detect polymorphisms related to response to medicines, such as metabolic and drug receptor or target characteristics and genomic profiles such as SNP Prints^{SM}, are minimal: the data that are obtained are quite limited and specific to the drug(s) being considered. No information about disease-causal or susceptibility genes is likely to be obtained. These tests, when validated, will be similar to routine laboratory tests such as blood typing, drug concentration monitoring and liver enzyme analyses. While health care providers would discuss the results with patients, there would be no need for genetic counseling and ongoing psychosocial support related to interpre-tation of the results, with rare exceptions.

The Secretary's Advisory Committee on Genetic Testing, an expert panel convened by the US National Institutes of Health Task Force on Genetic Testing, is working with the government and the FDA to develop terminology and guide-lines that more accurately reflect recent changes in genetic testing (Table 43.4). In the past, this group has focused mainly on mutational genetics and monogenic diseases and the need for government oversight in this area. This represents only one part of the spectrum encompassed by "genetic tests", however, and the major differences between tests that are specific to disease genes and those that are specific to genes involved in drug efficacy and safety have not yet been addressed (Roses, 2000b). Current information on this Committee's work can be found at its website: `<http:// www4.od.nih.gov/oba/sacgt.htm>`.

THE IMPACT OF PHARMACOGENETICS ON CLINICAL DRUG DEVELOPMENT

Historically, fewer than 10% of new chemical entities (NCEs) entering preclinical development are approved for clinical use, often because of unacceptable toxicity in animal studies or Phase I human trials or insufficient efficacy (Kleyn and

Table 43.4. Comparison of different types of "genetic testing".

Application	Disease genetics	Pharmacogenetics/medicine response tests
What is being tested	*Rare Mendelian (monogenic) diseases, "causal" genes *Complex common diseases (multifactorial), susceptibility genes	*Genes related to drug metabolism or action *SNP Prints^{SM} related to drug safety or efficacy
Potential benefits	Prediction of occurrence, diagnosis of disease; insights into disease mechanisms and development of new medicines	Optimal individual response to medicine
Potential risks	Informational risk to patient and family, with related ethical, legal and social issues (employment, insurance, etc.)	Low informational risk; data provided will relate only to individual response to specific medicines

Vesell, 1998). The cost of bringing a new drug to market is approximately $500 million; the costs of ADRs and treatment failures, discussed earlier, are staggering. The application of pharmacogenetic research and knowledge could result in streamlining and improving the clinical development process in several ways:

- by initial toxicogenomic screening of compounds to detect selective metabolism, disposition or action related to known polymorphic enzymes, transporters or targets,
- by enabling fewer subjects to be recruited into clinical trials, and
- by enhancing the efficacy and safety profiles of medicines in targeted populations.

Many pharmaceutical companies now routinely screen NCEs to see if they are metabolized selectively by known polymorphic enzymes, and development is discontinued or altered to include additional pharmacokinetic studies for many of those that are because of the potentially increased risk of serious ADRs or lack of efficacy in subpopulations of patients (Zuhlsdorf, 1998). The development and use of MRTs may serve to "rescue" some of these NCEs: if a cost-effective, valid and accessible predictive test is available to screen patients before the drug is prescribed, along with evidence-based guidelines for dose adjustments or drug avoidance, then many valuable medicines that in the past would have been abandoned may make it to market. The same may be true for approved medicines and even for some that have been withdrawn from market. For example, terfenadine (Seldane®) caused ADRs in patients who had a specific *CYP2D6* gene polymorphism and also were taking erythromycin— they were unable to metabolize terfenadine in this situation, which caused toxic accumulation of the drug in the body. The FDA worked with the pharmaceutical manufacturer to distribute appropriate warnings about the possible risks of its use with concomitant medicines, but the company and FDA decided that the drug's risk–benefit ratio did not justify its continued use. If a screening test to identify patients at risk for this problem had been available, it might have been possible to keep the

drug on the market while protecting some of those most likely to experience toxicity from it (Bhandari *et al.*, 1999).

Discussion of the potential impact of pharmacogenetics on clinical trial design is beyond the scope of this chapter, but it is clear that many pharmaceutical companies recognize its importance and are planning to initiate pharmacogenetic studies in the near future (Ball and Borman, 1997). Lichter and McNamara (1995) suggested one approach for incorporating pharmacogenetics into clinical trials:

- Perform preclinical identification of metabolic pathways and population screening for common DNA sequence variants of the relevant enzymes, transporters, receptors and target genes (and their homologues), as discussed above.
- Consider the ethnicity of study populations based on known differences in the frequency of specific polymorphisms.
- During Phase I trials, type subjects for the genes known to control the drug's metabolic pathway(s) to allow possible correlation of ADRs with genotype, and use this information as a basis for subject selection in Phase II and III studies.
- During Phase II trials, type any identified relevant polymorphisms in the entire study group. Also type the gene product and related targets in all subjects, allowing assessment of allele frequencies in the population and in responders vs. non-responders. Use these data as a basis for subject selection in Phase III trials.
- If useful genetic markers of efficacy or ADRs are identified during Phase II, the Phase III group could be expanded to include a cohort prescreened to include likely responders and those at low risk of ADRs.

This approach is limited by its reliance on identified candidate genes (genes selected on the basis of existing knowledge or an informed guess) and molecular pharmacology to identify drug–receptor interaction and down-stream signaling pathways, and unexpected associations (either causal or resulting from LD) may not be recognized.

Another approach that is being used already by some pharmaceutical companies and holds even greater promise as technological advances increase the accuracy, feasibility and cost-effectiveness of high-throughput whole-genome scanning, will involve collecting a single blood sample for DNA analysis from all consenting participants in selected Phase II and III clinical trials (after approval by the appropriate ethics review boards and provision of specific informed consent by subjects). This sample may be used to identify the occurrence of known polymorphisms affecting drug response, to evaluate candidate genes suspected of being involved in the disease or drug response and to assess patterns of SNP or haplotype occurrence related to efficacy or ADRs, allowing the creation of a SNP Print[SM] to screen potential subjects or patients (post-approval) for their likely response to the drug or determine heterogeneity of the disease in patients with similar phenotypes (Roses, 2000b).

Regulatory agencies might be concerned, appropriately, that the smaller numbers of patients in these streamlined clinical trials would be insufficient to detect rare ADRs (<1 : 1000) and that patients who did not receive or "pass" the recommended MRT for the drug would nevertheless receive it and be at increased risk of harm. However, rare ADRs are not likely to be detected even in the relatively large clinical trials that are conducted now; it certainly is not feasible to enroll the approximately 65 000 patients that would be required to be 95% confident of detecting three or more cases of an ADR with an incidence of 1 : 10 000 (Lewis, 1981). The major, albeit rare, ADRs associated with dexfenfluramine, zomepirac, benoxaprofen, troglitazone and terfenadine were not detected until after they reached the market. Extensive pre-approval safety testing in even larger populations is a possible solution, although, as noted above, it will be impractical to identify very rare ADRs in clinical trial study populations, and the increased cost and delayed time to market is likely to create significant financial barriers from the perspective of the pharmaceutical companies (and ultimately consumers and payers, to whom the cost will be passed along) (Roses, 2000a).

One solution to this problem would be an extensive, regulated post-approval surveillance system that incorporates the collection of pharmacogenetic data. Roses (2000b) proposes that hundreds of thousands of patients receiving a medicine would have filter paper blood spots taken (perhaps from the original blood sample used for the MRT) and stored in a central location. As rare and/or serious ADRs are reported and characterized, DNA from affected patients could be compared with that of control patients, allowing ongoing refinement of the MRT. There is increasing pressure to improve the inconsistent and largely unregulated current system of post-marketing surveillance, and many authors agree on the need to incorporate pharmacogenetic data in some form into a revised system (Edwards and Aronson, 2000; Nelson, 2000).

Another approach is one that would put increasing control of medical data in the hands of those most directly affected by it—consumers. In this scenario, an individual could choose to have a one-time blood sample taken for DNA analysis and stored at a tightly secured central repository. As research into disease-related genes, genetic risk factors and genetic associations with medicine responses progressed, the consumer or a designated representative (such as a health care provider) could request that the sample be analyzed using relevant MRTs (including SNP Prints[SM]) and other markers. This "bank" could serve as a central repository for the samples themselves and as a central database of information including well-established knowledge, current research and even opportunities for clinical trial subjects with specific conditions or genotypes. It could trigger genetic "alerts" to consumers who chose to provide a medical and family history as new research results potentially relevant to them became available. A host of ethical, legal and social issues would need to be addressed as part of this venture, but it presents one option for an efficient, centralized and consumer-controlled bank of health-related genetic expertise and information.

CONCLUSION

The results of pharmacogenetic research will impact the discovery, development and safe, effective use of medicines in several ways:

● Many diseases will be diagnosed based on genotype (underlying mechanism of disease) rather than phenotype (presenting signs and symptoms) alone, enabling health care providers to determine the optimal therapeutic approach.
● Health care providers will use SNP Prints[SM] and other MRTs as a basis for selecting the medicine and dose most likely to be efficacious and least likely to cause ADRs in individual patients.
● Identification of disease susceptibility genes will allow implementation of preventive measures or early treatment of specific diseases.
● New medicines will be designed to avoid or exploit specific polymorphisms of genes involved in disease susceptibility or drug metabolism, transport or action.

Many challenges remain to be overcome. The human genome is complex and dynamic, and although we have made great progress in unraveling its mysteries, it still holds many secrets. Diseases and responses to medicines are likely to involve many genes, each of which plays a specific role and interacts with other genes and the environment in complex, interdependent ways. Technological challenges involving statistics, bioinformatics tools, high-throughput sample processing, accuracy and cost still exist, although progress is being made in resolving them. In addition to these scientific and technological issues, we as a society have to deal with the many complicated ethical, legal and social questions that arise as a result of our increased understanding of our genetic heritage and our growing ability to affect it and alter its effect on us.

History has taught us that scientific knowledge and technological advances will continue; our human challenge is to apply what we learn skillfully and for the betterment of all humanity. Although the clinical relevance of progress in pharmacogenetics is just beginning to become clear, it holds great promise for improving health and quality of life for millions of people throughout the world.

REFERENCES

Arranz MJ, Munro J, Birkett J, Bolonna A, Mancama D, Sodhi M, Lesch KP, Meyer JFW, Sham P, Collier DA, Murray RM, Kerwin RW (2000) Pharmacogenetic prediction of clozapine response. *Lancet* **355**: 1615–16.

Ball S, Borman N (1997) Pharmacogenetics and drug metabolism. *Nature Biotechnol* **15**: 925–6.

Barosso I, Gurnell M, Crowley V, Agostini M, Schwabe JW, Soos MA, Maslen LI, Williams TD, Lewis H, Shafer AJ, Chatterjee VK, O'Rahilly S (1999) Dominant negative mutations in human PPAR gamma associated with severe insulin resistance, diabetes mellitus and hypertension. *Nature* **402**: 880–3.

Baselge J, Norton L, Albanell J, Kim YM, Mendelsohn J (1998) Recombinant humanized anti-HER2 antibody (*Herceptin*) enhances the antitumor activity of paclitaxel and doxorubicin against HER2/neu overexpressing human breast cancer xenografts. *Cancer Res* **58**: 2825–31.

Bhandari M, Garg R, Glassman R and Ma P (1999) The pharmacogenomics challenge. *In Vivo: The Business and Medicine Report* **March**: 36–41.

Bonnie A, Fijal MS, Hall JM, White JS (2000) Clinical trials in the genomic era: effects of protective genotypes on sample size and duration of trial. *Contr Clin Trials* **21**: 7–20.

Daly AK (1995) Molecular basis of polymorphic drug metabolism. *J Mol Med* **73**: 539–53.

Destenaves B, Thomas F (2000) New advances in pharmacogenomics. *Curr Op Chem Biol* **4**: 440–4.

Drysdale CM, McGraw DW, Stack CB, Stephens JC, Judson RS, Nandabalan K, Arnold K, Ruano G, Liggett SB (2000) Complex promoter and coding region β-adrenergic receptor haplotypes alter receptor expression and predict *in vivo* responsiveness. *Proc Natl Acad Sci* **97**: 10483–8.

Edwards IR, Aronson JK (2000) Adverse drug reactions: Definitions, diagnosis and management. *Lancet* **356**: 1255–9.

Evans WE, Horner M, Chu YQ, Kalwinsky D, Roberts WM (1991) Altered mercaptopurine metabolism, toxic effects and dosage requirement in a thiopurine methyltransferase-deficient child with acute lymphocytic leukemia. *J Pediatr* **119**: 985–9.

Evans WE, Relling, MV (1999) Pharmacogenomics: translating functional genomics into rational therapeutics. *Science* **286**: 487–91.

Farlow MR, Lahiri DK, Poirier J, Davignon J, Hui S (1996) Apoplipoprotein E genotype and gender influence response to tacrine therapy. *Ann NY Acad Sci* **802**: 101–10.

Gaedigk A, Tyndale RF, Jurima-Romet M, Sellers EM, Grant DM, Leeder JM (1998) NAD(P)H: quinone oxidoreductase: polymorphisms and allele frequencies in Caucasian, Chinese and Canadian native Indian and Inuit populations. *Pharmacogenetics* **8**: 305–13.

Garrod AE (1902) The incidence of alcaptonuria: a study in chemical individuality. *Lancet* **ii**: 1616–20.

Geller DS, Farhi A, Pinkerton N, Fradley M, Moritz M, Spitzer A, Meinke G, Tsai FT, Sigler PB, Lifton RP (2000) Activating mineralocorticoid receptor mutation in hypertension exacerbated by pregnancy. *Science* **289**: 119–22.

Gerdes LU, Gerdes C, Kervinen K, Savolainen M, Klausen IC, Hansen PS, Kesaniemi YA, Faergeman O (2000) The apolipoprotein E-4 allele determines prognosis and the effect on prognosis of simvastatin in survivors of myocardial infarction: a substudy of the Scandanavian simvastatin survival study. *Circulation* **101**: 1366–71.

Heils A, Teufel A, Petri S (1996) Allelic variation of human serotonin transporter gene expression. *J Neurochem* **66**: 2621–4.

Hoffmeyer S, Burk O, von Richter O, Arnold HP, Brockmoller J, Johne A, Cascorbi I, Gerloff T, Roots I, Eichelbaum M, Brinkmann U (2000) Functional polymorphisms of the human multidrug-resistance gene: multiple sequence variations and correlation of one allele with P-glycoprotein expression and activity *in vivo*. *Proc Natl Acad Sci* **97**: 3473–8.

Huizenga NATM, Koper JW, de Lange P, Pols HAP, Stolk RP, Burger H, Grobbee DE, Brinkmann AO, de Jong FH, Lamberts SWJ (1998) A polymorphism in the glucocorticoid receptor gene may be associated with an increased sensitivity to glucocorticoids *in vivo*. *J Clin Endocrinol Metab* **83**: 144–51.

Ingelman-Sundberg M, Oscarson M, McLellan RA (1999) Polymorphic human cytochrome P450 enzymes: an opportunity for individualized drug treatment. *Trends Pharmacol Sci* **20**: 342–9.

International Human Genome Sequencing Consortium (2001) Initial sequencing and analysis of the human genome. *Nature* **409**: 860–921.

Iyer L, Ratain MJ (1998) Pharmacogenetics and cancer chemotherapy. *Eur J Cancer* **34**: 1493–9.

Jonsson EG, Nothen MM, Gustavsson JP, Neidt H, Bunzel R, Propping P, Sedvall GC (1998) Polymorphisms in the dopamine, serotonin and norepinephrine transporter genes and their relationships to monoamine metabolite concentrations in CSF of healthy volunteers. *Psych Res* **79**: 1–9.

Kleyn PW, Vesell ES (1998) Genetic variation as a guide to drug development. *Science* **281**: 1820–1.

Kuivenhoven JA, Jukema JW, Zwinderman AH, de Knijff P, McPherson R, Bruschke AVG, Lie KI, Kastelein JJP (1998) The role of a common variant of the cholesteryl ester transfer protein gene in the progression of coronary atherosclerosis. *New Engl J Med* **338**: 86–93.

Lazarou J, Pomeranz BH, Corey PN (1998) Incidence of adverse drug reactions in hospitalized patients: A meta-analysis of prospective studies. *J Am Med Assoc* **279**: 1200–5.

Lewis JA (1981) Post-marketing surveillance: How many patients? *Trends Pharmacol Sci* **2**: 93–4.

Lichter J, McNamara D (1995) What's in a gene: Using genetic information for the design of clinical trials. *Curr Op Biotechnol* **6**: 715–7.

Liggett SB (2000) The pharmacogenetics of β-adrenergic receptors: Relevance to asthma. *J Allergy Clin Immunol* **105**: S487–92.

Lipworth BJ, Hall IP, Aziz I, Tan KS, Wheatley A (1999) β-2-adrenoceptor polymorphism and bronchoprotective sensitivity with regular short- and long-acting β-2 agonist therapy. *Clin Sci* **96**: 253–9.

Manasco P, Rieser PA, Pericak-Vance M (2000) Genes—Here today, gone tomorrow: a clinician's guide to genetic linkage and association studies. *The Endocrinologist* **10**: 328–34.

Mancinelli L, Cronin M, Sadee W (2000) Pharmacogenomics: the promise of personalized medicine. *Am Acad Pharmaceut Sci Pharmsci* **2**(1), article 4. Available at http://www.pharmsci.org

Meyer UA (2000) Pharmacogenetics and adverse drug reactions. *Lancet* **356**: 1667–71.

Muss HB, Thor AD, Berry DA, Kute T, Liu ET, Koerner F, Cirrincione CT, Budman DR, Wood WC, Barcos M, Henderson IC (1994) c-erbB-2 expression and response to adjuvant therapy in women with node-positive early breast cancer. *New Engl J Med* **330**: 1260–6.

Navis G, van der Kleij FG, de Zeeuw D and de Jong PE (1999) Angiotensin-converting enzyme gene I/D polymorphism and renal disease. *J Mol Med* **77**: 781–91.

Nelson R (2000) We need a postmarketing drug development process! *Pharmacoepidemiology and Drug Safety* **9**: 253–5.

Priori SG, Barhanin J, Hauer RN, Haverkamp W, Jongsma HJ, Kleber AG, McKenna WJ, Roden DM, Rudy Y, Schwartz K, Schwartz PJ, Towbin JA, Wilde AM (1999) Genetic and molecular basis of cardiac arrhythmias: Impact on clinical management, Parts I and II. *Circulation* **99**: 518–28.

Roses AD (2000a) Pharmacogenetics and future drug development and delivery. *Lancet* **355**: 1358–61.

Roses AD (2000b) Pharmacogenetics and the practice of medicine. *Nature* **405**: 857–65.

Sadee W. (2000) Using genetic information to optimize drug therapy. *Medscape Pharmacotherapy 2000*.

Available at `http://www.medscape.com/Medscape/pharmacology/journal/2000/v0.../pnt-mp7377.sade.htm`

Sousa AR, Lane SJ, Cidlowski JA, Staynov DZ, Lee TH (2000) Glucocorticoid resistance in asthma is associated with elevated *in vivo* expression of the glucocorticoid receptor β-isoform. *J Allergy Clin Immunol* **105**: 943–50.

Stipp D (2000) A DNA tragedy. *Fortune* **142**: 170–5.

Tan S, Hall IP, Dewar J, Dow E, Lipworth B (1997) Association between β2-adrenoreceptor polymorphism and susceptibility to bronchodilator desensitiza-tion in moderately severe stable asthmatics. *Lancet* **350**: 995–9.

Touw DJ (1997) Clinical implications of genetic poly-morphisms and drug interactions mediated by cyto-chrome P450 enzymes. *Drug Metabolism and Drug Interactions* **14**: 55–82.

White TJ, Arakelian A, Roh JP (1999) Counting the cost of drug-related adverse events. *Pharmacoeconomics* **15**: 445–58.

Zuhlsdorf MT (1998) Relevance of pheno- and genotyp-ing in clinical drug development. *Intl J Clin Pharmacol Ther* **36**: 607–12.

44

Keynote Clinical Lessons from Pharmacovigilance

DAVID H. LAWSON

Department of Clinical Pharmacology, Royal Infirmary, Glasgow, UK

INTRODUCTION

The history of predicting the future in medical sciences is fraught with difficulty. Almost invariably, major new developments lie just round the corner and are unforeseen by those working in the field. That said, I have always regarded the best guides to the future are the lessons gained from mistakes made in the past.

Unfortunately, the public perception of drug safety is not one of the triumph of science over disease. Rather it is one of vague unease and concern often aggravated by exaggerated and markedly adverse media publicity. At the time of writing (Spring 2001), adverse drug effects are again being trumpeted as a major cause of admissions to hospital. This is being emphasised with no regard to separating out those adverse reactions that are predictable (due to pharmacological effects and thus reflect inappropriate prescribing by doctors or inadequate adherence to clinical advice on the part of patients), from those that are idiosyncratic and thus unpredicted (due to intrinsic problems with medicines whether documented or as yet undiscovered). Nor is due attention directed towards the underlying disorders for which the medicines were prescribed and which themselves may have major consequences if left untreated. For example, more and more patients are subjected to heroic chemotherapy with the objective of prolonging existence in advanced neoplasia. Occasionally the therapy is effective, but more often it is associated with severe undesired effects, these being entirely predictable and an accepted risk by the prescriber (and hopefully the patient) at the time of initiating the chemotherapy. At the outset, the potential benefits may appear to be worth the risks. For many patients this turns out not to be so.

Similarly, the increasingly widespread use of prophylactic anticoagulation in patients with unstable rhythms with the objective of preventing life-threatening embolic phenomena is associated with a predictable burden of haemorrhagic complications, some of which are undoubtedly life-threatening. Were the media to address the reasons for the drug exposure as well as the consequences thereof, perhaps a more balanced approach to the subject could be undertaken. Unfortunately this is likely to be asking too much in our litigation-conscious society.

Pharmacovigilance. Edited by R.D. Mann and E.B. Andrews
© 2002 John Wiley & Sons, Ltd

Occasional sudden deaths from torsade de pointes in young individual recipients of antihistamine therapy has been another pressing cause for concern over the years. Despite this, there are little in the way of systematic efforts directed towards quantitating the frequency of such deaths. Identifying such patients and reviewing their treatment in the days and weeks preceding death could add valuable knowledge to our portfolio of information on this topic.

Another area of major current concern is the great parental anxiety about the potential hazards of the combined measles, mumps and rubella (MMR) vaccine. Clearly this is a problematic area. Vaccination is used to prevent illness, yet some of those vaccinated may experience minor (local) side-effects. Non-vaccinated children do not suffer any problems at the time when their peers are vaccinated. The reported associations between MMR vaccines, inflammatory bowel disease and autism have caused greatly increased concern about all vaccines in parents who have rarely seen the effects of mumps, measles, whooping cough or indeed most other contagious diseases in the raw. The overwhelming balance of evidence available at present indicates that this problem arises from a causal interpretation being placed erroneously onto an apparently random association. Such interpretations can cause enormous grief. They also cannot easily be rejected or proven wrong by the very nature of the information available to pharmacovigilators. Thus concerns of this type are likely always to be a part of the day-to-day experiences of those involved in this difficult and uncertain area. One key feature of most of these recent pharmacovigilance problems is the substantial rarity with which they occur as a consequence of the intrinsic properties of the medicine itself, as compared with the way in which it is used. I shall return to this topic in the concluding section of this chapter.

Finally, recurrent headline grabbing, but false, claims by the media of collusion between the pharmaceutical industry, drug regulators and advisory committees, such as the Committee on Safety of Medicines and Medicines Commission, serves greatly to heighten public concern in an area where the echoes of the thalidomide disaster are still audible.

If one then adds to the above concerns the epidemic of drug abuse that is hitting mainly the youth in western countries at the present time, the scene is set is for a major lack of understanding of the true benefits and risks of modern therapeutic medicines. *Patients at present seem to have higher expectations of new medicines than can realistically be realised, with lower thresholds for safety than is likely to be achievable without major new delays in licensing products.*

The public perception of a "pill for every ill" is, if anything, stronger over the last 10 years than in the past. There is a strong feeling that drugs should be safe. After all, they are tested for years by increasingly sophisticated mechanisms. The fact that at the time of marketing only a few thousand individuals with the disease of interest may have been exposed to the drugs at the dose for which they are licensed is not generally understood by the public. Moreover, individual members of the public have increasing desires to participate in decisions made about their health. More and more people insist on fully informed information about the risks of the disease from which they suffer, the benefits of therapy to be obtained, and the risks of such therapies. Whilst this is greatly to be lauded, it often places physicians in difficult situations, particularly where patients choose not to fully inform their physician about all their problems or about alternative therapies in which they are indulging. Should anything untoward happen, there is an inevitable tendency to blame the prescriber. Thus in the minds of many patients, the European Convention on Human Rights gives them complete justification for seeking information and making judgements on their own, independently of their physician. However, should things go wrong, there is a conspicuous absence of an equivalent European Convention on Human Responsibility. So any errors or misfortunes that arise are not seen as being, at least partly, those of the patient, but rather attributed in their entirety to the prescriber!

These topics raise an important problem in pharmacovigilance that has only recently begun to be recognised and dealt with. This is the question of acceptance of risk by the public. The former Chief Medical Officer of England (and before that of Scotland, Sir Kenneth Calman) has emphasised the need to have a public debate about this issue as it is clear that a substantial body of the general public (and possibly even some members of the professions) have at best a very hazy understanding of the concepts and magnitude of risks and benefits as far as they apply to disease and its medical treatment. Clearly pharmacoepidemiologists should be to the fore in supporting the necessary endeavours to initiate and sustain any such efforts aimed at improving this sad state of affairs.

PHARMACOVIGILANCE

Pharmacovigilance is all about the safety of drugs in their conditions of normal routine use. It does involve collection and analysis of information about drugs as they are used in a community. No longer is the major focus that of the randomised controlled clinical trial where a well-defined subset of the population is exposed under carefully controlled circumstances to a medicine of interest and followed for a defined duration thereafter. We now enter the area of observational studies with all the problems in interpretation that such observational studies entail. It is important to realise that the interpretation of observational data is much more complex than the interpretation of randomised controlled clinical trials. Such studies are, by their very nature, full of incomplete information and subject not only to controllable biases and distortions, but some are strictly unable to be interpreted because of insurmountable distortions. The various types of studies involved have been covered in earlier chapters in this book. They fall broadly into three categories:

1. The anecdotal study in which reports of suspected problems are solicited and analysed to see if they can give hints about possible drug-related problems, exemplified by the *spontaneous reporting schemes*.
2. More detailed observational studies, but still without appropriate comparator groups who are not exposed to the medicine of interest, e.g. *ad hoc follow-up studies*.

3. Controlled studies, including *follow-up and case–control studies*.

Some 15 years ago, giving the keynote address on pharmacoepidemiology and public health policy at the International Society of Pharmacoepidemiology meeting in Minneapolis, I made several points about this subject which I think are worthwhile repeating here. These are

1. It is the duty of pharmacoepidemiologists to ensure that spontaneous reports of suspected adverse reactions are used wisely in the full knowledge of their substantial limitations.
2. It is our duty as pharmacoepidemiologists to ensure that other sources of information are available which can be interpreted in a reasonably rapid time frame. Good data in six years is no substitute for usable data in six months or less.
3. Pharmacoepidemiology will not prosper if it develops as an intellectual subject which plots the history of why drugs fall from favour. It must be a live and contemporary subject, providing answers to current problems of drug use and drug safety in *real* time.

These aphorisms are as relevant today as they were when first spoken. They apply across the board to all types of studies. Thankfully we have made progress in the intervening years, albeit not as much as we would have liked.

SPONTANEOUS REPORTING SCHEMES

There is widespread agreement that spontaneous reporting schemes are here to stay. They are economical and embrace the entire population of patients and reporters. However, it is important to treat all such reports as hypotheses. Some will almost certainly be causally linked with the suspect drug, whereas others will turn out not to be so. With the increase in acceptance of reports from pharmacists and nurses in addition to doctors, the balance may vary somewhat from region to region and from one group of reporters to another. It is important that standardised procedures are adopted to review and analyse all such spontaneous reports. In so doing, there is a danger that the output from any review could be made available without the benefit of careful clinical and pharmacological expertise and input with serious consequences to all concerned. The rule here is to appreciate that the raw information from spontaneous reporting schemes are anecdotes—no more and no less. They have to be treated as such. Sophisticated analyses of anecdotal data are justified if great care is taken with the subsequent interpretation, otherwise more harm could arise than good. Careful review of all reported suspect reactions to a particular medicine may point to a sub-population at especial risk. Such reviews can rarely be automated, but require careful, time-consuming analysis by trained, experienced observers. Such people are in short supply; nevertheless, they are extremely valuable in the context of logical interpretation of spontaneous reporting schemes.

The development of Augmented Spontaneous Reporting Schemes whereby potential reporters are contacted about details of outcomes after specific medicines have been prescribed in the hope that they will respond in greater numbers and with better quality information, is to be encouraged. These schemes are best developed in New Zealand and by the Drug Safety Research Unit in Southampton. The present author believes that these schemes should be encouraged and developed further in the coming decade. They are not without their problems, however. This is especially so in United Kingdom at present where there is a severe epidemic of concern about confidentiality of medical information within the public psyche. Whilst no one would disagree with the need to maintain confidentiality when dealing with information on illness, and all would support the need for great care in this area, nonetheless there are circumstances in which the need to link information from several different sources is necessary to ensure appropriate interpretation of the data. This is most marked in the case of cancer registry data, but is also a clear feature of many pharmacovigilance issues.

The problem becomes particularly acute when we observe the controversy about patient confidentiality in the United Kingdom at the present time. The regulatory authority for prescribers (the General Medical Council (GMC)) has been extremely legalistic in its approach to patient confidentiality. Led by its President, a distinguished retired general practitioner, the GMC has been draconian in its emphasis of the need for total patient confidentiality. Whilst at first sight this seems entirely reasonable and laudable, the areas of research referred to above could be seriously damaged by such an approach: in particular, observational studies such as cancer registries and drug safety monitoring studies are uniquely vulnerable since both require coordination of disparate data sources (e.g. demographic data, drug prescription data, hospital records and general practice records) to form a relevant patient record. In the absence of adequate *anonymous* patient registration numbers to bring these records together, names and addresses may be required solely to coordinate such information. If this can only be undertaken by receiving individual patient consent, an unknown proportion of patients (possibly up to 30%), will for one reason or another be unable or unwilling to give such permission. Thus the value of the resulting data set is dramatically reduced as it no longer constitutes a random sample from the population. Moreover, in the case of prospective databases involving literally millions of patient-years of observations, the practicalities of obtaining patient approval to use names and addresses solely to permit record linkage with the objective of furthering public health objectives of potential benefit to all people in the land, seem at first sight almost insurmountable as well as being prohibitively expensive. Are we then to cease this type of research? Surely the answer to this must be a resounding "No"!. We must find other more practical ways of achieving the desired end of maintaining quality research into drug safety and into cancer surveillance whilst fulfilling the need for confidentiality for all patients. I would suggest that a reasonable position to adopt would be one in which it was a recognised duty on patients receiving treatment in the National Health Service to accept that their information would be used for routine monitoring purposes, including disease incidence and prevalence studies and studies into the safety of medicines. Such studies will require records to be linked across several areas, and names and addresses may be needed for this purpose. At all times such confidential information would be kept to the minimum necessary and would be used solely for this purpose. Any breach of this confidentiality would be dealt with severely by fines or suspension of a licence to practice. To this writer's knowledge, there is no record of any confidential information being placed in the public domain from such data sets. Thus the obsessive concentration on confidentiality to the exclusion of all other facets of this issue is likely to do substantial harm to world-class research if the issue of *post hoc* anonymisation cannot be adequately and economically addressed. The value of such systems is proportional both to their duration in existence and to their continuity. Any breach in either of these two areas could have serious long-term consequences for the value of their work.

Although I have addressed the confidentiality issue early in this review, it applies to all pharmacovigilance work. *Briefly, anonymised records should be the usual type of information used by pharmacovigilators and pharmacoepidemiologists; however, there are times when, for the public good and because anonymised information is not readily available, named records will be required for linkage purposes. With suitable safeguards in place and enforced, such records should become a part of participation in NHS treatment and at the same time participation in future research in this crucial area.*

DISEASE REGISTRIES

For many years it has been known that a number of disorders are at particularly high risk of being drug-induced. Calls have been made to commence registries for such disorders, similar to the initiatives on aplastic anaemia following the chloramphenicol problem or the registry of vaginal adenocarcinoma in young women which proved so useful in identifying high dose stilboestrol in pregnancy as a culprit. These calls have yet to lead to action. It seems that this has been an opportunity missed. Perhaps someone will review the position in the near future, as I believe that a number of such registries could prove to be valuable additions to the pharmacovigilance arena as well as providing additional information about the natural history of the selected key disorders in the twenty-first century.

FOLLOW-UP STUDIES

In the era before large automated data sets became available for pharmacoepidemiology research, a number of *ad hoc* studies were mounted to look at the safety aspects of specific drugs. These studies had undoubted problems, and were generally expensive to mount and to conduct. Nonetheless they served to provide quantitation for several interesting risks, refute others, and they also helped to improve our understanding of methodology in this arena. They were however reported as being unhelpful to members of the UK Medicines Control Agency in their periodic safety assessments of licenced medicines. In a paper published in the *British Medical Journal* (Waller *et al.*, 1992; 304: 1470–1472) individuals from the MCA and the Committee on Safety of Medicines effectively published their obituary. It was clear that from then on no future developments would be seen in that area of study, and such has proven to be the case. Whether it was wise of a regulatory agency to take this course of action is debatable, particularly when the details of the criticisms of individual studies was notably lacking in the article cited. This author believes that regulators should generally remain aloof from issuing guidance on methodology until such time as the issues are clear-cut and generally accepted by experts within the field. We are now left with the main source of information in this area being the multi-purpose databases.

MULTI-PURPOSE DATABASES

Large data sets based on demographic information, disease occurrences and prescribing information are now available from several sources for use by trained and competent observers. We have extensive populations, particularly in the United States, Canada and the United Kingdom, for whom routine information about demography, drug exposure and disease experience are available in reasonably standardised formats. We have skilled analysts available to review such data sets for important causal associations between drugs and events. These information sets are extremely powerful tools and must be used with skill and great care lest the results reported turn out to be erroneous. In such circumstances great damage could be done both to public health and also to the data sets themselves. It is therefore crucially important that investigators ensure the validity of their observations by careful scrutiny of at least a sample (if not all) of the basic records. To rely solely on computer codes for disease identification without returning to verify basic written records is, in the opinion of this author, likely to lead to serious potential for error. Failure to undertake basic validations could easily lead to untold collateral damage to the reputation of individual medicines, and indeed to the parent data set itself.

Recently there have been some examples of conflicting conclusions emanating from different investigators reviewing the same topic from within the largest database in the United Kingdom, the General Practice Research Database. This may seem surprising at first sight. However, it must be clearly understood that the world-wide experience in this exciting area is confined to relatively small groups of investigators, as there are formidable logistical problems to overcome in entering and conducting research on these data resources. For example, drug-, symptom- and disease-codes tend to change with time during the years of data accrual. This is not territory for the amateur or the unwary! One simply cannot go to these extremely complex information systems and expect to perform high-quality research overnight. The issues are usually technically challenging and epidemiologically extremely complex.

Classical epidemiology is well used to dealing with fixed properties of individual patients, such as sex, height, weight, parity, smoking habits, etc. or one-off exposures to toxic substances, such as chemicals or infective agents. It is not so comfor-

table dealing with intermittent exposures at varying doses such as is customarily the case in drug epidemiology studies. There are some areas where the exposure status can be somewhat constant. Examples of these would be the use of oral contraceptives and hormone treatments (replacement therapies with oestrogens, insulin, thyroxine, etc.). Even here, however, patients regularly change individual preparations and great care must be taken to ensure accuracy and fairness in data interpretation. In other areas intermittent exposures are the norm.

In embarking upon a drug safety study in a large database, the investigator must clearly specify the hypothesis to be tested. (Such databases are so complex as to be generally unsuitable for hypothesis-generation except under very confined circumstances arising usually within an individual study.) Once one has defined the hypothesis, exposure and outcome status have to be assessed accurately. The nature of the study design has to be identified. Is it a follow-up study, a case–control study, or will it be a nested case–control study within a large group of subjects exposed to a individual medicine or class of medicines?

Failure of clarity at this stage could doom the study from the onset. Investigators interested in a particular hypothesis can often be mesmerised by the apparent abundance of information available to them. They should keep in mind that it is crucial to restrict themselves to appropriate comparisons. Thus if one is looking at the effect of, say, hormone replacement therapy on osteoporosis, the relevant outcome measure available in such databases is generally a fracture. However, not all fractures are relevant. Indeed, most are irrelevant to the hypothesis, as they will have an obvious and sufficient cause, such as a road traffic or other accident, an underlying neoplasm or pre-existing bone disease. Similarly, not all exposures to hormones are relevant. For example, it would seem unlikely (biologically implausible) that a single prescription for such treatment would be relevant to the outcome of interest. Trained epidemiologists are used to thinking of chance, bias and confounding as explanations for any associations they see in data. Although the items mentioned above are forms of bias, they tend to be obscure to all but those trained in the complexities of pharmacoepidemiology. Yet they are crucial issues to consider before one embarks on a seemingly large and promising study. Reflect that a negative outcome to a project could be because the study drug does not cause the outcome of interest. However, it could also arise from the fact that there is so much "noise" in the system that an investigator cannot not see the true link between drug and disease when it is in front of him because of inappropriate inclusions in the disease and drug exposure categories and inappropriate inclusions and exclusions in the comparator population. Finally, there is the problem of missing information found in all systems, yet requiring particularly careful handling in a multi-purpose database. Such information rarely leads to a false-positive conclusion, but it could result in missing a key finding. The main safeguard here is familiarity with the data set itself.

I have spent some time on this topic because I fear that the availability of more and more powerful information systems could lead to an epidemic of poorly undertaken studies that would reflect badly on the fledgling science of pharmacoepidemiology. This would be a matter of great regret, as the subject is of major importance for the future safety of patients, prescribers, dispensers and manufacturers alike. All have different perspectives, yet all share a common goal of getting the safest medicines to the appropriate patients at the right dose and at the right time. For a guide to some of the less obvious pitfalls in this type of research see the recent paper by Jick and colleagues in the *Lancet* (1998; 352: 1767–1770).

The development of pharmacovigilance is now at a critical stage. With powerful new tools at our disposal we have at last the opportunity to provide the public with some of the reassurances it requires from the industry and the professions. Ironically, it has taken over 35 years since David Finney originally recommended this approach in a seminal article in the *Journal of Chronic Diseases* (1965; 18: 77–98). It is crucial that we now rise to this challenge with enthusiasm and skill, seizing the opportunities that present themselves to us in these powerful information systems and surmounting the local difficulties relating to anonymisation of data sets, scientific rigour and credibility. For once we in the United Kingdom are in possession of a world-beating facility for research in the form of the General Practice Research Database, due solely to the foresight of its founding practitioner, the large numbers of collaborating general practitioners, and the analytic skills of the supporting Drug Surveillance Program.

OVER-THE-COUNTER AND ALTERNATIVE MEDICINES

Multi-purpose databases generally concentrate information collection upon prescription medicines. Over-the-counter (OTC) and alternative medicines are excluded or dealt with in a nonstandard manner. Whilst OTC medicines usually have been reviewed in detail when they were prescription medicines, the same cannot be said for alternative medicines such as herbal and homeopathic preparations. Many of these have been found to be associated with serious health hazards in the past and some have also been found to interact with prescription medicines. We need some method other than relying solely on spontaneous reporting systems to be reassured that these preparations are indeed as safe as we believe them to be. The resulting system need not be as all embracing as the large databases; however, the work needs to be done and done both rapidly and cost-efficiently in the near future.

NEW PRESCRIBERS

The large databases are best developed in the United Kingdom because of its unique feature of the general practitioner being the gateway through which patients progress to specialist care. Were the system to change and others such as nurses or pharmacists begin to prescribe in measurable numbers, these systems could become less effective. As this is likely to occur in the near future, for reasons that are entirely laudable and in patients' interests, there will have to be careful thought directed towards the best ways in which the relevant information can be captured economically to ensure the continuing maintenance and viability of the databases. This can most readily be achieved by channeling records of all prescriptions through a patient's practitioner, thereby ensuring not only continuity of records but also safety in therapy.

EVIDENCE-BASED MEDICINE

Evidence-based medicine is the new buzz term used to describe that which virtually all prescribers have been striving for throughout their professional lives. With better evidence from large clinical trials, there is increasing information to suggest that additions of several more medicines to the base package of treatment can result in better outcomes. What is not known is the effect of adopting this approach in real life. Will patients comply with all the additional medicines or will they attempt to reduce and rationalise the number of pills they have to take? If the latter, will they take the most important ones or will they take a random selection such that they end up worse off than before? So far, the large databases have been used primarily to study the effects of medicines on patients. They have rarely been used to study prescribers' or patients' behaviour. For obvious reasons, this area is complex. It could also be perceived as being potentially threatening to the very practitioners who supply the data in the first place! Nevertheless, I believe that these problems could easily be surmounted by ensuring adequate anonymisation for prescribers, and indeed this has been a feature of some of the large databases throughout their existence. Practitioners have nothing to fear about such developments if they are conducted in an inquiring mode rather than in a potentially inquisitorial mode. Indeed, they could learn substantial amounts from them. I await the results of these analyses with interest.

HOSPITAL DRUG MONITORING

Drug safety monitoring started with detailed studies of suspected adverse drug effects in hospitalised patients. Recently most pharmacovigilance work of an observational nature has been confined to domiciliary practice, because the number of drugs used and the number of underlying conditions experienced by patients are generally fewer there than in hospitals. This leads to easier interpretation of data but does leave a gap in our knowledge of the safety of drugs whose use is confined to the hospital setting, such as anaesthetics and several third-line antibiotics. There will need to be some efforts directed from time to time towards correcting these omissions, probably by *ad hoc* studies in hospitals such as have been undertaken by the Boston Collaborative Drug Surveillance Program in the 1970s and 1980s, and the Medicines Evaluation and Monitoring Organization in Dundee.

Such studies would be facilitated by more widespread use of computerised prescribing systems in hospitals. Their benefit would be enhanced greatly were such systems to be linked directly with patients' general practice records. This is entirely practicable if the will, finance and issues of patient confidentiality can be resolved.

GENOME RESEARCH AND PHARMACOVIGILANCE

The large pharmacovigilance databases have been and, in my view, will continue to be remarkably useful in focusing on safety issues of individual drugs or family of drugs. Nonetheless, in the twenty-first century this will not be sufficient on its own to justify their expansion and increasingly widespread use. Some have been in existence for over 10 years and hence have a significant risk of detecting any drug-induced neoplasias, which could be lurking in the undergrowth, for those exposed to long-term therapies. The only significant area in which this seems to have occurred to date, apart from very rare tumours in users of regular hormone therapies, is with the long-term immunosuppressed patients. This is good news insofar as it goes. The power of the databases to recognise tumour formation in long-term recipients of individual medicines or classes of medicines would be greatly enhanced were they to include a sizeable sub-population for whom genetic footprints were known. Such an advance is now coming within our grasp. Whilst a number of groups are looking at setting up new surveillance systems to include genetic profiles in the information they capture, the real prizes are likely to be won by grafting this additional information on to existing large data sets in which long-term studies have already been undertaken. The pay-off from this research is likely not only to be a greater understanding of the links between the genome and adverse drug events, but also a better understanding of tumour genesis in the population at large. Were these issues to be clarified, it is theoretically possible that a proportion of susceptible individuals could be advised to avoid certain drugs before they have ever been exposed to them. One suspects this will take several decades to achieve, but it could have the overall benefit of reducing individual risks of adverse events and prolonging the useful life of those drugs that have problems in a specific small sub-set of the population of recipients, but are otherwise acceptably safe and of good reputation. Clearly, such a development could only go ahead with the full approval of participating individuals. Nonetheless, it will also require societal debates if it is to experience seamless progress to its desired end. Genome research has significance for the population, but it also has important relevance to individual participants. The legal implications of acquiring knowledge about one's genetic fingerprints cannot be ignored. It is not merely a matter for the individual immediately involved, but also a matter for the entire family involved. The consequences for individuals seeking life insurance, a mortgage, paying maintenance, etc. are potentially large and must be considered carefully before we embark on such monitoring projects.

RESPONSES TO RISKS

One of the problems that has concerned me over the years is the relatively restricted nature of interventions available to Drug Regulatory Authorities in the event that a licensed medicine turns out to have unsuspected toxicity. These are suspension, revocation or modification to the summary of product characteristics. In these situations the perceived need to take action in relation to the risk from the product is often greater than the apparent risk itself warrants. There is an understandable tendency to emphasise risk and forget about benefit. An example of this would be the manner in which the on-going controversy about the risks of the third generation oral contraceptive pills and thromboembolic disease. As well as being of great intrinsic interest, this example emphasises that not all risks relate to new or nearly new drugs. Pharmacovigilance needs to remain alert to the potential problems of drugs at all stages in their development. Another example of a relatively old drug running into problems in the past was nomifensine, an effective antidepressant in which evidence came to light about the risks of acute haemolysis under unusual circumstances of use. Given the relatively long standing nature of the medicine itself, the company involved found it easier to withdraw it from sale than risk litigation by continuing use with adequate warnings. Was this the right decision? What happened to the long-term recipients who were receiving benefits from this drug? Did they transfer to an older antidepressant, or to a newer one (for which we had no comparable information), or discontinue treatment? What were the outcomes in relation to recurrence of depression, suicides and adverse effects to replacement therapies? Unfortunately, we do not know the answers to these questions. Clearly, the company involved in manufacturing nomifensine was not going to fund such a study. The issue seems to me to be a public health one and thus to require public funding. Perhaps with the development of multi-purpose databases we will be better at managing such an event in future. I hope so, but the question remains unanswered at present.

I believe that the need for post-withdrawal surveillance studies in large databases is clear and is clearly a duty that devolves on the public purse. I hope the need will occur infrequently!

CONCLUSIONS

The future for pharmacovigilance and pharmaco-epidemiology should be bright. That there is a need for this type of information is without doubt. The original vision of Professor Finney that it should be possible to uncover most significant drug-induced disorders by systematic analysis of routine information collected as part of everyday clinical practice is on the verge of fulfilment. Funding is a chronic problem for workers in the field. The pharmaceutical industry cannot be expected to fund all this effort. So far it has taken the lion's share of the initiative. Research Councils and others involved in the public conduct of affairs also need to contribute if the systems we have evolved to date are to realise their full potential. Hopefully, the twenty-first century will see an improvement in this area compared with the closing years of the previous decade. The signs are good with the Medicines Control Agency in the United Kingdom contributing substantially to the development of the General Practice Research Database in the last three years.

Index